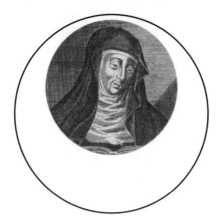

HISTORICAL ENCYCLOPEDIA OF NURSING

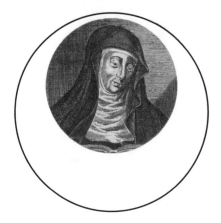

HISTORICAL ENCYCLOPEDIA OF NURSING

Mary Ellen Snodgrass

ABC-CLIO

Santa Barbara, California
Denver, Colorado
Oxford, England

Figures 1, 2, and 3 by Raymond M. Barrett, Jr.

Library of Congress Cataloging-in-Publication Data
Snodgrass, Mary Ellen.
    Historical encyclopedia of nursing / Mary Ellen Snodgrass.
        p.   cm.
    Includes bibliographical references and index.
    Summary: An encyclopedia covering the history of nursing, spanning topics from abortion to World War II.
        ISBN 1-57607-086-7 (alk. paper)
        1. Nursing—History—Encyclopedias.   [1. Nursing—History—Encyclopedias.]   I. Title.
RT31.S66   1999
610.73'0921—dc21   99-042670

05   04   03   02   01   00   99   10   9   8   7   6   5   4   3   2   1

ABC-CLIO, Inc.
130 Cremona Drive, P.O. Box 1911
Santa Barbara, California 93116-1911

Typesetting by Letra Libre, Inc.

This book is printed on acid-free paper ∞.
Manufactured in the United States of America.

For Dr. Harry King and Rosemary King, R.N.,
compassionate healers

Some day, the Red Cross will triumph over the cannon. The future belongs to the nurse, to the little grey sister, to all helpful powers, however humble; for two allies are theirs, suffering humanity and the merciful God.

—Charles Wagner, quoted in Mabel Boardman's
Under the Red Cross Flag at Home and Abroad *(1915)*

You are a warrior against death and suffering, a technician of the highest degree; you are a mother, a sister, a best friend, a psychiatrist; you are a teacher, a magician, a sounding board, a secretary, a fortuneteller, a politician, but most of all, you are a loving human being who has chosen to give that love in one of the best ways you can.

—Echo Heron, Intensive Care: The Story of a Nurse *(1987)*

Contents

HISTORICAL ENCYCLOPEDIA
OF NURSING

Preface

The plan of *Historical Encyclopedia of Nursing* is to present the backgrounds and careers of noted healers along with eras of conflict and social change, particular healing methods of ethnic groups, innovations in treatment, and the war on disease. For ease of use, I have provided overviews of ancient times, the Middle Ages and Early Renaissance, and the nineteenth and twentieth centuries. A focal world summary of midwifery establishes its importance to well-being and human survival. In addition to broad spans of time, detailed essays on periods of conflict illustrate the emergence of military medical preparedness following the Spanish-American War; creation of mobile army surgical hospital (MASH) units for the Korean War; nursing under communism and Nazi domination; and battlefield strategies during the Revolutionary War, two world wars, and Vietnam War. Other articles typify the work of such familiar figures as Dr. Elizabeth Blackwell, the United States' first female doctor, Sister Elizabeth Kenny, and Mother Teresa along with less familiar names—Naomi Deutsch, Esther Hasson, Elizabeth Cellier, Luisa Rosada, Mother Angela Gillespie, Tsahaí Haíle Selassíe, Ruth Lubic, Mary Agnes Jones, and Lillian Wald. Particular cadres of nurses come under the headings of Cadet Nurse Corps, Navy Nurse Corps, Red Cross, public health nursing, and *curandera*. Philosophies of nurse care are the source of essays on hospice, disease, and abortion.

Significant to my approach to history is an intentional deviation from works that reduce nursing to political acts, military promotions, and labor movements. Although my text includes the beginning of the Victorian Order of Nurses, American Nursing Association, and Town and Country Nurses, the substance of my work favors the contributions of individuals. For proper grounding in nursing history, I studied the total picture from numerous histories, the best being Philip Kalisch and Beatrice J. Kalisch's book *The Advance of American Nursing*. I have relied on first-person narratives to convey the sense impressions of events:

- the taste of buffalo meat and impure pond water in Manila's Santo Tomás prison compound
- the sound of strafing and machine gun fire along the Marne
- the feel of soaked chest dressings and crushed limbs in ground troops evacuated from Khe Sanh
- the sight of amputated legs and arms stacked under a tree near Union and Confederate field stations at Gettysburg

- the smell of ether, feces, and putrefaction in operating theaters in Santiago, Cuba, and among yellow fever victims in Philadelphia's Bush Hill pest house

Such eyewitness accounts enrich interviews with Clara Hale and Elizabeth Kenny; exhortations of Mother Teresa; professional texts by Florence Nightingale, Margaret Sanger, Hildegard of Bingen, and Lavinia Dock; and the diaries and journals of Martha Ballard, Confederate head nurse Kate Cumming, corpsman Walt Whitman, and the anonymous author of *Mademoiselle Miss.* The most astounding stories derive from surprisingly good reads:

- Álvar Núñez Cabeza de Vaca's *Castaways*
- Mary Jane Seacole's *Wonderful Adventures of Mrs. Seacole in Many Lands*
- Cornelia Spencer's *The Last Ninety Days of the War in North Carolina*
- Amy V. Wilson's *A Nurse in the Yukon*
- Shirley Lauro's *A Piece of My Heart*
- Thelma M. Schorr and Anne Zimmerman's *Making Choices, Taking Chances: Nurse Leaders Tell Their Stories*
- Lynda Van Devanter and Joan A. Furey's *Vision of War, Dreams of Peace: Writings of Women in the Vietnam War*
- Mary Breckinridge's *Wide Neighborhood: A Story of the Frontier Nursing Service*
- Winnie Smith's emotion-charged *American Daughter Gone to War: On the Front Lines with an Army Nurse in Vietnam*

I researched essential historical, military, and scientific data and current events in biographies, films and videos, monographs, newspapers, magazines, journals, and the Internet as well as in interviews with specialists, particularly AIDS nurse Helen Miramontes, women's rights crusader Judith Widdicombe, and Dr. W. Grimes Byerly, a retired army colonel who helped shape the MASH concept in Vietnam.

To assist the student, classroom teacher, nursing instructor, researcher, medical professional, reference librarian, and general reader, I have organized essays alphabetically and appended cross-references, source lists, art, and illustrations for more specific information about such matters as the Crimean War, the structure of field medicine in World War II, and the function of a MASH unit. The text precedes a brief timeline of landmarks in nursing history and a lengthy source list, which is divided into major works written by and about healers; books; articles, interviews, and monographs; and Internet sources. A comprehensive index offers

- names (Agnodice, Rhazes, St. Elizabeth Seton, Francis de Sales),
- specific elements (forensic nursing, Hadassah, lazaretto, school nursing, *Hakuiaisha,* Christ rooms, Lamboréné, Air Force Nurse Corps),
- related issues (homosexuality, genital mutilation, New Age healing, witchcraft, *Roe v. Wade,* forceps),
- historical eras (Crusades, Depression, Middle Ages),
- diseases (Spanish influenza, leprosy, AIDS, tuberculosis),
- medications (coca, herbs, vaccination, quinacrine),
- ethnic groups and tribes (Jewish healers, Native American healers),
- hospital ships (*Solace, Red Cross, Refuge, Red Rover*), and
- publications (*American Journal of Nursing,* "Nursing Beyond the Year 2000," *So Far from the Bamboo Grove, Malleus Maleficarum*).

After compiling these facts and drawing conclusions about the people who pioneered nursing protocols, I have gained new respect for the world's healers. The adventure of medical breakthroughs has given me a broader perspective on human accomplishment. I look forward to sharing my work with readers.

—*Mary Ellen Snodgrass*

Acknowledgments

Beth Bradshaw and Carol Camenga,
    reference librarians
Janey Deal, archivist
Patrick Beaver Library
Hickory, North Carolina

Dr. W. Grimes Byerly, retired MASH surgeon
Hickory, North Carolina

Brenda Chenosky
Vancouver Public Library
Vancouver, British Columbia

Peter Dargin, author and researcher
New South Wales, Australia

Avis Gachet
Wonderland Books
Granite Falls, North Carolina

Frances Hilton
Chapter One Books
Hickory, North Carolina

Karen Martinez, AHEC reference librarian
Catawba Memorial Hospital
Hickory, North Carolina

Burl McCuiston, reference librarian
Lenoir-Rhyne College
Hickory, North Carolina

Helen Miramontes, critical care nurse
Santa Clara, California

Diana Norman, author and researcher
Datchworth, England

Lynne Bolick Reed and Wanda Rozzelle,
    reference librarians
Catawba County Library
Newton, North Carolina

Renee Rodin
MacLeod's Books
Vancouver, British Columbia

Mark Schumacher, reference librarian
Walter Clinton Jackson Library
University of North Carolina
Greensboro, North Carolina

Helen Sherwin
Nursing Archives
Boston University
Boston, Massachusetts

Judith Widdicombe, founder
Reproductive Health Services
St. Louis, Missouri

Introduction

A history of nursing reveals the soul of human civilization. By its nature, nursing blends landmarks in healing with multiple strands of advancement, discovery, and innovation. However complex the job of nursing in current times, its rudiments spring from the simple acts of easing fears of a mother in childbirth, calming a tearful toddler, treating an injured neighbor, and comforting a dying elder. From prehistory, these humanitarian deeds have evolved into medical milestones:

- Aesculapius's instruction to Greek temple healers
- Hippocrates' study of symptoms
- Hildegard of Bingen's application of herbalism through a visiting nurse program
- St. Vincent de Paul's creation of religious healing societies
- Anne Hutchinson's Christian midwifery in Puritan New England
- Angélique du Coudray's invention of a realistic birthing model
- Harriet Tubman's wayside ministrations to slaves fleeing bondage
- Florence Nightingale's institution of England's battlefield nurse corps

- Dorothea Lynde Dix's supervision of Union nurses during the American Civil War
- Clara Barton's establishment of the American Red Cross
- Lillian Wald's influence in the creation of the U.S. Children's Bureau
- Margaret Sanger's design of the United States' first birth control clinic
- Dr. Marie Stopes's introduction of birth control to working-class London
- Mary Breckinridge's vision of a frontier nurse program
- Annie Dodge Wauneka's battle against tuberculosis on southwestern U.S. Indian reservations
- Mother Teresa's insistence on humane care for India's underclass
- Sister Elizabeth Kenny's innovative treatment of polio
- Dr. Cicely Saunders's influence on the hospice movement
- Elisabeth Kübler-Ross's publication of *On Death and Dying*
- Dr. Luther P. Christman's insistence on gender equity for nurses

A network of such accomplishments in the name of nurse care dots the globe, linking

Sister Dulce's mission to Brazil's poor and Geneviève de Galard's courageous stand at an underground fortress in Dien Bien Phu, Vietnam, with Clara Hale's nurturance of addicted babies in her Harlem apartment; Mary Ann Bickerdyke's mothering of Union troops in Chattanooga, Tennessee; Father Damien's martyrdom among Hawaii's lepers; Susan La Flesche Picotte's dedicated treatment of the Omaha in Nebraska; Tsahaí Haíle Selassíe's public health initiative in Ethiopia; Lottie Moon's mission to Tengchow, China; Edith Cavell's rescue of Allied soldiers from Nazi-held Brussels, Belgium; and Clara Maass's bravery during human tests that linked yellow fever to the *Aedes aegypti* mosquito after the Spanish-American War. Unnamed practitioners have performed last rites and baptism; upgraded the nutrition of fellow prisoners of war at Andersonville, La Cabaña Prison Fortress, and Bataan; welcomed fellow traumatized veterans at "the Wall"; written letters and performed songs for Japan's blind and disabled; cooked wholesome soups and broths for India's outcasts; and trekked by mule, canoe, and cart into the outback to carry medicines and comfort to peoples on the margins of civilization.

For all its altruism, nursing history cannot retreat into paeans of glory. In its resolve to end suffering, the basics of medical practice have acquired overtones of struggle and contention within pure science, ecology, religion, law, philanthropy, human rights, race and gender equity, and the strategies of war. It is not surprising that the controversial elements of human caregiving nettle keepers of the status quo. An entrenched traditionalism doubts the efficacy of smallpox vaccination and the value of home births; questions unlicensed midwives and nuns who practice medicine outside convents; ridicules herbalism and therapeutic touch; derides the Hispanic tradition of the *curandera* and the Orient's dependence on acupuncture; forbids Catholic, Jewish, and Quaker midwives from practicing among Protestants; and criminalizes women's health clinics and contraceptive information

in the U.S. mails. Like all human efforts, medicine contains its share of dark deeds. Beyond controversy lie reprehensible events in nursing history: genital mutilation of female newborns and toddlers in some Islamic and African nations; attendants fleeing victims of the Black Death, leprosy, and AIDS; Caucasian medical authorities rejecting nonwhite volunteers; male bureaucrats marginalizing female professionals; conquerors posing as healers in New World colonies; Nazi nurses participating in euthanasia, genocide, and medical experiments at the Auschwitz death camp; and communist nurses tormenting dissidents at detention centers masked as psychiatric facilities. These landmarks remind the historian that medicine is not exempt from the corruption that shadows dynamic events in world affairs.

Significant to eras of suffering are humanists whose selfless acts outweigh the crimes of pernicious, destructive forces. Against the image of Nanna Conti in Hitler's Germany and scavengers of organ transplants in China are army and Red Cross nurses at Anzio, Bataan, and Dachau. Opposite conquistadores and colonialists spreading European diseases in Central America and among the Cree and Mohawk of Canada are Catholic sisters who set up the Hôtel Dieu in Montreal and Quebec. Counter to racists who enforced sterilization on the underclass are trauma nurses who acted as sexual assault nurse-examiners to treat rape victims and who treated refugees from the Boxer Rebellion and casualties of the Irish Rebellion and the 1995 bomb blast that rocked Oklahoma City. Outnumbering midwives who scarify and excise the genitalia of young Sudanese girls in the name of patriarchy are professional nurses worldwide teaching hygiene and nutrition and vaccinating children for the Peace Corps, World Health Organization, UNICEF, religious mission boards, Sisters of Charity, and Doctors without Borders.

The totality of nurses' good deeds and creativity overwhelms any account of medicine's worth. Since the groundswell of medical advancement in the 1850s, nurses have revamped battlefield rescue, equalized medical care among social and economic strata, reprieved the dying from loneliness and isolation, and spread lifesaving information about birth defects, trachoma, consumption, polio, and AIDS. Major crises in the past 150 years have produced nursing heroes in hospices at the Crimea; on hospital ships off Cuba and Korea; in inner-city routes among squalid tenements in New York City and Salvador de Bahía, Brazil; in tent aid stations on the Russian front; on planes bound for Zaire's Ebola outbreak; at polio and tuberculosis camps in North Carolina and Alabama; on mission boats up the Amazon Basin; and in MedEvac helicopters over Vietnam and Kuwait. Strong women, the backbone of nursing, have forced patriarchy into decline in the military, municipal hospitals, mission boards, and the Vatican. Within the cadre of female nursing authorities, men have returned to claim equal status

as caregivers. As the warrior-monks and baymen of the past supported regiments marching to the Holy Lands and naval convoys secured American waters, male nurses have risen to honorable positions in critical care wards, asylums for the insane, trauma centers, rural clinics, submarine sick bays, and home health programs for the elderly.

The proof of nurses' multiple benefits to humanity lies in their ubiquity. Wherever human figures struggle, plan, invent, or labor, the caregiver tends to physical and emotional needs. Essential to providing quality preventive medicine and treatment are the practitioner's adaptability and willingness to serve. Future challenges in Third World countries, urban centers, and combat zones map nurse training for the twenty-first century. Whatever tomorrow's demands—unknown contagion, breakdown of social structures, violence, and natural disaster—nursing will reshape, realign, and replot the most humane methods of uplifting humankind.

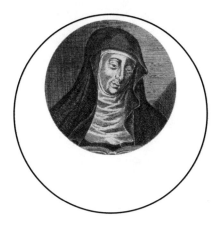

HISTORICAL
ENCYCLOPEDIA
OF NURSING

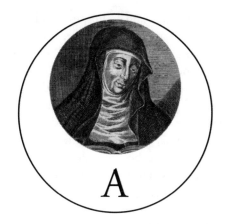

A

Abortion

In the twentieth century, no topic so challenged the health care community as the bioethics regarding a woman's choice to terminate a pregnancy, which many nations have traditionally followed and others labeled as infanticide and a mortal sin. In the United States, abortion on demand was legalized on January 22, 1973, after the Supreme Court overturned a severe Texas law in the case of *Roe v. Wade*. To feminists, no court ruling has made so profound a change in government limitations on freedom. The nursing profession, heavily dominated by women, was drawn into the fray as the theoretical and moral battlegrounds came down to a pro-mother, pro-child face-off.

Heavily clouded by religious dogma, conservative cant, and governmental statutes in Europe and the United States, the abortion issue led to a climate of suspicion and unrest at all levels of society and among professionals in the media, education, law, religion, and medicine. On the pro-life side, England's LIFE nurses rejected abortion, citing as deterrents the death of the fetus, in particular, one capable of survival outside the womb, as well as the mother's possible loss of reproductive ability and a lifetime of grief and guilt. The opposing side, represented by the National

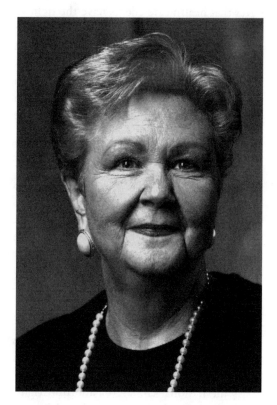

Judith Widdicombe, pioneer of women's rights to safe and legal abortion (photo courtesy of Judith Widdicombe)

Abortion Campaign (NAC), focused on mental and physical risks to pregnant women and on a wide range of woman-centered needs, particularly privacy issues, unbiased counseling, nursery care, adoption counseling, and maternity facilities.

Beset by protesters shouting Bible verses, waving photos of aborted tissue, and accusing abortion providers of murder, nurses on both sides of the issue steered a fearful path, like the *weise Frauen* (wise women) and *Engelmacherinnen* (angel makers) of Weimar Germany in the 1930s who had to choose between Nazi policy and pricks of conscience. American health professionals continued to perform abortions, which were legal, but which incensed certain subversive patriot clans and fundamentalist groups, particularly some Roman Catholics and Protestant evangelicals. In 1989, the American Nurses Association (ANA) clarified its stand: "ANA believes that health care clients have the right to privacy and the right to make decisions about personal health care based on full information without coercion. Also nurses have the right to refuse to participate in a particular case on ethical grounds. However, if a client's life is in jeopardy, nurses are obliged to provide for the client's safety and to avoid abandonment" ("Position Statements," www.ana.org).

Subsequent commentary from ANA's board of directors characterized abortion as a "symptom of social failure" and placed nurses on the side of "a fair and equitable health care delivery system," which the ANA labeled an American right. Of particular concern for ANA was the concerted legal whittling away of patient access to gynecological care, particularly the young and the poor, and a court-created adversarial atmosphere that might inhibit women at all social and economic levels from seeking legal termination of unwanted pregnancies.

As the national climate of abortion rights changed from criminal to legal, a Missouri nurse quickly developed a local program. Founder and president of Reproductive Health Services in St. Louis, Missouri, Judith McWhorter Widdicombe launched a drive for a constitutional amendment to nullify a 1986 state law limiting abortion. A mother of two sons, registered obstetrical nurse at a Catholic hospital, and volunteer counselor for a suicide hotline, she had reason to connect the need for legal abortion services with the desperation of women wanting to die. She also had tended patients brought to emergency rooms after unqualified abortionists had lacerated and infected them during illegal, unsanitary, and life-threatening abortions. Until the law could catch up with need, Widdicombe helped set up an underground system in cooperation with a professor at Washington University.

Immediately after the Supreme Court legalized abortion, Widdicombe directed clients to New York, where health care centers were already in place to receive clients. Drawing on the warmth and medical efficiency of a competent staff, she and nurse Vivian Rosenberg launched Missouri's first abortion clinic in a twelve-story building only minutes from an emergency room. Widdicombe determined that the Russian vacuum extraction method suited her clientele. Simpler than scraping the uterus with a curette, the method required only two minutes' application without general anesthetic and offered safe tissue extraction and less trauma and endangerment of the patient. After determining that the Supreme Court's ruling overrode state law, she opened the clinic in May. In place of brutal abortion mills, Widdicombe's service, directed by B. J. Isaacson-Jones, offered quality health care and an option for women despairing to the point of self-destruction.

In 1998, Cynthia Gorney published *Articles of Faith: A Frontline History of the Abortion Wars,* a dialectic that targeted Widdicombe's devotion to freedom of choice and the opposing campaign of Sam Lee, lobbyist for Missouri Citizens for Life and author of the 1989 challenge to Reproductive Health Services. Among the facts that Gorney uncovered in her research was the emergence of one thousand Protestant ministers who, since 1968, had operated a national abortion underground. Another group, Chicago's Jane Collective, coordinated an all-women effort to aid women during crisis pregnancies.

Reducing the shrill debate over abortion has been the introduction of mifepristone, a medicinal abortifacient used in France, Sweden, and the United Kingdom. Commonly known as RU-486, the pill was developed in France. French medical authorities tested RU-486 at Broussais Hospital in Paris in 1984, and decreed it the moral property of women in 1988. Preferred by French patients over the more intrusive surgical abortion, the drug, used in combination with a prostaglandin called misoprostol, expels amniotic sacs from the wall of the uterus. In a Paris hospital, nurses displayed a tiny sac to each woman who chose the abortifacient. An amorphous bit of tissue about the size of a grain of rice, it deflates trauma resulting from fears that the patient has opted to kill an infant.

In April 1997, protests directed at the pill's distributor, the Population Council, by American antiabortionists forced the manufacturer, Roussel Uclaf, offshoot of Hoechst, to halt distribution in the United States. According to Jane Gallagher, director of the American Civil Liberties Union Reproductive Freedom Project, that concerted uproar is the work of extremists whose agenda is to ban all abortions. To counter scarcity of RU-486, Dr. Edouard Sakiz, retired chairman of Roussel, promised the French Movement for Family Planning and Planned Parenthood to keep searching for a manufacturer. The likelihood of an American sponsor for the drug dimmed in June 1998, when Congress voted against Food and Drug Administration approval.

In the mounting backlash by right-wing fundamentalists during the 1990s, violence and obstruction continued to trouble professional abortion providers. In 1992 alone, there were sixteen arsons, thirteen attempted arsons or bombings, and one bombing at abortion clinics, with damages amounting to more than $2 million. One clinic nurse took a strong antiabortion stand on July 9, 1995. Registered nurse Brenda Pratt Shafer sent her congressman, Tony Hall (D-Ohio), a first-person account of the controversial partial birth abortion procedure, performed in 1993 at the Women's Medical Center in Dayton, Ohio. Most offensive to Shafer's ethics was the doctor's termination of a six-month pregnancy by inserting scissors in the fetus's head, then suctioning brain matter from the cranium. In conclusion to her letter, Shafer urged Hall to support a bill banning a procedure she equated with infanticide. An immediate rebuttal to Shafer's graphic description came from Christie Gallivan, head nurse of the center, who declared that Shafer had been employed only three days and that she would not have been trained for second-trimester dilation and extraction. Additional rebuttals came from Congresswomen Patricia Schroeder, Sheila Jackson Lee, and Zoe Lofgren, who declared Shafer's letter erroneous and misleading.

On January 29, 1998—a week after the twenty-fifth anniversary of *Roe v. Wade,* the landmark decision guaranteeing a woman's right to an abortion—a security guard was killed and head nurse and counselor Emily Lyons was crippled, scarred, and almost blinded by a bomb blast at Birmingham's New Woman All Women Health Care Center, established in 1987. The incident, the first fatality at a U.S. abortion center, resembled two unsolved abortion clinic bombings the previous year in Atlanta. The escalation of protest into stalking, breaking and entering, shootings, communicating threats by mail and telephone, arson, and outright murder altered the work of nurse to activist. In reference to her own nearly fatal experience, Lyons commented, "I believed in what I did. . . . Some people questioned if I was ashamed of what I did, and the answer is 'no'" (Bragg 1998, 2A). In the April/May 1999 issue of *Ms.* magazine, Lyons posed for a full-length view of her damaged legs. When asked if she would testify to terrorism at abortion clinics, she replied, "I've been blown up. I cannot be intimidated"("In Praise of Women" 1999, 65).

See also: African-American Nurses; Midwifery

Sources

Abrams, Lynn, and Elizabeth Harvey, eds. *Gender Relations in German History: Power, Agency and*

Experience from the Sixteenth to the Twentieth Century. Durham, N.C.: Duke University Press, 1997.

"ACLU Urges FDA to Approve Mifepristone for Early Medical Abortion." http://www.aclu.org/news/n071996a.html.

Benshoof, Janet. "Beyond *Roe,* after *Casey:* The Present and Future of a 'Fundamental' Right." *Women's Health Issues* (fall 1994): 162–168.

Bragg, Rick. "Despite Bombing, Clinic Goes On." *Charlotte Observer,* June 20, 1998, 2A.

"Condition Upgraded for Nurse Severely Injured in Bombing." http://www. boston.com/dailynews/wirehtml/033/Condition_upgraded_for_nurse_severe.htm.

Galloway, Paul. "Book Turns Down Volume to Look at America's Sometimes-Uncivil War over Abortion." http://www.arlingtonnet/news/doc/1047/1:BPAGE13/1:BPAGE13020198.html.

Gorney, Cynthia. *Articles of Faith: A Frontline History of the Abortion Wars.* New York: Simon and Schuster, 1998.

Grimes, D., et al. "An Epidemic of Antiabortion Violence in the United States." *American Journal of Obstetrics and Gynecology* (1991): 1266.

Guash-Melendez, Adam. "The Truth about the Testimony of Nurse Brenda Pratt Shafer." http://www.cais.net/agm/main/nurse.htm.

Heath, Melanie. "Nurses for LIFE." *Nursing Times,* December 13, 1979, 2145–2146.

"In Praise of Women." *Ms.* (April/May 1999): 62–71.

McKeegan, Michele. "The Politics of Abortion: A Historical Perspective." *Women's Health Issues* (fall 1993): 127–131.

Montgomery, Lori. "Despite Popularity, RU-486 May Disappear." http://www.bergen.com/more-news/475861997062807.htm.

"NARAL Factsheet—Mifepristone (RU 486) and the Impact of Abortion Politics on Scientific Research." http://www.naral.org/publications/facts/ru486fin.html.

"One Nurse's Experience on Partial Birth Abortion." http://www.fril.com/~buchanan/dorie/abrtpage.htm.

"Position Statements." http://www.ana.org/readroom/position/social/screpr.htm.

Radford, Barbara. "Antiabortion Violence: Causes and Effects." *Women's Health Issues* (fall 1993): 144–151.

Scouller, Alison, Mary Smith, and Barbara Nelson. "Nurses for a Woman's Right to Choose." *Nursing Times,* December 13, 1979, 2144–2145.

Shafer, Brenda. "Nurse Is Eyewitness to Horrifying Partial-Birth Abortion Procedure." http://www.fc.net/~garti/newsletter/sep95/nurse.html.

Soltis, Andy. "Cop Killed and Nurse Hurt in Bombing at Ala. Abortion Clinic." http://www.nypostonline.com/news/3345.htm.

"Statement Concerning Mifepristone." http://www.now.org/foundationreproduc/ru486tes.html.

"Surge in Political Power." http://www.umsl.edu/services/library/womenstudies/1990s.htm.

Weatherford, Doris. *American Women's History.* New York: Prentice Hall, 1994.

Widdicombe, Judith, telephone interview, April 22, 1998.

African-American Nurses

American history gives little credit to its first black nurses, the plantation nannies, healers, herbalists, and midwives who attended patients of all races and who functioned in free society after emancipation, often for no pay or recognition. Lay midwifery in Georgia slave quarters derived from practices of slaves' African forebears. The designation of plantation midwife, freighted with responsibility

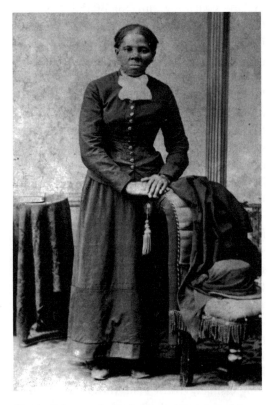

Harriet Tubman, who worked as a nurse and cared for Confederate prisoners and ex-slaves (Library of Congress)

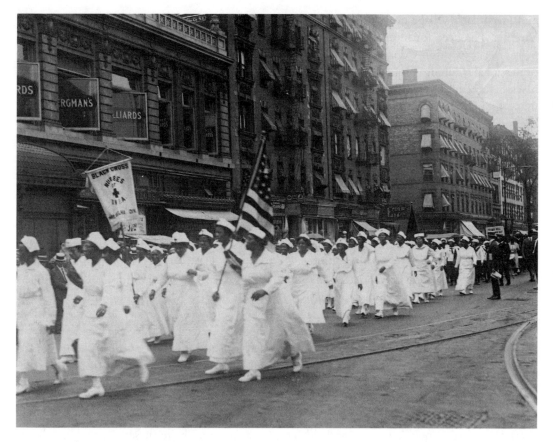

Black Cross Nurses march through Harlem during the opening of the thirty-day world convention of the Universal Negro Improvement Association, 1 August 1922. (Corbis/Underwood & Underwood)

and trust, carried a womanly esteem, for the next generation of slaves and the master's investment depended on quick thinking and steady hands to "catch babies." In the estimation of one Virginia doctor, in the years preceding the Civil War, black midwives attended 50 percent of the state's white women. And a pre-emancipation death notice printed in a Charleston paper recognized "One of our faithful nurses, Soye, the property of William Ravenal, Esq." (Boardman 1915, 77). Other nameless black nurses were donated like chattels to Confederate medical corps by patriotic owners.

According to *Lamps on the Prairie: A History of Nursing in Kansas* (1942), one of the early free black settlers in Kansas was practical nurse–midwife Lyda Baker, who worked in Topeka in the 1800s and was honored with a memorial window at the Topeka African Methodist Church. Another doughty survivor, Mary McCray, fled slavery in Wilson County, Tennessee, in 1861 and, with her sister Henrietta Frances, volunteered as a Union nurse in Nashville. After recovering from the smallpox contagion that killed Henrietta, Mary McCray worked at Hospital No. 11 in the smallpox unit. In 1903, she joined the National Association of Civil War Nurses and remained faithful to her calling until her death in 1932, when she was buried with military honors.

Two freedom fighters, Sojourner Truth and Harriet Tubman, earned additional credit for nurse care. The first, Isabella Van Wagenen, better known as Sojourner Truth, worked as a nurse-counselor at the Washington Freedman's Relief Association, Freedman's Hospital, and Freedman's Village in Arlington Heights, Virginia. The need for more black nurses impelled her to petition Congress for additional professional training programs. The second black heroine of the era, Harriet "Moses" Tubman, escaped plantation bondage in Dorchester County, Maryland, in 1849. She assisted other runaways, including her sister and two children, and supervised a route on the Underground Railroad that rescued more than eight hundred slaves. Primarily a soldier and antislavery agent, she assisted Union forces as spy, scout, and raider. Her postwar career placed her at the front of the women's rights movement. In 1944, Eleanor Roosevelt christened the Liberty Ship Harriet Tubman in her honor; in 1978, the United States Post Office issued a commemorative stamp lauding Tubman's courage.

The subsequent generation produced the first civilian black nurse, Mary Eliza P. Mahoney, who was free-born on May 7, 1845, in Dorchester, Massachusetts, to Mary Jane Stewart and Charles Mahoney. After fifteen years as domestic, cook, laundress, and aide at New England Hospital for Women and Children, she entered as a student and graduated at age thirty-four. After registering with the Massachusetts Medical Library, she worked as a one-on-one critical care nurse for three decades in New Jersey, Washington, D.C., and North Carolina. In 1911, she directed the Howard Orphan Asylum for Black Children in Long Island. To establish the National Association of Colored Graduate Nurses (NACGN), she opened the first convention in August 1909 with a welcoming speech and accepted the post of chaplain. In a notable public appearance on behalf of black nurses, she led a delegation to a White House reception hosted by President Warren G. Harding and his family.

Mahoney died of breast cancer on January 4, 1926, at the hospital where she trained. A monument in her honor stands at Woodlawn Cemetery in Everett, Massachusetts, a site revered by the Chi Eta Phi nursing sorority. On the tenth anniversary of her death, the NACGN established the Mahoney Award for outstanding female nurses who foster racial integration. Her alma mater named one of its departments the Mary Mahoney Health Care Clinic. Forty years later, her name was added to the roll of the Nursing Hall of Fame.

Parallel to the work of Mahoney were other initiatives to establish black nurses as health professionals. Both Celia Saxon and Celia Mann of Columbia, South Carolina, left bondage to serve as midwives. Bridget "Biddy" Mason, a slave born of African, Choctaw, and Seminole ancestry on a plantation in Hancock County, Mississippi, on August 15, 1818, received training in midwifery and served the John Smithson and Robert Smith families. Carried into Indian territory when her owner joined a Mormon migration, she lived in Utah until 1851, when Smith settled in San Bernardino, California. In the latter half of the nineteenth century, she demanded manumission from her corrupt owner in a court action that established rights of blacks transported to the West. She thrived as a nurse-midwife in service to Dr. John S. Griffin in a multicultural community in Los Angeles. On November 16, 1989, the city declared Biddy Mason Day, and authorities unveiled a timeline in memory of her philanthropic contributions and wise nurse care among Indian, Hispanic, and Anglo residents.

Another former slave, Susie Baker King Taylor, provided the only written account of a black female participant in the Civil War. She was born August 5, 1848, on Wight Island near Savannah, Georgia, and fled by boat with her family to St. Catherine's Island at the beginning of the Civil War. From literacy skills gained from white children, in 1856 she opened a school on St. Simon's Island. Although laws forbade slaves to learn to read and write, she taught forty refugee children each day and tutored adults at night. The project ended as war threatened locals, who were evacuated to Beaufort, South Carolina. As a laundress and volunteer nurse, Taylor was assigned to a black troop, Company E, the First South Carolina Volunteers, and tended casualties at Beaufort's Camp Saxton base hospital. In summer 1863, she accompanied Clara Barton on hospital rounds during the Civil War, an era she described in her memoirs, *Reminiscences of My Life in Camp* (1902). Into the late 1880s, Taylor maintained her loyalty to Union war veterans by helping to launch the Women's Relief Corps.

These forerunners of modern nurses legitimized the nursing profession, which derived from the plantation tradition of black nurses, and pioneered the establishment of schools for women of color, beginning in 1886 with Spelman Seminary in Atlanta. More facilities followed with varying degrees of success. Adah Thoms's study of nursing programs for blacks reveals facts about the establishment date, size, and number of graduates from thirty-six schools, as shown in Table 1.

The data, although sketchy in places, reveal a trend toward modest educational opportunities in southern states, followed by a surge in the Midwest and larger teaching facilities in New York, Philadelphia, and Washington, D.C., three cities with a substantial black population. As a result of these start-up programs, by 1928, nearly twenty-eight hundred black nurses were ready to enter medical service.

The military had its own upsurge of admissions to nursing programs. By 1898, the need for enlistees in the Navy Nurse Corps rose during the medical crisis that accompanied the Spanish-American War. Five female graduates of the Tuskegee Institute served in Cuba and one black male nurse in the Philippines. To relieve the yellow fever epidemic that threatened thousands of soldiers, Namahyoke Curtis searched New Orleans for immune staff members to care for patients. In July, she was successful in locating thirty-two. Two years later, she aided Clara Barton and the Red Cross during the flood in Galveston, Texas. Curtis was honored with a military burial at Arlington National Cemetery in 1935.

During a Spanish influenza epidemic at Camp Sherman, Ohio, in 1911, the question arose of hiring black nurses. At a meeting between the surgeon general's staff and the American Red Cross on December 5, the surgeon general determined that the greatest obstacle was the shortage of separate housing, which racism dictated in the decades preceding integration. By June 1917, the problem recurred when the surgeon general considered assigning black nurses to a special service in Iowa. When a separate world war unit was established at Camp Sherman, the nine professionals who formed the initial cadre of black nurses attached to the American Red Cross—Aileen Cole, Susan Boulding, Lillian Spears, Jeanette Minnis, Sophia Hill, Marion Brown, Jeannette West, Clara Rollins, and Lillian Ball—performed more than medical service. The matron reported, "They really were a credit to their race, for they did valuable service for our patients and it was a service that patients appreciated. I now find myself deeply interested in the problems of all colored nurses and believe in giving them such opportunities as they can grasp for advancement" (Thoms n.d., 164). The experiment proved so successful that a second detachment began work in December 1918, a second blow to resistance to nonwhite staff.

One by one, other pioneering efforts took black nurses out of segregated settings to place them at the forefront of medical initiatives:

- Beginning in New York City on October 3, 1900, Jessie Sleet Scales, a Canadian from Stratford, Ontario, served the Charity Organization Society as the United States' first black public health nurse. Her nine-year record of quality care ended questions of a discriminatory hiring policy for the agency and encouraged white authorities to offer positions for more nonwhite professionals.
- A vigorous advocate for black nurses, Carrie E. Bullock trained at Scotia Seminary Normal Department, Concord, North Carolina. After working at Provident Hospital in Chicago, she served the city's Visiting Nurses Association. Her

Table 1: Nursing Programs for African Americans

Name	Location	Year Established	Bed Capacity	Number of Graduates
Brewster	Jacksonville, Fla.	1902	34	63
Burrell Memorial	Roanoke, Va.	1915	50	25
Burwell Infirmary	Selma, Ala.	1927	26	0
Charity	Savannah, Ga.	1901	42	unknown
Dixie-Hampton	Hampton, Va.	1891	65	281
Douglass	Kansas City, Ks.	1898	25	30
Dunbar	Detroit, Mich.	1918	65	6
Flint Goodridge	New Orleans, La.	1896	60	137
Fort Worth Negro	Fort Worth, Tex.	n/a	n/a	n/a
Fraternal	Montgomery, Ala.	1919	35	14
Freedmen's	Washington, D.C.	1894	260	439
Grady	Atlanta, Ga.	1917	250	80
Great Southern Fraternal	Little Rock, Ark.	1919	48	8
Georgia Infirmary	Savannah, Ga.	1926	80	unknown
Hale	Montgomery, Ala.	1889	35	unknown
Harlem	New York, N.Y.	1923	350	72
Hospital & Training School	Charleston, S.C.	1897	20	127
Hubbard	Nashville, Tenn.	1900	140	138
John D. Archbold	Thomasville, Ga.	1925	111	unknown
Kansas City General	Kansas City, Mo.	1911	150	86
Lincoln	New York, N.Y.	1898	330	493
Mercy	Philadelphia, Pa.	1907	100	136
Piedmont (TB training)	Burkeville, Va.	1918	150	25
Prairie View	Prairie View, Tex.	1918	50	34
Provident	Baltimore, Md.	1926	36	unknown
Provident	Chicago, Ill.	1891	65	226
Red Cross	Louisville, Ky.	n/a	n/a	n/a
Royal Circle	Little Rock, Ark.	1921	85	4
St. Agnes	Raleigh, N.C.	1896	100	172
St. Phillips	Richmond, Va.	1920	140	27
Tuggle Institute	Birmingham, Ala.	1925	25	unknown
Tuskegee Institute	Tuskegee, Ala.	1892	75	125
United Friends	Little Rock, Ark.	1920	25	6
University—Lamar Wing	Augusta, Ga.	1893	260	unknown
Waverley Fraternal	Columbia, S.C.	1924	50	2
Wheatley Provident	Kansas City, Miss.	1910	65	30

honors include election as president and delegate in 1927 to the National Association of Colored Graduate Nurses, for which she edited and published the monthly *National News Bulletin*.

- Bullock's contemporary, Elizabeth Tyler, the first colored nurse at the Henry Street Visiting Nurse Service in New York, also integrated the Phipps Institute in Philadelphia, the State Health and Welfare Commission of Delaware, and the New Jersey Tuberculosis League.
- Sadie Stewart Hobday of St. Helena Island became the first black nurse–social worker. Based in Tulsa, Oklahoma, in 1919, she conducted tuberculosis, pre-

natal, and child welfare clinics and held health weeks at a makeshift clinic in a large church. In nine years, Hobday's work opened the way for two full-time positions—a black public health officer and a dentist.

- Another pioneer, Pauline Bray Fletcher, Birmingham's first black registered nurse, relieved the suffering of young consumptives at a camp opened in Kelly Ingram Park in 1926.
- A nursing administrator and educator from Palestine, Texas, and superintendent of nurses at Homer G. Philips Hospital in St. Louis, Missouri, Estelle Massey Riddle assumed the post of educational director of the Freedmen's Hospital in Washington, D.C., and launched a drive for qualified students in 1931. She appointed a task force to investigate nurse training in the South. Her efforts resulted in federal grants to communities in need. Because of her dedication to high standards, in 1943 she was named a consultant to the National Nursing Council for War Service.
- An administrator from Tuskegee, Alabama, Margaret Thomas, R.N., directed a nurse-midwifery preparatory program, the Tuskegee School of Nurse Midwifery. Opening on September 15, 1941, in cooperation with the Alabama State Department of Health with funds from the Children's Bureau, the school joined forces with the John A. Andrew Memorial Hospital to provide care for mothers with birthing difficulties and sick infants. Carrington Owens, a black nurse-midwife, took charge of the school, which produced thirteen graduates in 1943. A less successful program intended to help poor blacks began at the Flint Goodridge Hospital in New Orleans, Louisiana. Directed by Kate Hyder, R.N., the school operated from 1942 to 1943 and closed for lack of participation.

Following the success of private nursing schools, the military made parallel strides toward less prejudicial hiring policies. When Lucile Petry Leone began recruiting 135,000 members for the U.S. Cadet Nurse Corps, she included on her staff Rita Miller Dargan, a black nurse and consultant from New Orleans chosen to solicit black volunteers. Because generous grants to nursing schools forced an end to segregation, white schools began scrapping discriminatory admission policies and recruiting black applicants. By the final months of World War II, twenty-six hundred black nursing students had enrolled and forty-nine nursing schools were integrated, yet the Navy Nurse Corps remained segregated.

A quiet rebel and author of *No Time for Prejudice: A Story of the Integration of Negroes in Nursing in the United States* (1961), Mabel Doyle Keaton Staupers confronted entrenched racism by supporting equal rights for black nurses and established a private hospital in Harlem where black professionals could work without denigration or bias. A native of Barbados, she earned her degree from Freemen's Hospital School of Nursing in Washington, D.C., and worked as a private duty nurse, health care surveyor, and secretary of the Harlem Tuberculosis Committee. For twelve crucial years during the struggle to integrate the military nurse corps, with the support of Eleanor Roosevelt, Staupers pressured army surgeon Norman Kirk and Secretary of War Henry Stimson to accept black military nurses.

On January 25, 1945, the Navy Nurse Corps acceded to public support by admitting its first black nurse, Phyllis Mae Daley, who took the oath of office March 8, 1945. A second black enlistee, Edith M. DeVoe, entered the service the next month and, in 1948, became the first black nurse to transfer to the regular navy. Mabel Staupers, the quiet force that brought about the transformation of the all-white military nurse corps, continued to labor inside organized nursing as secretary of the NACGN, which ceased to exist in 1948 after black nurses were welcomed into the

American Nurses Association. Her efforts earned her the Spingarn Medal, an alumni award from Howard University, and a citation from New York mayor John Lindsay.

The last half of the twentieth century brought black nurses into positions of authority. A strong voice for equality in opportunity came from Mary Elizabeth Lancaster Carnegie, who obtained a degree in nursing school administration from the University of Toronto. In addition to serving as dean of the nursing school at Florida Agricultural and Mechanical College in Tallahassee, Florida, she edited *Nursing Outlook* and *Nursing Research* and worked on the editorial boards of the *American Journal of Nursing*. In 1973, she focused attention on the need for better preparation with the article, "ANF Directory Identifies Minorities with Doctoral Degrees," which was the impetus for a grant from the National Institute of Mental Health to aid black nurses in obtaining Ph.D.'s. An inductee to the American Academy of Nursing, in retirement she furthered the cause of medical history with an overview, *The Path We Tread: Blacks in Nursing Worldwide, 1854–1984* (1986), and an autobiographical sketch in *Making Choices, Taking Chances: Nurse Leaders Tell Their Stories* (1988).

Crucial to the fight for women's health and reproductive rights is Faye Wattleton, a former maternity nursing instructor at Miami Valley Hospital of Nursing in Dayton, Ohio. From public health work, she moved into minor roles in Planned Parenthood Federation of America and, in 1978, advanced to the presidency. During the antichoice backlash of 1977, she fought the fundamentalist Right to Life initiative with radio and television talk show appeals. Chief among her goals for family planning was the distribution of diaphragms, birth control pills, and intrauterine devices among sexually active teens. Of the cruelty of the Hyde Amendment, which ended Medicaid abortion funding to the poor in 1976, Wattleton said, "The women who came to my hospitals under less than dignified circumstances were not affluent. That girl in

Harlem who died was not affluent. . . . *That's* when I became aware of the political significance of these people. If [Congress] really cared about equity and fairness in life they would say that as long as abortion is legal in this country, poor people should have the same access as the rich" (Smith 1993, 577).

Cool and composed, Wattleton stood her ground and offered rational solutions to controversial social issues, especially the high rate of teen pregnancies. During the Reagan-Bush administration, she forced the media to divulge attempts to dismantle women's health programs and to limit the accessibility of abortion. Her 1986 book, *How to Talk to Your Child about Sex,* sold more than thirty thousand copies. Her career in extending equal protection of reproductive rights to all women earned her the 1986 Humanist of the Year Award.

In the military, Brigadier General Hazel Winifred Johnson, a twenty-four-year veteran from West Chester, Pennsylvania, achieved a notable position of authority. In 1979, she became the first black woman in American military history to be promoted to general. A graduate of Harlem Hospital School of Nursing, Villanova University, and Columbia University, she earned a Ph.D. from Catholic University of America. She advanced to head the Army Nurse Corps, a staff of seven thousand nurses in the regular army, reserves, and national guard. Her command encompassed fifty-six community hospitals, eight medical centers, and 143 clinics in the United States and five other countries. Her honors include a Legion of Merit, Army Commendation Medal with oak leaf cluster, Distinguished Service Medal, and Meritorious Service Medal.

In 1987, President Ronald Reagan appointed another famous black woman as chief of the Army Nurse Corps, Brigadier General Clara Mae Leach Adams-Ender, who grew up sharecropping tobacco in Willow Springs, North Carolina. A nurse specializing in medical surgical nursing and holding two M.S. degrees, she worked as a maid and hairdresser while completing her studies at North Carolina A&T State University. In 1976, she became the first nurse to complete a degree in the art and science of military operation from Command and General Staff College in Fort Leavenworth, Kansas. The first woman to earn an Army Expert Field Medical badge, she is the second black chief of operations, following Hazel Johnson, who held the post from 1979 to 1983. In 1990, as commander of Ft. Belvoir in Fairfax County, Virginia, General Adams-Ender became the first nurse to manage a major army base. When discussing the history of the military medical corps, she claimed that sexism was more of a hindrance to nurses in the military than racism. Her responsibilities have placed her over recruitment, selection, assignment, and retention of nurses and general personnel management, a charge affecting a staff of forty thousand worldwide. During the Gulf War, she directed twenty thousand army nurses and twenty-five thousand medical personnel and rose to the highest rank attained by a female member of the army. She earned a Distinguished Service Medal, Meritorious Service Medal, Army Commendation Medal, and the Legion of Merit. In 1995, after retirement from the army, she joined CAPE Associates as chief executive officer and produced a video, "Caring about People with Enthusiasm," an inspirational message about management, quality, and productivity.

See also: Civil War; Disease; Hale, Clara; Seacole, Mary Jane

Sources

Boardman, Mabel. *Under the Red Cross Flag at Home and Abroad.* London: J. B. Lippincott, 1915.

Bois, Danuta. "Mary Eliza Mahoney." http://www.netsrq.com/~dbois/mahoney-me.html.

Campbell, Marie. *Folks Do Get Born.* New York: Rinehart, 1946.

"Caring about People with Enthusiasm." http://cause-www.colorado.edu/information-resources/ir-library-abstracts/vic0027.html.

Carnegie, M. Elizabeth. *The Path We Tread: Blacks in Nursing Worldwide, 1854–1994.* New York: National League for Nursing Press, 1995.

Cheers, D. Michael. "Nurse Corps Chief." *Ebony* (June 1989): 64–66.

"Clara Adams-Ender." http://www.army.mil/cmh-pg/anc/18_Ender.html.

"Gen. Adams-Ender Now Top Woman in Army as Head of Ft. Belvoir in Va." *Jet,* October 21, 1991, 8.

"The General Is a Lady." *Ebony* (February 1980): 44–47.

"Harriet Tubman." http://www.acusd.edu/!jdesnet/tubman.html.

———. http://www.davison.k12.mi.us/projects/women/tubman.htm.

———. http://www.techline.com/~havelokk/harriet.html.

"Hazel W. Johnson." http://www.army.mil/cmh-pg/anc/18—Johnson.html.

Hine, Darlene Clark. *Black Women in White.* Bloomington: Indiana University Press, 1989.

Hine, Darlene Clark, Elsa Barkley Brown, and Rosalyn Terborg-Penn, eds. *Black Women in America: An Historical Encyclopedia.* Bloomington: Indiana University Press, 1993.

Hurmence, Belinda. *Before Freedom: 48 Oral Histories of Former North and South Carolina Slaves.* New York: Mentor Books, 1990.

Jordan, Denise. *Susie King Taylor.* Orange, N.J.: Just Us Books, 1994.

Kalisch, Philip, and Beatrice J. Kalisch. *The Advance of American Nursing.* Boston: Little, Brown, 1978.

Lamps on the Prairie: A History of Nursing in Kansas. Emporia.: Kansas State Nurses' Association, 1942.

"Mabel Keaton Staupers." http://www.nursing-world.org/hof/staumk.htm.

"Mary Eliza Mahoney." http://www.njrsingworld.org/hof/mahome.htm.

Schorr, Thelma M., R.N., and Anne Zimmerman, R.N., eds. *Making Choices, Taking Chances: Nurse Leaders Tell Their Stories.* St. Louis: C. V. Mosby, 1988.

Sheldon, Kathryn. "A Brief History of Black Women in the Military." *Precinct Reporter,* April 18, 1996, 2–6.

Sherr, Lynn, and Jurate Kazickas. *Susan B. Anthony Slept Here: A Guide to American Women's Landmarks.* New York: Times Books, 1994.

Shoemaker, Sister M. Theophane. *History of Nurse-Midwifery in the United States.* New York: Garland Publishing, 1984.

Smith, Jesse Carney. *Epic Lives: One Hundred Black Women Who Made a Difference.* Detroit: Visible Ink, 1993.

———. *Notable Black American Women.* Detroit: Gale, 1992.

Sterne, Capt. Doris M. *In and Out of Harm's Way: A History of the Navy Nurse Corps.* Seattle, Wash.: Peanut Butter Publishing, 1996.

Thoms, Adah B. *Pathfinders: A History of the Progress of Colored Graduate Nurses.* New York: Kay Printing House, n.d.

"Women in the Military." *Essence* (April 1990): 44–45.
Yost, Edna. *American Women of Nursing.* Philadelphia: J. B. Lippincott, 1947.

Ancient Times

Medical texts, which were among the earliest documents retrieved from prehistory, tended to ascribe ancient healing to one figure, the priest-physician, and to limit nursing to male attendants or temple women. Across European and Asian cultures, the practice of incubation, or sleeping in holy places, was linked with miraculous cures and with dreams that provided keys to restorative practices. This psychic method occurred at the oracle of Dionysus at Phocis, where the god cured disease by revealing to dreamers the remedies for their ills. The Egyptians accorded care of the sick to three gods. Strongest among the triad was Isis, nurturing mother, joined in healing ceremonies by her son Horus, her disciple. Osiris, Horus's father, ruled over the soul as it migrated from the body of the deceased into the afterlife. Artistic representation of the Egyptian healing family on murals and decorative scrolls presented a picture of tender devotion to the sick.

In more substantial form, written historical evidence of postmythic nurse care offered a sketchy timeline of early medical advancement. Around 2650 B.C., the court physician Imhotep so impressed King Zoser (or Djoser) that he became one of the few Egyptian mortals to be deified and reigned as god of medicine. His disciples welcomed the sick as well as barren women, who sought his aid at numerous temples. At about this same time, the Emperor Shen Nung, a noted Asian herbalist, founded Chinese medicine. Over two thousand years later, his decoctions, both beneficial and poisonous, appeared in China's first medical text, the *Pen Tsao* (Herbal). Additional healing treatment was recorded in Emperor Huang-ti's *Neiching* (Medicine) (ca. 2575 B.C.), which instructed the physician to look, listen, ask questions, and feel for signs of illness. Acupuncture, massage, moxa (com-

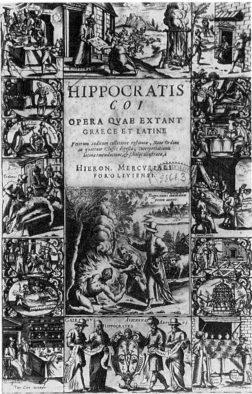

Title page showing the various roles of a physician from Opera Quae Extant Graece et Latine, *a sixteenth-century edition of the text by Hippocrates (U.S. National Library of Medicine)*

bustion of herbs against the skin), and herbal application of seaweed, ma huang, and ginseng were also part of ancient traditions, which practitioners of alternative medicine embraced in the mid-to-late twentieth century. No mention of a hospital occurred in Chinese history until 651 B.C., when Son Gand Wu referred to the Halls of Healing. Noted healers began appearing in texts in the first century B.C., with the recorded treatments of Ts'ang Kung, innovator Chang Chung-ching in the second century A.D., and a contemporary, Hua T'O, a surgeon skilled with anesthesia. Late in the spread of Buddhism from China to Korea and Japan, the oriental figure of Kwan-Yin (also Kwannon), a goddess of mercy and patron of childbirth, appeared in art as a nurturing benefactress cradling a child.

To the west, ancient medical workers made parallel progress from superstition to hands-on care. Egyptian papyri dating to 3000 B.C. indicate a systematic treatment of disease through a synthesis of magic and worship. The Ebers Papyrus, found at Luxor and dated to 1500 B.C., contained a treasury of ancient Egyptian spells, incantations, and eight hundred simples. Sumerian clay tablets from the town of Nippur excavated in southern Iraq recorded additional commentary on medical use of myrtle, thyme, pear, fig, myrrh, and barley. An Assyrian cuneiform tablet of the seventh century B.C. from King Ashurbanipal's library at Nineveh in northern Iraq revealed botanical information about the application of 250 healing remedies to specific symptoms.

The Jews were the first to mention nurses as caregivers of the sick by calling for healing and visiting patients as a community obligation. To distinguish the healer from priests, Hebrew texts referred to the nurse as a general practitioner, a secular figure. According to the Babylonian Talmud, nurse care as one of the ten ethical duties was an outgrowth of the third book of the Torah. In Leviticus 19:18, the law commands, "And you shall love your neighbor as yourself" (Dorff 1988, 35). From this specific obligation came Jewish visitation societies and prayers for the sick. Late in the twelfth century, Rabbi Moses Maimonides, a Spanish clinician and personal doctor of Sultan Saladin, was one of many doctor-rabbis over two millennia. He allied piety with medical scholarship and practice in a life devoted to godly service. His dual career embodied the explicit instruction of Deuteronomy 30:19–20: "I call heaven and earth to witness against you this day: I have put before you life and death, blessing and curse. Choose life—if you and your offspring would live—by loving the Lord your God, heeding His commandments, and holding fast to Him" (Dorff 1988, 36). Simultaneously with the Torah and Talmud, India revered its own professional writings, particularized in the Atharvaveda (or Ayur Veda), compiled about 700 B.C. A twenty-volume medical text on health and longevity, it outlines a series of six hundred incantations to accompany such herbal remedies as lotus root and physical prevention and treatment of disease.

In the gray area separating Greek mythology from history, the first doctor was Aesculapius (also Asklepios or Asclepius), a human doctor who rose in stature to a revered cult figure about 600 B.C. as the deified son of Apollo, the Olympian god of healing. His Eastern parallel, Arabus, son of Apollo and Babylone, taught medicine in Arabia. Aesculapius trained in medicine under Chiron the centaur and remained a favorite of Greek deities until he overstepped his healing art by bringing a dead man back to life. At the Delphic Oracle, petitioners prayed to Aesculapius to avert plague or epidemic, a very real and terrifying stalker in Greek history. The fullest account of a patient seeking treatment in the temple of Aesculapius occurred in the *Sacred Tales* of Aelius Aristides, a second-century Greek hypochondriac who lived at Smyrna in Lydia, due east from Athens on the modern-day coast of Turkey. In well-documented first-person testimony, he centered his affairs in the diagnosis and cure of a long string of physical ailments.

One vivid account of a terrible outbreak of fever occurred in the historian Thucydides' *The Peloponnesian War,* a six-book overview left unfinished at his death about 399 B.C. In Book 1, he describes a raging malady and the social breakdown that resulted from its virulence. In reference to caregivers, he spoke of the frustration that accompanied treatment: "Some died from want of care, but so did others who were receiving the greatest attention. No single remedy was established as a specific; for what did good to one did harm to another. . . . More often the sick and the dying were tended by the pitying care of those who had recovered, because they knew the course of the disease and were themselves free from apprehension" (Thucydides 1963, 75).

Aesculapius shared his powers with two daughters. Hygieia (also spelled Hygea,

Hygeia, or Hygia), goddess of health and mental acuity, and her counterpart, Panacea (or Panaceia) the all-healer, goddess of cures and treatments, symbolized contrasting medical states. In their honor, ancient people established Aesculapian shrines in sunny hillside healing centers at Kos and Pergamum and propitiated the great doctor with gifts to his daughters, through whom the sick hoped to return to health. A central healing shrine at Epidaurus developed into a health spa, where the sick took mineral waters, bathed, slept in holy quarters, and sought attendance from Aesculepiads, the temple's religious attendants. These figures are the first public nurses named in ancient lore. From this era derives the *iamata,* or recorded cures and miracles inscribed on the colonnade, and the caduceus, the winged, serpent-entwined walking staff of Aesculapius, which became the emblem of Hygieia, who fed snakes from a cup as a symbol of regeneration and physical renewal.

More substantive information about healing and nurse care is available from plentiful sources. References to Greek prehistory in early manuscripts retain the community respect for caregivers and name men and women as healers: for example, Apollonius of Rhodes's *Argonautica* (ca. 260 B.C.), which describes how the ship *Argo* sailed to the Black Sea bearing its own medic, Eurybates (or Eribotes), who treated Oileus for a wound inflicted by the Stymphalian birds. In the Western world's most revered war narrative, the *Iliad* (ca. 850 B.C.), Homer cited Aesculapius's sons Machaon and Podaleirius as army doctors. The Greek historian Pausanias enlarged on the family trade in the fifth century B.C. with mention of Machaon's son Polemocrates. Two female practitioners appear in Homer's texts: Helen of Troy, who dispensed nepenthe, a soporific, and Hakameda, a female combat nurse, the first mentioned in European literature. Likewise, he detailed wartime surgery and first aid rendered by fellow warriors.

The Golden Age of Greek literature added to the store of data about early nurse care. The tragedian Euripides gave a leading role to the nurse in *Hippolytus* (428 B.C.) and had her tend the frenzied Phaedra. As Theseus's queen sickens with an unwholesome love, it is the nurse who supports and comforts her and speaks the concern of a bedside caregiver:

> It's better to be sick than nurse the sick.
> Sickness is a single trouble for the sufferer:
> But nursing means vexation of the mind,
> and hard work for the hands besides.
>   (Euripides 1960, 186–189)

After Phaedra's suicide, it is the nurse who supervises the other servants in laying out her patient's body.

Contemporaneous with Euripides' stage plays was the evolution of empirical healing and scientific discovery devoid of the Aesculapian worship and superstitions of past ages. The father of medical arts, Hippocrates of Kos, founded a system of *klinikos,* a patient-centered medicine. Central to his system was *vis medicatrix naturae* (the healing force of nature), which rejected magic and omens and looked for the causes of disease in the patient's anatomical condition, whether from poor hygiene, contaminated food, contagion, lack of exercise, or other natural occurrence (Bean 1963, 56). The young interns who studied under Hippocrates performed the nurse's duties of bathing, dressing wounds, and observing symptoms firsthand, which formed the basis of Hippocrates' diagnoses.

Late in the fourth century B.C., Lycurgus, the Athenian statesman, orator, and lawgiver, described in detail the disposal of a newborn. As reiterated by the biographer Plutarch in *Lives of the Noble Greeks* (ca. 100 A.D.), the decision whether a child should be tended or abandoned as unworthy was left to the father and the elders of the tribe. If the child's constitution proved hardy, it was passed to the care of nursemaids, who bathed it in wine rather than water to give it a wholesome complexion and temperament. Lycurgus extolled the caution of Spartan nurses, who left infants unswaddled to toughen them. Averse to

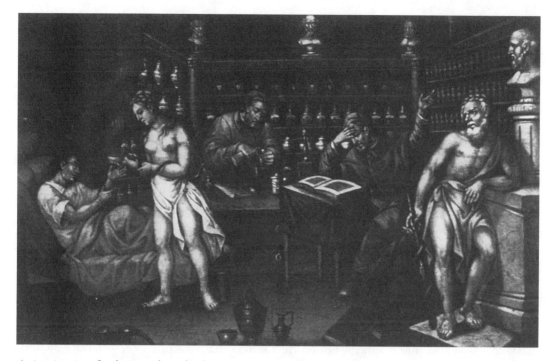

An interior view of a pharmacy shows the physician, the pharmacist, and a patient being attended to by Hygeia, the patron goddess of the pharmacy. Aesculapius, leaning against a bust of Hippocrates, observes the scene. (U.S. Library of Medicine)

the Mediterranean custom of binding children to a swaddling board papoose-style, the Spartan nursery keepers let babies thrive unconstrained to expose them to the elements and taught them not to fear the dark, whimper or refuse food, or mind being left alone. For this regimen, parents in other countries prized and sought out the Spartan nurse for family service.

The first *maia,* or midwife, in the Western world and founder of women's health initiatives, Agnodice (also Agnodike or Hagnodike), whose name translates as "pure before justice," is an obscure figure in Greek folk history. As described in the first century A.D. by Roman mythographer Hyginus, staff librarian to the Emperor Augustus, she established the traditions of female practitioners who supported women in contraception, fertility, pregnancy, abortion, childbirth, postpartum recovery, and lactation. According to Latin reference texts, Agnodice lived in Greece in the early third century B.C. and most probably had children of her own, a re-

quirement in Athens for practitioners of midwifery. To circumvent an Athenian ban on broader medical training for women, she cut her hair and enshrouded her feminine features in men's clothing. Thus freed of prejudice against women, she studied under Herophilus the Chalcedon, the renowned anatomist, obstetrician, textbook author, and specialist in internal medicine who taught and practiced dissection in Alexandria, Egypt, around 285 B.C. He probably taught her the latest techniques, for example, use of a cranial augur to perform embryotomy.

The writings of Plato typify the work of Agnodice's peers. Like them, she probably dispensed medication, attended laboring women at the birthing stool, concocted herbal recipes to speed labor and reduce pain, removed the "afterburden," and performed abortions, likely by the insertion of pessaries or herbal suppositories into the vagina. Aristotle augmented knowledge of this era of midwifery with his picture of the ideal practitioner: a sturdy, god-fearing woman of middle age, clean and healthy of body, steady of hand, strong-willed, and patient. Over all the fearful sufferings of women, midwives invoked the guidance and blessing of Hera and Artemis, two beneficent, pro-female deities.

History indicates that Agnodice became a great favorite of women seeking quality gynecological advice and care. During her practice, an incident regarding a woman refusing aid from a male doctor forced her to lift her chiton and reveal her gender to establish rapport with the patient. The act corroborates Hippocrates' claim in *De Morbis Mulierum* (On Women's Diseases) that prudish female patients hesitated to confide in or cooperate with male doctors. Athenian physicians blocked competition from Agnodice by labeling her a lecher. They claimed that she seduced and corrupted patients and asserted that women feigned illness to gain her lewd ministrations. Specifically, she was charged with practicing medicine under false pretense and with committing adultery with Agisilea, wife of Areopagites.

It was the loyalty of women that saved Agnodice. In court, she again lifted her garment to disclose female genitalia. If convicted of the men's charge of illegally entering medical study, she faced a death sentence. In a show of support, patients came to Agnodice's rescue, clamoring for her release and spurning their assembled husbands as enemies of women's health. According to legend, the unity of women won out over the fusty all-male medical establishment. Athenian lawmakers altered community statutes by lifting the ban on freeborn female practitioners and extended government stipends for licensed midwives.

In the following millennium, Hindu healers followed the example of Hippocrates by producing a standard medical text *Charaka* (or Caraka) (120 A.D.). Composed by a physician of the same name, the work advanced a holistic system of treatment to restore balance of mind and body. The author insisted that nurses be decent, skillful, and compassionate. According to the text, they should spare physicians by accepting all basic manual labor, whether cooking, changing bed linens, or lifting, repositioning, bathing, and massaging patients. Nearly three centuries later, Susruta (or Sushruta), an Indian surgeon, described symptoms, complex surgical procedures, instruments, anesthesia, and medicaments, which his colleagues used in amputation, cautery, trepanation, cataract removal, plastic surgery, and skin grafting.

Parallel to the growth of medical knowledge to the east, the citizens of the early Roman Empire, ever the pragmatists, accepted care from any healer, *sive masculus sive femina* (whether male or female) (Marks and Beatty 1972, 42). A systematized nurse care among the destitute suited the Roman municipal planners of a well-run city. They established *valetudinaria* (nursing homes) for slaves and separate hospitals for war casualties in which slave nurses practiced medicine under the orders of Greek doctors, themselves prisoners of war whom the Romans, nonetheless, respected. Catalogued in *De Re Medicina* (About Medicine), the encyclopedia of first-century scholar Aurelius Cornelius Celsus, are eight surviving books of medical history. In addition to surgery and pharmacology, he describes prevailing concepts of psychiatry and nutrition.

Perpetuating the Aesculapian cult under the aegis of Salus, the personification of health, the Romans preserved the wisdom of the Greek healing arts and evolved their own noted practitioners. A realistic text from the Roman Empire derives from an army surgeon and botanist, Pedanius Dioscorides, who traveled about the Mediterranean shore as a member of Nero's military staff in the first century A.D. By sampling and studying animal, plant, and mineral products, he compiled a five-volume work on pharmacopoeia, *De Materia Medica,* which remained in use until the seventeenth century. One of the prominent treatments was *salix,* the Latin word for willow, a source of aspirin widely available wherever the army camped and applicable to fever, swelling, and pain.

Also a recipient of Greek expertise, the Islamic world developed nurse care by applying the medical notations of Hippocrates, who developed individualized treatment regimens based on patient observation. To his classical protocols, the Arabs added their knowledge of chicory, oxymel (a syrup of honey and vinegar), balsam, spinach, saffron, and camphor and the application of mercury to skin ailments suffered by desert dwellers. To maintain good health among early bedouins, Arab doctors countered the constant onslaught of dehydration from scarce water; flying insects; and internal parasites, including bilharziasis, roundworms, and guinea worms; and battled septic conditions that encouraged epidemics. In prehistory, healers applied folk medicine and superstitions to ailments, crotchets, moods, and passions. Islamic followers of Hippocrates linked obtrusive symptoms to imbalances, overproduction, and depletion of the four body humors—blood, phlegm, yellow bile, and black bile, which correspond with the emotional states of jocularity, indolence, envy, and anger. For treatment of contagious disease, nurse-practitioners valued camel's milk and urine, honey, henna, salt, sulphur, and cupping as general treatments for outbreaks of smallpox, leprosy, dysentery, trachoma, conjunctivitis, malaria, and tuberculosis.

In the golden age of Islamic medicine, there was no direct mention of nursing staffs. The era's medical authority, Rhazes, an eminent physician of Baghdad, extracted from the Greek texts of Hippocrates and Galen the elements of anatomy and physiology unknown to Arab doctors, who were forbidden to dissect human corpses. In Rhazes's initial monograph, *A Treatise on the Small Pox and Measles* (910 A.D.), he provided the medical world with the first precise description of two persistent plagues. His major work, *The Compendium* (ca. 925 A.D.), recorded patient histories that reveal his diagnostic skill. A century later, the Arab world augmented Rhazes's innovations with the advice of Avicenna, author of *Canon of Medicine* (ca. 1025). A well-read scholar, he based his text on the classical medical writings of Aristotle, Dioscorides, and Galen, earning for himself the sobriquet of "the Persian Galen." Avicenna's comprehensive medical encyclopedia was so thorough and innovative that it remained in print in Europe into the seventeenth century.

The advent of Islamic hospital nurse care derives from three developments: the work of Caliph Harun al-Rashid, founder of a Baghdad facility in the ninth century, a subsequent tenth-century Baghdad hospital established by Caliph al-Muktadir, and the practice of Maimonides. Valuable insights of Islamic medicine fill the treatises that Constantinus Africanus transported to Salerno, Italy, in 1060, upgrading the Italian medical profession. By the late thirteenth century in Arab facilities in Cairo, Baghdad, Alexandria, and Damascus, nurse care, provided only by males, had evolved in separate wards, which focused on fevers, wounds, women's needs, and trachoma and other eye diseases. Pharmacies offered individualized blends to heal sickness and maintain wellness. Teaching hospitals consisted of lecture halls and medical libraries and employed settlement workers to reestablish convalescing patients in normal life.

See also: Christian Nursing; Disease; Hospice; Midwifery; Native American Nursing

Sources

Aikman, Lonnelle. *Nature's Healing Arts: From Folk Medicine to Modern Drugs.* Washington, D.C.: National Geographic, 1966.

Baly, Monica E. *Nursing and Social Change.* New York: Routledge, 1995.

Bean, William B., M.D. "Medicine's Forgotten Man—the Patient." *Nursing Forum* (1963): 46–69.

Bell, Robert E. *Dictionary of Classical Mythology.* Santa Barbara, Calif.: ABC-CLIO, 1982.

———. *Women of Classical Mythology: A Biographical Dictionary.* Santa Barbara, Calif.: ABC-CLIO, 1991.

Bowder, Diana, ed. *Who Was Who in the Greek World.* New York: Washington Square Press, 1982.

Brainard, Annie M. *The Evolution of Public Health Nursing.* Philadelphia: W. B. Saunders, 1922.

Cavendish, Richard, ed. *Man, Myth and Magic.* New York: Marshall Cavendish, 1970.

Dock, Lavinia, and Isabel M. Stewart. *A Short History of Nursing.* New York: G. P. Putnam's Sons, 1938.

Dolan, Josephine A., R.N. *History of Nursing.* Philadelphia: W. B. Saunders, 1968.

Dorff, Elliot. "Judaism and Health." *Health Values* (May-June 1988): 32–36.

Durant, Will. *The Life of Greece.* New York: Simon and Schuster, 1939.

Ellis, Peter Berresford. *Celtic Women: Women in Celtic Society and Literature.* Grand Rapids, Mich.: William B. Eerdmans, 1995.

Euripides. *Hippolytus* in *Greek Tragedies* Vol. 1. David Grene and Richmond Lattimore, eds. Chicago: Phoenix Books, 1960.

Finnegan, Rachel. "The Professional Careers: Women Pioneers and the Male Image Seduction." *Classics Ireland.* http://www.ucd.ie/~classics/Finnegan95.html.

Fischer-Kamel, Doris Sofie. "The Midwife in History with Special Emphasis on Practice in Medieval Europe and in the Islamic World." Monograph. University of Arizona, 1987.

Franck, Irene, and David Brownstone. *Women's World: A Timeline of Women in History.* New York: HarperPerennial, 1995.

Griffin, Gerald Joseph, and H. Joann King Griffin. *Jensen's History and Trends of Professional Nursing.* St. Louis, Mo.: C. V. Mosby, 1965.

Hammond, N. G. L., and H. H. Scullard, eds. *The Oxford Classical Dictionary.* Oxford: Clarendon Press, 1992.

Hurd-Mead, Kate Campbell. *A History of Women in Medicine: From the Earliest Times to the Beginning of the Nineteenth Century.* Haddam, Conn.: Haddam Press, 1938.

James, Peter, and Nick Thorpe. *Ancient Inventions.* New York: Ballantine Books, 1994.

Jamieson, Elizabeth, and Mary F. Sewall. *Trends in Nursing History.* London: W. B. Saunders Company, 1949.

Kalisch, Philip, and Beatrice J. Kalisch. *The Advance of American Nursing.* Boston: Little, Brown, 1978.

Kent, Jacqueline C. *Women in Medicine.* Minneapolis, Minn.: Oliver Press, 1998.

Lefkowitz, Mary. *Women's Life in Greece and Rome.* Baltimore: Johns Hopkins University Press, 1992.

Magic and Medicine of Plants. Pleasantville, N.Y.: Reader's Digest, 1986.

Marks, Geoffrey, and William K. Beatty. *Women in White.* New York: Charles Scribner's Sons, 1972.

Marland, Hilary, ed. *The Art of Midwifery: Early Modern Midwives in Europe.* London: Routledge, 1993.

McKown, Robin. *Heroic Nurses.* New York: G. P. Putnam's Sons, 1966.

Nikiforuk, Andrew. *The Fourth Horseman: A Short History of Epidemics, Plagues, Famine and Other Scourges.* Toronto: Penguin, 1992.

Plutarch. *Lycurgus* in *Lives of the Noble Greeks.* Edmund Fuller, ed. New York: Laurel Classic, 1959.

Snodgrass, Mary Ellen. *Voyages in Classical Mythology.* Santa Barbara, Calif.: ABC-CLIO, 1994.

Thucydides. *The Peloponnesian Wars.* New York: Washington Square Press, 1963.

Ullmann, Manfred. *Islamic Medicine.* Edinburgh: University Press, 1978.

"Under the Knife: A History of Medicine." http://musejhu.edu/demo/performing_arts_journal/18.2skipitares.html.

"Women in Medicine." http://www.med.virginia.edu/hs-library/historical/antigua/stext.htm.

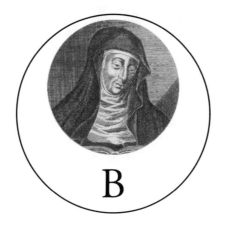

B

Ballard, Martha

Martha Moore Ballard, a multiskilled general practitioner, herbalist, midwife, and visiting nurse from Kennebec, Maine, typifies the career and social position of the town nurse in the three decades following the American Revolution. Laurel Thatcher Ulrich, a history professor at the University of New Hampshire at Durham, reshaped and expounded on Ballard's daybook of experiences over a twenty-seven-year period in *A Midwife's Tale: The Life of Martha Ballard, Based on Her Diary, 1785–1812* (1990). The text opens in Ballard's fiftieth year and touches on the hardships incurred by an itinerant healer in the nation's early years. She was born in 1735 in Oxford, Massachusetts, and trained through practical experience. The wife of Ephraim Ballard, a surveyor, mapmaker, and miller, she knew the anguish of debt, which brought her husband an eighteen-month term in jail in 1804–1805. In addition to bearing nine children and burying three in a little over three years, she performed the daily woman's work of readying flax for weaving, bartering for vegetables, brewing beer and vinegar, baking and cooking, slaughtering, making soap and candles, and monitoring the minutiae of colonial housekeeping.

As a health professional, Ballard began delivering babies in July 1778, thus setting up a source of steady income for herself among local females, regardless of race or social status. Her birth records are meticulous for the times and include the name of the father and the condition of mother and child. In one description of teamwork at a social or community childbirth, she concludes with the rewards to the dominant midwife: "Mrs Sewall was ill till 3 hour pm when shee was through divine asistance made a Living Mother of a Living Son, her 3d Child. Mrs. Brooks, Belcher, Colman, Pollard & Voce assisted us. . . . Colonel Sewall gave me 6/8 as a reward. Conducted me over the river" (Ulrich 1990, 94–95). Her amassed data show that she safely delivered 768 babies to 814 parturient women, averaging thirty-three deliveries annually. In only two instances was she obliged to call in a physician, one a delivery botched by another midwife.

As was typical of midwives throughout history, Ballard earned community esteem as an observer and spokesperson. A difficult time occurred locally in 1789, when her testimony at a rape trial put her at the center of controversy over a capital crime. Concerning her role at the Vassalboro trial, she wrote, "The 26 instant I called to mind Mrs. Foster saying

Colonel North had positively had unlawful concors with a woman which was not his wife and I Begd her never to mentin it to any other person. I told her shee would Expose & perhaps ruin her self if shee did" (Ulrich 1990, 117). Obviously a confidante of the abused woman, Ballard listened patiently and compassionately, keeping wise counsel and rendering advice consistent with her milieu. In private commentary, she appended the particulars of the rape, committed by a man of stature who was eventually exonerated.

In addition to obstetrics, Ballard tended human and animal patients, laid out corpses for burial, and gathered and dried her own herbs for syrups, tinctures, salves, teas, ointments, poultices, gargles, and emulsions. On April 4, 1801, she described her observations at an autopsy: "The left lobe of the lights were found to be much inflamed, the intestines allso in which were 4 intersections, an inflamation of the kidneys and Blather. There were not a single worm Contained in the boddy. . . . The gaull blather was larg and very full" (Ulrich 1990, 236). From her immersion in the dissection of internal organs, she left to attend a woman in labor and stayed the night. For a woman in her mid-sixties, Ballard functioned well and sustained an interest in human health and welfare.

Over rain-swelled creeks and rivers by canoe, through ice and snowbanks, and on horseback down shadowy country lanes, Ballard visited the sick. Usually on foot, she returned from a busy practice to keep her daybook, gather firewood, and see to her family's needs. When weariness precipitated illness from May 22 to 23, 1798, Ballard, then sixty-three years old, took to her bed and wrote, "I Eat a little cold puding and Cold milk twice in the coars of the day and perform part of my washing. I Laid myself on the bed in the bedroom was not able to rise from ther. . . . How many times I have been necasatated to rest my self on the bed I am not able to say. God grant me patience to go thro the fatages of this life with fortitude looking forward to a more happy state" (Ulrich 1990, 226). When called

to a deathbed, she nursed the patient as though performing a Christian duty. Of Parthenia Pitts's demise, she writes: "She Expird in a very short space without a strugle Except distress for Breath. We have reason to hope our loss [is] her gain" (Ulrich 1990, 253). The unsentimental account of Ballard on the edge of Maine's outback ennobles a nurse-midwife dedicated to helping her neighbors and to fulfilling a religious mission.

See also: Gender Issues in Nursing; Midwifery; Nineteenth-Century Nursing

Sources

Marland, Hilary, ed. *The Art of Midwifery: Early Modern Midwives in Europe*. London: Routledge, 1993.

Ulrich, Laurel Thatcher. *A Midwife's Tale: The Life of Martha Ballard, Based on Her Diary, 1785–1812*. New York: Alfred A. Knopf, 1990.

Barton, Clara

One of the many patriotic nurses and laywomen who volunteered during the Civil War, nurse Clarissa "Clara" Harlowe Barton expanded her involvement in humanitarianism by searching for missing soldiers and by founding the American Red Cross. While heading the organization for twenty-two years, she treated suffering as close to home as the Johnstown Flood and as distant as Armenia. Through her persistence, the United States abandoned isolationism and, in March 1882, signed the Geneva Convention, an international agreement that bound its sixteen member nations to abstain from attacks on medical transport, supply trains, buildings, and staff and to care for sick and wounded combatants without regard to allegiance, nationality, or race.

Significant to the history of Barton's altruism is the thirty-five-volume diary she kept of her family background and two published memoirs, *A Story of the Red Cross* (1904) and *The Story of My Childhood* (1907). Born December 25, 1821, in Oxford, Massachusetts, she was the fifth child of a farm couple, Sarah and Stephen Harlowe, who operated a sawmill. She learned of army life from her father, a veteran of the Indian wars, and got home training in patient care while tending her invalid brother David. Barton was a superintendent of schools and teacher in Bordentown, New Jersey. On her suggestion, a local district offered free schooling to the poor. She augmented the method's success by opening a second school building to accommodate more children. From 1854 to 1857, she worked as a copyist in the patent office in Washington, D.C. When the Civil War broke out, her father urged her to go to the front, "anywhere between the bullet and the hospital" (Ward 1988, 15).

Nicknamed the "Angel of the Battlefield," Barton applied native ability, moral purpose, and discretion to the job of patient care. An independent volunteer with the Sixth Massachusetts Regiment, she was appalled at the men's suffering when the first wounded arrived in Baltimore in April 1861 and were transported to the Capitol and bedded down on the Senate Chamber floor. She ran an ad in the *Worcester Spy* for more volunteer nurses, whom she assigned as needed.

As nursing superintendent for the Army of the James, Barton accompanied troop transports and nursed at the front during the battles of Cedar Mountain, Bull Run, Antietam, Fredericksburg, Charleston, Fort Wagner, Petersburg, Chantilly, and the Wilderness. The Cedar Mountain engagement introduced her to the terrors of combat nursing. For five days, she made do with three hours of sleep. At the Second Battle of Bull Run in August 1862, she and Almira Fales faced three thousand wounded lying in the sun at the Fairfax railroad station with nothing but two water buckets, five tin cups, a kettle and stewpan, two lanterns, four knives, three plates, and a tin casserole. Dodging shells, Barton drove a mule wagon to dressing stations. She garnered discarded jars, bowls, tumblers, and cans to carry soup or coffee to survivors and, within two days, packed them off to convalescent wards by train.

At Antietam on September 17, 1862, where twenty-three thousand fell in combat,

Barton anticipated the battle by four days and arrived by mule convoy. After reconnoitering through field glasses, she ferried supplies through corn rows to dressing stations, where doctors had little more than corn shucks to use as bandages. A steady hand with a lamp at the surgical table, she administered chloroform and managed instruments. As shells burst overhead, jostling patient and surgeon, she wrung blood from her petticoats to lighten the hem. While attending a soldier, she bent to his request just as a bullet passed through her sleeve and killed the man instantly. With a pocketknife, she removed a minié ball from another casualty's cheek. To ferry crackers to hungry men, she pinned a square of cloth together at the corners to form an apron pocket. Among her other rewards to convalescing soldiers were discreet gifts of whisky, wine, and tobacco. At the end of her service at Antietam, she departed by mule wagon and slept soundly as a guard drove her back to Washington, D.C.

The Battle of Fredericksburg placed Barton at the center of another sea of wounded. From the improvised aid hospital in Lacy House, on December 13, 1862, she answered the call of surgeon J. Clarence Cutter, who named her specifically to nurse the fallen of the 21st Massachusetts Regiment. After crossing a bridge under fire where a bullet ripped her sleeve, she displayed a talent for imposing administrative calm by attending black and white Union and Confederate victims of a disorderly rout and dispatching wounded men to tents, churches, hotels, and private residences. Unruffled, she passed unchallenged through an unruly area controlled only by martial law.

On September 15, 1863, Barton's battlefield ministrations ended after she received notice that she was no longer needed. Dispirited, she returned to Washington to a whirl of social engagements and honors. In March 1864, she met President Abraham Lincoln and flourished under media attention yet longed to return to action. Rescued from boredom by General Benjamin F. Butler, she assumed the title of superintendent of the Department of Nurses for the Army of the James. To carry out her post, she acquired an unlimited pass and personally nursed the sick at Point of Rocks, Virginia. She worked at hospitals in Richmond and Morris Island, secured supplies, and remained at Andersonville Prison to tend patients for six weeks after General Robert E. Lee's surrender.

With authorization on March 11, 1865, a week before his assassination, Lincoln appointed Barton as supervisor of the office of missing soldiers, making her the first woman to operate a U.S. government bureau. The simple letter read:

To the Friends of Missing Persons:
Miss Clara Barton has kindly offered to search for the missing prisoners of war. Please address her at Annapolis, giving her name, regiment, and company of any missing prisoner.
[Signed] A. Lincoln (Ross 1956, 86)

With $15,000 from her own bank account, she hired a crew of grave diggers to locate the missing at the prison in Andersonville, Georgia. Guiding her were captured Confederate records and a list kept by Dorrence Atwater, a prison clerk. After exhuming four hundred Confederate and 12,800 Union bodies, she identified thousands of unmarked graves and corrected gravestone inscriptions improperly quoted from the Bible. By advertising names in post offices and placing ads in newspapers, she tracked down twenty-two thousand men and published the names of the war dead and the location of their graves. Still moved by the need for frontline nursing, she lectured on her experiences.

While taking a needed rest cure in Europe in 1869, Barton encountered another altruistic cause, the International Committee of the Red Cross, a humanitarian effort initiated by Jean-Henri Dunant five years before. Although the era's patriarchy denied women full participation in the Red Cross, she joined the group, which functioned during the Franco-Prussian War of 1870, and traveled to battle-grounds in Strasbourg, Paris, Lyons, Belfort, and Montpellier. Decorated by the Emperor and Empress of Germany with the Iron Cross of Merit and by the Grand Duke and Duchess of Baden with the Gold Cross of Remembrance, she returned to the United States in 1875 with plans for a national effort to supply impartial national disaster relief wherever victims appealed for help.

Six years later, on May 20, 1881, with Barton as president, the American Red Cross became a reality. Within three months, the Clara Barton Chapter No. 1, which is still in service, took shape at St. Paul's United Lutheran Church in Dansville, New York. In 1882, President Chester A. Arthur and a senate approval made the organization official. At a speech delivered to the International Council of Women in Washington, D.C., on April 1, 1888, she spoke of the kind of volunteerism she expected from the Red Cross: "I walked its hospitals day and night. I served its camps, and I marched with its men, and I know whereof I speak. The German, the Frenchman, the Italian, the Arab, the Turko, and the Zouave were gathered tenderly alike and lay side by side in the Red Cross palace hospitals of Germany. The royal women, who today mourn their own dead, mourned the dead of friend and foe" (Holland 1896, 61).

After directing battlefield relief during the Spanish-American War, she remained as head of the Red Cross until it reorganized on June 16, 1904. Her travels took her to the 1881 Michigan forest fires, the 1888 Florida yellow fever epidemic, and the 1889 Johnstown flood, during which the Red Cross aided twenty-five thousand victims. She was in Russia during the famine of 1892; in South Carolina for the hurricane and tidal wave in 1893–1894; in Turkey after the Armenian massacres in 1896; in Cuba providing postwar relief in 1898–1899; in Galveston, Texas, during the hurricane of 1900, where she worked for six weeks; and in Butler, Pennsylvania, during the 1904 typhoid epidemic. That year, at age eighty-three, she resigned her post to Mabel T. Boardman.

Barton retired to Glen Echo, Maryland, where she maintained her diary until 1910. She died of pneumonia on April 12, 1912. Her last words were an apology for groaning, which shamed her. Veterans escorted her funeral procession to Memorial Hall in Oxford, where her body lay in state under the silk pennant of the Women's Relief Corps. Red roses covered her casket as it was committed to the earth. Linked with Florence Nightingale as the two prominent caregivers of the nineteenth and twentieth centuries, Barton earned widespread acclaim for greatheartedness, modesty, and innovative administration. The Detroit *Free Press* proclaimed her the "most perfect incarnation of mercy the modern world has known" and declared her philanthropy "an intrinsic part of world civilization" (Ross 1956, 290).

The nation treasured Clara Barton as a symbol of determination and resolve. In 1910, in an article for *American Magazine,* journalist Ida Tarbell lauded her selflessness. The encomium saluted Barton's valor but championed above all her evenhandedness toward suffering people of any nationality. A memorial and shelter in Evansville, Indiana, celebrate service during the 1884 Ohio River flood, America's first organized disaster relief, during which Barton boarded the first Red Cross relief ship, the *Josh V. Throop,* to search for survivors. The Glen Echo home houses her medals and personal items. The battlefield at Antietam commemorates her many kindnesses with a marble slab and brick red cross. At the Andersonville National Cemetery, a memorial was established in 1915, the first to honor a civilian volunteer.

See also: Civil War; Red Cross

Sources

Boylston, Helen. *Clara Barton.* New York: Random House, 1955.
"Civil War Nurses." http://www.wayne.esu1.k12.ne.us/civil/morris.html.
"Clara Barton." http://www.redcross.org/hec/pre-1900/cbarton.html.
Denney, Robert E. *Civil War Medicine: Care and Comfort of the Wounded.* New York: Sterling Publishing, 1995.
"Discovered Historical Documents Uncover the First Official Missing Persons Investigator, Clara Barton." http://www.pimall.com/nais/n.barton.html.
Dolan, Josephine A., R.N. *History of Nursing.* Philadelphia: W. B. Saunders, 1968.
"A History of Helping Others." http://www.redcross.org/pa/lancaste/history.htm.
Holland, Mary A. Gardner, comp. *Our Army Nurses.* Boston: Lounsberry, Nichols and Worth, 1896.
McKown, Robin. *Heroic Nurses.* New York: G. P. Putnam's Sons, 1966.
Pryor, Elizabeth Brown. *Clara Barton: Professional Angel.* Philadelphia: University of Pennsylvania Press, 1987.
Ross, Ishbel. *Angel of the Battlefield.* New York: Harper and Brothers Publishers, 1956.
Sherr, Lynn, and Jurate Kazickas. *Susan B. Anthony Slept Here: A Guide to American Women's Landmarks.* New York: Times Books, 1994.
Sterne, Capt. Doris M. *In and Out of Harm's Way: A History of the Navy Nurse Corps.* Seattle, Wash.: Peanut Butter Publishing, 1996.
Ward, Geoffrey C. "Queen Barton." *American Heritage* (April 1988): 14–15.

Bickerdyke, Mary Ann

Mary Ann Bickerdyke was perhaps the most colorful, officious, and thoroughly documented civilian heroine to rise to the challenge of the Civil War. When she began work in the first months of combat, soldiers were already dying in alarming numbers from exposure, neglect, filth, and disease. During the spring of 1861, dysentery, pneumonia, and typhoid sapped the military as surely as a well-managed siege. The only attendants for the sick were convalescing soldiers, who shared tents with the wounded and contracted their fevers. When Dr. Edward Beecher informed his congregation of abhorrent conditions at the Cairo, Illinois, camp, the president of the Ladies' Aid Society proposed Bickerdyke, a pillar of morality, charity, and good will. She immediately accepted the post as a Christian duty.

From childhood, Bickerdyke was known for a can-do spirit. Born in Mount Vernon, Ohio, on July 19, 1817, to Hiram and Anna Rodgers Ball, she was motherless from infancy and lived with an uncle, Henry Rodgers. When the family settled in Cincinnati, she attended Oberlin College. She studied nursing privately with Dr. Reuben Mussey but had to leave school prior to graduation because of a typhus epidemic, during which she worked at the Cincinnati and Hamilton County hospitals. At age twenty-nine, she married a widower, Robert Bickerdyke, and raised their three children as well as the four children from his first marriage. The family was living in Galesburg, Illinois, when her husband and infant daughter died.

Bickerdyke supported her two sons by opening a practice in physio-botanic medicine. She was a staff herbalist at the local hospital when she accepted a charge to deliver relief supplies to the Cairo camp. She departed on June 8, 1861, aboard an all-night stage for Fort Defiance. Next morning, she surveyed the regimental hospital—three tents erected in a muddy field, straw pallets, flies, excrement, and sweaty patients lying in a heap. Dressed in serviceable calico and apron, she went to work. By bribing recruits with promises of better chow, she and aide Andy Somerville of Iowa set them to building washing facilities. She personally stripped and washed each patient in hogsheads filled with hot water and brown laundry soap, then stripped and shaved them to remove lice. Fitted out with clean linens and bedclothes, they rested on clean straw after she shoveled mud from their billets and burned old pallets and army blankets. Hopeful and contented, they ate from her picnic basket of fried chicken and home-cooked bread and vegetables. To weaker patients, she spoon-fed a watered-down toddy of whisky and brown sugar.

A noncommissioned nurse, Bickerdyke rejected the offer of a one-day pass and engaged a room at a boarding house while she cleaned and supplied the field hospital and staffed it with men commandeered from the guardhouse. Aiding her was Mary Jane Safford, the "little angel of Cairo" and, ultimately, professor of women's diseases at Boston University School of Medicine, whom Bickerdyke taught the art of camp nursing. From a woodstove in her quarters, Bickerdyke produced home-cooked delicacies and dietetics for the sick; in camp, she trained company cooks to make the most of army rations of salt pork and beans and unclaimed food parcels from home. To supplement scant funds, she advertised for volunteer nurses and donors of supplies. From the rapidly spoiling boxes that arrived at the depot, she salvaged edible food and rationed out nonperishable jams, honey, and baked goods. By October 1861, she was receiving supplies from the Chicago office of the newly organized U.S. Sanitary Commission. To halt pilfering, she dosed an enticing dish of stewed peaches with a tartar emetic and threatened to use rat poison if the staff did not stop stealing food meant for patients. By November, her systematic stocking and efficient management produced a model hospital.

When Ulysses S. Grant's troops moved south in early February 1862 to St. Louis, Missouri, and Louisville, Kentucky, Bickerdyke followed on the *City of Memphis,* one of the five river steamers converted into hospital ships. For ten days after the Battle of Fort Donelson, Tennessee, she had no time to change clothes as she received farm carts, wagons, and stretchers bearing men nearly frozen in the mud. Immediately sponged clean, dressed in fresh linens, and fed, casualties brightened at her touch and welcomed soup, crackers, coffee, and whisky. When their needs were satisfied, she took basket and supplies and visited each field hospital and then worked into the wee hours searching the battlefield for overlooked survivors. A horde of volunteers attempted to keep up with her but departed the next morning from the grim sight of so much suffering.

Bickerdyke unofficially attached herself to Grant's army and continued along the Mississippi River to Pittsburg Landing, Tennessee, performing the same job at numerous locations. Safford aided Bickerdyke in tending the sick at the confluence of the Ohio and Mississippi rivers. By the time the Union battle train reached Savannah, Tennessee, the local sanitary commission legitimized her efforts by naming her a government agent. Rebuffed by local doctors, she withdrew temporarily from the sick and set up wash pots for boiling the blood-soaked laundry that had accumulated. She petitioned the Sanitary Commission in Chicago for tubs, kettles, washing machines, irons, and mangles as a means of salvaging garments and linens from the scrap heap.

By the time wounded began arriving from Shiloh (or Pittsburg Landing) in April 1862, Bickerdyke, wrapped in a Confederate overcoat, stood on the dock and handed out crackers, hot soup, tea, and panada, an invalid's gruel made of brown sugar and crumbled hardtack stirred into whisky and hot water. To a surgeon challenging her authority to serve, she replied that she worked at the command of the Lord God Almighty. Her amazing energy is obvious from one day's laundry in September 1862, when she cleaned 3,595 pieces of wash: 1,532 undershirts, 200 shirts, 175 underpants, 400 handkerchiefs, 6 pairs of pants, 600 towels, 112 blankets and quilts, 478 pillowcases, 22 pillows, and 70 mattress covers, all washed in the woods, rinsed in a stream, and dried on branches. At sight of an overlooked patient or a moment of self-indulgence among her staff, she rebuked them for dereliction of duty.

In January 1863, Bickerdyke, aided by the trusty Somerville, superintended the army pest house at Fort Pickering outside Memphis, Tennessee. To clean the building of corpses and infected bedding, she summoned men who had survived smallpox and began burning, scrubbing, and whitewashing. With fifty black helpers, she set up a laundry in the basement and rescued soiled blankets earmarked for burning. A similar assignment in the Memphis Gayoso Hospital pitted Bickerdyke against typhoid, scurvy, and pneumonia. She worked without Safford, who had suffered nervous collapse from overwork and returned to Cairo, but replaced her with Eliza Chappell Porter, a volunteer who cut through military red tape. On a twenty-day furlough, Bickerdyke escorted several hundred amputees to Illinois, promising to return with fresh eggs and milk. On the return trip from Chicago, she silenced critics by rounding up one hundred cows and one thousand hens for the Union cause.

When Vicksburg fell to the Union army on July 4, 1863, following a two-month siege, Bickerdyke was jubilant over the victory and General William Tecumseh Sherman's statement that she outranked him. As permanent hospital aide to "General Billy," she escorted veterans on a transport to Paducah, Kentucky, and left the train to tend three wounded veterans sheltering in a shed. After locating tea, crackers, and jelly, she tore cambric nightgowns into bandages, treated infections, and redressed each wound. The next morning, she flagged a train to Paducah and settled the trio at a convalescent center. She and Boston nurse Mary Livermore worked with other volunteers to plan a soldier's home in Cairo and visited families of casualties Bickerdyke had tended in the South, one of whom she rescued from eviction and penury. Returned to combat duty, she marched with Sherman's army to Chattanooga, stopping to treat blistered feet when soldiers' boots wore out.

At the Battle of Lookout Mountain, Tennessee, Bickerdyke used bed warmers made out of bricks from an old chimney to comfort two thousand serious surgical cases and amputees. She pampered the men with her personal toddy recipe laced with captured Rebel moonshine, hundreds of peach pies, and five hundred loaves of bread, a day's baking in a converted brick chimney. During the dismal Christmas of 1863 spent in the field at Chattanooga, she whipped up molasses taffy for every soldier and commandeered laborers from the Pioneer Corps to saw a log breastwork into firewood. When an officer arrested her for burning a military fortification, she retorted that keeping patients warm was more important than preserving wooden breastworks. A week later, she greeted thirteen ambulances from Ringgold, Georgia, bearing pitiable cases through a windy, freezing night. She assisted surgeons in treating men chilled to stiffness, many of whose limbs had to be amputated to save their lives. By March she was so exhausted that she returned north for a three-week rest.

After General Sherman's orders sidetracked supplies in Chattanooga, Bickerdyke helped pack army ambulances, filling in every available niche with necessaries, and then demanded that Sherman allot the hospital two carts per day to and from the Nashville depot. Part of the need resulted from her call to patriotic civilians for pickles to counter scurvy. The request brought in pickled beets and cucumbers, chowchow, sauerkraut, and canned fruit. Arriving at Resaca, Georgia, on May 14, 1864, she and Eliza Porter found a single surgeon operating under a tree and patients spread out over the meadow, their bodies bound with torn shirttails. The two women performed battlefield magic, setting up a kitchen to dispense soup and coffee.

As the army slashed its way to Kingston, Altoona Pass, Kennesaw Mountain, and Marietta, Bickerdyke turned way stations into receiving wards for the wounded. A pragmatic herbalist, she replaced limited medicines with blackberry cordial for diarrhea, jimsonweed for pain, and bloodroot and wild cherry for stimulants. When food stores diminished, she led raiding parties to seize chickens, pigs, corn, milk, eggs, nuts, and vegetables. Using revival tents, she superintended a tent city in Atlanta that earned the name "Mother Bickerdyke's Circus." As men recovered enough to be moved, she and Mary Livermore ferried them north on a series of round trips by rail.

During Sherman's final assault on the South, he furloughed Bickerdyke along with the other female nurses and volunteers on the last train before the Union army burned the depot. At an impromptu speech to an admiring women-only audience in Brooklyn, New York, she lectured on the horrors of battlefield amputations, vermin, and filth. She shamed fashionable listeners into donating three trunk loads of muslin petticoats to the cause. The impromptu dropping of petticoats prefaced the poignancy of Andersonville Prison, whose inmates she visited in Wilmington, North Carolina, on her return voyage down the At-

lantic coast. She and other volunteers swathed wretched, underfed men in strips of Brooklyn's finery. For the first time in months, they lay under clean linens, sipped soup and lemonade, and ended their first decent meal with oranges and tapioca pudding. In a spare moment, Bickerdyke gladdened families with letters bearing news of survivors.

Settled in Beaufort, North Carolina, on April 9, 1865, when Lee's surrender ended the war, Bickerdyke quickly dispatched 90 percent of two thousand convalescents to friends and family. While in Washington, D.C., to receive sixteen thousand Tennessee Army veterans, she cabled New York for help. On her name alone, she got her request and welcomed a special train loaded with staples. Into the night, she served up bacon, steak, potatoes, and onions accompanied by bread, butter, and coffee. By morning, she had started rolling out crusts for apple pies.

Renowned for high standards of nutrition and cleanliness, Bickerdyke earned respect for discretion in maintaining military secrets of siege locations and times. She established over three hundred field hospitals and nursed casualties on nineteen battlefields, once dressing a wound with the lace from her nightgown. A favorite of Sherman's, she earned his respect and the sobriquet "Mother Bickerdyke" from his troops. On May 24, 1865, as the Union army paraded before White House reviewing stands, she mounted a horse saddled with a captured Confederate sidesaddle and joined Brigadier General John Logan at the head of the Fifteenth Corps. Her work continued until the last discharge on March 21, 1866, when she borrowed $10,000 from a banker to return three hundred Union veterans by rail to Kansas. She retired from the military and began nursing convalescing veterans and lobbying for GAR (Grand Army of the Republic) pensions, homesteads, and the funding of the Mother Bickerdyke Home for war widows and Union nurses.

On July 19, 1897, the Union Veterans of Kansas declared her eightieth birthday "Mother Bickerdyke Day." At her death from stroke on November 8, 1901, in Bunker Hill, Kansas, she retained a revered status among veterans and civilians. Mourners at the family plot in Galesburg, Illinois, honored her grave with a granite stela. A dramatic statue at the Galesburg courthouse, completed three years later, depicts her holding a cup for a casualty to drink from. Her fame continued into World War II, when the freighter *S.S. Mary A. Bickerdyke* ferried troops to the Pacific theater.

See also: Civil War

Sources

Baker, Nina Brown. "Cyclone in Calico." *Reader's Digest* (December 1952): 141–162.

"Civil War Nurses." http://www.wayne.esu1.k12.ne.us/civil/morris.html.

Denney, Robert E. *Civil War Medicine: Care and Comfort of the Wounded.* New York: Sterling Publishing, 1995.

Dolan, Josephine A., R.N. *History of Nursing.* Philadelphia: W. B. Saunders, 1968.

Holland, Mary A. Gardner, comp. *Our Army Nurses.* Boston: Lounsberry, Nichols and Worth, 1896.

Kalisch, Philip, and Beatrice J. Kalisch. *The Advance of American Nursing.* Boston: Little, Brown, 1978.

Lamps on the Prairie: A History of Nursing in Kansas. Emporia.: Kansas State Nurses' Association, 1942.

McKown, Robin. *Heroic Nurses.* New York: G. P. Putnam's Sons, 1966.

Sherr, Lynn, and Jurate Kazickas. *Susan B. Anthony Slept Here: A Guide to American Women's Landmarks.* New York: Times Books, 1994.

Blackwell, Dr. Elizabeth

One of the world-class feminists, along with Florence Nightingale, Lucretia Mott, Lucy Stone, and Susan B. Anthony, Elizabeth Blackwell was a champion of women's rights, a combatant of venereal disease, a proponent of sex education, the first female physician in the United States, and a pioneer in the training of obstetrical nurses. A native of Counterslip, England, she was born February 3, 1821, to Quaker parents—Hannah Lane and Samuel Blackwell, a sugar refiner and lay minister. Confident and scholarly from childhood, she read widely from writers of the period. After a fire razed the family refinery

when Blackwell was eleven, the Blackwells resettled in Long Island, New York, and supported abolition. Their children attended private school and enjoyed horseback riding, opera, theater, art, and tutoring in modern foreign languages.

The family suffered financial reverses and moved to Cincinnati in 1838. After Blackwell's father died that summer, she and her sisters, Anna and Marianne, opened a girls' boarding school. Elizabeth went alone to Henderson, Kentucky, to found a second school. When her friend Mary Donaldson lay dying of cancer, Blackwell decided to study medicine as a means of improving women's lives. Because of misogyny in the medical profession, she read privately and studied with Dr. Samuel H. Dickson of Charleston, South Carolina. After a lengthy search for an appropriate medical college, she gained admittance to Geneva Medical School in Geneva, New York. She was scornfully dubbed "the doctress" and lived apart from male students. With Quaker aplomb, she ignored public scorn and maintained the decorum and sobriety common to the women of her sect. On her own, she studied in the syphilis ward of the Philadelphia Almshouse and focused on the treatment of typhus. In January 1849, she graduated first in her class, earning a medical degree. Immediately after, the school barred women as students.

Continuing her training at the Collège de France and La Maternité in Paris, Blackwell was accidentally infected in one eye with diseased tissue during surgery on an infant. She realized the necessity of removing the eye, which cost her the binocular vision necessary to a career in surgery. She recovered and was fitted with a glass eye. While studying at St. Bartholomew's Hospital in London, she learned the sanitation measures introduced by Florence Nightingale, her friend and colleague. On her return to Cincinnati, Blackwell was still shunned by the medical establishment; nonetheless, she lectured to attentive audiences on the need for exercise, cleanliness, and a simple diet for women and compiled her texts in a compendium, *The Laws of Life with Special Reference to the Physical Education of Girls* (1852).

When no hospital would offer privileges, Blackwell left Ohio and set up a New York dispensary near Tompkins Square, an immigrant slum, in 1853. The hospital was the nation's first staffed entirely by women. Joined by her sister, Dr. Emily Blackwell, an anesthetist specializing in childbirth, and Marie "Dr. Zak" Zakrzewska, a German midwife, in 1857 Dr. Elizabeth Blackwell opened the New York Infirmary for Women and Children, a lying-in hospital on Bleecker Street, which featured an operating theater, obstetrical department, and three wards. Zakrzewska, who treated some three thousand patients in the clinic's first year, supported the clinic by soliciting donors throughout Boston and Philadelphia.

During the 1860s, Blackwell wrote down the specifics of medical training for young women. In "Letter to Young Ladies Desirous of Studying Medicine," published in *The English Woman's Journal* in February 1860, she advised aspiring medical students to serve as hospital nurses to learn about disease. She remarked on improvements to the nursing corps in London hospitals: "I have ascertained that a lady can enter in such a capacity as I here recommend, without injury to health, and, with a little womanly tact and real earnestness in the work, this residence may be made a most valuable time of study" (Lacey 1987, 458). She added that maternity work was essential, but warned of "many old midwife prejudices and practices clinging to that institution which you can better discriminate and avoid" (Lacey 1987, 459).

During the Civil War, Blackwell broadened her work as tutor by superintending nurse preparation for the newly commissioned United States Sanitary Commission. Her guiding principle was the example of her friend Florence Nightingale, veteran of the Crimean War. Receiving candidates at New York hospitals, Blackwell expanded the role of women in the medical professions by training nurses for battlefield aid stations. By 1868, her New York–based training facility had established a hygiene department and developed into the Woman's Medical College, which eventually became part of Cornell University. The infirmary survives as Beth Israel Medical Center.

Near the end of her career, Blackwell founded the National Health Society and the London School of Medicine for Women. As professor of gynecology, until age eighty-six she trained doctors, nurses, and midwives. Nearly thirty-five years before her death on May 31, 1910, in Hastings, England, she declined from bronchitis and liver disease but regained her strength with travels in Europe, stringent vegetarianism, and writing. She published *Counsel to Parents on the Moral Education of Their Children,* a call for better sex education. In 1885, she completed *The Decay of Municipal Representative Government,* followed by a collection of lectures, *Essays on Medical Sociology* (1902). Dr. Emily Blackwell survived her sister by only a few months.

Sources

Apple, Rima D., ed. *Women's Health, Health and Medicine in America: A Historical Handbook.* New Brunswick, N.J.: Rutgers University Press, 1992.

Austin, Anne L. *The Woolsey Sisters of New York.* Philadelphia: American Philosophical Society, 1971.

Baker, Rachel. *The First Woman Doctor.* New York: Scholastic Books, 1987.

Brown, Jordan. *Elizabeth Blackwell.* New York: Chelsea House, 1989.

"Civil War Nurses." http://www.wayne.esu1.k12.ne.us/civil/morris.html.

Denney, Robert E. *Civil War Medicine: Care and Comfort of the Wounded.* New York: Sterling Publishing, 1995.

Dolan, Josephine A., R.N. *History of Nursing.* Philadelphia: W. B. Saunders, 1968.

Ehrenreich, Barbara, and Deirdre English. "Witches, Midwives, and Nurses: A History of Women Healers." New York: Feminist Press, 1973.

Felder, Deborah G. *The 100 Most Influential Women of All Time: A Ranking Past and Present.* New York: Citadel Press, 1996.

Gay, Kathlyn, and Martin K. Gay. *Heroes of Conscience.* Santa Barbara, Calif.: ABC-CLIO, 1996.

Kent, Jacqueline C. *Women in Medicine.* Minneapolis, Minn.: Oliver Press, 1998.

Lacey, Candida Ann, ed. *Barbara Leigh Smith and the Langham Place Group.* New York: Routledge and Kegan Paul, 1987.

Latham, Jean L. *Elizabeth Blackwell: Pioneer Woman Doctor.* Champaign, Ill.: Gerrard, 1975.

Marks, Geoffrey, and William K. Beatty. *Women in White.* New York: Charles Scribner's Sons, 1972.

Ross, Ishbel. *Child of Destiny: The Life Story of the First Woman Doctor.* New York: Harper, 1949.

Sabin, Francene. *Elizabeth Blackwell: The First Woman Doctor.* Mahwah, N.J.: Troll Associates, 1982.

Sherr, Lynn, and Jurate Kazickas. *Susan B. Anthony Slept Here: A Guide to American Women's Landmarks.* New York: Times Books, 1994.

Smith, Dean. "A Persistent Rebel." *American History Illustrated* (January 1981): 28–36.

Snodgrass, Mary Ellen. *Crossing Barriers: People Who Overcame.* Englewood, Colo.: Libraries Unlimited, 1993.

Breckinridge, Mary

Mary Breckinridge, R.N., a sophisticated health professional with background gained in Europe and major medical centers in the United States, chose to make her mark on nursing history with a radical proposal. She formed a team of "nurses on horseback" to treat the poor of inaccessible backwoods Kentucky, where there was no resident physician. A champion of Lillian Wald and the Children's Bureau, she was open-minded about innovative social initiatives run by women. Her program, the Frontier Nursing Service (FNS), was the first organized U.S. outreach to mothers and children. Through careful gathering of data, she proved the value of treating mountain inhabitants at home and of educating them to care for themselves by eating healthfully, practicing good hygiene, and getting immunizations.

Born in 1877 in Memphis, Tennessee, Breckinridge came from patriotic stock, including a grandfather who was a Civil War general and another who was vice president of the United States. While her father served in St. Petersburg, Russia, as U.S. ambassador, she and her sister learned German and French from their governess, attended Czar Nicholas II's coronation, and boarded at a school in the Swiss Alps. After completing finishing school in Stamford, Connecticut, Breckinridge married an attorney. From 1907 to 1911, she attended St. Luke's Hospital School of Nursing in New York. The loss of her twins, Polly and Breckie, impelled her to help others produce healthy children.

Trained in public health under Anne Strong and Mary Beard, Breckinridge served the American Committee for Devastated France from 1919 to 1923 and assisted the organization of public health nursing, but stopped short of accepting a city post. Introduced to the European concept of nurse-midwifery, she altered the direction of her career. From 1924 to 1925, she completed a course at the York Road Lying-in Hospital in London, studied Sir Leslie McKenzie's highlands and islands district midwifery practice in Scotland's Outer Hebrides, and earned her certification in midwifery at the British Hospital for Mothers and Babies in Woolrich, England. On her return to the United States, she was eager to put her observations to use in isolated areas. She chose mountain people because of their record of early marriage and high birth rates and because Appalachian coves and hollows were typically served only by herb doctors and mountaineer "granny women," whose ignorance jeopardized the people they intended to save.

Breckinridge advocated a system similar to the quality midwifery she had seen in the British Isles, New Zealand, and Australia. Under her leadership, the decentralized FNS nurse-midwifery program began in Leslie County in southeastern Kentucky on May 28, 1925. Grounding her principles on European models, she and Rose McNaught, a British instructor in nurse-midwifery, opened their clinic in 1925 in a log dwelling at Wendover. They covered 1,000 square miles with a population of 29,572. The first Kentucky support committee numbered sixty-three, six of whom were doctors.

Encompassing areas not served by rail or highway required travel by horseback or mule in darkness and varying weather and trail conditions. To make the best use of the small staff, Breckinridge divided the outpost into six districts—Beech Fork, Possum Bend, Red Bird, Flat Creek, Brutus, and Bowlington. She assigned each worker to live with a teammate in the heart of the district and, supplied by a 30-pound saddlebag, to treat whatever health needs they encountered. Couriers transported those requiring hospitalization to Hazard or Lexington. Most families paid for the service; five dollars covered their needs during the year. The rest of the funding she sought from local endowments. For four decades, she oversaw a crusade for mother and child as practitioners galloped—and eventually drove a Model A Ford and jeep donated by Edsel Ford—to remote coves outside the range of established medical practice. An informal motto guided decisions about fording streams or braving snow and ice: "If the father can come for the nurse, no matter what the weather, the nurse will always get to the mother" (Shoemaker 1984, 23). Initiated as the Kentucky Committee for Mothers and Babies, the project reduced the rate of infant and maternal deaths in rural areas to less than that in the general populace.

Breckinridge's staff survived many a spill, slide, and snakebite. One of the devoted immigrant nurses, Nancy O'Driscoll, had served royalty and spent three years in Malta and Constantinople before making Kentucky her home in 1930. She practiced nurse-midwifery without complaint and died on the job from a burst appendix. Breckinridge herself refused to be intimidated by Prohibition-era tensions that pitted federal agents against moonshiners, who were known to shoot at strangers prowling their land. With typical insouciance she demanded, "Why should I have minded endangering my life in the Prohibition era when the lives of younger people than I were forfeited every year?" (Breckinridge 1952, 249). True to her ideals, she survived the minor inconveniences but was sidelined in November 1931 after a fall from her horse fractured a vertebra.

In the 1930s, low funding limited the project's growth and forced the closure of one clinic, but Breckinridge's brainchild weathered the Depression because staff agreed to subsistence pay, longer hours, and no vacations. Radio appeals brought in donations of milk and cod liver oil for thousands of mountain children whose family's cows were depleted by drought. The Red Cross assisted the unemployed. In 1935, the FNS offered institutional care at the Hyden Hospital and Health Center, a twelve-bed facility staffed by eight nurse-midwives and two additional nurses who received patients with injuries too severe for itinerant personnel to treat. Badly needed, it was the only hospital in three counties. In support of his former pupil, Dr. Leslie McKenzie and Lady McKenzie attended the dedication ceremony. In the project's second stage, Breckinridge recruited courier assistants and, on November 1, 1939, began training local women at the Frontier Graduate School of Midwifery at Hyden to replace the British nurse-midwives, who returned to England at the beginning of World War II.

Nurse Breckinridge remained on the job until her death in 1965. Loving hands decorated her casket with ivy, mountain laurel, and yellow rosebuds; mountaineers came from distant hollows to honor her. Overall, the success of her program derived from its nearness to people in need, who were no more than 6 miles from qualified nurses. Recipients delighted in improved health services for themselves and their children. Within the first decade, the service grew to include a social worker, surgeons, and dentists. In 1987, the Kentucky Coalition of Nurse Practitioners and Nurse Midwives supported Breckinridge's mission to establish excellence in health care among the underserved. The success of frontier nursing influenced programs in Canada, New Zealand, Asia, Africa, and South America.

Sources

Breckinridge, Mary. *Wide Neighborhood: A Story of the Frontier Nursing Service.* New York: Harper and Row, 1952.

"The Frontier Nursing Service." http://www.achiever.com/freehmpg/kynurses/fns.html.

"Frontier School History." http://www.midwives.org/history.htm.

"History of Nurse-Midwifery in the U.S." http://www.acnm.org/educ/fenmhist.htm.

Kalisch, Philip, and Beatrice J. Kalisch. *The Advance of American Nursing.* Boston: Little, Brown, 1978.

"Mary Breckinridge, 1881–1965." http://www.ana.org/hof/brecmx.htm.

McKown, Robin. *Heroic Nurses.* New York: G. P. Putnam's Sons, 1966.

"Notes on Advanced Nursing." http://www.search.com/Infoseek/1,135,0,0200.html.

Sherr, Lynn, and Jurate Kazickas. *Susan B. Anthony Slept Here: A Guide to American Women's Landmarks.* New York: Times Books, 1994.

Shoemaker, Sister M. Theophane. *History of Nurse-Midwifery in the United States.* New York: Garland Publishing, 1984.

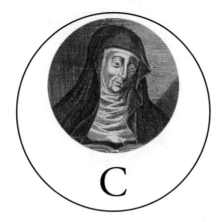

Cadet Nurse Corps

The possibility of a protracted conflict in Europe, Africa, and the Pacific during World War II inspired the Federal Security Agency to study potential nurse shortages. A conference of professionals from major hospitals and nursing associations concluded that 20 percent of U.S. nurses were already enrolled in the military. The staggering shortage of nurses to meet civilian needs resulted in a bill submitted by Ohio representative Frances Payne Bolton to establish tax-supported education for a national nursing reservoir in the United States known as the Cadet Nurse Corps. To qualified high school graduates with good grades and excellent health, the proposed corps would offer free thirty-month training plus textbooks, uniforms, and a monthly living allowance of $15–30 to volunteer students from seventeen to thirty-five years of age. The theory behind the corps was practical—to attract young women early in their careers and make better use of their professional service for either military or civilian purposes for the duration of the war. The bill passed into law on June 15, 1943.

For the first time in history, nursing got heavy publicity. Immediately, posters and billboards went up nationwide featuring eager, wide-eyed faces. Schools and guidance counselors distributed attractive pamphlets to potential cadets. On the cover, models wore snappy gray and white uniforms designed by Molly Parnis and berets styled by Sally Victor. Each jacket was decked with gold buttons, red epaulets, and the cadet sleeve insignia—a red Maltese Cross on white background, which earned the wearer reduced bus and train fares. Membership was divided into three levels—precadet for the first nine months, junior cadet for the succeeding period of fifteen to twenty-one months, and senior cadet status for the remaining term until graduation. The concluding months preceding board certification were spent in clinical practice. Under the U.S. Public Health Service, the Division of Nurse Education took shape, with Surgeon General Thomas Parran as supreme commander.

The Cadet Nurse Corps was overwhelmingly successful. Its founders selected Lucile Petry, dean of Cornell University, to direct the corps and head an advisory committee to set national nursing standards. In June 1944, in Washington, D.C., Surgeon General Parran presented to Petry the official Cadet Nurse Corps flag, which featured its insignia at top center. To speed recruitment and fill gaps, she promised R.N. degrees and commissions in the army or navy. She set goals at sixty-five

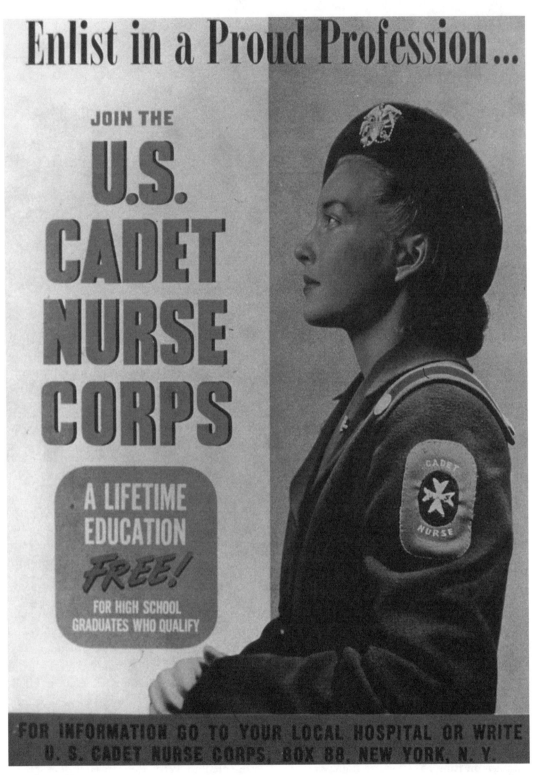

A recruitment flier for the U.S. Cadet Nurse Corps dated 1943 (U.S. Library of Medicine)

thousand volunteers within a year and sixty thousand in the second year, for a total of 125,000 reserve nurses. Although no one could predict when the war would end or when cadets would complete their commitment, the combination of Petry's enthusiasm and public patriotism produced 135,000 volunteers. In the words of former cadet Charlene Edwards Medenwald, "It was wartime and it seemed the only patriotic thing to do. Also the financial benefits seemed terrific at the time" ("The Cadet Nurse," www.armstrong.son.wisc.edu, 1).

The increase in nursing students and intensified training of the Cadet Nurse Corps put additional strains on nursing schools and faculties, which profited from scrutiny and upgrading. To meet requirements, some schools farmed out students. For example, at the University of Wisconsin, students completed the necessary three months of maternity observation at the Chicago Lying-in Hospital. To provide sufficient sites, the Lanham Act of 1941 set aside $17 million to build residences, classrooms, and laboratories. By 1945, nearly 52 percent of the U.S. Public Health Service budget was spent on educating these cadets. Overall, 179,000 woman passed through the corps. Some, such as Mary Beckman at Riley General Hospital in Springfield, Missouri, worked in military or veterans hospitals, and others entered the U.S. Public Health Service, Bureau of Indian Affairs, or such specialties as psychiatry, orthopedics, surgery, pediatrics, and polio wards.

After V-J Day, President Harry Truman set October 15, 1945, as the end of admissions for new cadets. By 1948, when the corps was disbanded, Congress had allocated $160 million for the education of 125,000 graduates. Additional moneys sent fifteen thousand nurses to postgraduate courses. During this ebullient era, the number of young women choosing nursing as a profession grew rapidly. In subsequent years, nursing schools and faculties had to adapt when the numbers lessened as interests and needs developed in directions other than medicine.

In addition to boosting career opportunities for women, the Cadet Nurse Corps made significant inroads against segregation. Basing her decision on the success of private nursing schools, director Petry included on her staff Rita Miller Dargan, a black nurse and consultant from New Orleans chosen to solicit black volunteers. In all, two thousand black women wore the familiar gray-and-white uniform. In addition, the GI Bill helped veteran nurses to complete their training with higher degrees, thus increasing their presence as head nurses and nursing school faculty. Except for one holdout, the Navy Nurse Corps, the Cadet Nursing Corps marked the end of nursing school discrimination against nonwhites.

Sources

"The Army Nurse Corps in World War II." http://www.island.net/~times/timesdir/T4/nurses.htm.

"The Cadet Nurse: 'The Girl with the Future.'" http://armstrong.son.wisc.edu/~son/dean/alumni/vol6cad.html.

Carnegie, M. Elizabeth. *The Path We Tread: Blacks in Nursing Worldwide, 1854–1994.* New York: National League for Nursing Press, 1995.

Hine, Darlene Clark. *Black Women in White.* Bloomington: Indiana University Press, 1989.

Hine, Darlene Clark, Elsa Barkley Brown, and Rosalyn Terborg-Penn, eds. *Black Women in America: An Historical Encyclopedia.* Bloomington: Indiana University Press, 1993.

"Images from the History of the Public Health Service." http://ftp.nlm.nih.gov/exhibition/phs_history/137.html.

Kalisch, Philip, and Beatrice J. Kalisch. *The Advance of American Nursing.* Boston: Little, Brown, 1978.

Schorr, Thelma M., R.N., and Anne Zimmerman, R.N., eds. *Making Choices, Taking Chances: Nurse Leaders Tell Their Stories.* St. Louis: C. V. Mosby, 1988.

Sheldon, Kathryn. "A Brief History of Black Women in the Military." *Precinct Reporter,* April 18, 1996, 2–6.

Sherr, Lynn, and Jurate Kazickas. *Susan B. Anthony Slept Here: A Guide to American Women's Landmarks.* New York: Times Books, 1994.

Smith, Jesse Carney. *Epic Lives: One Hundred Black Women Who Made a Difference.* Detroit: Visible Ink, 1993.

———. *Notable Black American Women.* Detroit: Gale, 1992.

Sterne, Capt. Doris M. *In and Out of Harm's Way: A History of the Navy Nurse Corps.* Seattle, Wash.: Peanut Butter Publishing, 1996.

"The Wichita Black Nurses Association." http://www.wichitawellness.org/wbna.html.

Yost, Edna. *American Women of Nursing.* Philadelphia: J. B. Lippincott, 1947.

Cavell, Edith

During World War I, President Woodrow Wilson maintained U.S. neutrality until two shocking events occurred—the sinking of the British liner *Lusitania* in May 1915 and the execution of nurse Edith Cavell for helping Allied soldiers hide in Brussels, Belgium, and escape to Allied territory. Having outwitted the German command by assisting hundreds of Allied soldiers, she was fully aware of enemy scrutiny but failed to identify a mole who revealed the names of Cavell and others to the German high command. At the end of World War I, survivors extolled among the heroes of the battlefield the name of Edith Cavell, the Clara Barton of Belgium.

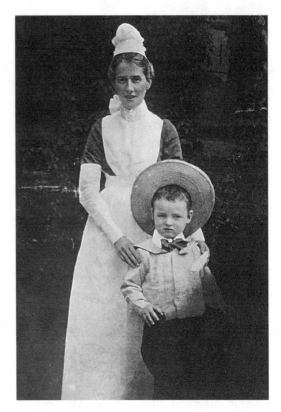

A 1919 photograph of Edith Louisa Cavell (Corbis/Bettmann)

The founder of a nursing school in Brussels, Cavell had learned altruism from infancy. Born December 4, 1865, into a religious family, she profited from being the daughter of the vicar of Swardeston, who tutored her and three younger siblings at home. She grew up serious and disarmingly sober for a youngster. While attending a local school in her teens, she mastered French, the key to a post as governess to the François family in Brussels, who employed her in 1890 to tend and teach the fashionable *l'éducation à l'anglaise* (English education) to their son Georges and daughters Hélène and Evelyne.

Pressing family business called Cavell back to England. At age thirty, she nursed her father through serious illness, a duty that sparked an interest in medicine. She took three months' training at Fountain Hospital in Lower Tooting and completed a degree from the London Hospital Nurses' Training School before donning the blue silk veil, blue coat, and elbow-length cape of her class. She volunteered to tend young victims of a ty-

phoid epidemic at Maidstone and trained beginning nurses in treating patients housed in three hospital tents, where twenty-eight died in a week. In a second assignment, she served London's St. Pancras Infirmary as night superintendent. In 1904, she began instructing practical nurse trainees at Shoreditch Infirmary, where she advanced to assistant matron.

Cavell's experiences prepared her for the staff position at Brussels's Berkendael Institute offered by Dr. Antoine Depage, a Belgian surgeon seeking nonsectarian nurses for a municipal program based on the Nightingale model. Marguerite François Graux, one of Cavell's former charges, nominated her for the post. Called L'École Belge Pour Infirmières Diplomées (The Belgian School for Graduate Nurses), the institution drew trainees from Germany, France, and Holland. Strict and self-confident, Cavell began classroom teaching on October 1, 1907, following the English system and, during brief furloughs home, enticed more promising British girls to her classes. As head nurse, she established a routine of cleanliness and order, the hallmarks of the Nightingale method. At the institute and at St. Gilles Hospital, she assisted surgeries while students viewed from the amphitheater. By 1914, her students were serving private homes, hospitals, and schools.

World War I altered Cavell's orderly plan of advancement as a nursing educator. As the arrival of German forces in Belgium on August 20, 1914, encroached on normal life, she calmed the staff by maintaining composure at wild rumors of sieges and imminent death. Within five days, curfews emptied the streets of private citizens. She and her colleagues visited a canteen set up by Madame Carton de Wiart on the Quai du Bois à Brûler to question refugees. Substantiated stories of German atrocities against civilians alarmed the nurses, particularly the slaughter of Belgians to cover up Germans' friendly fire against their own men.

In September, following a battle at Mons, Herman Capiau, an engineer from Wasmes, petitioned Cavell to hide two English soldiers, Sergeant Meachin and Colonel Bodger. She admitted them to a ward until they had convalesced and found guides to lead them to Holland. Recruited by architect Phillippe Baucq to help Prince Reginald de Croy, the Comtesse de Belleville, and others search the area for British, Belgian, and French survivors and hide them until they could be spirited out of German territory, she offered her aid and learned the password, "yorc," which is Croy spelled backward. She provided money, forged identification papers, and gave directions to two hundred fugitives, often as many as thirty-five at a time. When she ran out of ward space, she lodged men in the cellar, furnace room, or private residences.

Under clandestine conditions, Cavell cooked and washed for the hidden soldiers and personally steered some to meetings with other agents to complete the escape. Eventu-

ally, she took Sister Elizabeth Wilkins into her confidence, yet concealed names so that Wilkins would not share the danger. Other nurses guessed that their matron was involved in spy work, a likely conclusion after Cavell traveled under cover of night in an ambulance to retrieve two seriously wounded soldiers from a private home. Aided by Princess Marie de Croy, a Red Cross nurse, in the absence of a surgeon, Cavell operated on one man's gangrenous thigh wound to remove bullets.

After the German authorities chose her nursing facility to convert into a Red Cross hospital, Cavell continued treating wounded casualties, regardless of their nationality. The German doctor, addressing her as "Madame la Directrice," complimented her goodness and excellent services. In secret, she grew bolder and retrieved postcards from "Cousin Lucy" in Holland, which indicated that rescued men were thriving. Against Sister Wilkins's advice, she deliberately ignored a directive from the German *Kommandantur,* which instructed nurses to report the name, nationality, and condition of all male patients to the command center.

Through informants, Cavell's pro-Allied sympathies came to the attention of the German high command. The *Polizei* placed the nursing home under surveillance and, in her absence, ransacked every room, closet, and niche. Somehow, they overlooked her notebook, a straightforward account of her compatriots' illicit activities. Near the end of July, Princess Marie de Croy and Louise Thuliez advised Cavell that thirty Allied soldiers were in danger. Guided to the nursing home in small groups, they hid in the cellar. An infiltrator, Gaston Quien, posing as an Alsatian volunteer, penetrated the secret network. On July 31, 1915, stormtroopers arrested Baucq but failed to capture the Prince de Croy, who escaped to Holland.

The collapse of Cavell's secret system left her an opportunity to flee, but she chose to continue her work. By early morning, the police had apprehended her and also Sister Wilkins, whom they released that afternoon.

After interrogation, investigator Otto Meyer sent Cavell to St. Gilles Prison. On August 8, he and two lieutenants tricked her into acknowledging names, dates, and associates to save herself from punishment. After an October trial, under the German Military Code, the court sentenced to death four spies— Phillippe Baucq, Louise Thuliez (the Comtesse de Belleville), Louis Severin, and Edith Cavell.

Without demur, Cavell accepted the penalty, rejecting advice to plead for a commutation or reprieve. In the time she had left, she wrote a touchingly personal farewell to the staff, stating: "If any of you has a grievance against me, I beg you to forgive me. I have perhaps been too severe sometimes, but I have loved you all much more than you thought" (Armstrong 1965, 181). Despite intervention from the Spanish and American embassies, on October 12, the firing squad at the Tir National carried out the executions. She had rejected a blindfold but heard through closed eyes the refusal of a Rhinelander to shoot a woman. Both soldier and nurse died on the spot.

On May 15, 1919, English officials exhumed Cavell's remains from Tir National. King George V and his queen honored Cavell with a service at Westminster Abbey. She was reinterred at Norwich Abbey. The Edith Cavell–Marie Depage Institute in Brussels preserves her name, and the skill of actress Anna Neagle in the dramatic film *Nurse Edith Cavell* (1939) reenacts a war heroine's idealism and martyrdom. Frequented by nurses bearing bouquets, a statue in St. Martin's Place near Trafalgar Square in London depicts Cavell in long cape and carries the date and place of her execution: "Brussels—Dawn— October 15—1915" (McKown 1966, 145). The inscription honors Cavell with a quotation: "Patriotism is not enough. I must have no hatred or bitterness for anyone" ("Edith Cavell" 1997, 1).

Sources

Armstrong, Dorothy Mary. *The First Fifty Years: A History of Nursing at the Royal Prince Alfred Hospital, Sydney, from 1882–1932.* Sydney: Royal Prince Alfred Hospital Graduate Nurses' Association, 1965.

"Edith Cavell." http://www.thehistorynet.com/BreitishHeritage/articles/1997/05972_text.htm.

Elkon, Juliette. *Edith Cavell, Heroic Nurse.* New York: Julian Messner, 1956.

Kalisch, Philip, and Beatrice J. Kalisch. *The Advance of American Nursing.* Boston: Little, Brown and Co., 1978.

McKown, Robin. *Heroic Nurses.* New York: G. P. Putnam's Sons, 1966.

Sterne, Capt. Doris M. *In and Out of Harm's Way: A History of the Navy Nurse Corps.* Seattle, Wash.: Peanut Butter Publishing, 1996.

Cellier, Elizabeth

A seventeenth-century London midwife, Elizabeth Cellier of St. Clements Danes provided women with competent health service. One contribution to medical science from her early work was the data she collected from 1642 to 1662. Her records note that over the course of these two decades, 6,000 women seeking the care of midwives died in childbirth, 5,000 produced stillbirths, and 13,000 chose abortion. Her subjective commentary blamed 65 percent of fetal deaths on incompetent practitioners. To reduce mortality rates for mothers and children, she dreamed of systematizing midwifery through a confederation of 2,000 practitioners and a college of midwifery.

Cellier, a Catholic convert and wife of French Catholic businessman Peter Cellier, was one of many visiting nurses and health professionals whose career suffered from political vicissitudes and religious oppression in London, Europe's first major Protestant city. Churchmen began to control midwifery following the Act of Uniformity of 1662, which removed licensing rights from barber-surgeons and placed midwives under the supervision of bishops of the Church of England. After 35 years of practice, Cellier's work foundered because of the Popish Plot of 1678—a nonexistent conspiracy that Titus Oates concocted to stir up anti-Catholic feeling. According to the London Sessions Records of April 10, 1678, during the Protestant backlash John Atterbury, his wife, and their three children attacked Cellier, inflicting life-threatening wounds. Following the unexplained death of the investigating magistrate, Sir Edmund Berry Godfrey, on October 17, 1678, five Catholic lords were executed along with laymen and Jesuits.

Cellier's subsequent malignment appears to have grown out of routine professional visits. For example, while calling on Catholics in Newgate Prison in January 1679, she offered to attend a woman who appeared to be in labor but then learned that she was actually a Catholic suffering under torture. Months later, Thomas Dangerfield, a notorious liar, falsely implicated Cellier in the Meal Tub Plot of October 26, 1679, by linking her to a group of potential regicides. He alleged that she had concealed an informant's documents; the justice of Middlesex retrieved lists of traitors against Charles II and alleged rebel rendezvous from a meal tub in her kitchen. However, the courts found Dangerfield guilty of perjury and sentenced him to the pillory. Although Cellier was acquitted on June 11, 1680, detractors labeled her the "Popish Midwife."

In the aftermath of the scurrilous affair, Cellier published "Malice Defeated," a 44-page apologia that blamed the crown for believing rumormongers and for sanctioning anti-Catholic torment. The subtitle illuminates Cellier's purpose: "A Brief Relation of the Accusation and Deliverance of Elizabeth Cellier, Wherein her Proceedings both before and during her Confinement, are Particularly Related, and the Mystery of the Meal-Tub fully discovered. Together with an Abstract of her Arrangment and Tryal, written by her self, for the satisfaction of all Lovers of undisguized Truth" (Marland 1993, 43). Among her statements was a call for midwives to keep secret their professional skills, which the bishops sought to control. The document led to another trial at the Old Bailey, in which jurors at the earlier trial recanted or altered their testimony out of spite because she refused to pay them. Cellier received a sentence of three ses-

sions on the pillory and a fine of £1,000 for libelous publications, which were burned.

Cellier suffered an outpouring of scorn and ridicule. A cottage industry in vicious doggerel broadsides depicted her as a Catholic plotter disguised as a simple midwife. Anonymous or pseudonymous versifiers accused her of drinking, consorting with the devil and with a bawd, Mother Creswell, using her knowledge of female anatomy to perform lewd acts, and carrying on wanton adulteries with a Spaniard and a black menial. One bit of yellow journalism named her as a chief conspirator who intended to set herself up as Archbishopess of England and a saint with the intention of peddling splinters of the pillory as holy relics. A broadside titled "The Scarlet Beast Stripped Naked" castigated her as a second Pope Joan, a reference to a medieval transdresser who was named pope of Rome.

In 1687, Cellier offered King James II a plan for a royal hospital to care for foundlings and abandoned children, but he ignored her petition. When she insisted on an audience, he ordered her pilloried and her documents burned. On May 10, 1687, he commuted her sentence. The timing was propitious, for she recirculated the proposal during a period of concern for James's wife, Mary of Modena, who had suffered four miscarriages and the death of four infants. The king advanced Cellier's ambitions by agreeing to charter a midwives' union. On January 16, 1688, while his wife flourished in anticipation of a healthy birth, Cellier published "To Dr. . . . an Answer to his Queries, concerning the College of Midwives." The document fought a concerted effort by the Hugh Chamberlen obstetrical group to stereotype midwives as ignorant bumblers. Under Cellier's plan, members of the midwives' union would pay a £5 fee and annual dues of £5 and practice according to the Bills of Mortality. The setup would provide a lying-in hospital and midwife training center with a governess, secretary, and twelve matron-assistants to tend poor women and foundlings and to prevent the murder of bastard infants. In addition to course work, the hospital would publish lectures on midwifery and distribute them free to enrollees.

Critics saw Cellier's proposal as a female plot to monopolize the trade of midwives. They failed to acknowledge her true aim—to prevent infanticide and the resulting executions of mothers by instituting higher professional standards through midwife certification. Midwife testimony to her practice of an honest and honorable calling suggests that Cellier earned the respect of her peers. To prove the tradition and historical basis of female collectives, she cited the work of the Greek Agnodice, the first midwife mentioned in Western literature, and examples from pre-Roman Britain and afterward, when women assembled at the temple of Diana to improve health through the goddess's intervention. Perhaps because the king was deposed and replaced by William III, the grand dream of a college of midwives passed from history in 1688, when Elizabeth Cellier was last mentioned.

Sources

"Freedom of the Press, an Annotated Bibliography." http://www.lib.siu.edu/cni/leter-c1.html.

Lyons, Albert S., M.D., and R. Joseph Petrucelli, M.D. *Medicine: An Illustrated History.* New York: Abrams, 1987.

Marks, Geoffrey, and William K. Beatty. *Women in White.* New York: Charles Scribner's Sons, 1972.

Marland, Hilary, ed. *The Art of Midwifery: Early Modern Midwives in Europe.* London: Routledge, 1993.

Rostenberg, Leona. *Literary, Political, Scientific, Religious and Legal Publishing: Printing and Bookselling in England 1551–1700.* New York: Burt Franklin, 1965.

Christian Nursing

The transformation of Rome from a pagan capital into the Catholic world center brought a phenomenal change in nursing care for the sick and dying. In the first century A.D., the Roman system of slave nurses tending the sick was replaced by godly attendants who, in emulation of St. Luke, the beloved physician and disciple of Jesus, set up *diakonia* (Christ

rooms) for pilgrims, indigent locals, and victims of epidemics. Christian women welcomed nursing as a way to follow Christ's example of succoring those in need. A male contingent, the brotherhood of nurses known as the Parabolani, treated plague victims in Alexandria, Egypt, in the late third century and saw to dignified burial of the dead.

A handful of nurses from the early Christian era are known by name, including Olympias of Constantinople, the governor's widow. St. Paul named a nurse of his acquaintance, Phoebe (or Phebe) of Cenchrea, Greece, who had tended him among her many patients. Others whose names survive are those revered for Christian piety and kindness:

- A late third-century settlement worker, Flavia Helena, mother of the Emperor Constantine and August Empress of Rome, was later known as St. Helena for her construction of shelters for indigent pilgrims and for opening a *gerokomion* (a nursing home for the elderly).

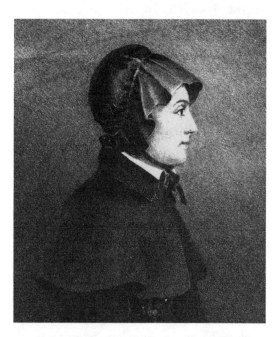

A lithograph of Elizabeth Ann Bayley Seton, founder of the American Sisters of Charity of St. Joseph in Baltimore (Library of Congress)

- Helena's contemporaries, St. Cosmas and St. Damian, were Arab twins brought up as Christians who served humanity in Asia Minor as allied doctor and apothecary. They, along with St. Pantaleon, the emperor Galerius's personal physician, died in the religious persecutions invoked by Diocletian.

- In the fourth century, Flacilla, an emperor's wife, worked daily in a makeshift Byzantine hospital washing the elderly and infirm, changing linens, rehabilitating the handicapped, and serving nourishing gruel.

- The first nursing instructor, St. Marcella, was a Roman matron who converted her Aventine palace into a monastery near the end of the Roman empire. In her nursing school, disciples learned to tend the sick. One of these followers, St. Paula, was a scholarly noblewoman from the distinguished Scipio and Gracchi families. To express her piety, she sailed to Bethlehem in Palestine in 385 A.D. to establish a *xenodochium* (hospice for pilgrims who were too ill or infirm to find their way home). With her band of nurses, she demonstrated the Christian virtues of humility, nurturance, and service to the poor. At Paula's death, her daughter Eustochium continued the mission.

The fourth century was the beginning of permanent community hospitals. St. Zoticus established one in Constantinople. Another opened in 350 A.D. at Edessa in northern Greece, where St. Ephrem superintended three hundred beds for critically ill plague victims. St. Alexis followed his example in the fifth century. The building eventually served a medical school as its clinic. According to St. Jerome, at the height of this era of medical outreach, Rome acquired its first hospital. In 390 A.D., Fabiola, a Roman altruist, opened the Nosocomium, the first Christian hospital, in her palace. As a hospice for the critically ill, the facility offered bedside care and feeding carried out by Fabiola herself. The unusual aristocratic volunteer, she worked in the slums; established a hospice at Ostia, Rome's seaport; and applied her personal wealth to benefit the poor and malnourished as well as those suffering loathsome diseases. According to St. Jerome's eulogy for Fabiola, her personal touch inspired love among those she bathed, bandaged, and fed.

Additional Christian hospices sprang up at the same time as Fabiola's hospital, beginning with the Basilias of Caesarea, a major harbor of Palestine. Founded in 370 A.D. by Bishop Basilias of Caesarea and his sister Macrina, it served as a model municipal facility and challenged monks to augment piety with good works. At its heart was a chapel, surrounded by individual cells for patients and servants, workshops, laundries, and kitchens. A staff of visiting nurses combed the city for people in need of transportation to the hospice. Among the staff were volunteers from aristocratic and royal families who attended to housekeeping, cooking, supplying oil for lamps, comforting women in labor, treating sick children, teaching trades to the handicapped, and dressing wounds. More facilities sprang up around the Mediterranean, namely, St. John Chrysostom's hospitals in Constantinople and John the Almoner's missions in Alexandria.

In the early Middle Ages, monks opened Europe's first hospitals—small monastic treatment centers and pharmacies in *infirmitoria*, which flanked sources of pure water and herb gardens. Another group of shelters for lepers, Maudlin houses, took their name from a corruption of the name of Mary Magdalene, a follower of Christ. Other way stations, raised in honor of St. Stephen, the first Christian martyr, were called *martar* houses. Locations of early hospices tend to be named Spittle, Spiddal, Spital, or some combination with the word, for example, Spittal Park, Spitalfield, or Spittal House, all derived from the word "hospital"; another verbal mark of religious communities is some combination of "palmer," the early designation for a pilgrim to the Holy Land. Mention of lepers and their care dot the

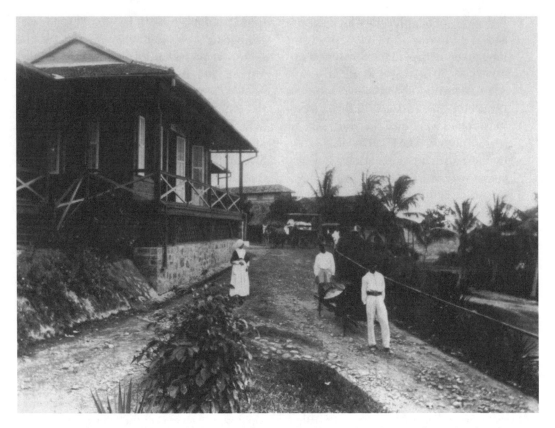

A view of the Ancon Hospital showing the quarters of the Sisters of St. Vincent de Paul (U.S. Library of Medicine)

writings of William Caxton, Charlemagne, Thomas Malory, Geoffrey Chaucer, Raphael Holinshed, and William Shakespeare because of the significance of contagion to a loathesome and disfiguring disease.

Leprous patients included members of the religious community, local worshippers, and wanderers and pilgrims. Whether suffering true Hansen's disease or other cutaneous maladies such as leukoderma, scale, or elephantiasis, the leper was, from ancient times, forbidden access to temples, inns, fairs, and markets. Equipped with bells, rattles, and clappers, the victim had to announce an arrival to a municipality and abstain from drinking water, using communal bathing facilities, and, according to the writ *De Leproso Amovendo* (Concerning the Removal of Lepers), even breathing the air that others breathed. Historically, St. Patrick, patron saint of Ireland, is credited with washing leprous sores at his own home in 432 A.D.

Also in the fifth century, nomadic companies of lepers sought out St. Bridget's abbey in Kildare, where she provided treatment. Likewise, St. Columba and St. Fechin are both credited with nursing lepers, perhaps with *aquavit* and *usquebeatha,* the original Irish whisky.

The establishment of a hospice for unsightly disease, particularly leprosy, was a true example of Christian love and compassion, which the state traditionally honored by rescinding taxes and municipal fees. The recipients earned the designation *pauperes Christi* (Christ's poor). In Caesarea, St. Basil expanded his hospital with a lazer house, or leprosarium. Dedicated to St. Lazarus, it is the earliest *hospitaller* in Christendom, the first venture into an area of disease that had long terrified and puzzled the populace. Other missions to diseased patients followed the example of Christ by succoring the poor and despised:

- Begun in 1095, a brotherhood known as the Order of Antonines dedicated their labors to the treatment of erysipelas, a streptococcal infection. They opened receiving centers throughout Europe, thus isolating the diseased to contain contagion.
- In 1145, under the auspices of Pope Innocent III, the Holy Ghost Hospital opened at Montpellier, France, and sponsored additional hospices in Europe.
- The Misericordia, a masked band of Italian laymen, initiated an ambulance and first aid service in 1244. From headquarters in the Piazza del Duomo in the heart of Florence, the brothers, garbed in black robes and hoods, maintained their twenty-four-hour rescue operation into the twentieth century.
- Around 1348, the Alexian brotherhood, founded by Tobias of Mechlin, Belgium, opened an ascetic European beggar house, and began a mission to indigent sufferers. A testimonial from the fourteenth century remarks on citizen respect for the humble monks who "sit up with the sick of all kinds of infirmities, waiting on them by day and night until death, rendering them the services necessary, comforting them in all good things and assisting them in their agony against the attacks of the devil" (Kauffman 1976, 130). As a final gesture of love and mercy, the monks dressed the corpses, transported them to the cemetery, and buried them.
- A Jesuit convert to Christianity in Shanghai, known only as Candida, baptized and renamed in the sixteenth century, purchased land to develop into a foundling home.
- In 1633, St. Vincent de Paul and St. Louise de Marillac founded the Daughters of Charity as a means of upgrading hospital care.

The opening of mission fields and religious colonies in the New World transmitted European concepts of Christian teaching and healing to American communes. In 1605, the first European nurse in the Americas, Marie Rollet Hébert Hubou, joined the Jesuit colony hospital at Port Royal, Nova Scotia, and in 1617, she served as nurse to the diseased patients of her husband, apothecary-surgeon Louis Hébert. In 1629, Jesuits and sick bay corpsmen at Port Royal, performed the first Christian nursing on plague victims. By 1639, a more substantial program began at the Hôtel Dieu in Quebec, where Mère Marie de St. Ignace, Anne Lecointre de St. Bernard, and Marie Forestier de St. Bonaventure de Jésus set up a ward for contagious patients. In September 1641, Jeanne Mance, the New World's first lay hospital nurse-missionary, began practicing her altruism in Canada. The founder of the Hôtel Dieu in Montreal, she was born in Langres, France, in 1606, and followed the first convoy of nuns who had set out on August 1, 1639, to open a Hôtel Dieu in Quebec. Although unskilled at hospital work, Mance, with the financial backing of Madame de Bullion, established the Montreal hospital in 1644. She nursed the Iroquois and other local tribes and comforted white settlers during Indian raids through three decades of frontier healing. A monument sculpted by Philip Hébert at the Place d'Armes depicts Mance dressing the hand of an Indian child.

With the dissolution of monasteries and confiscation of church holdings by the English crown during the Protestant Reformation, many hospitals passed to the control of municipalities. Care deteriorated with the hiring of incompetent, untrained, and poorly paid attendants and unskilled administrators. The height of shame for these institutions occurred during epidemics, particularly the Great Plague of London in 1665, when attendants refused to risk infection by handling the sick and dying. In England and the United States, uncloistered medical missionaries often worked alone or in small cells. One such person, Elizabeth Haddon Estaugh, a Quaker from London who emigrated to New Jersey in June 1700 after coming under the influence of William Penn, opened her home to the needy. She made her own salves, tended local Indians, and opened the meeting house at Newtown to wayfarers. During the winter, she carried medicines and provisions by sled to the homebound. Her benevolence, continued over half a century, prompted local people to name the town of Haddonfield after her.

Much of eighteenth- and nineteenth-century religious work followed the pattern of medieval nursing, providing emergency care during epidemics and dispatching delegations of home nurses to tend the homebound.

- During the 1703 smallpox outbreak and 1710 yellow fever epidemic in Quebec, the sisters of the Hôtel Dieu devoted themselves to patient care, losing some nuns from close contact with contagion. Subsequent challenges to their mission included a disastrous hospital fire in 1755 and wartime demands in 1759 as the British fought to retain Canadian territories. Joined by the Ursulines, they served both orders by treating Canadian patients during the transition from French to British masters.
- In New Orleans in 1727, Mother Marie Tranchepain de St. Augustin shepherded Ursuline nuns from France to set up the Ursuline Academy, a multiracial girls school. In addition, they established shelters for the destitute and a hospital. In 1730, Sister Anne Leroy founded Les Filles du Bon Sauveur de Caen (Maidens of the Good Savior of Caen) as visiting nurses to the homebound sick and elderly and teachers of poor girls and deaf mutes.
- The creation of missionary orders throughout Europe and the United States brought two forms of nursing—visiting nurses to private homes and hospital care, the latter demonstrated by the Sisters of St. Joseph, Sisters of Charity, and Ursulines, who established care centers. In 1810, Elizabeth Ann Bayley Seton, founder of the American Sisters

of Charity of St. Joseph in Baltimore, moved her cell to Emmitsburg, Maryland, to serve the community. As Mother Seton and later St. Elizabeth Ann Seton, she traveled over the Allegheny Mountains and down the Ohio and Mississippi rivers to St. Louis, where she established the first Catholic hospital in the United States. Her outreach to lepers, convalescents, the elderly, deaf-mutes, and maternity cases accepted all races and creeds. In 1878, six members of the Sisters of Charity of Holly Springs, Mississippi, treated hundreds of yellow fever victims, providing skilled nurse care until they, too, died of contagion.

- In Ireland in 1820 and 1833, the Sisters of Charity and of Mercy opened a hospital in Dublin. Simultaneously, in St. Louis, the Sisters of St. Mary earned the nickname of "smallpox sisters" for their assistance during epidemics.
- In the 1830s, Margaret Barrett Prior, a saintly missionary, visited the sick in homes and, in 1840, at Sing Sing Prison, in Ossining, New York.
- In 1832 Mother Mary, a Hispanic nun fleeing from Cuba, set up an orphanage and freedman's school at the Oblate Sisters of Providence, Maryland, the first black Catholic mission in the United States. During a cholera outbreak, she and her staff treated local patients.
- In 1889, the Catholic Sisters of St. Francis, led by Sister Mary Joseph Dempsey, completed St. Mary's Hospital, a segment of the renowned Mayo Clinic in Rochester, Minnesota. A statue of nursing instructor Edith Graham Mayo, the area's first professional nurse, stands on the grounds.

A spontaneous juncture of Christianity with healing occurred in Lourdes, a French town in the Hautes Pyrénées on the Gave de Pau River. Like the shrine of St. Winifred in North Wales, the area became a Christian gathering spot after a simpleminded asthmatic villager, Bernadette Soubirous, began falling into trances. She explained her rapt behavior between February 11 and July 16, 1858, as religious ecstasy from eighteen appearances of *une petite demoiselle* (a small maiden), identified as the Virgin Mary. At a nearly inaccessible spot called Massabielle, where Bernadette had gathered firewood, she unearthed a spring and ate wild cress.

After the trickle from the Virgin's spring mounted to twenty-seven thousand gallons a day, local fervor sparked religious pilgrimages among the peasantry of Marseilles, La Touraine, and La Franche-Comté to seek comfort and healing from the waters of the grotto. As word of miraculous cures spread, Lourdes became a world center of piety and adoration. However, unlike Fatima's shrine in Portugal, Croagh Patrick in Ireland, the shrine of St. Dympna (or Dymphna) in Gheel, Belgium, and the isle of Iona off Scotland, Lourdes appealed specifically to sick and handicapped people. In towns throughout Europe, religious healers organized trains to carry the sick to Lourdes. Daily, they traveled down the main esplanade, along a walkway depicting Stations of the Cross, and on to the sacred grotto.

To save the phenomenon of Lourdes from shoddy fakery and showmanship, by 1882 a medical office began asking rigorous questions of each person reporting an instance of ecstatic healing. A shrine erected at the direction of the apparition evolved into three subsequent chapels, each built on top of its predecessor. Over time, sixty-five miracles have been documented. Thirty-six years after the first basilica was erected, Lourdes earned church approval. In 1912, Catholic officials established a community dedicated to Our Lady of Lourdes; in 1933, Bernadette Soubirous, who in 1866 had taken holy orders among the Sisters of Charity at the Convent of Notre Dame at Nevers, was canonized as Saint Marie-Bernarde. In the twentieth century, the largest resulting structure, the Basilica of St. Pius X, was built to accommo-

date thirty thousand seekers of holy comfort and healing.

In the early days of pilgrimages as now, *hospitalières* (volunteer nurses) greeted arrivals at the train station or in the lobby, then turned their care over to trained staff known as *les Soeurs de Notre Dame des Sept Douleurs* (the Sisters of Our Lady of the Seven Sorrows). Since the late nineteenth century, the church has provided hospital lodging and food at its three hospices. To coordinate candlelight rosary processions and individual visits to the shrine, Catholic priests began greeting sufferers with towels and monitoring their entry into the shrine and grotto, where aides helped the sickest to kneel at the altar, light votaries, and then bathe their wounds and failed limbs and sip cups of pure water from the spring. Physicians examined *les malades,* the frailest sufferers, to determine whether bathing in the cold waters was advisable. On the way to Massabielle, *brancardiers* (volunteer attendants) assisted wheelchair and litter cases first to sick bays in one of the hospitals, then to the underground church, to the grotto, and into the *piscine* (pool). Porters and nurses remained with pilgrims until they could absorb the curative powers attributed to the spring. Medical staff validated and recorded first-person testimonials of immediate cures to mind and body, improvements in health and well-being, or reconciliation to earthly suffering.

On the other side of the globe, a moving example of volunteer caregiving derived from the selflessness of Father Damien, known worldwide for his devotion to lepers. Born Joseph De Veuster on January 3, 1840, in Tremeloo, Belgium, he attended business classes at Braine-le-Comte, then abruptly altered the direction of his life toward religious service. At age nineteen, he entered the Sacred Hearts Congregation in Louvain and adopted the name of a martyred physician. Before taking orders, he arrived in Hawaii in 1863 as an outbreak of Hansen's disease (leprosy) swept through the native population. After ordination in 1864, he mastered the Hawaiian language and devoted his energies to a parish at Kohala. Under the decree of King Kamehameha V, authorities banished the diseased to an isolated quarantine settlement in Kalawao. Accessible only by boat, the steep cliffs became a virtual prison where victims and their families were sequestered beginning in 1868. Lacking contact with doctors, the maimed victims lived without hope, receiving bundles of clothing and food delivered to their barren shore.

In 1873, Father Damien volunteered as nurse-missionary and served outcast lepers by treating misshapen bodies, binding ulcers, ministering to despair, and building coffins and preparing the graves of Hawaii's pariahs. Eleven years after his arrival, he, too, contracted the disease. Nursed by Franciscan sisters dispatched by Mother Marianne Cope and by a Vermont native, Ira Barnes Dutton of the Sacred Hearts Brotherhood, Damien remained in service up to his death at age forty-nine and was buried at St. Philomen's Church among his fellow outcasts. On April 15, 1889, he was acclaimed a latter-day Christian martyr. After removal of his body in 1936 to a tomb in his hometown, he became an international model of Christian nurse care. Additional statues stand in Hawaii's capitol and in National Statuary Hall in Washington, D.C. In 1977, his name was elevated in the first of three steps toward sainthood.

During a nineteenth-century burgeoning of world missions, nurse-altruists carried their healing charity to Asia. China had its introduction to nurse training through medical missionaries. The first to brave social bias was Dr. Peter Parker, who set up a mission hospital in Canton in 1835, where nursing staffs were limited to dressing wounds. In 1877, Lottie Moon, a Baptist missionary to Tengchow, observed relief efforts among hungry, sick peasants during a famine and reported the dire situation in home mission newspapers. From her example, Virginian Jessie Pettigrew decided to volunteer as the first trained nurse assigned by the Baptist Foreign Mission Board. Her service in Hwanghsien in the early 1900s resulted in the construction of the Warren Memorial Hospital, a field effort supported largely by the First Baptist Church of Macon, Georgia. The structure and staff survived the Boxer Rebellion, in part because Moon warned the staff to hide the skeleton they used for classes to keep the Chinese from trumping up charges of cannibalism or totemism. When overwork, age, and a tumor on her head threatened Moon's work in March 1913, Pettigrew dispatched her to P'ingtu, where mission nurse Florence Jones treated her for infection and malnutrition. By 1914, China's first college-trained nurse, Elizabeth McKechnie, had organized the China Nurses' Association with the help of Elise Chung Lyon, China's first *hu-shih* (trained nurse), and two native association officers—Lillian Wu, president, and Mary Shih, secretary.

In 1983, Marian Stringer reported to *Nursing Mirror* on a visit to a typically low-key Christian outreach—the Christian Medical Centre, a community nursing service at Rennie's Mill on Junk Bay outside Hong Kong. Begun in 1963 and funded by the Community Chest, the facility served Taiwanese refugees and, in two decades, advanced to nearly ninety patients a day. The staff, headed by Anita Ho, consisted of six nurses, two aides, and an amah (servant). Daily, a doctor visited from nearby Haven of Hope Hospital, which had began as a small missionary sanitarium for tubercular patients. In addition to dressing wounds, giving injections, and performing minor stitching and lancing, workers provided dental care, a baby clinic, attention to some three hundred elderly patients, methadone treatment, and home-help service and meals. In addition to medical care, the staff offered supervised recreation, gospel teaching, community nursing service, and nurse training. The Christian atmosphere and wards named "Faithfulness," "Love," and "Joy" set the service apart from government hospitals.

Japan was late to extend such opportunities. It owes its first Christian hospital to Dr. John Berry, a medical missionary who established the International Hospital in Kobe in

1872. It expanded eleven years later, adding a school of nursing to train Japanese women, who encountered a strong social taboo against females engaging in hospital work. Inaugurated by the United States' first registered nurse, Linda Richards, the project flourished, opening the way for a new career for women. After the hospital passed to Japanese management, a parallel facility, St. Luke's Hospital, founded in 1904 by the Protestant Episcopal Church, thrived under the management of Araki San, its U.S.-trained superintendent of nurses. Within five years, Japanese nurse trainees had one hundred schools to choose from. The surge in Asian nursing facilities influenced Dr. Mary Cutler's establishment of the East Gate Hospital for Women in Seoul, Korea, in 1886. Staffed by Elizabeth Webster, Emily Heathcote, and Anna P. Jacobson, the hospital grew to include the country's first nursing school, begun in 1905 by Margaret Edmunds. A second school, which Esther L. Shields established at Seoul's Severance Hospital, increased the number of choices for trainees wishing to enter the medical market.

Simultaneously, medical missionaries entered Thai society, which welcomed hospital service more warmly than other Asian nations. The opening of the government-run Siriraj Hospital in Bangkok in 1888 preceded the building of twelve mission hospitals. The queen merged the royal school of midwifery with a nursing school established by the Siamese Red Cross in 1912. Princess Mandaroba, Red Cross president, managed nursing at the Chulalongkorn Hospital, a facility sponsored by the Ministry of Education and named for the previous Siamese king, who was influenced by his Welsh teacher, Anna Leonowens, to abolish slavery. Two American nurses, Alice Fitzgerald and Mildred Porter, developed a curriculum to ensure quality ward care. As of 1927, Thailand's nurses formed a single union with native midwives and compiled the first Thai nursing texts.

Sri Lanka and India also embraced Western medical arts. The General Hospital of Colombo, Sri Lanka, opened in 1878, and Franciscan nuns began teaching natives the rudiments of patient care. Nurse Mary Scott established the first Sri Lankan nursing school. By 1928, Lady Stanley had organized the Association for Promoting Nursing as a Profession in Sri Lanka. India elevated nurse care by adopting the Nightingale model, bolstered by the Lady Dufferin Fund of 1885, which opened Western schools to female trainees. Building on mission hospitals—Madras Hospital, Bombay's Cama Hospital, and the Canning Home, established by the Sisters of St. John the Baptist—the nation's medical facilities began drawing native trainees late in the century. Also raising standards of health were the visiting nurses of the Indian Red Cross Society, founded in 1920.

The Arab world adopted Western medicine through missions with hospitals in Tehran, Tabriz, Hamadan, and Urumia. In Baghdad, Iraq, the one-thousand-bed Royal Hospital was founded in 1833 under the supervision of an English head nurse. Nurse May Evans earned a royal decoration for excellence in service to the Iraqi Health Service; similar dedication by nurse Emma Cushman in Konia and Istanbul, Turkey, and Corinth, Greece, aided orphans and prisoners during World War I. In Armenia, Catherine Tucker inaugurated a Near-East Relief program with coursework in public health. Jane Van Zandt supervised a Beirut nursing school in 1905. Professionals graduating from her program found work in the Middle East, South America, and England.

The Caribbean also profited from mission work and altruism. At the beginning of the twentieth century, Amy Pope opened the Municipal Hospital in San Juan, Puerto Rico, and established medical translator Pilar Cabrera as head nurse. Ellen T. Hicks and Dr. Costas Diaz organized St. Luke's Hospital in Ponce, a training center that has supplied the island with qualified nurses. To the west in Panama City, the Sisters of Charity managed a leprosarium on the island of Pala Seca and staffed St. Thomas Hospital, which opened a nursing school in 1908.

Foreign medical missions enticed many to pledge their lives to populations without churches in distant lands even though home mission fields still lacked attention. In 1891, Maria Francesca Cabrini, a native of Lombardy, Italy, later known as Mother Cabrini, gave up her yearning to serve in China's mission fields when Pope Leo XIII assigned her to run a foundering Italian hospital on East 129th Street in New York City, operated by the Fathers of St. Charles Borromeo. Without experience, she located two residences to take patients, a temporary setup that required her fellow nuns to cut sheets from bolts of muslin and import meals from a nearby restaurant.

As the mission thrived in the area's Italian immigrant ghetto, Mother Cabrini determined it should be named Columbus Hospital in honor of Christopher Columbus, a Genoese hero. The growing staff of Italian-speaking novices welcomed the order name of Sisters of Columbus and moved their busy medical outreach to less cramped facilities on East 20th Street. By 1905, Cabrini expanded the project to a second Columbus Hospital in Chicago, where Italian-speaking nurses tended grateful patients. Additional hospitals in Seattle and New York continued her work among the nation's newcomers and spread to Peru, Argentina, Brazil, Nicaragua, and Panama. Felled by malaria at age sixty-seven, Mother Cabrini left a vast network of fifteen hundred nuns in sixty-seven chapter houses. She was canonized in 1946 as the first American saint and patron of refugees and immigrants.

Like Mother Cabrini, Rose Hawthorne Lathrop, a native of Lenox, Massachusetts, and daughter of novelist Nathaniel Hawthorne, was a devout Catholic but did not enter charitable work as a trained nurse. As a writer, she published *A Story of Courage* (1894), the history of the Visitation nuns in the Georgetown district of Washington, D.C. In 1895, she ended turmoil in her personal life by volunteering to treat cancer patients at the Blackwell's Island charity hospital in New York City. Prepared with only three months of ward nursing and study of malignant tumors, she set up a home nursing network in the Lower East Side slums, supported by the sale of her jewelry, a donation from poet Emma Lazarus, and publicity from the *New York Times*. She flourished at the task of bandaging unspeakably fetid tumors and distributing clothing and supplies to suffering outcasts. Her rented rooms, shared with nurse Alice Huber, grew into a small clinic, where Lathrop dosed terminally ill patients with cheer, affection, and pain relief.

In 1900, the two volunteer nurses joined the Order of St. Dominic as sisters Mary Rose (Alice) and Mary Alphonsa (Rose). Mother Alphonsa moved St. Rose's Free Home to a donated residence in Westchester County, later named Rosary Hill Home. She raised money by issuing a tract called *Christ's Poor* (1901). After Mother Alphonsa's death on July 9, 1926, Sister Mary Rose continued their joint mission by establishing the Servants of Relief for Incurable Cancer and other receiving homes for cancer patients, including Our Lady of Good Counsel in St. Paul, Minnesota; Holy Family and Sacred Heart in Cleveland, Ohio; Our Lady of Perpetual Help in Atlanta, Georgia; and the Rose Hawthorne Lathrop Home in Fall River, Massachusetts.

The growth of medical missions through the Americas, Europe, the Pacific, and parts of Asia left the African heartland as a vast unserved frontier. The first European missionaries to arrive in South Africa in the late nineteenth century were usually Catholic priests, Benedictine and Anglican nuns, and Protestant married couples, with the man serving as evangelist and the woman as nurse and teacher. Among those dispatched from the London Missionary Society and the Rhenish Mission, Sister Henrietta began a one-year on-the-job training program at Kimberley in 1877 to spread nurse care over British colonies and territories in South Africa. Her mission was to improve the fragmented medical service provided to the underclass.

The first professional nurses in South Africa were German Red Cross staff, who arrived at Windhoek, Namibia, around 1896. German Catholic Sisters joined them in 1903, adding piped-in water; increasing their general hospital to forty-six beds; and providing sterilization, a mortuary, wards, and an operating theater. During this pioneer effort, Sister Winkelman died of typhus, becoming the first of many to succumb to Africa's rampant ills. The staff also had to guard against diphtheria, malaria, leprosy, measles, bubonic plague, tuberculosis, and syphilis. Branching out with mission stations, the order dispatched Sister Emma Bohle to Rehoboth in central Namibia in 1907 and provided a German midwife. Bohle's mission prefaced the opening of a lying-in clinic, Elizabeth Haus, named in honor of its patroness, Duchess Elizabeth of Mecklenburg.

Dr. Selma Rainio, a Finnish doctor, augmented the staff in 1908 and served Oniipa, Namibia, as nurse-midwife, pharmacist, and the only doctor to the northwest, in the area around Onandjokwe. Her patient load grew to forty Owambans daily. In 1935, she welcomed the support of auxiliary nurse Rakel Kapolo, one of the first Owambo nurses to receive training at Onandjokwe. Kapolo operated her own clinic to the north at Eenhana. Other missionary nurses opened small bush hospitals run by the Finnish Medical Mission Society and the Dutch Reformed Church. Isolated by place and social conditions, they faced the additional barrier of language where differences in bush dialects hampered communications.

Gradually, humanitarian work spread inward from the South African coast. As the only medical personnel available to local people, the nursing sister stationed at Kavango set up clinics in remote sections. The daily case load of such pioneer nurses was a daunting list—seasonal fevers, leprosy, malaria, typhoid, and puerperal fever, the endemic diseases that plagued the nation and lowered survival rates far below European standards. With sanitation, immunization, and mid-

wifery as high priorities, nurse-missionaries reduced mortality rates for mothers and children. The hazards of outback nursing cost them five members—four to accidents and one to a veld fire. At Kaokoveld, Namibia, in the 1960s, Sister Marie Brink of the Dutch Reformed Mission became a local legend for her skill at diagnosis and treatment and her improvised ambulance service, from which porters moved on foot to ferry isolated patients across the dunes by litter.

West Africa's mission field opened at the beginning of the twentieth century. In Liberia, Agnes P. Mahoney, a nurse-missionary at the Metropolitan Hospital, began her ministry in 1901, followed by nurse-educator Agnes Ward. In 1921, Mother Mary Martin of Glenageary, Ireland, a nurse-midwife and founder of the Medical Missionaries of Mary, volunteered at the Catholic mission in Calabar, Nigeria. Against Vatican orders, her disciples specialized in surgical and obstetrical nursing. The mother cell flourished in Ireland and spawned a student house in Dublin and a novitiate and maternity hospital in Collon and Drogheda. For her work, Martin earned the 1963 Florence Nightingale Medal of the International Red Cross and was named the first female honorary fellow of Ireland's Royal College of Surgeons.

In Uganda, Teresa Kearney, an idealistic missionary known as Mother Kevin, ran an open-air dispensary at Nsambya, which developed into a permanent shelter at Nakifuma. In 1913, she sponsored a second hospital in Busoga, which tended the native bearers injured while serving the British army during World War II. To introduce European methods to local women, in 1921, she launched a course for native midwives, the beginning of a Ugandan birthing service. By the end of the century, her native house, known as the Little Sisters of St. Francis, had grown from eight postulants to several hundred and branched out into Kenya with nursing schools, a leprosarium, wellness clinics, orphanages, and a school for the blind. At her death on October 17, 1957, Ugandans interred their beloved

"Flame-in-the-Bush" at Nkokonjeru and honored her memory by adding the word Kevina to their language as a synonym for a hospital or charity.

An unsung nurse of the African mission field, Hélène Bresslau Schweitzer, joined her husband, Dr. Albert Schweitzer, in training in 1906 before journeying to French Equatorial Africa to build Lambaréné, their world-renowned medical clinic on the Ogowe River just south of the Equator, accessible only by canoe. The surgical and clinical hospital at Lambaréné surprised observers by its primitive state—malodorous, pocked with the excrement of goats and chickens, and flanked by two privies and an open sewer underneath. To encourage the trust of sick natives, Dr. Albert Schweitzer chose to treat patients African-style. The general nursing and housekeeping staff consisted of families of the patients, who supplied linens and washed and cooked for the whole family outside bungalow wards.

In a steamy jungle amid poisonous snakes, the Schweitzers settled in an abandoned chicken coop and immediately began dispensing a meager trove of medicines. Much of their pharmacy was destroyed by humidity, mold, and insect contamination. After constructing a four-room hospital, they set about practicing general medicine, primarily first aid and treatment of leprosy, malaria, and sleeping sickness among natives. At their first surgery on August 15, 1913, she swabbed with antiseptics and applied anesthesia as Dr. Schweitzer performed a successful hernia repair in a surgical suite designed for hens and roosters.

Imprisonment during World War I halted the Schweitzers' work until November 1917, when Dr. Schweitzer returned to their home in Strasbourg while Hélène sought treatment for tuberculosis. In 1925, he led two nurses and two doctors back to Lambaréné to resurrect the jungle ministry and treat the sick. In 1939, Hélène Schweitzer fled Nazi atrocities in Europe and reunited with her husband in Africa, where they trained native workers in nurse care and medical technology. Altruistic volunteers from many parts of the world joined Schweitzer without remuneration. Because of the heat, humidity, and swarming insects, volunteer staff members, nurses, and doctors required a leave of absence after a year or two of work. For his perseverance in the name of humanitarianism, in 1952 Schweitzer earned the Nobel Peace Prize; by 1958, their daughter, medical technologist Rhena Eckert, was ready to take her mother's place. Both Dr. Albert and Hélène Schweitzer were buried at the original hospital compound.

As demonstrated by the Schweitzers' experience, European politics reached far into the continent of Africa. The onset of World War I in 1914 caused Africa's mission hospitals to convert to military facilities, which received staff doctors, dentists, nurses, and aides to meet the needs of combat. Local services came under heavy demand during the epidemic of Spanish influenza from 1918 to 1919. One Irish nurse, Albertina M. Walker, supervised an emergency center for flu victims and remained on duty in Windhoek, Namibia, for three weeks without relief. Her courage and tenacity earned her a £300 gratuity and a ward named in her honor. Round-the-clock nursing duties took the life of Mary Anne "Breeza" Nelson, who dropped dead in the ward after serving the garrison and prison camp at Aus, Namibia. She was the only civilian nurse in southern Africa to be buried in a military cemetery with full honors. The area's progress stalled at the beginning of World War II, when German nurses were reassigned to the military fronts.

One far-reaching alteration in medical service derived from staff shortages during World War I. Left with local staff, Africans began to depend on native nurses. Officially, patient segregation ended with an edict from local authorities that nursing staff would treat all races and nations, including the beaten Germans and victorious English. One native nurse, Margaret Mosiane, advanced from Oranje Hospital in Bloemfontein to a small hospital in Windhoek. To facilitate her job as the only medical staff, she planted shade trees and tended the donkeys that transported patients. As the quality of medical work increased, nurse Karin Kirn of Owamboland published *Theory and Practice of Nursing* (1935) in the Oshindonga language.

African-American nurses joined the African mission field in the 1920s. Nahketa A. Williams, R.N., completed training at Lincoln Hospital School of Nursing in the Bronx, New York, in 1920 and accepted appointment from the Methodist Episcopal board of missions to a teaching and nurse-missionary post in Krutown, Liberia. She ran a school and dispensary to treat Kru tribe members suffering tropical diseases and assisted French and German clinics in Monrovia. In French Equatorial Africa, Laura M. Bayne, R.N., added her skills to the pioneering black nursing mission from the United States. Having obtained her first job after graduating from the New England Hospital in Boston, she fled racism from an otherwise all-white staff at the Government Hospital in Panama by joining New York City's public health staff. Nine years later, she felt called to serve in Bangassou. Dispatched by the Mid-African Mission Board in 1926, she was the only black nurse in central Africa. After four years, she sought postgraduate study at Harlem Hospital and returned to treat lepers, the most pathetic of Africa's sufferers. In a speech delivered October 21, 1927, she recalled hopeful scenes, and declared: "One often spends the night in a native hut helping to bring into the world a new babe, instead of resting quietly in bed. Only God can give wisdom and strength to endure the life there" (Thoms n.d., 197–198).

As World War II ended, the Anglican Mission and Catholic Mission introduced on-the-job nurse training among natives, thus shifting management from whites to indigenous peoples. The late 1940s brought two more pioneers to South Africa: I. I. Ruuska, an operating room nurse from Helsinki, and Eila Muukonen, a nurse-radiographer stationed at Cape Town. In 1946, Ilma Kaisa Esteri Laitenen, a decorated World War II hero, became the first official nurse-instructor in the territory. When local medical care transferred subsidized religious institutions to state ownership, midwife and nurse educator Antoinette Zandagh Bremer, a graduate of the University of Pretoria, assisted as in-service trainer and ombudsman. Traveling the back roads of South Africa, she relied on instinct and pragmatism to solve medical quandaries unique to Africa. Her contributions and those of others enlivened the records of Magrietha Muller Williams, medical historian for South Africa's first eight decades of health service.

To the northwest, Kakata, Liberia, acquired its own pioneer, Ellen Miama Moore, who set up a $100,000 maternity center. To end the bloody business of tribal midwifery and the gris-gris superstitions spread by witch doctors, she contacted Bishop Samuel A. Grimes of the Pentecostal Association of the World and, in 1939, began a difficult odyssey toward certification. In 1946, the fruit of her work, the Samuel Grimes Maternal and Child Welfare Center, served patients along the main highway of Liberia and drew on staff from the nearby Firestone Hospital, which purchased a mobile maternity unit for her trainees' use on the company's rubber plantation. Expectant mothers placed their feet in makeshift rattan stirrups; beds propped on boxes and cribs hacked from kerosene tins and set on concrete blocks cradled the orphans Moore rescued. Premature infants survived in cribs warmed by hot water bottles. In addition to infant delivery and care, Moore set up prenatal clinics and child-welfare days. Her parenting classes, which welcomed prospective fathers and mothers, were equipped with anatomical mannequins demonstrating physical changes during pregnancy and birth. In village visits, Moore spoke Vai, Bassa, and pidgin English during examinations and encouraged families to boil water and practice home hygiene.

Just as African missions spread inland, medical missionaries moved into the interior of South America. Nebraskans Leo and Jessie Halliwell carried their Seventh-Day Adventist mission along Brazil's Amazon Basin in 1921 on a floating clinic called the *Luzeiro,* which is Portuguese for "bearer of light." Among natives ravaged by elephantiasis, yaws, hookworm, trachoma, malaria, leprosy, and malnutrition, they treated over two thousand patients. According to Halliwell, the area accommodated two medical systems: "On one hand are the witch doctors with their trances and incantations. On the other, in our clinics and those the government has been setting up along the river, are penicillin and the latest antibiotic drugs" (Halliwell 1959, 14). In 1929, they began a second posting to Baía, Manaus, and Belém, which confronted them with medical emergencies ranging from infected thorn and stab wounds to snakebite and parasitic skin lesions. In a rare instance of emergency surgery, nurse Jessie Halliwell amputated a gangrenous toe. The Halliwells returned in 1956 for a third tour of duty in Paraguay and Brazil and, in 1958, earned a government citation, the Brazilian Cross.

A contemporary of the Halliwells, Sister Dulce, born Maria Rita Lopes Pontes on May 26, 1914, became a volunteer nurse in Salvador de Bahía, Brazil. Like Mother Teresa in India, in 1952, Sister Dulce was moved by pitiful life-threatening conditions on city streets outside her home. While teaching at the College of the Immaculate Conception in Itapagipe Town, she began seeking wandering waifs, the elderly homeless, and transients dying in the streets. In an aristocratic section of town, she established an emergency clinic by breaking into an abandoned building, pulling together makeshift beds, and rescuing sixty street people suffering from malnutrition, anemia, tuberculosis, and cancer. After the health department evicted her patients, she transferred them to protective arches outside a nearby church, then moved once again to a padlocked market.

Sister Dulce's street mission survived like the poor, on chance donations and day-to-day pragmatism. Each morning, she petitioned local merchants for food so she could return to her patients with some form of lunch.

Gaining on-the-job training as a practical nurse, she learned how to succor foundlings and treat fever and gangrene. The next eviction sent her and the one hundred patients in her care to lean-tos in the alley alongside the convent until she could commandeer the compound's chicken coop. While petitioning the government for aid, she acquired a Volkswagen van to use in scouring the streets for the sick, elderly, and destitute. At local hospitals, she gathered in the incurables whom ward staff ejected to make room for patients who would survive.

An American auto parts dealer, William Brokaw, summoned Sister Dulce to help a pathetic woman lying unconscious in the street. Through his connections with other businessmen and diplomats, her work came to the attention of American philanthropists. On donated land, in 1960, she built a 150-bed sanitarium, the Albergue Santo Antonio (Shelter of St. Anthony). Within a year, she, her staff of four volunteer nuns, and Dr. Frank Faifa of Chicago treated thirty-seven thousand needy Brazilians. When funds ran low, she met President Getulio Vargas in the street and showed him her mission to Salvador's destitute citizens. For a personal donation, he earned a line in her Golden Book of donors. In the 1960s, she expanded the outreach by counseling roaming delinquents and distributing food to the hungry. Her medical mission sponsored receiving centers in the Alagados slum. The city of Los Angeles, California, adopted Salvador de Bahía as a partner city and welcomed Sister Dulce on her North American tour. Her honors include Nathan Havestock's flattering biography, *Give Us This Day: The Story of Sister Dulce, Angel of Bahía* (1965), and recognition as the Poor's Mother and the Bahía's Saint.

In Asia, nurse-missionaries like Sister Dulce carried their own brand of humanism and Christian outreach to unstable areas. On February 1, 1968, during the Tet offensive, Betty Ann Olsen, a native of the Ivory Coast and staff nurse for the Christian Missionary Alliance, was captured in the fourth year of service to the leprosarium at Ban Me Thuot, Vietnam. During a concerted Viet Cong reprisal in Dar Lac Province, she was nabbed during an evacuation mission and caged at a prison camp, surviving on daily servings of rice soup and boiled manioc. Rescue pilots scoured the area, sniffing out abandoned campsites swept clean as prisoners were shuttled steadily northward over mountainous jungle terrain. Chained to two other prisoners, Olsen suffered exposure, fatigue, dysentery, and malnutrition yet managed to treat agricultural adviser Michael Benge for cerebral malaria and infection. The third prisoner's death in July 1968 reduced the burden as Vietnamese prisoners forced their remaining pair of captives into constant resettlement from Tay Ninh Province to Quang Duc. Repeated blows from rifle butts and diarrhea from partially cooked bamboo shoots killed Olsen on September 29, 1968. Her name joined those of other selfless missionaries killed in Southeast Asia.

See also: African-American Nurses; Ancient Times; Civil War; Disease; Gillespie, Mother Angela; Hildegard of Bingen; Hutchinson, Anne; La Flesche Picotte, Susan; Medieval and Early Renaissance Nursing; Public Health Nursing; Richards, Linda; Teresa, Mother

Sources

Allen, Catherine B. *The New Lottie Moon Story.* Nashville, Tenn.: Broadman Press, 1980.

Baly, Monica E. *Nursing and Social Change.* New York: Routledge, 1995.

Berrill, Jacquelyn. *Albert Schweitzer: Man of Mercy.* New York: Dodd, Mead, 1956.

Boeynaems, Libert H. "Father (Joseph de Veuster) Damien." *Catholic Encyclopedia.* http://www. knight.org/advent/cathen/04615a.htm.

Brainard, Annie M. *The Evolution of Public Health Nursing.* Philadelphia: W. B. Saunders, 1922.

Buckley, William F. "A Visit to Lourdes To Be a Pilgrim." *National Review,* August 9, 1993, 33.

Clarke, Richard F., S.J. *Lourdes, Its Inhabitants, Its Pilgrims, and Its Miracles.* New York: Benziger Brothers, 1888.

Clement, J., ed. *Noble Deeds of American Women with Biographical Sketches of Some of the More Prominent.* Williamstown, Mass.: Corner House, 1975.

Cohn-Sherbok, Lavinia. *Who's Who in Christianity.* Chicago: Routledge, 1998.

Cousins, Norman. *Albert Schweitzer's Mission: Healing and Peace.* New York: W. W. Norton, 1985.

Day, A. Grove. *Hawaii and Its People.* New York: Duell, Sloan and Pearce, 1960.

Deen, Edith. *Great Women of the Christian Faith.* Westwood, N.J.: Barbour, 1959.

Dock, Lavinia, and Isabel M. Stewart. *A Short History of Nursing.* New York: G. P. Putnam's Sons, 1938.

Dolan, Josephine A., R.N. *History of Nursing.* Philadelphia: W. B. Saunders, 1968.

"Father Damien de Veuster." http://www.damien. edu/damien/father.html.

Goodnow, Minnie. *Nursing History.* London: W. B. Saunders, 1942.

———. *Outlines of Nursing History.* Philadelphia: W. B. Saunders, 1940.

Griffin, Gerald Joseph, and H. Joann King Griffin. *Jensen's History and Trends of Professional Nursing.* Saint Louis, Mo.: C. V. Mosby, 1965.

Halliwell, Leo. *Light in the Jungle.* New York: David McKay, 1959.

Hastings, James, ed. *Encyclopedia of Religion and Ethics.* New York: Charles Scribner's Sons, 1951.

Hufton, Olwen. *The Prospect Before Her: A History of Women in Western Europe, 1500–1800.* New York: Vintage Books, 1995.

"In Honor of Sister Dulce." http://psg.com/ ~walter/irmadulc.html.

Jamieson, Elizabeth, and Mary F. Sewall. *Trends in Nursing History.* London: W. B. Saunders, 1949.

Kauffman, Christopher J. *Tamers of Death: The History of the Alexian Brothers.* New York: Seabury Press, 1976.

Kerr, Janet, and Jannetta MacPhail. *Canadian Nursing: Issues and Perspectives.* Toronto: McGraw-Hill Ryerson, 1988.

Kuykendall, Ralph S., and A. Grove Day. *Hawaii, a History.* Englewood Cliffs, N.J.: Prentice-Hall, 1961.

Lee, Gerard A. *Leper Hospitals in Medieval Ireland.* Dublin: Four Courts Press, 1996.

Marshall, George, and David Poling. *Schweitzer.* Garden City, N.Y.: Doubleday, 1971.

Mathews, Basil. *The Book of Missionary Heroes.* New York: George H. Doran, 1922.

McHenry, Robert, ed. *Liberty's Women.* Springfield, Mass.: G. C. Merriam, 1980.

McKown, Robin. *Heroic Nurses.* New York: G. P. Putnam's Sons, 1966.

Mellish, J. M. *A Basic History of Nursing.* Durban, South Africa: Butterworths, 1984.

Moore, Judith. *A Zeal for Responsibility: The Struggle for Professional Nursing in Victorian England, 1868–1883.* Athens: University of Georgia Press, 1988.

Myers, Pamela. *Building for the Future: A Nursing History 1896–1996.* Chiswick, London: St. Mary's Convent, 1996.

O'Ceirin, Kit, and Cyril O'Ceirin. *Women of Ireland: A Biographical Dictionary.* Galway: Tir Eolas Newtownlynch, 1996.

Sherr, Lynn, and Jurate Kazickas. *Susan B. Anthony Slept Here: A Guide to American Women's Landmarks.* New York: Times Books, 1994.

Smaridge, Norah. *Hands of Mercy: The Story of Sister-Nurses in the Civil War.* New York: Benziger Brothers, 1960.

Spiritual Wonders of Europe (video). British Virgins: Palm Plus Produkties, 1997.

"St. Elizabeth Ann Seton." http://www.catholic. org/saints/saints/elizabethannseton.html.

———. http://www.knight.org/advent/cathen/ 137391a.htm.

Stringer, Marian. "Junk Bay Bus to Hope." *Nursing Mirror,* November 2, 1983, 38–39.

Thatcher, Virginia. *History of Anesthesia, with Emphasis on the Nurse Specialist.* New York: Garland, 1984.

Thoms, Adah B. *Pathfinders: A History of the Progress of Colored Graduate Nurses.* New York: Kay Printing House, n.d.

"Two Brave Women." http://www.sunlink.net/~bud/ dak8f.htm.

van Dyk, Agnes. *A History of Nursing in Namibia.* Windhoek: Gamsbert Macmillan, 1997.

Wallin, Rev. Msgr. Kevin. "A Visit to Lourdes." http://www.spirituality.org/issue10/10page04. html.

Woodward, Kenneth L. *Making Saints.* New York: Simon and Schuster, 1990.

Civil War

Although not unexpected after decades of wrangling over the issue of slavery, the American Civil War was a national cataclysm. Within four years—from April 12, 1861, to April 9, 1865—the internal conflict generated thousands of deaths and casualties, including Yankees and Rebels, blacks and whites, and a sizable number of noncombatants. Preceding the creation of the American Red Cross by twenty years, the war swept eastern, Mississippi Valley, and southern battlefields in which there were no preparations for emergency, either civil or military. The respective medical corps of North and South were poorly staffed for surges of incoming trauma

victims and for long-term care of invalids, amputees, and tubercular and blind prisoners of war. The South suffered from its failure to weed out the weak and unfit from the ranks. As the demand for Confederate soldiers grew urgent, by July 1863, the Adjutant and Inspector General issued a stipulation that "no able-bodied white man between the ages of 17 and 45 or detailed soldiers fit for field duty, will be retained in any capacity in or about hospitals, but will be returned to their commands" (Cunningham 1986, 77). Surgeon Edmund Burke Haywood of General Hospital No. 7 in Raleigh, North Carolina, complained that the job called for professional staffing rather than recuperating soldiers or men commandeered from the guardhouse. The situation exacerbated the frantic call for nurses and ward masters. By 1864, General Robert E. Lee himself established a commission to study the shortage of hospital staff.

A surprising fact of American military strategy and preparedness was the deplorable state of medicine and sanitation, which had advanced little since the end of the American Revolution eighty years before. Surgery had made advances, but nursing was in its infancy. Shortages of medicines, anesthesia, and supplies resulted from slow or inaccessible transportation and inadequate sources. For volunteers, the horror of mass amputation without morphine produced a nightmare of poignant scenes in which they anchored patients on cots and field tables for the necessary severance of limbs. Many workers proved too young, emotionally unsteady, or physically unfit for the task. Significant causes of loss were septic conditions in camp hospitals, transport vessels, and field dressing stations. In the years preceding Joseph Lister's research into bacterial infection, nurses placed patients on used bedding and pillows and washed sponges and bandages in well and creek water before returning them to use, thus spreading corruption to patients and staff, rendering even minor treatment deadly.

Immediately after the attack on Fort Sumter in the harbor of Charleston, South

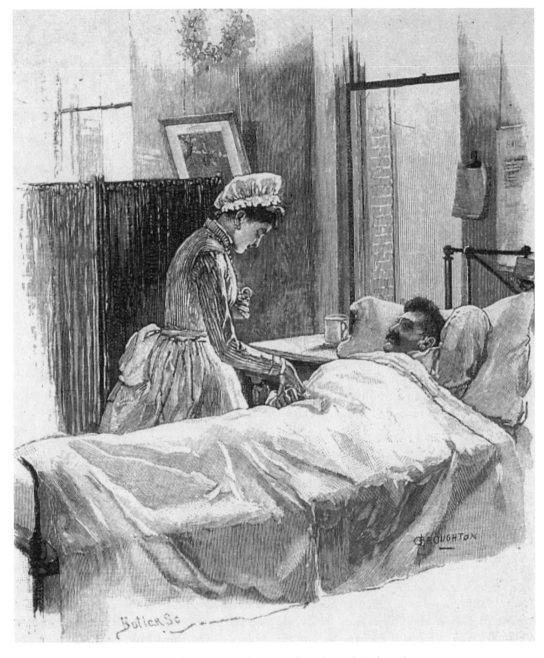

"The gentle misses ministering to the soldiers," a scene from a Civil War hospital (Archive Photos)

Carolina, on April 12, 1861, the war turned Washington, D.C., into a military camp. Tents, barracks, and supply dumps sprang up; improvised hospitals in churches, hotels, schools, government buildings, and residences housed and treated men who were either wounded in battle or felled by infectious diseases, primarily pneumonia, measles, mumps, dengue fever, enteritis, and dysentery. Amid muddy streets clogged with army transports, corpsmen ferried patients to the least crowded facility, where local women supplied food from their kitchens as well as blankets, bandages, dishes, and cutlery. For

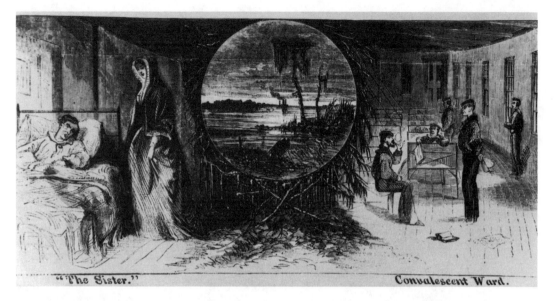

"The Sister."   Convalescent Ward.

This wood engraving depicting three scenes on board the Civil War hospital ship Red Rover *first appeared in* Harper's Weekly *in 1863. (U.S. Library of Medicine)*

Washington's limited volunteer nursing staff, duties included padding crutches, laundering patient clothing, quelling vermin, and hand-feeding invalids, all tasks that untrained people could perform. In nearby Charlottesville, Virginia, the Young Men's Christian Association sent male nurses to staff a wayside shelter near the railroad. Overall, the work of nursing remained a man's job: in the entire Civil War, no more than 20 percent of the staff was female.

The best known of the Civil War's volunteer nurses were those who detailed their struggles in journals and wrote letters home to family, friends, and news gatherers, thus preserving their valor and skill at improvisation. Volunteer Walt Whitman, poet and author of war reportage, published *Specimen Days and Collect* (1883), which contained the freelance articles that evolved from his hospital visits in Washington, D.C. In December 1862, he managed a trainload of wounded bound for Washington, the beginning of his role as wound-dresser and aide. He served for three years, caring for some eighty thousand patients, the source of his lyric *Memoranda during the War* (1876), in which he described the rhythm and emotion of his work:

I onward go, I stop,
With hinged knees and steady hand to dress
    wounds,
I am firm with each, the pangs are sharp yet
    unavoidable,
One turns to me his appealing eyes—poor boy!
    I never knew you,
Yet I think I could not refuse this moment to
    die for you,
if that would save you.
(Kalisch and Kalisch 1978, 53)

Without pay, he carried a pass from the Christian Commission to the dressing stations, convalescent wards, and veterans assemblies, where he was welcome for bearing tobacco, jelly, oranges, dried fruit, fruit syrup, pickles, and rice pudding.

On his numerous visits, Whitman spotted substandard treatment, lack of order and cleanliness, and inadequate diet. At Armory Square Hospital, he earned the surgeon's praise for accomplishing good among demoralized soldiers and writing letters to families. In a letter to his mother, he mused: "It is curious, when I am present at the most appalling things—deaths, operations, sickening wounds (perhaps full of maggots)—I do not fail, although my sympathies are very much excited, but keep singularly cool; but often hours afterward, perhaps when I am home or out walking alone, I feel sick and actually tremble when I recall the thing and have it in my mind again before me" (Marinacci 1970, 220–221). Among his most significant war memoirs is an account of the aftermath of the Battle of Chancellorsville, Virginia, fought May 1–4, 1863.

Among female nurses in the Confederacy, Kate Cumming and Sally Louisa Tompkins took leadership roles by managing the hospitals. A native of Edinburgh, Scotland, Cumming disobeyed her parents and, in 1862, went to northern Mississippi to join the South's nurse corps. As matron in charge of nurses, she and her colleagues struggled to treat casualties from the Battle of Stone River at Murfreesboro, Tennessee, from December 31, 1861, to January 2, 1862. Commissioned a captain in the Confederate cavalry by President Jefferson Davis, Tompkins, a native of Poplar Grove, Virginia, was the only official female officer. Like her contemporaries, Tompkins was swept into the war effort. Following the First Battle of Bull Run, fought at Manassas, Virginia, July 21, 1861, "Cap'n Sally" converted her Richmond residence into the twenty-two-bed Robertson Hospital. In the words of her nephew, "As medicines were contraband of war, her treatment for all diseases was air, light, turpentine and whiskey, all home products. If these failed, her panacea was prayer and the Bible" (Boardman 1915, 75). By war's end, Tompkins's temporary facility had served 1,333 patients with only seventy-three deaths. She earned a reputation for cleanliness and maintained the lowest death rate, around 7 percent, even though she accepted desperate cases. At her death in 1916, she was honored with a full military funeral and a headstone dedicated by the Daughters of the Confederacy. Mabel Boardman, chief of the Red Cross, lamented that Tompkins "cannot be canonized in the Episcopal Church but only saints can do the work she did" (Boardman 1916, 75).

In the North, a more complex nursing hierarchy began taking shape. As of July 14, 1862, the surgeon general's office in Washington, D.C., set up an all-female nurse corps under superintendent Dorothea Lynde Dix, aided by Louisa Lee Schuyler of the Women's Central Association of Relief. The government allotted one nurse for each ten beds per hospital, to be supplied by the United States Sanitary Commission. Each building was marked by a yellow flag bound in green with a large "H" in the center. The use of untrained female staff was essential to stem catastrophic loss of life. Many workers were local women, particularly wives, daughters, and sisters of soldiers, who were featured in a series of illustrations for the September 6, 1862, issue of *Harper's Weekly.* The pen-and-ink collage, entitled "The Influence of Woman," pictured women at work:

- Sedate ladies, in long flowing skirts and neat peplum tops with hair pinned to the nape of the neck, mend shirt collars and socks.
- Under guard, a group of laundresses hand-wash and dry nightshirts at a military camp.
- A lone nurse in cap and aproned work dress takes dictation from a wounded man.
- A nun in habit and winged wimple attends the bedside of a suffering patient.

Whether anticipating the prim, ladylike tasks of nurturing and comforting or the more realistic demands of hospital drudgery, the typical volunteer performed all levels of nursing chores, from the more genteel spoon-feeding, Bible reading, and will writing to stripping and scrubbing casualties, lice removal and boiling of uniforms and bedding, assisting with surgery, and tagging the dead for burial. Their duties called for baking, cooking, lifting, hauling, scrubbing, ironing, and rolling bandages. To free their hands, they followed the example of Katharine Wormeley, a Newport nurse who created one of the war's images of pragmatic nurse care by tossing over her shoulders twin flasks of brandy and broth tied with ribbon. Other practical staff members filled their apron pockets with needed bandages, scissors, and treats for despairing patients.

When accepted by Dix into the United States Sanitary Commission, volunteer nurses received written regulations concerning age, marital status, and behavior. She admitted no nurses in hoop skirts or finery. Likewise, Confederate matrons preferred simplicity. Louisa Susannah Cheves McCord discouraged women of fashion from working at her hospital in Columbia, South Carolina, and encouraged only Sisters of Charity. Diarist Mary Chesnut remarked: "When [McCord] saw them coming in angel sleeves displaying all of their white arms, and in their muslin, showing all of their beautiful white shoulders and throats, she felt disposed to order them off the premises. That was no proper costume for a nurse" (Woodward 1981, 414).

McCord's fashion plates were soon in the minority. The exigencies of war, which blockaded ports and halted supply trains, quickly divested southern women of fashionable dress, leaving them tattered and out at elbows by the end of the conflict. Nurses learned to patch and mend smocks, aprons, stockings, and shoes to eke out the last bit of wear from serviceable garments.

The job of Civil War ward nurse is anchored in American history alongside the tasks of stretcher bearer, corpsman, dietitian, and hospital aide. Written accounts of nursing chores appear in letters, journals, and published poetry, fiction, and reflection, such as Mary A. Gardner Holland's compendium *Our Army Nurses* (1896). A collection of brief memories written by eyewitnesses, the vignettes bear the mark of Victorian refinement, for few women spoke candidly about battlefield terror and omitted or avoided comment on hospital smells, makeshift sewage removal, gruesome wounds, and three-to-a-bed overcrowding in patient wards. Individual authors produced more detailed studies. Mobile, Alabama, novelist Augusta Jane Evans Wilson, the first female author to earn over $100,000, published *Beulah* (1869), a popular novel derived from her wartime nursing experiences. Frances Watkins Harper's novel *Iola Leroy: Or, Shadows Uplifted* (1892), one of the first by a black American writer, details the adventures of a mixed-blood slave from emancipation to employment as a Civil War nurse.

A thoughtful relief worker from New Brunswick, Canada, Sarah Emma Evelyn Edmonds, one of the Civil War's known transdressers, served in a Michigan regiment under the name Frank Thompson and fought at the battles of Bull Run and Fredericksburg, Virginia. Lest the disguise be discovered in a hospital, she deserted her army post after contracting malaria. As a nurse for the Christian Commission, she served at Harpers Ferry, Virginia. She married and settled in Texas, where she wrote a fictionalized autobiography, *Nurse and Spy in the Union Army* (1865), a sophisticated memoir dedicated to the sick and wounded of the Army of the Potomac and filled with some of the era's most acute dramas and meticulous reflections. Beginning in the spring of 1861, she tells of her journey from Baltimore to Washington, where she witnessed the first stream of casualties. Following the troops to Manassas, Virginia, in July, she observed firsthand the shelling that maimed and dismembered bodies. She served the Union army by speeding to Centerville to locate fresh lint and brandy. On return, she found carnage: "Men tossing their arms wildly calling for help; there they lie bleeding, torn and mangled; legs, arms and bodies are crushed and broken as if smitten by thunderbolts; the ground is crimson with blood; it is terrible to witness" (Edmonds 1865, 43). At the nearby stone church, she passed a heap of severed limbs and entered the sanctuary to comfort the dying. During the early days of her spying missions in the South, she duplicated her efforts for Confederate soldiers whom she encountered beyond enemy lines.

Edmonds's work required much time in the saddle. An intrepid equestrienne, she stayed on the move, halting only to snatch a nap and rest her mount. Her fearless expeditions as an army courier kept her constantly in service, frequently in disguise as she spied on southern bivouacs and returned with head counts and news of supply lines. Among Union casualties at Harrison's Landing, Virginia, she intentionally kept up cheery banter with the men and accepted her share of triage: "We had our patients divided into three classes; one was our working department, another our pleasure department, and a third our pathetic department. One we visited with bandages, plasters and pins; another, with books and flowers; and the third, with beef tea, currant wine, and general consolation" (Edmonds 1865, 250).

At Vicksburg, Edmonds sought out the most horrifying mutilations to nurse and soothe and was impressed by men without arms or legs who maintained a valiant will to survive. The scarcity of comforts reduced her ministrations to pouring water on crusted limbs and fanning men to soothe their troubled sleep and rid their wounds of flies. To better assist the medical corps, she quelled her disgust at distorted corpses trampled in mire and "the hum and hissing of decomposition" (Edmonds 1865, 369). At war's end, she offered the highest praise for refined ladies who were able to rise above the loathsome nature of hospital nursing to tend the wounded. Shortly after enrolling officially in the army, she died and was buried in Washington Cemetery in Houston, Texas.

At war's end, Alabaman Kate Cumming wrote *The Journal of Hospital Life in the Confederate Army in Tennessee* (1866), particularizing the carnage of the Battle of Shiloh, Tennessee, which produced 23,700 casualties from April 6 to 7, 1862. She and her southern colleagues placed themselves in treacherous situations in which many nurses died from disease, extremes of weather, staphylococcus infection, impure water, drowning, and rail and steamer accidents. Still ladies in conscience and conduct, they defended themselves against moral outrage, thieves, rapists, and pompous members of the high command. On their own, women like Cumming wrote reams of letters to friends and charitable organizations soliciting butter, dried fruit, candles, bedding, and bandages as the South slowly fell to its knees.

The largest contingent of nurses consisted of the impartial nuns from Catholic and Anglican sisterhoods—the Anglican Order, Daughters of Charity, Sisters of Charity, Sisters of Mercy, Sisters of St. Joseph, Sisters of St. Vincent, the Holy Cross order, Sisters of St. Dominic, Ursuline Sisters, Franciscan Sisters of the Poor, Sisters of Our Lady of Mount Carmel, Sisters of Providence, and Sisters of Our Lady of Mercy. In *My Story of the War* (1887), nurse Mary A. Livermore remarked, "The world has known no nobler and no more heroic women than those found in the ranks of the Catholic Sisterhoods" (Gollaher 1995, 414). The quiet grace of nuns tenderly debriding and dressing wounds, assisting surgeons, and presiding over tents and wards of the sick and dying was a high point of the war's volunteer effort. A moral, disciplined force lauded in *Medical and Surgical History of the War of the Rebellion, 1861–1865* (1888), Catholic sisters halted gambling, swearing, and carousing; made men write their families and groom themselves; and rewarded them like mothers with treats dispensed from habit pockets. When the situation called for morale boosting, nuns could read, recite, sing, and write poetry as well as console and pray. Their influence ranged from these more personal efforts to the establishment of an orphanage in Albany, New York, and administration of a charity hospital in New Orleans, Louisiana.

Familiar with self-denial and taking orders without question, the Catholic sisterhood kept less detailed records as they posted impersonal reports to the mother superior and wrote modest accounts of their charities in convent journals for their order's archives. Frequently unidentified by name, they remained faithful to traditional vows of poverty, chastity, and obedience, the hallmarks of Christian service. For the South, the Sisters of Charity of St. Francis de Sales Infirmary in

Richmond, the Confederate capital, was a haven after the Battle of Bull Run, when five thousand casualties spilled out from field dressing stations into churches, homes, and temporary shelters. Sometimes with no more than a withering glance or nod, the nuns tactfully overrode prejudice against female nurses, expanding their undertaking from feeding and measuring dosages to general hospital work. Assisted by male corpsmen, often convalescents not in the best condition, many nuns became everyday heroines, such as Sister Valentine Latouraudais, who comforted the profoundly wounded and administered extreme unction. Others served diluted communion wine as a stimulant, and bilingual sisters translated for German soldiers. When the Union high command gave up their naive hope of suppressing the southern rebellion in three months, recruiters established training camps of enlistees to man the lines. Parallel to their efforts, Sister Euphemia Blenkinsop launched a search for skilled and unskilled nurses to supply wartime hospitals. Traveling under flag of truce from Emmitsburg to Annapolis, Maryland, and on to Petersburg and Richmond, Virginia, she was returning convent boarding students to their homes when she encountered the aftermath of a train boiler explosion and treated the injured as best she could.

In Harpers Ferry, Virginia, on April 18, 1861, Catholic sisters prepared for a major conflict. Traveling by stagecoach from the mother house, they passed through Union lines and among barrels of gunpowder that dotted the bridge. After the initial attack, they authorized a call for more nuns, which Sister Euphemia's outreach supplied. Among their lay staff in Washington, D.C., was poet Walt Whitman. Early in 1862, sisters accompanied an Ohio surgeon on board a hospital ship. They cheerfully staffed abandoned hotels and chapels and readied warehouses for the influx of wounded. The mark of their skill at comfort was the addition of bright curtains, altars and shrines, and plants and bouquets among the makeshift hospital furniture, often made from packing crates and out-of-service caissons.

On June 19, 1862, seven nuns from New York's St. Catherine's Convent, traveling by ship and tug, established a treatment center at a looted hotel in Beaufort, North Carolina. Without candles or beds, the "North ladies" requisitioned brooms, kerosene lanterns, and laundry tubs from the War Department and threatened to quit if they were refused. When the supplies came, the women worked harmoniously at upgrading the treatment center and comforting the men. Mother Paul Lennon, one of four nuns who returned to the mother house for rest, died from exhaustion. On September 6, 1862, a federal hospital in Frederick, Maryland, was overrun by Confederate scouts. For a week before their recall to the mother house, the Sisters of Charity remained under guard to treat four hundred casualties who inundated the meager facility. To increase efficiency, the nuns summoned local volunteers as aides.

At an enlistment center in Indianapolis, Indiana, the Sisters of Providence fought pestilence that ravaged the overtaxed camp. Convent housekeepers scrubbed and aired linens at the rickety City Hospital and made up beds in cattle stalls. When General William Tecumseh Sherman's men began arriving from Louisville, Kentucky, and Jeffersonville, Indiana, the nuns greeted them with order, solace, and hot food. The dead rooms received the fallen with dignity, a sight that comforted families. In Vincennes, Indiana, the nuns duplicated their triumph to aid typhoid victims, whom local people shunned. Sister Athanasius performed distinguished service to quarantined men, crossing a hazardous plank bridge with provisions and laundering blankets into the night.

At Camp Curtin near Harrisburg, Pennsylvania, the Sisters of St. Joseph overcame abysmal conditions by cleaning and disinfecting the hospital interior and posting a sentry at the kitchen to prevent pilfering. In an island of order amid military chaos, the nuns managed medical wards, allotted drugs, and charted patient progress. They refused to marginalize the dying and attended all with gentleness and Christian kindness. In Wheeling, West Virginia, Sisters of St. Joseph offered the military the order's hospital, chartered in 1856. To a stream of ambulances, hospital ships, and cattle trains, Mother de Chantal and her staff gave up their own sleeping quarters and worked around the clock, napping in a corner of the chapel with mounds of leaves for pillows.

Land-based treatment centers profited from floating hospitals in February 16, 1862, after the Battle of Fort Donelson, Tennessee, where General Ulysses S. Grant's forces seized Confederate fortifications on the Cumberland River. Initially slow and ineffective, evacuation craft ferried the wounded up the Mississippi River to St. Louis, Missouri; Paducah, Kentucky; and Mound City and Cairo, Illinois. Staffing the vessels were volunteers who coped with haphazard conditions. Armed with lanterns, nurses disembarked to tend victims in barns, huts, stables, and tents. Sister Felicitas Dorst, the provincial vicar of the Franciscan Sisters of the Poor, took two nuns, two postulants, and a laywoman to staff the *Superior,* which patrolled the area from Cincinnati, Ohio, downriver to Pittsburg Landing, Tennessee. Their work consisted of setting up feeding stations, rolling bandages, packing lint, and stuffing mattresses with straw for the nine hundred beds that covered the ship and adjacent barrack barges. On a tour of the Tennessee River, the nuns rescued casualties abandoned on marshy shores, where they were beset by insects.

A second coordinated boat lift occurred after the ten-hour Battle of Shiloh. Sisters of Mercy staffed the *Empress,* accepting men of both armies; the Sisters of St. Joseph served the *Whilden* and the *Commodore,* poorly supplied hospital ships that required constant improvisation to house, feed, and treat unforeseen influxes of casualties. Stretcher-bearers covered decks, stairs, and gangplanks with an overflow of patients, numbering seven hundred on one vessel. To save the ships from

hostile fire, the nuns assembled on deck to display their habits as proof of their humanitarian intent. They soaked hardtack in buckets of water and hot milk and sprinkled the mush with sugar to make an appetizing meal. Their ingenious mixture of molasses, ice, and water created a refreshing drink in the absence of tea, coffee, oranges, and lemons.

A valuable source of nurse care came from the Sisters of Charity in Emmitsburg, Maryland, established by Elizabeth Ann Bayley Seton in 1810 and patterned after the French Daughters of Charity founded in 1633 by St. Vincent de Paul and St. Louise de Marillac. In the gray-blue robe and white cornette of their parent organization, the "cornette sisters" or "white caps," along with the Sisters of Charity in New York and Cincinnati, earned respect and recognition for their battlefield and epidemic work, even under heavy fire and interdiction. The sisters quietly treated, dressed wounds, and comforted, pinning to pockets the names and addresses of those who couldn't speak for themselves. When a call from Harpers Ferry, Virginia, reduced the staff by three nuns, the others doubled their efforts to meet the needs of casualties.

One immigrant nun from Limerick, Ireland, Mary Anthony O'Connell, later known as Sister Anthony of the Sisters of Charity in Emmitsburg, Maryland, took charge of a Cincinnati house and orphanage, founded the city's first visiting nurse program, and directed St. John's Hotel for Invalids, formerly an old boarding school. During the Civil War, she trained nurses and corpsmen and served at the front at Camp Dennison, Ohio; Winchester, Cumberland, Stone River, Pittsburg Landing, and Nashville, Tennessee; Richmond, Virginia; Gallipolis, Ohio; and Lynchburg and Culpeper Courthouse, Virginia. As assistant surgeon to Dr. George Blackman on the banks of the Tennessee River, she met the impossible conditions of heavy rain, too few stretcher-bearers, and tents and a log house carpeted with soggy hay, where she received the most pressing cases. Working amid the stench of unburied corpses, she and her colleagues persevered and followed the army up-river to Corinth, Mississippi. Along the way, they prayed to the Holy Mother to spare their hospital ship from harm. In the war's aftermath, Sister Anthony returned to Cincinnati to build a better hospital, named the Good Samaritan, and opened St. Joseph's Foundling and Maternity Hospital, which she managed until her retirement in 1880.

In June 1863, at Emmitsburg, 10 miles from Gettysburg, Pennsylvania, the St. Joseph's convent of the Daughters of Charity met the demands of the decisive battle between generals George Meade and Robert E. Lee. According to the reflections of Sister Marie Louise, community secretary, who shared quarters with Mother Ann Simeon, the nuns awoke to the sudden appearance of the Union army, which shortly decamped to be replaced by Rebel forces. Mother Ann supplied an omnibus of food, bandages, and stimulants, which rolled into the blockaded battlefield under a flag of truce. In the first days of July, war dead filled the Catholic church, where nuns tended many infected with tetanus. Reinforcement sisters from Baltimore brought coffee, tea, jelly, and ham. They supplied the wounded with bedding, clothing, and combs to remove vermin. In honor of three weeks of intense nursing and care, the diocese erected a statue to Notre Dame des Victoires (Our Lady of Victories), protectress of St. Joseph's valley.

Less dramatic scenes occurred in religious orders throughout the embattled area. Near Springfield, Kentucky, the Dominican Sisters of St. Catherine kept their academy open through influxes of troops from both armies. To assure the convent of wagon transportation, Sister Columba and her students prevented scavengers from stealing their horses. At the Battle of Perryville, fought 10 miles west of Danville, Virginia, sisters worked all night on a muddy battlefield to rescue casualties, carry spring water to their receiving station, and bathe wounds. They augmented General Don Carlos Buell's short supplies,

cooked and laundered, and transformed academy dormitories into wards.

During the Union siege of the Confederate stronghold at Galveston, Texas, in 1862, Ursulines, led by Mother St. Pierre Harrington, offered the convent school for a hospital. When shelling endangered the buildings, the nuns raised a creamy yellow flag, fashioned from a sister's flannel petticoat, to designate a hospital sanctuary open to both sides. The staff abandoned their safety to search for casualties beyond the post by lantern light and welcomed Union, Confederate, black, Hispanic, and white soldiers. Amid the chaos of the Union capture, school and worship continued. In Baltimore, Maryland, Sister Tyler of the Protestant Episcopal Church demanded admittance to a police station to retrieve wounded Massachusetts volunteers. She superintended hospitals in Maryland and Pennsylvania and the Naval School Hospital in Annapolis, where the pathetic prisoners from Andersonville and Belle Isle prisons were rehabilitated.

Among the sisters who died in service were those who suffered fevers and disease. Sister Mary Consolata Conlon, a Daughter of Charity from Boston, served the base hospital on the Pamunkey River in Virginia. During the evacuation of patients on June 25, 1862, the beginning of the Seven Days' Battle, she loaded transports and made up bunks to receive the most severe cases. After the two-week maneuver, Sister Consolata volunteered for worse conditions at Point Lookout, Maryland. Working night duty, on July 30, 1862, she succumbed to fever while praying for dying patients. Soldiers provided her a military funeral.

Another victim, Sister Fidelis of Holy Cross at St. Mary's Convent, South Bend, Indiana, nursed under the supervision of Mother Angela Gillespie at the hospital in Mound City, Illinois. A makeshift affair thrown together in unfinished warehouses, the hospital depended on the services of seven sisters, who shared one bed, one chair, and a laundry table. Averaging seven deaths per day, the hospital absorbed several thousand wounded from the Battle of Fort Donelson, fought in freezing February weather in 1862. Sister Fidelis treated frostbite and worm-infested wounds. Flooding forced the nuns to evacuate patients from the first floor to the third and to ferry ambulatory patients down-river to the care of Holy Cross sisters in St. Louis, Missouri. On her deathbed from chills and fever, Sister Fidelis confided that she had never seen the exterior of the building because she arrived by night and, for six months, had never left. Her body was rowed from the building and borne to South Bend, Indiana, for burial at St. Mary's Convent.

As with the many unnamed nuns, the roster of secular Civil War nurses is largely composed of forgotten or unidentified Mary Sues, Belindas, and Annas who received no pay or credit for their heroism. Among those who earned the nation's praise were people whose names and deeds belong in the annals of nursing history, including the following examples.

In *Hospital Sketches,* a candid memoir published in three installments in *Commonwealth* from May 22 to June 26, 1863, *Louisa May Alcott* published her personal letters originally intended for her family. Speaking through the fictional persona of Nurse Periwinkle, she gave vivid glimpses of nurse care in the foul confines of Union Hotel Hospital, a former Georgetown tavern in Washington, D.C. She described the men as "torn and shattered . . . riddled with shot and shell . . . borne suffering for which we have no name" (Sterne 1996, 5). From December 1862 until January 21, 1863, Alcott performed night duty, which taxed her strength with feeding, cleansing and dressing wounds, sewing bandages, and answering calls of patients from the Battle of Fredericksburg. Delirious with typhoid fever and pneumonia, she collapsed and was returned home to recuperate. The rigors of nursing and disease left her with hallucinations, hysterics, and forbidding memories, but her reportage lauds Dorothea Dix— "Long may she wave!"—and matron Hannah

Stevenson, the military nurse who inspired Alcott to volunteer (Saxton 1977, 264).

A native of Peoria, Illinois, *Lizzie Aiken,* nurse to the head surgeon of the 6th Illinois Cavalry, followed the regiment to Shawneetown the winter of 1861. For her devotion to the twenty to eighty casualties arriving daily, grateful patients named her "Aunt Lizzie." The attending surgeon credited her with saving more than four hundred men.

A worker for the Christian Commission, *Arabella Barlow* served in the thick of fighting at the Battle of Antietam, Maryland, on September 17, 1862, and at Gettysburg in early July 1863. While attached to General Winfield Scott Hancock's command, she dashed across enemy lines while both sides were firing. Wherever her husband was deployed, she offered her aid until her death from camp fever in 1864. After her husband, Frank Barlow, was elected New York attorney general, he remarked on Arabella and other volunteer nurses: "The time will come when the finest monument in this country will be built to the memory of the women of the Civil War" (Boardman 1915, 73).

Like Arabella Barlow, Confederate nurse *Fannie Beers* followed her husband, August P. Beers, as his unit ranged from New Orleans to Richmond. She was named matron of Buckner Hospital in Gainesville, Alabama, and nursed soldiers through a smallpox epidemic at Lauderdale Springs, Mississippi. In 1888, she recounted her exploits in an autobiography, *Memories,* which cites mule meat as standard ration.

Amy Morris Bradley, who accompanied the 3rd Maine Volunteers to Washington, D.C., treated casualties in Manassas, Virginia. She took charge of the 5th Maine Regiment hospital at Camp Franklin, Virginia. As the only nurse, she had to rely on untrained soldiers and slaves as hospital aides. Of the loss of her first patient, she wrote, "We have our Charley packed in salt and saltpeter. There is a hothouse nearby, so I have purchased some delicate flowers and placed them around his pale face. How beautiful he looked asleep in Death!" (Denney 1995, 58).

Nicknamed "Child of the Regiment," *Kady Brownell* accompanied her husband, R. S. Brownell, into the 1st Rhode Island Volunteers and, in July 1861, attended the casualties at Manassas. While taking over the job of the regiment's fallen standard bearer, she was wounded in action.

Florena Budwin, a Union transdresser, fell into enemy hands and was imprisoned in Florence, South Carolina. After a physician discovered her masquerade, Budwin donned female clothes and aided wounded prisoners.

Charleston's star diarist, *Mary Chesnut,* lived across the street from Lucy Mason Webb's hospital, at Clay and 12th streets, where Chesnut observed the heavy demands on limited facilities. She joined volunteers Mary Henry Jones and Martha Milledge Carter to ferry supplies to casualties. She hand-fed patients typical southern fare for invalids—rice and gravy, hominy, and milk-soaked bread.

North Carolinian *Carrie Cutter,* the first female nurse to enlist in the South, died at age eighteen while bringing supplies to casualties. As troop ship attendant aboard the *Northerner* at Roanoke Island, Virginia, she worked alongside her father, a Confederate surgeon, and succumbed to a typhoid epidemic while attending soldiers.

A matron of the 18th Corps Hospital in September 1864, *Harriet P. Davie* of Barnstead, New Hampshire, tried to join the military but settled for nursing as second-best. She served at the Second Battle of Bull Run in late August 1862. After capture by Confederate forces, she earned a pass to tend casualties on both sides.

In La Vergne, Tennessee, spy *Mary Kate Patterson Davies* concealed medicine for Confederate hospitals in her riding skirt and in a hidden niche under her buggy seat. A compatriot, Virginia Bethel Moon, used a similar ruse. In 1863, while smuggling opiates in her bustle, parasol, and hoop skirts, Davies was arrested but returned to her job of nursing Southern casualties.

Anna P. Erving, of Hagerstown, Maryland, nursed the heavy load of casualties at Gettysburg, Pennsylvania, both in field and hospital. She served the National Corps of Civil War Nurses as an eyewitness to volunteer nurse care by publishing her experiences on the battlefield and in the hospital in *Reminiscences of the Life of a Nurse in Field, Hospital and Camp during the Civil War* (1904). Of Antietam, she recalled local women collecting useful items and then going out to relieve the overwhelming number of casualties. Left alone when others fled, she remarked, "I braced myself for the task and at sunrise I was on the spot. As many as could be put into the little church were carried there and attended to at once" (Erving, www.snymor. edu). Working under a white flag of truce, she treated the wounded of North and South.

Isabella Morrison Fogg, of Calais, Maine, was one of a contingent of volunteers who departed from the Maine Soldier's Relief Agency in Washington, D.C., to be near her son Hugh with the 6th Maine Regiment. Outside Sharpsburg, Maryland, she, Charles C. Hayes, and Harriet Eaton washed, fed, and treated the wounded and sick left behind in tents and outbuildings. In her report to the agency, she stated: "Here the sick are in a fearful condition, in every old house and church and hundreds on the ground. You no doubt think your ladies in Washington are doing a great work, but I can assure you, if they were here, they would find the stern reality of want, privation and extreme suffering ("Antietam," www.state.me.us). She toured aid stations at Kedarsville, Harpers Ferry, Russell Spring, Smoketown, Bakersville, and Burketsville. While serving with the U.S. Christian Commission on the Ohio River in 1865, she permanently injured her spine in a fall through an open hatch on the hospital ship *Jacob Strader* and was awarded a federal pension.

Helen Gilson exemplifies unheralded volunteer service. An enlistee with the Army of the Potomac, she nursed Union casualties at the war's major battles and earned the men's respect for quiet grace and a sweet singing voice during the Peninsula Campaign of 1862.

While still in her teens, *Cornelia Hancock,* a Quaker nurse from Tenafly, New Jersey, and founder of the Laing School for Negroes in Charleston, South Carolina, and Philadelphia's Children's Aid Society, was numbered among the United States's Florence Nightingales. In her correspondence, published in 1956 as *South after Gettysburg: Letters of Cornelia Hancock, 1863–1868,* she recorded the filth and hunger she shared with the wounded at Gettysburg and Fredericksburg. In Washington, D.C., she tended black refugees and earned a pass that carried her to Wilderness, Virginia, with General Ulysses S. Grant's cortege. Army bands honored her by playing "The Hancock Gallop" (Sherr and Kazickas 1994, 291).

On July 4, 1863, after the Battle of Gettysburg, *Mrs. John Harris* reported that she left Baltimore for Pennsylvania with stimulants and chloroform, a mid-nineteenth-century innovation, and penetrated as far as possible into the stream of casualties and among operating theaters erected in the open air to offer the best light.

The wife of a brigadier general, *Harriet Foote Hawley* accompanied him with the 7th Connecticut Regiment and served mostly in the South. She worked at a Beaufort, North Carolina, hospital and in South Carolina and Florida; after the war, she tended prisoners from Andersonville, Georgia.

Nicknamed "the South's Florence Nightingale," *Juliet Ann Opie Hopkins* managed three hospitals in Richmond, Virginia, after illness sidelined her husband, the chief administrator. While retrieving casualties from the battlefield at Seven Pines, Virginia, on May 21, 1862, she sustained a wound that left her permanently handicapped. After returning to her home state of Alabama in 1864, she managed a medical facility at Camp Watts. The state honored her by printing her portrait on 25 cent coins and $50 bills. At her death in Washington, D.C., on March 9, 1890, she was interred in Arlington National Cemetery with military honors.

A Pennsylvania native, *Mary Morris Husband* established a home hospital to treat one of her two sons, who became ill in service. As a member of the United States Sanitary Commission, she nursed the wounded aboard a hospital transport under bombardment and served in Washington, D.C., until war's end.

Hannah E. Judkins, from Skowhegan, Maine, worked alongside thirteen other nurses at St. John's College Hospital in Annapolis, Maryland. Her response to paroled prisoners is typical: "Pen cannot describe the first boat-load of half-starved, half-clothed, thin, emaciated forms whose feet, tied up in rags, left footprints of blood as they marched along to be washed and dressed for the wards. In many cases their minds were demented, and they could give no information as to friends or home, and died in that condition, their graves being marked, 'Unknown'" (Holland 1896, 423).

Commissioned by Dorothea Dix, *Lucy L. Campbell Kaiser* of St. Charles, Illinois, served at the siege of Vicksburg, Mississippi, and the Battle of Springfield, Virginia. Of the patients' plight, she complained: "The fact was I could not get enough food; butter out, sugar out, no crackers, poor bread, tough beef, no vegetables, no candles; in fact, the commissary was bare, and the officers in town on a drunk" (Holland 1896, 180).

Sallie Chapman Gordon Law, a North Carolina patriot and volunteer nurse, established the twelve-bed Southern Mothers' Hospital in Memphis, Tennessee, in 1861. After the Battle of Shiloh in April 1862, she expanded the hospital's capacity to manage hundreds of Confederate casualties. To keep her assets out of Union hands, she spent her all cash for opium, morphine, and quinine and transported the drugs through enemy lines to rebel headquarters. After the surrender, she established the Southern Mothers' Association to honor Civil War dead.

Mary Ashton Rice Livermore, a Boston temperance leader, suffragist, and originator of nursing training in the United States, joined the United States Sanitary Commission in 1861. Aided by Jane Hoge and Eliza Chappell Porter, she founded the Soldiers' Aid Society and personally gathered supplies, food, and clothing, carried them to the front, and distributed them to field stations. To assist Dorothea Dix, Livermore recruited nurses and aides and organized bazaars to collect linens and medical equipment, which comprised two-thirds of the total amassed for the Union army. In *My Story of the War* (1887), Livermore's incisive commentary preserved much of the exploits of Mary Ann Bickerdyke, Livermore's head nurse and dear companion.

Commissioned into the Union army nurse corps in 1862, *Louisa Maertz* of Quincy, Illinois, escorted sick soldiers to hospitals and helped establish Soldiers Home in New Orleans, Louisiana. In 1865, she was one of many to attend survivors of Andersonville Prison, where the only nurse care had been provided by parolees.

Iowan *Nannie C. Martin* enlisted in 1864 and served Hospital No. 6 in New Albany, Indiana, and Crittenden Hospital in Louisville, Kentucky, where she organized a lint gathering program and invited three hundred convalescents to a traditional Christmas dinner. In 1903, she addressed a convention of the Nurses' Associated Alumnae on the concept of professional nursing.

Emily V. Mason, matron of Richmond's Winder Hospital, supervised a five-thousand-bed facility spread over 125 acres. As dietitian at the Confederacy center, she produced fifteen turkeys, 150 chickens and ducks, a barrel of corned beef, 240 pies, a barrel of cider, plus rice custard, pudding, oysters, and eggnog for the holiday meal on December 25, 1862. Near the end of the war, she was lucky to have a gill (4 fluid ounces) of sorghum and pint of cornmeal per person per day and half-rations of flour, bacon, and lard. She resolved complaints from the men who tired of eating dried peas and threw them on the wall and quelled a riot when two hundred inmates tore down the hospital bakery.

In Shepherdstown, Virginia, in September 1862, volunteer nurse *Mary Bedinger Mitchell* viewed the Confederate column advancing on Antietam and the returning casualties, who filled corncribs, cabins, barns, and farm sheds. Her notes describe amateur nurses washing wounds, stanching blood flow, splinting broken bones, and holding instruments and basins during crude amputations.

A noteworthy nurse-administrator for the Confederacy, *Ella King Newsom* volunteered in December 1861 at Bowling Green, Kentucky, and rose to the position of hospital supervisor. While serving in Corinth, Mississippi, at the Tishomingo Hotel after the bloody Battle of Shiloh on April 6–7, 1862, she noted, "Every yard of space on the floors, as well as all the beds, bunks and cots were covered with the mangled forms of dying and dead soldiers" (Cunningham 1986, 49). By war's end, she had served in similar posts in Chattanooga and Nashville, Tennessee, and Atlanta, Georgia.

In Lynchburg, Virginia, *Lucy Wilhelmina Otey,* a sixty-year-old nurse and mother of seven Confederate soldiers, established the Ladies' Relief Hospital in the old Union Hotel, a nonmilitary facility staffed entirely by volunteers. Nursing excellence earned the hospital its reputation for the best place to send difficult cases.

In 1863, activist *Emily Elizabeth Parsons* superintended nurses at the army hospital in St. Louis, Missouri. Although weakened by the rigors of combat nursing, she raised funds in 1867 for Massachusetts's Mount Auburn Hospital, where an office complex is named in her honor.

A Jewish widow, *Phoebe Yates Levy Pember,* served as chief matron of the eight-thousand-bed Chimborazo Hospital in Richmond, Virginia, a facility equal to a small medical town. It was the largest military hospital in American history and consisted of five divisions, 150 buildings, and peripheral rehabilitation tents plus a goat and cow farm, five soup kitchens, five icehouses, Russian bathhouses, a bakery, and a brewery. Pember's career headaches included unwise political appointments, hunger, and erratic delivery of supplies, which arrived up the James River via traders from Lynchburg and Lexington. She battled drunken attendants and rats while treating more than fifteen thousand Confederate soldiers. She managed to delight the inmates on December 25, 1863, with a seasonal meal accompanied by twenty-four gallons of eggnog. According to Pember's journal, *A Southern Woman's Story* (1879), a hindrance to supervision was the influx of families who came to tend wounded sons, husbands, and brothers and who required room and board during their sojourn at the hospital. Over Pember's years of service, the hospital, with the assistance of 256 slave nurses, treated seventy-six thousand casualties. She earned the regard of patients when she found time to cook them special dishes to whet failing appetites. In April 1863, following the skirmish at Drewry's Bluff, she noted that the men were so exhausted from forced marches, loss of sleep, and trench warfare that they did not stir during operations performed without anesthesia. Her despair at the fall of the Confederacy by June 1864 forced her to admit that starving soldiers made unpromising candidates for surgery: "Poor food and great exposure had thinned the blood and broken down the system so entirely that secondary amputations . . . almost invariably resulted in death, after the second year of the war" (Cunningham 1986, 224).

Mary Phinney, Baroness von Olnhausen, received her placement directly from Dorothea Dix. Assigned to Mansion House Hotel in Alexandria, Virginia, she found the surgeon determined to thwart Dix. Phinney begged for a transfer but, at Dix's order, remained and eventually thrived as matron and head of her own nurse corps.

In January 1864, *Felicia Grundy Porter,* a native of Nashville, Tennessee, organized the Women's Relief Society of the Confederate States to supply prostheses for all war casualties.

Nurse *Hannah Anderson Chandler Ropes,* a fifty-three-year-old Maine native on staff at the Union hospital in the Georgetown section of Washington, D.C., awoke on the night of July 6, 1862, to a deluge of wounded. She recalled, "From the broad open entrance into the hall to the base of the staircase, there, bent, clung, and stood, in dumb silence, fifty soldiers, grim, dirty, muddy, and wounded" (Denney 1995, 131). She was one of many volunteers to die of typhoid.

Honored by a statue in Arlington Cemetery, *Sarah S. Sampson,* a hospital nurse in Washington, D.C., gathered supplies and medicine for field hospitals. After the war, she established the Bath Military and Naval Children's Home, which cared for orphans of Civil War veterans.

In May 1861 at a female seminary in Williamsburg, Virginia, *Letitia Tyler Semple,* daughter of a former president, opened a seventy-five-cot hospital.

A vigorous Confederate nursing supervisor, *Lurinda C. Smith* served in sight of Lookout Mountain, Tennessee, and amassed kitchen dishes and utensils from donated spoons, tin cups, and crockery. With the true sentiment of an eyewitness, she recalled, "Lookout Mountain was where they rolled loose rock down on the enemy. I couldn't keep from crying to see so much killing, and the wounded everywhere begging for water. That was a battlefield one cannot forget" *(Lamps* 1942, 63).

A widow from Kansas, *Mary A. Sturgis,* an associate of Mary Ann Bickerdyke, enlisted with the 6th Illinois Cavalry and began work at Camp Butler in Springfield in November 1861. Traveling with the regiment from there to Paducah, Kentucky, and Memphis, Tennessee, she earned praise for administration of the Adams Block Hospital, which she stocked from her own goods and donations garnered from locals.

Fanny M. Titus-Hazen was one of many nurses who combined treatment with Christian compassion. She wrote: "During the summer, June, July, August, and September, our heads, hands, and hearts were taxed to the utmost; so much to do, so many claiming our sympathy, so many to tell that soon they must answer the last bugle call, and cross to the beautiful shore" (Holland 1896, 471).

Dr. Mary Edwards Walker, a graduate of Syracuse Medical College, enlisted in the

Union army as a physician, but was rejected by the Union Medical Corps, which refused female applicants. Dressed in a man's uniform, she moved about battlefields and assisted emergency work at Warrenton, Virginia, where the hospital was served capacity loads of casualties. She worked as surgical nurse, rehabilitation assistant, and spy at Fredericksburg, Bull Run, and Chickamauga and, to offset the necessity of field amputations, transferred serious cases to Washington, D.C., for specialized care that saved injured limbs. On the streets of the capital, she organized a Women's Relief Association to aid impoverished women tending members of their families.

By January 1864, Walker's skill won her an appointment as assistant surgeon attached to the 52nd Ohio Infantry. She selflessly crossed enemy lines to treat soldiers as well as civilians suffering typhoid fever or needing a midwife. On one of these missions, she was captured. From April 10 to August 12, 1864, she remained in Castle Thunder, a filthy jail in Richmond, Virginia. She was exchanged for Confederate medical personnel and was the only woman during the Civil War to receive the Congressional Medal of Honor for Meritorious Service, conferred by President Andrew Johnson. The remainder of her career she spent at a women's prison in Louisville, Kentucky, an orphanage in Clarksville, Tennessee, and the Central Women's Suffrage Bureau of Washington.

While serving transport ships on the Potomac, *Annie T. Wittenmyer* of Keokuk earned the nickname "Iowa's Angel of the Civil War" (Sherr and Kazickas 1994, 151). As described in her memoir, *Under the Guns: A Woman's Reminiscences of the Civil War* (1895), she survived numerous nearby hits by bullets and shells. To assure supplies, she maneuvered a load from Pittsburg Landing to Vicksburg while under siege. During shelling at the surrender to Union troops on July 4, 1863, she distributed food despite danger to her person. General Ulysses S. Grant commented, "No soldier on the firing line gave more heroic service than she rendered" (Sherr and Kazickas

1994, 244). In 1864, she revolutionized government hospital diet by managing kitchen sanitation and serving nourishing menus rather than army issue gruel and hardtack.

Georgeanna M. Woolsey, one of the first to volunteer in the New York area, was assigned to Washington, D.C. She recorded the courage of refined ladies who silenced their qualms to scrub floors, shift patients in their beds, or assist in amputations. Angrily, she added that surgeons and male administrators deliberately forced nurses into unfit accommodations and burdensome tasks usually reserved for men to terrify them or force them to flee. Working under a mentor, Deborah Hughes, Woolsey described her as one of the hardy: "A faithful, gentle woman, enduring all kinds of hardships, coarse unappreciativeness from the surgeons, vulgar tyranny from the matron . . . hardly ever sitting down, sometimes late into the night, watching with them, falling asleep in her chair sometimes, so catching a nap to fit her for the next day" (Austin 1971, 43). After Hughes's death in a train-carriage accident, Woolsey recounted widespread mourning for a loving, gentle nurse.

Commissioned in September 1861 to the makeshift infirmary in the unfinished patent office, Woolsey bedded patients on rough scaffolding and smoothed bed linens with broom handles. Surrounded by wood shavings, machinery, laths, and plaster, she and other staff members treated a raging typhoid epidemic. Off-duty, they amassed pastries, brandy, champagne, cordials, beef tea, lemons, arrowroot, cocoa, and farina. For convalescent men, they scoured neighborhoods for books, slates and chalk, pens and paper, mittens, and socks. With her sister Eliza, Georgeanna Woolsey quartered aboard the *Wilson Small* while serving as nurse-at-large, then rose to the rank of charge nurse aboard the *Daniel Webster,* a steamer leased on April 25, 1862, to patrol the James and Potomac Rivers for isolated casualties. Woolsey encountered the Sisters of Charity, who staffed General Hospital at White House, the Virginia home of General Robert E. Lee.

Postwar care kept nurse volunteers on the job, particularly to rehabilitate amputees and former Union prisoners of war, who suffered as the South declined. In reference to the prison in Salisbury, North Carolina, Cornelia Phillips Spencer reported in *The Last Ninety Days of the War in North Carolina* (1866, 24): "Their men died by thousands in our semitropical climate, because we were powerless to relieve them with either food or medicine." Significant to the rapid decline was the wretched state of railroad service after Sherman's notorious looting and destruction. In defense of her homeland, Spencer adds: "We knew the condition of those prisoners while we were mourning over the destitution of our own army. The coarse bread served at our own meagre repasts was made bitter by our reflections."

In New York, Jane Stuart, Georgeanna Woolsey, and Abby Woolsey joined others in a decade-long effort to organize convalescent services in New York hospitals, including readings, strolls at the zoo, and an hour's ride in a Central Park carriage. As nursing director, Jane improved the service of New York's Presbyterian Hospital. Abby published an overview, *A Century of Nursing with Hints toward the Organization of a Training School* (1876), a handbook on training centers. Georgeanna Woolsey launched a nursing school in New Haven, Connecticut, and contributed to *A Handbook of Nursing for Family and General Use* (1879), modeled on Dr. Victoria White's *A Manual of Nursing* (1878).

As matron of thirty-five patients in Ward 4 of West Building Hospital, Baltimore, Maryland, Jane M. Worrall recorded dismal scenes: "The cots filled with rebel prisoners, badly wounded, who in turn were exchanged for Union men from Libby Prison. A more distressing sight could not be imagined. They were in a dying condition, nearly starved. Five died within twenty-four hours. Those who could talk told me they had not had water to wash their faces and hands for three months; and if a bone was thrown to them they would fight for it like dogs. They were all brought on stretchers, and it was only with the best of care that any of them were saved" (Holland 1896, 186).

In the war's aftermath, women, both professionals and volunteers, continued their commitment to victims, refugees, and noncombatants. At the request of General Sherman, Sister Augusta Anderson, mother general of the Holy Cross order, left Overton Hospital in Memphis, Tennessee, to take charge of a postwar facility in Cairo and care for eight babies orphaned by a smallpox epidemic. At night, the children slept in her cot while she sewed garments for them. She reunited seven of the children with relatives and smuggled one child out of isolation by hiding him under her habit. A war heroine, Mother Angela Gillespie, hospital administrator, author, and educator, accepted General Ulysses S. Grant's request to establish convent nurses at the military hospital at Paducah, Kentucky. Clara Barton, head of the nurse corps for the Army of the James, expanded her involvement in emergency aid with the establishment of the American Red Cross. By the end of the war, the government saw the wisdom of opening nursing schools to supply the nation before the next crisis.

See also: Barton, Clara; Bickerdyke, Mary Ann; Blackwell, Dr. Elizabeth; Cumming, Kate; Dix, Dorothea; Etheridge, Anna Blair; Gillespie, Mother Angela; Navy Nurse Corps

Sources

"Antietam Aftermath: The Stern Reality of Want." http://www.state.me.us/sos/arc/archives/military/civilwar/foggyarn.htm.

Apple, Rima D., ed. *Women's Health, Health and Medicine in America: A Historical Handbook.* New Brunswick, N.J.: Rutgers University Press, 1992.

"Aunt Lizzie Aiken from Peoria." http://www.rsa.lib.il.us/~ilwomen/files/03/htm1/aiken.htm.

Austin, Anne L. *The Woolsey Sisters of New York.* Philadelphia: American Philosophical Society, 1971.

Bell, Irvin Wiley. *Embattled Confederates.* New York: Harper and Row, 1964.

Boardman, Mabel. *Under the Red Cross Flag at Home and Abroad.* London: J. B. Lippincott, 1915.

Breeden, James O. "Confederate General Hospitals." *North Carolina Medical Journal* (February 1992): 110–119.

"Civil War Nurses." http://www.wayne.esu1.k12.ne.us/civil/morris.html.

Cumming, Kate. *A Journal of Hospital Life in the Confederate Army of Tennessee from the Battle of Shiloh to the End of the War.* Louisville, Ky.: John P. Morton, 1866.

Cunningham, H. H. *Doctors in Gray: The Confederate Medical Service.* Baton Rouge: Louisiana State University Press, 1986.

Denney, Robert E. *Civil War Medicine: Care and Comfort of the Wounded.* New York: Sterling Publishing, 1995.

Dolan, Josephine A., R.N. *History of Nursing.* Philadelphia: W. B. Saunders, 1968.

Donahue, M. Patricia. *Nursing, the Finest Art.* St. Louis: C. V. Moody, 1985.

Duncan, Louis C. *The Medical Department of the United States Army in the Civil War.* Washington, D.C.: Surgeon General's Office, 1914.

Dyer, Brainard. "The Treatment of Colored Union Troops by the Confederates, 1861–1865." *The Journal of Negro History* (July 1935): 273–286.

East, Charles, ed. *Sarah Morgan: The Civil War Diary of a Southern Woman.* New York: Touchstone, 1991.

Edmonds, S. Emma. *Nurse and Spy in the Union Army: The Adventures and Experiences of a Woman in Hospitals, Camps, and Battlefields.* Philadelphia: W. S. Williams, 1865.

Erving, Anna P. *Reminiscences of the Life of a Nurse in Field, Hospital and Camp during the Civil War.* http://www.snymor.edu/pages/library/local_history/sites/letters/annie.htmlx.

Fessler, Diane Burke. *No Time for Fear: Voices of American Military Nurses in World War II.* East Lansing: Michigan State University Press, 1996.

Gollaher, David. *Voice for the Mad: The Life of Dorothea Dix.* New York: Free Press, 1995.

Gragg, Rod, ed. *The Illustrated Confederate Reader.* New York: Harper and Row, 1989.

Greenbie, Marjorie Barstow. *Lincoln's Daughters of Mercy.* New York: G. P. Putnam's Sons, 1944.

Holland, Mary A. Gardner, comp. *Our Army Nurses.* Boston: Lounsberry, Nichols and Worth, 1896.

Hyman, Paula, and Deborah Dash Moore. *Jewish Women in America.* New York: Routledge, Chapman and Hall, 1997.

Kalisch, Philip, and Beatrice J. Kalisch. *The Advance of American Nursing.* Boston: Little, Brown, 1978.

Kent, Jacqueline C. *Women in Medicine.* Minneapolis, Minn.: Oliver Press, 1998.

Lamps on the Prairie: A History of Nursing in Kansas. Emporia.: Kansas State Nurses' Association, 1942.

"Louisa Lee Schuyler." http://www.allsoulsnyc.org/UUsofnote/Louisa-Lee-Schuyler.html.

Lowry, Thomas P. *The Story the Soldiers Wouldn't Tell: Sex in the Civil War.* Mechanicsburg, Penn.: Stackpole Books, 1994.

Marinacci, Barbara. *O Wondrous Singer! An Introduction to Walt Whitman.* New York: Dodd, Mead, 1970.

Marvell, William. *Andersonville: The Last Depot.* Chapel Hill: University of North Carolina Press, 1994.

"Mary Edwards Walker." http://www.northnet.org/stlawrenceaauw/walker.htm.

———. http://www.wayne.esu1.k12.ne.us/civil/mary.html.

McKown, Robin. *Heroic Nurses.* New York: G. P. Putnam's Sons, 1966.

Moore, Frank. *Women of the War: Their Heroism and Self-Sacrifice.* Hartford, Conn.: S. S. Scranton, 1866.

"Mother Angela Gillespie." http://women.eb.com/women/articles/Gillespie_Mother_Angela.html.

Oates, Stephen B. *Woman of Valor: Clara Barton and the Civil War.* New York: Free Press, 1994.

O'Ceirin, Kit, and Cyril O'Ceirin. *Women of Ireland: A Biographical Dictionary.* Galway: Tir Eolas Newtownlynch, 1996.

Saxton, Martha. *Louisa May: A Modern Biography of Louisa May Alcott.* Boston: Houghton Mifflin, 1977.

Schroeder-Lein, Glenna R. *Confederate Hospitals on the Move: Samuel H. Stout and the Army of Tennessee.* Columbia: University of South Carolina Press, 1994.

Sharpe, William D. "Introduction." *Confederate States Medical and Surgical Journal.* Metuchen, N.J.: Scarecrow Press, 1976.

Sherr, Lynn, and Jurate Kazickas. *Susan B. Anthony Slept Here: A Guide to American Women's Landmarks.* New York: Times Books, 1994.

Smaridge, Norah. *Hands of Mercy: The Story of Sister-Nurses in the Civil War.* New York: Benziger Brothers, 1960.

Spencer, Cornelia Phillips. *The Last Ninety Days of the War in North Carolina.* New York: Watchman Publishing, 1866.

Sterne, Capt. Doris M. *In and Out of Harm's Way: A History of the Navy Nurse Corps.* Seattle, Wash.: Peanut Butter Publishing, 1996.

Straubling, Harold E. K. *In Hospital and Camp: The Civil War through the Eyes of Its Doctors and Nurses.* Harrisburg, Pa.: Stackpole Books, 1993.

Sutherland, Daniel E., ed. *A Very Violent Rebel: The Civil War Diary of Ellen Renshaw House.* Knoxville: University of Tennessee Press, 1996.

Thatcher, Virginia. *History of Anesthesia, with Emphasis on the Nurse Specialist.* New York: Garland, 1984.

Underwood, J. L. *Women of the Confederacy.* New York: Neale Publishing, 1906.

"Women's Philanthropic and Charitable Work." http://www.harpweek.com.

Woodward, C. Vann, ed. *Mary Chesnut's Civil War.* New Haven, Conn.: Yale University Press, 1981.

Woolsey, Jane Stuart. *Hospital Days: Reminiscence of a Civil War Nurse.* 1870. Edinburgh, Scotland: Edinburgh Press, 1996.

Communism, Nursing under
Russia

The advent of communism altered profoundly the status and performance of nurses and other medical personnel in affected countries worldwide. War and preparations for war against the capitalist world involved nurses along with other civil and military personnel. For lab technologists in Russia, hellish research in biological warfare in the 1930s dehumanized the Soviet medical world as the People's Health Commissariat turned its research initiative over to the Red Army Biochemical Institute. By the summer of 1935, at the Volga field station and in Ostashkov, experimenters were field-testing tularemia, leprosy, cholera, dysentery, typhoid, paratyphoid, and tetanus. On the Siberian-Mongolian border, tests on plague, anthrax, and cholera preceded human experimentation on dissidents and Japanese prisoners of war. During World War II, the fifteen members of the Union of Soviet Socialist Republics (USSR) drew on female nurses for demanding and dangerous wartime jobs, including handling poisonous or hazardous materials. In the winter of 1941–1942, Russians suffered a catastrophe during the Nazi siege. Medical personnel and services, demoralized, their ranks decimated by the war, struggled against cold, inadequate housing, disease, starvation, and bombardment, all of which reduced Leningrad's citizenry from 2.5 million to 500,000 people.

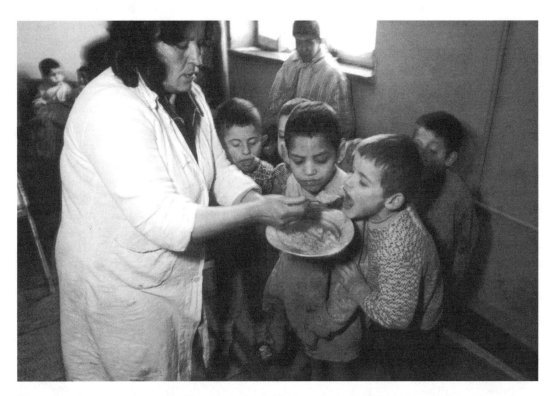

Hungry boys cluster around a nurse holding only one bowl of food at a hospital in Albania for mentally handicapped children, 1992. (Corbis Peter Turnley)

After the war, application of medical procedures as prison punishment created one of Soviet communism's most damning eras. Reports of inhuman treatments and debilitating medicines evoked the terrors of the Nazi Holocaust under Josef Mengele. A Ukrainian peasant, Petro Grigorenko, who was jailed at a penal psychiatric unit in 1964 for criticizing the Soviet regime, reported undergoing a two-hour encephalogram, a procedure that usually took ten minutes. The protracted graphing dented his scalp and left his feet swollen and dangling. During his hospitalization, ten more punitive psychiatric units took shape at Kazan, Leningrad, Sychyovka, Alma-Ata, Oryol, Chernyakhovsk, Dneprepetrovsk, Sverdlovsk, Blagoveshchensk, and Poltava-Kiev. According to medical student Elinor Lipper, an eleven-year victim of Soviet prison camps, the "invalid camp" at Mariinsk in central Siberia was a savage institution "where [handicapped] prisoners were permitted to die slowly" (MacKenzie and Culbertson 1992, 270). Sadistic hierarchies at these camps blurred the line between militia and medical workers by assigning military rank and uniforms to head nurses.

An essay entitled "Punitive Medicine" (1980) by Alexander Podrabinek, a Muscovite paramedic whom the KGB illegally smuggled to Siberia and incarcerated at the Serbsky Central Scientific Research Institute of Forensic Psychiatry, surveyed special psychiatric hospitals and general psychiatric hospitals for dissidents whom authorities cleverly labeled "socially dangerous mentally ill." He described prison cells and dreary exercise courtyards. Patients who refused to report for work detail were reclassified as deteriorating and suffered rounds of torturous injections, isolation, beatings, shock therapy, or straitjackets as punishment. He specifically named nurses, orderlies, and attendants as well as doctors who stole their patients' food, engaged in sexually perverse attacks on elderly or vulnerable patients, locked them up with paid informers, or left them at the mercy of murderous psychotics. An insidious form of corporal correction was the wrapping of patient-prisoners in wet sheets, a crippling torment that could last from hours to months and result in extreme filth, bedsores, warped joints, and atrophied muscles. Podrabinek's eyewitness accounts tell of staff who harmed victims by various means—transfer to the "violent" ward; capricious, vindictive injections; or dosing with handfuls of capsules containing haloperidol, aminazine, trifluoperazine hydrochloride, insulin, or sulfazine. Certain paramedics drove a special black Volga on house calls to inflict torment on dissidents in their homes. Podrabinek claims that, on December 31, 1975, two orderlies beat political prisoner Georgy V. Dekhnich "at the request of Margarita V. Deyeva, a nurse, whom he had called 'a commie bitch.' Shortly before this, Dekhnich had had an ulcer perforation. After the beating, the stitches came apart. No one called the doctor, and the nurse, Deyeva . . . said: 'By morning, we won't be bothered by him anymore.' In the morning, Dekhnich died" (MacKenzie and Culbertson 1992, 297). Former patient-prisoners reflected that, if they could choose, they would prefer losing their physical health in a labor camp to the destruction of intellect and emotions in one of these institutions masquerading as a mental health facility.

While these atrocities were occurring, the average Soviet nurse faced an economic and professional decline. During the Soviet glory days in the early 1960s, the population enjoyed cheap energy, housing, and transportation but suffered food shortages that embarrassed the boastful communist government and thwarted their efforts to impress capitalist countries with the efficiency of Marxism. For nurses in Latvia, postwar assimilation into a vast Ministry of Health cost them privileged status and a living wage. Governed by the multilayered National Health Service, the nation's comprehensive nursing bureaucracy paid for student training and offered uniforms and a monthly stipend of 30–40 rubles. From these beginners, the medical profession developed a predominantly female staff—doctors

(70 percent), midwives, nurse–ambulance attendants, and *feldschers,* a hybrid nurse-doctor or nurse-practitioner. Surgeons were usually male. Under the provincial head nurse, underlings earning 130 rubles a month staffed three-bed wards or worked in polyclinics, which provided on-site screening, treatment, and home visits for up to 180,000 patients per institution.

On the surface, late twentieth-century Soviet nursing paralleled the achievements of the faceless, robotized Soviet military. For example, at Dr. Svyatoslav Fyodorov's assembly line radial keratotomy clinic, nurses prepared up to eighty patients a day and cycled them through surgery to reduce myopia. The systemization of nurse care proved effective in a major catastrophe, a nuclear explosion at the Chernobyl power station on April 26, 1986. In this terrifying instance, the mechanized health care system triumphed against heavy odds. Medical workers activated an emergency plan developed in the late 1960s. The most seriously injured of 100,000 Ukrainians contaminated by the meltdown were transferred to Hospital Number 6 in Moscow. It is remarkable that only eighteen hundred casualties were admitted, of whom thirty-one died, primarily from organ damage and burns. The treatment for exposure, including bone marrow transplant, chemotherapy, intravenous feeding, and treatment with antibiotics and antiviral agents, required round-the-clock staffing by nine hundred nurses, twelve hundred doctors, three thousand physician's assistants, and seven hundred medical students.

On the whole, however, by the early 1990s, as communism waned, impressive innovations in health care theory fell far below implementation. According to Moscow's head nurse Larisa Svirenko, as of 1996, the city had thirty-seven nursing schools, a nursing council, and a twenty-member board composed of head nurses from the largest hospitals. Under this lock-step plan, the nursing profession lost the warmth and compassion of Eastern Orthodox *zelsirdiga masa* (sisters of mercy), who

had run religious hospitals and hospices before the Russian revolution of 1917. The newly created title of *medmasa* (medical sister) presaged a loss of humanity, a central theme of Alexander Solzhenitsyn's best-selling novel *Cancer Ward* (1968). Bulletin board notices reminded staff of unrelenting officialism, which curtailed nurses' opportunities to individualize treatment. Overall, there was a shortage of qualified staff who were further limited by creaky centrifuges, old-fashioned rubber tubing, glass syringes, and outdated record-keeping and sterilizing methods. To their detriment, state-mandated nursing colleges came under the control of doctors and produced substandard medical workers whom patients accused of fatigue, cynicism, and indifference. In the words of Leopold Tyrmand, "As a result, a new Communist citizen learns from the beginning that it is more sensible not to rely on the state's service, but to take care of oneself" (1972, 22).

Because of low pay, unreasonable workloads, and the demands of multiple cultures and languages and ethnic diets, nursing morale plummeted. Government nurses earned 40 percent of the average worker's salary. To survive, about 50 percent moonlighted in a parallel for-fee medical service, which only the wealthy could afford. In proletarian hospitals, lack of pharmaceuticals reduced medical staff to using folk remedies, cupping, and leeches. Isolation from the worldwide medical community, absence of technological advancements such as computerized axial tomography (CAT) scans, and worsening conditions—infant mortality rates, the spread of acquired immunodeficiency syndrome (AIDS) from unsanitary clinic conditions, death from cardiovascular disease, high incidence of alcoholism, increase in lung disease from smoking and air pollution, and decline in overall life expectancy—dragged nurse care in the former Soviet Union to the level of that in Third World countries. Thus, the decline in health standards became one of the strongest arguments against the communist experiment.

China

China was even more devastated than the USSR by a violent wrenching of its medical system. Although philanthropic hospitals, leprosaria, and homes for the blind and insane flourished in the 1860s, the concept of nursing in China dated to 1884, when an American, Elizabeth McKechnie, set up the first Nightingale system in Shanghai. Ella Johnson, also American, opened a nursing school in 1888, the year that the word *KanHu* (nurse) was added to the language. Catholic and Protestant missionary societies quickly learned that the number of Chinese converts increased in regions served by Christian nurses. In 1914, McKechnie and Elise Chung Lyon formed the China Nursing Association (CNA) and six years later began publishing a professional journal. In the 1920s, when Xiangya Hospital and Yanjing University developed nursing programs, women's medical curricula flourished.

By 1949, when communist chairman Mao Tse-tung introduced reforms, the nation had 32,600 nurses. His original complaints about China's medical care was that too much attention was paid to cities and that traditional medical care had been neglected. Three years later, he closed all nursing schools, including the Peking Union Medical College, which had offered B.S. degrees in nursing since 1922. Communist bureaucracy took control of medical care, banished Western methods, disbanded the CNA, and introduced a military-style health cadre. While reducing parasitic infestation and tuberculosis, the regimented effort virtually wiped out smallpox, cholera, typhus, typhoid fever, plague, and leprosy along with opium addiction and venereal disease. By 1957, around 390,000 hospitals were serving the cities, but outlying areas still suffered neglect.

In 1965, near the end of the Socialist Education Movement, new directives from the Ministry of Public Health moved control of primary care and preventive medicine to families and regional clinics. In 1974, mobile teams and one million paramedics, known as "barefoot doctors," spread throughout the countryside to reiterate the need for self-reliance and family-style nursing rather than dependence on expensive medical gadgetry and hospital stays. Under this program, the quality of care fluctuated, depending on the expertise of local staff and family willingness to follow directives. In 1982, nearly sixteen million women and four million men underwent voluntary sterilization in a government-mandated effort to stabilize population growth, which outpaced available medical facilities. Although nursing programs reopened at Tianjin Medical College and Beijing Medical University under Chairman Deng Xiaoping's modernization strategy in the mid-1980s, China struggled to recover from a severe nursing shortage, inadequate training, isolationism, and endemic disease and substandard service in rural collectives.

In the 1990s, human rights issues clouded Chinese communist gains just as they had in the Soviet Union. Chinese atrocities came up for debate in the United Nations Committee against Torture in 1993. Three years later, Shanghai-born American humanitarian Harry Wu—who had spent the years 1960–1979 wrongfully detained in a Chinese prison—broadcast communist abuses in prisons and labor camps through interviews, public appearances, and a book, *Troublemaker: One Man's Crusade against China's Cruelty.* One startling disclosure was the government system of executing prisoners to harvest and sell corneas, kidneys, and other organs for transplant. Wu compared the extermination of one Chinese population to salvage another to Nazi medical experiments on dissidents and prisoners during the Holocaust. The Chinese, he alleged, had covertly begun the practice in 1979 but had made no formal policy on the use of organs from condemned criminals until 1984. Against the callously streamlined practice—declaring prisoners brain-dead, harvesting organs, then executing the involuntary donors—Wu recoiled: "My stomach turned. An entire segment of Chinese society was being turned into grave robbers, desecraters of the dead" (Wu 1996, 154–155).

To determine the procedure for himself, Wu visited First University Hospital at West China University of Medical Sciences in Chengdu. As with the Russian radial keratotomy surgeries, the work of nurses and surgeons honed the well-rehearsed process to only ten hours, compared to twenty in the United States. When Wu's documentary appeared on BBC television, Chinese officials protested accusations of ghoulish harvesting methods but offered no refutation of the practice of removing organs from living prisoners before executing them. In subsequent investigation in 1995, Wu studied doctors and nurses performing involuntary abortions on women who had already borne one child. He condemned the sale of harvested fetuses to pharmaceutical labs for grinding and processing into fertility and potency tonics. Wu's advocacy realigned Western thinking about the morality of Chinese communism and its effect on world medical practice.

Cuba

As happened in Russia and China, the precipitous nature of revolution had similar effects on nursing in Cuba. After Fidel Castro overthrew the hated dictator General Fulgencio Batista in 1959, Cuba, the newest communist state, made its own rapid shifts in nurse training. The era's medical chaos derived from the self-exile of nearly 50 percent of Cuban doctors and nurses to the United States, while faculty at the medical school of the University of Havana dropped 87 percent. To ensure medical progress, Castro's government took over schools, lowered educational standards, and staffed Isle of Pines Prison and Calixto García Hospital with Marxist-Leninist nurses, mostly imported from Iron Curtain countries or recruited from a pool of hastily trained island blacks. With a minimum of course work, ambitious nurses could become doctors. According to John Martino—an American electronics expert falsely detained at La Cabaña Prison Fortress in July 1959 and held until September 1962—poorly staffed prison infirmaries could do little for detainees wounded by sadistic guards: "There was no alcohol in the infirmary, no bandages, nothing with which to suture wounds, no sulpha, or antibiotics. The victims were left untended. The wounds festered" (Martino 1963, 138). He learned that 10 percent of the prisoners had tuberculosis; more suffered fungal infection.

One Cuban nurse-detainee, Reynaldo Soto Hernández, earned a reputation for humanism and noncompliance with the communist ban on protest of human rights violations. A prison poet and human rights activist for the Comité Cubano Pro Derechos Humanos (Cuban Committee for Human Rights), he was arrested, tried, and sentenced on the same day for "dangerousness." Jailed at the Prisión Provincial de Ciego de Avila, he was refused reading material and family visits, denied medical care for skin and ear infections, and threatened with transfer to a distant prison for criticizing prison conditions and summary executions. For his humanistic poetry in *Habitaciones* (Rooms), he won the 1994 provincial poetry prize in Ciego de Avila.

Time was not on the side of Castro as he hustled more communist innovations into action. Throughout Cuba, substandard medical workers fought an outbreak of gastroenteritis among the babies of Marianao and plunged into the 1962 epidemic of syphilis and gonorrhea without penicillin, Aureomycin, and other antibiotics. To stem rampant venereal disease, Dr. Rafael de la Palma, chief of the Cuban public health department, reported that the country had no choice but to import inferior drugs from the USSR. For all the surface Cuban-Russian camaraderie during the island's dismantling of capitalism, Russian supervision of hospitals resulted in dissension among native staff, who despised their overseers for favoring high-level patients over the Cuban proletariat.

In 1978, Fred Ward, an American writer on assignment from *National Geographic*, spent seven months examining the changes that communism had wrought in Cuba. Because Castro had lived so intimately with the peasantry of the Oriente section of the island during the guerrilla stage of his takeover, as head of state, he was determined to uplift an outback peasantry deprived of education, medical service, running water, and electricity. From the beginning of his tenure as dictator, he made public health and preventive care the cornerstone of a policy to improve life for the poorest Cubans. Although the enrichments Castro had envisioned were tentative, in the early 1960s, the transformation of public health grew out of the nationalization of private practices, pharmacies, clinics and dental offices, and for-profit hospitals.

Eventually, upgraded health care under Castro became a reality, outdistancing similar programs in Vietnam, North Korea, China, and the Soviet bloc. Immediately after coming to power, he tackled malnutrition, infant and maternal mortality, communicable disease, impure water, and poor hygiene. To provide nurses, he pushed the number of nursing schools from six to thirty-four. By 1967, his prevention plan had virtually eradicated malaria and diphtheria; in 1973, polio all but disappeared. In 1974, statistics recorded a drop of 73 percent in tuberculosis deaths. That same year, maternal deaths fell to 56 per 100,000, the lowest in Latin America.

Within a decade of the Cuban revolution, the Rural Service reflected demographics by stripping Havana of its glut of medical staff, instituting industrial nursing in cigar and sugar factories, and spreading fifty hospitals, 150 dispensaries, and 340 polyclinics over the countryside. At each polyclinic, individual doctors teamed with a nurse and several medical students and residents to offer families CAT scans and magnetic resonance imaging (MRI), organ transplant, in-vitro fertilization, sonograms and prenatal diagnoses, and neonatal care. In one example—the east coast town of Chivirico—a small hospital staffed by Havana obstetrician-gynecologist Dr. Robert Gandarilla and ten nurses delivered babies to women who had not previously come to a hospital for care. To assist nursing staff in administering and recording immunizations, Committees for the Defense of the Revolu-

tion listed people needing shots and oral polio immunization and stockpiled necessary supplies. The Cuban Women's Federation encouraged women to seek Pap smears and breast exams. The streamlining worked, boosting Cuban life expectancy and establishing to the capitalist world that communism did indeed take the working class to heart.

Current Trends

In recent years, exchange programs to the communist world began the overdue process of familiarizing the rest of the world with nurse care and hospital procedures in Cuba, China, and former republics of the USSR. According to a team from the American Public Health Association touring Cuba in 1995 and 1996, the small island, one of the most seriously strapped medical communities under communism, recovered its pre-Communist reputation for health care among developing countries and competed through discipline and innovation with industrialized nations. Following the heady days of the revolution in 1959, the government-controlled education system set up free training programs in each province. Consequently, the ratio of nurses to patients rose to 0.62 nurses per hospital bed. Castro's medical impetus improved access to clinic, mammography vans, and emergency service, even in rural areas. One rural practitioner, Diolaida Guzman, who served families near Baracoa, explained to visitors the nurse's role in routine hygiene supervision and treatment of hypertension, both essential to improving life for Cuban families.

Visitors were quick to point out that these programs were not without failings. Despite gains, Cubans continued to suffer malnutrition and disease. Following the disastrous Bay of Pigs invasions on April 12, 1961, American partnership in Cuban recovery officially ended. Cuba's total isolation from textbooks, journals, clinics, and research facilities in capitalist countries impeded exchange of ideas concerning more efficient nurse care and modernized preventive techniques. Furthermore, trade embargoes and the loss of Soviet trade subsidies after the demise of the Soviet Union limited supplies of foodstuffs, antibiotics, chemotherapy drugs, mammography film, multiple vitamins, and chlorination equipment. In the absence of allopathic medicines, thermal bathing experienced a resurgence at forty locations; *medicina verde* (green medicine), based on traditional herbs, flourished among nonwhite Cubans, particularly followers of the Santeria cult. The island's low level of technology forced a return to community-based public health initiatives, in which public health nurses went from house to house vaccinating all citizens against twelve infectious diseases. In 1996, the American Association for World Health discovered delayed diagnosis, declining treatment and surgeries, and increases in water-borne disease and concluded that "only the excellence of the system and the extraordinary dedication of the Cuban medical community have prevented infinitely greater loss of life and suffering" ("Jewel" 1998, 29).

Since 1984, significant improvements have elevated Cuba's medical reputation worldwide.

- Its Medicina General Integral (General Integral Medicine) program has extended emergency service and family practice in internal medicine, pediatrics, and obstetrics and gynecology by placing staff near a *consultorio* (clinic) in the communities they serve.
- An outbreak of human immunodeficiency virus (HIV) among war heroes returning from service in Angola in the mid-1980s resulted in an unusual system of containment at restrictive sanitariums.
- From 1991 to 1993, medical workers treated fifty thousand Cubans during an epidemic of optic neuritis and polyneuropathy arising from malnutrition, which eased in 1994 after the economy improved.
- At Hermanos Almeijeiras Hospital in Havana, Cuba's upscale referral center,

operating room nurses remain in demand for extensive transplant surgeries (cornea, heart, heart-lung, kidney, pancreas, liver, and bone marrow) for patients selected by a computerized matching system.
- The Cuban government offered its expertise to its fellow communists in the Soviet Union by treating more than four thousand children afflicted with leukemia after the 1986 nuclear accident at Chernobyl.

For all this medical progress, as Cuba suffered from failed crops and trade embargoes, Castro's communist regime failed to counter a resurgence of malaria, tuberculosis, pellagra, lice, and chicken pox. Much of the capitalist world took note of strong U.S. anti-Castro policies during the Clinton administration and condemned tactics that targeted women and children, the elderly, and the poor.

Capitalist visitors to China found similar weaknesses in medical service under communism. As witnessed by a delegation of orthopedic nurses from the Citizen Ambassador Program of People to People International to the People's Republic of China in 1996, the typical Chinese nurse staff combated problems endemic in the world's largest population, fastest-developing economy, and most polluted nation. Chinese nurse-trainees studied both modern and ancestral methods of preventing illness by controlling diet, temperature, and emotions. However, in comparison with their Western counterparts, they lacked up-to-date methodology and equipment and were forced to recycle and improvise. A sliver of progress for China began in 1958 with Project Hope, a Virginia-based philanthropic outreach dedicated to upgrading health care through self-sustaining medical training. Spread to five continents, the organization focused on China and, in 1984, began targeting universities. Western philanthropists spread primary care programs to Beijing, Shanghai, Xian, Hangzhou, and Chengdu. According to associate director of nursing Leslie Mancuso, project leaders asked the Chinese to identify their needs, which are greatest in nurse care. Project Hope nursing program director Marcia Petrini credited the CNA with rapid retraining of one thousand nurses, who are already applying newly acquired strategies and health care data to local needs. The inauguration of pediatric services at the nonprofit Shanghai Children's Medical Center in 1996 promoted the use of state-of-the-art techniques and provided modern equipment while continuing the original goal of training more nurses for service.

According to a 1996 article in *AORN Journal,* a twenty-seven-member visiting team of operating room nurses learned how in-country clinical practice, infection control, and academic training served China's 1.2 billion citizens. Hosted by the China Association for Science and Technology, perioperative nurses from the United States, Canada, and Australia visited members of the CNA at its headquarters in Beijing, and learned that the first post-Mao school opened in Tianjin in 1984. Because of the intervening shortage of nurse-educators, faculties relied on practitioners whose education predated the revolution and imported skilled personnel from Thailand, Hong Kong, and other countries. Visitors found the seven-year-old Medical College of Nursing at Xian Medical University in Shaanxi Province a prospering facility—clean, well-lit, and equipped with reference library, computer science lab, and operating room and intensive care units. Visitors noted impressive electronic models of the nervous and circulatory systems but were dismayed at outdated journals and scanty reference materials primarily in English. The school's one hundred nursing students could choose from associate, five-year B.S., or M.S. degrees. Still founded on the communist model, regimentation discouraged students from asking questions during professional presentations and offered no continuing education.

Visitors concluded that Chinese nurses had much to learn. Representatives of the 190,000 members of CNA were unfamiliar with universal precautions against hepatitis, a prevalent problem for the Chinese. Surgical nurses acquired their jobs through demonstration of excellence during a two-year period of medical-surgical experience. Those who prospered in their specialty were expected to reeducate and observe procedure in varied settings, including outside China. Perioperative nursing was a separate attainment, which they acquired on the job in a three-month program. Visitors were appalled that gloving for surgery was sometimes omitted, for example, during laryngoscopy, and that gloves were processed for several reuses. Because of the scarcity of disposables, nurses prepared needles and sutures individually. Operating room nurses, who had to retire at age forty, were surprised to discover over-forty visitors still active in the profession. Outsiders noted that forced retirement did not apply to male surgeons, who earned further disdain from nurses for their arrogance and disrespect of women professionals. The visitors were nonplussed to learn that, under communist equalization of salary, nurses and surgeons received similar pay.

According to nurse-consultant Cynthia C. Spry of Irvine, California, during observation at several Chinese hospitals, visitors noted differences in quality of service. Nursing staff operated a mix of modern and outdated equipment, such as a tank, hose, and reusable face mask as well as epidural injection for anesthesia. The number of instruments was much smaller than equipment packs found in the United States. Laparoscopic surgery was still in its infancy. Also, Chinese surgical teams lacked surgical technologists.

At Quang An Men Hospital in Beijing, a renowned oncology treatment center, staff combined traditional Chinese medicine and pharmacology with Western practice. Staff treated side effects of radiation and chemotherapy, chronic pain, and insomnia with massage, acupuncture, acupressure, moxibustion, implantation of seeds in the ear, and other herbal remedies. Nurses seeking a full license in holistic medicine—ancestral harmony-seeking methods dating back thirty-five hundred years to the Shang dynasty—had to complete standard training and practice several years before taking an additional one hundred hours of study. They could perform these folk-based methods only under supervision of a doctor.

Near the end of the twentieth century, conditions for Chinese nurses showed promise.

- In 1997, Interhealth Canada China established a cooperative—the Beijing/Toronto International Hospital Project, which began work on an up-to-date eighty-bed hospital. The bilateral health initiative offered staff full-time telemedical communication with Ontario's Hamilton Health Sciences Centre.
- In 1998, China began combating the threat of AIDS to nurses from contaminated blood supplies by banning a system of paid donors.
- U.S. President Bill Clinton assisted Chinese nursing staff in June 1998 by offering low-interest loans to upgrade medical equipment.

These strides indicate that the Chinese government maintains a serious commitment to state-of-the-art health care for its citizens.

The situation in the USSR worsened after the demise of communist control, when lack of staff lowered standards at teaching institutions, individuals worked twenty-four-hour shifts, and nursing salaries fell to the official poverty level of 120 rubles a month. The European Region Committee of the World Health Organization (WHO) reported that economic collapse threatened the health of each former republic. To maintain morale, women like head nurse of Riga Hospital Number 4 Lucija Lapina, president of the Latvian Red Cross Nurses Association, cherished oral history and tattered copies of professional journals dating to the 1930s. The gesture suggested the dearth of up-to-date information that nurses can consult in solving the problems of the twenty-first century.

Capitalist outreach to the disintegrating postcommunist world has been a godsend as the former Soviet nations struggled against devastating pollution, hunger, aging hospital equipment, and an inadequate staff of some 2.6 million nurses. Following the creation of a National Council of Nurses in 1989, member states—Armenia, Kazakhstan, Kyrgyzstan, the Russian Federation, Turkmenistan, and Uzbekistan—asserted the priority of nursing and midwifery to all former communist nations. According to the recommendations of the World Health Assembly of 1992, each nation was assigned to develop a plan for nurse care centering on better pay and upgraded working conditions. With headquarters at Alma-Ata, Kazakhstan, the WHO Collaborating Centre for Primary Health Care and Nursing led the necessary networking among member states, which were still working out relationships between disparate peoples who had only recently been fellow communists.

Chief nurse of the Soviet Union Helen Kashirina encouraged a WHO program that brought nine Soviet nurses to Britain for study. She applauded the exchange of ideas gleaned from Western progress. Most debilitating to fellow professionals was limited training, which at that time allowed a sixteen-year-old to enter a state-paid three-year nursing program. In its tenuous state, Russian nursing also lacked graduate degree programs, nursing research, in-service training, and refresher courses. Under glasnost (opening) and perestroika (restructuring), the nation's nurses anticipated unheard-of triumphs: improved prestige and working conditions, independence from physicians, and negotiated wages.

Because Soviet nurses were unfamiliar with the hospice concept of care for the dying, in 1991 journalist Victor Zorza and British hospice workers helped launch the Soviet Hospice Society, which began aiding terminally ill patients from the wooden hut that served as its Leningrad headquarters. Although the facility was primitive, the society offered clean bedding and wholesome food to twenty-five patients. Donors from outside Russia provided staff salaries, medicine, and equipment. Supported by the Cancer Relief Macmillan Fund (CRMR), British nurses Anne Brown, Ann Dent, and Ann Nash taught thirty Russian nurses the psychology of dying and palliative care, established policy, and set up on-site and home-care services. Two of their pupils hoped to carry their training to a developing hospice movement in the Ukraine. In retrospect, Nash commented, "It was very new to the Russian nurses—to plan, to act, and to evaluate. It added a whole new dimension to their care" (Trevelyan 1991, 17).

Additional international medical partnerships raised nursing standards through varied cooperatives:

- Beginning in 1988, Russian émigré nurses brought their language skills and bicultural understanding to North American hospitals, where they were retrained for employment throughout the world.
- In 1991, three weeks after Latvia gained its independence, Zaiga Kalnins, a Latvian-born U.S. citizen, served as a visiting professor at the nursing department of the Latvian Medical Academy. Her observations on the end of oppressive conditions under communism and the emancipation of nurses provided insight into transcultural nursing in former Soviet bloc countries.
- In 1992, the American International Health Alliance linked nurses in Kyrgyzstan with the University of Kansas Medical Center. The purpose of their partnership was cultural and professional exchange to upgrade nursing administration programs and nursing education.
- From 1992 to 1996, the Canadian Society for International Health dispatched nurses on short-term residencies to bolster Ukrainian health programs. In addition to aiding hospital staff, the outsiders brought advanced technology, improved skills, and initiated degree nursing programs to elevate the Ukraine's 110 nursing schools to international standards. Canadians enumerated numerous failings: only four college-based training centers and four-year programs, practicum limited to two years, absence of professional organizations and networking, and schools run by physicians. To reform a deplorably outmoded situation, in 1992, Canadian nurses led by Gerri Nakonechny, dean of health and community studies at Grand MacEwan Community College, joined the Ukraine's Ministry of Health to revise curricula and select nurses from Lviv for on-site training in Canada. In September 1995, Nakonechny coordinated a professional conference in Chernivtsi and subsequent workshop for four hundred Ukrainian nurses on policy development and implementation. As a result, participants intensified nursing education and founded a national nursing association.

Sources

Allen, A. "Old Enemies Practice Teamwork . . . Health Problems That Exist in Russia." *Journal of Post-Anesthesia Nursing* 9, no. 4 (1994): 247–249.

Anthony-Tkach, C. "Nursing and Health Care in the Soviet Union." *Nursing Forum* 22, no. 2 (1985): 45–52.

Baj, R. "Integrating the Russian Émigré Nurse into U.S. Nursing." *Journal of Nursing Administration* 25, no. 3 (1995): 43–47.

Baldinger, Pamela. "Training the Care Givers." *China Business Review* (July-August 1992): 34–36.

Bernal, H., et al. "Community Health Nursing in a Former Soviet Union Republic: A Case Study of Change in Armenia." *Nursing Outlook* 43, no. 2 (1995): 78–83.

"Calling for a Nursing Revolution in Eastern Europe." *World Health* (November-December 1993): 28–37.

"Canadian Nursing Professionals Help Update Ukraine's Health Care." *Ukrainian Weekly,* June 23, 1996, 9.

Carr, Mary. "Kindness and Consideration." *Nursing Mirror,* November 2, 1983, 26–28.

Castledine, George. "Proud Sunset over Leningrad." *Nursing Mirror* 156, no. 7 (1983): 22.

Chen, Kaiyi. "Quality versus Quantity: The Rockefeller Foundation and Nurses' Training in

China." *Journal of American–East Asian Relations* (spring 1996): 77–105.

Dennis, L. I. "Soviet Hospital Nursing: A Model for Self-Care." *Journal of Nursing Education* 28, no. 2 (1989): 76–77.

Erickson, John. "Night Witches, Snipers, and Laundresses." *History Today* (July 1990): 29–36.

Falcoff, Mark. "Is It Time to Rethink the Cuban Embargo?" *Latin American Outlook*. http://www.aei.org/lao/lao8875.htm.

Gale, Dr. Robert Peter, and Thomas Hauser. *Final Warning: The Legacy of Chernobyl*. New York: Warner Books, 1988.

Gioiella, E. C. "Russia: The Soviet Health Care System for the Aged." *Journal of Gerontological Nursing* 9, no. 11 (1983): 582–585.

Halpin, Tony. "Cover Story: Disaster and Recovery; Two Years Later, a Shattered Nation Picks Up the Pieces at a Crawling Pace." *Armenian International Magazine,* January 31, 1991, 8.

Harris, Robert, and Jeremy Paxman. *A Higher Form of Killing: The Secret Story of Chemical and Biological Warfare*. New York: Hill and Wang, 1982.

"Jewels in the Crown." *New Internationalist* (May 1998): 27–29.

Kahl, Jurgen. "Psychology Comes to China." *World Press Review* (November 1992): 48.

Kalnins, Irene, and Zaiga Priede Kalnins. "Latvian Nurses Depart from Soviet Ways." *Nursing Outlook* (March-April 1991): 64–68.

Kalnins, Zaiga Priede. "Nursing in Latvia from the Perspective of Oppressed Theory." *Journal of Transcultural Nursing* 4, no. 1 (1992): 11–16.

Karosas, L. M. "Nursing in Lithuania as Perceived by Lithuanian Nurses." *Nursing Outlook* 43, no. 4 (1995): 153–157.

Kent, Heather. "Canada-China Hospital Being Developed." *Canadian Medical Association Journal,* November 15, 1997.

Lago, José F. "A First Approximation Design of the Social Safety Net for a Democratic Cuba." http://info.lanic.utexas.edu/la/cb/cuba/asce/cuba4/healsys2.html.

Mackenzie, Ross, and Todd Culbertson, eds. *Eyewitness: Writing from the Ordeal of Communism*. New York: Freedom House, 1992.

Martin D. L. "The Development of the Profession of Nursing in Kyrgyzstan." *Journal of Multicultural Nursing and Health* 3, no. 1 (1997): 6–10.

Martino, John. *I Was Castro's Prisoner: An American Tells His Story*. New York: Devin-Adair, 1963.

Meisner, Maurice. *Mao's China: A History of the People's Republic*. New York: Free Press, 1977.

Moody, Linda E. "Glasnost, Perestroika, and Health Problems of the 1990s." *Journal of Holistic Nursing* (March 1992): 47–62.

Nayeri, Kamran. "The Cuban Health Care System and Factors Currently Undermining It." *Journal of Community Health* (August 1995): 321–335.

"Nurses and Human Rights." http://www.amnesty.org/ailib/aipub/1997ACT/A7500297.htm.

"Paid Blood Donors Banned with AIDS Spreading Fast." *Seattle Post-Intelligencer,* October 1, 1998.

Pasquali, Elaine Anne. "Santeria." *Journal of Holistic Nursing* (December 1994): 380–391.

Ryan, T. Michael, and Ray Thomas. "Trends in the Supply of Medical Personnel in the Russian Federation." *Journal of the American Medical Association,* July 24, 1996, 339–342.

Sado, Monica. "The Good, the Bad and the Different." *Nursing Mirror,* November 2, 1983, 24–26.

Schwab, Peter. "Cuban Health Care and the U.S. Embargo." *Monthly Review* (November 1997): 15.

Solzhenitsyn, Alexander. *Cancer Ward*. New York: Farrar, Straus and Giroux, 1968.

Spence, Jonathan D. *The Search for Modern China*. New York: W. W. Norton, 1990.

Spry, Cynthia C. "A Western OR Delegation to the People's Republic of China." *AORN Journal* (March 1996): 525–533.

Trevelyan, J. "Bringing Hope: Hospice Care in the Soviet Union." *Nursing Times,* January 16, 1991, 16–17.

———. "Nursing Sisters." *Nursing Times,* May 30, 1990, 16–17.

Tyrmand, Leopold. *The Rosa Luxemburg Contraceptives Cooperative: A Primer on Communist Civilization*. New York: Macmillan, 1972.

Turton, Pat. "After Chernobyl." *Nursing Times,* May 28, 1986, 27.

Waitzen, Howard, et al. "Primary Care in Cuba: Low- and High-Technology Developments Pertinent to Family Medicine," *Journal of Family Practice* (September 1997): 250–259.

Ward, Fred. *Inside Cuba Today*. New York: Crown Publishers, 1978.

Wei Ke. "Chinese Hospitals Get U.S. Loans." *China Daily,* June 23, 1998.

Wienke, Kay. "Health Care Chinese Style." *Orthopaedic Nursing* (May-June 1996): 39–48.

Wu, Harry. *Troublemaker: One Man's Crusade Against China's Cruelty*. New York: Times Books, 1996.

Cumming, Kate

A respected Confederate nursing matron, Kate Cumming merited praise for her nurse care with the Army of Tennessee. By way of introducing her eyewitness account of the Civil War, *A Journal of Hospital Life in the*

Confederate Army of Tennessee from the Battle of Shiloh to the End of the War (1866), she explained that charges of maltreatment of Union prisoners forced her to reveal experiences that refuted any notion of malevolence against enemy wounded. A facile diarist, she balanced each day with hope and offset ward work with treks into the countryside to see landmarks such as Lookout Mountain, Tennessee, and the gardens of Atlanta, Georgia. In troubled moments, she vented disquiet over the South's rebellion and battled with her conscience the area's sin of slavery.

Born in 1835 in Edinburgh, Scotland, Cumming emigrated with her family to Mobile, Alabama, and identified with southern causes and philosophy. As the Civil War began, she was moved by the example of two friends who served under Florence Nightingale in the Crimea. After hearing a speech delivered by a nursing recruiter, the Reverend Benjamin M. Miller, she determined to enlist as a military nurse. Cumming disobeyed her family members, who were repulsed by the impropriety of a refined lady treating soldiers. In April 1862 after the Battle of Shiloh, she joined forty other women on a train to Corinth, Mississippi, to enroll in the nurse corps and serve as matron of the hospital opened at the Tishomingo Hotel, a facility so disordered that amputated limbs lay scattered about the compound.

The decline of the Confederate army and starvation across the South left Cumming and other nurses in dire situations. On April 11, 1862, she expressed shock at the wretchedness and horror of war. The next day, she reported, "We have to walk, and when we give the men anything, [must stand] in blood and water; but we think nothing of it at all . . . I have been busy all day, and I can scarcely tell what I have been doing; I have not taken time even to eat, certainly not time to sit down" (Gragg 1989, 63). She complained that the nurse staff changed every few hours and that the hospital authorities followed no system. That night, she fell asleep among the baggage on a stack of boxes and, on a subsequent night, was happy to have sawdust and straw to rake up into a makeshift mattress.

At the beginning of her service, Cumming, like Dorothea Dix, praised the best in nurses and disdained the worst. She admired the Sisters of Charity for deft care of patients and for working under terrible conditions without complaint. When single laywomen entered the corps as a form of diversion or as a means of hunting beaux, she scribbled in her journal in annoyance that anyone could find a combat zone an entertainment or a suitable source of husbands. On September 4, 1862, Cumming arrived in Chattanooga, Tennessee, one of the worst scenes of misery and deprivation, and took some comfort in comparing medical chaos to the scene that greeted Florence Nightingale at Scutari during the Crimean War. Five days into the job, Cumming, stung by complaints that proper ladies did not go to hospitals, addressed southern women directly: "Have we not thousands who, at this moment, do not know what to do to pass the time that is hanging heavily on their hands?" (Cumming 1866, 45). She remarked that from the beginning of history, women have had the special task of relieving suffering and reasoned that, if the situation were too harsh for young women, then young men should also withdraw from combat.

In October 1862, Cumming chafed at the lack of trained nursing staff and the lack of clean garments for exchanged prisoners, who had been wearing the same unlaundered clothing for over a month. As matron in charge of nurses at Newsom Hospital, she and her staff struggled to treat casualties from the Battle of Stone River and the Capture of Murfreesboro, Tennessee, fought from December 31, 1862, to January 2, 1863. Along with aides Susan E. D. "Grandma" Smith and Fannie Beers, Cumming worked from 4:00 A.M. until midnight to ready a row of warehouses and to treat 350 casualties, many of whom acquired gangrene after admission. One by one, she named and described her most troubling cases and remarked on the valor and restraint of men facing death from dysentery, grievous wounds, and the trauma of amputation. Some patients arrived from the field with their wounds dressed in strips of tarps and old tent cloth.

Cumming's honest reportage captures the anguish of war nursing. On February 10, 1863, she felt demoralized and complained that the damp, uncomfortable hospital was so cheerless that, were it not for the patients, she could not tolerate the work. In better spirits a month later, she detailed the ingredients of batter cakes and named a recent serving of spiced pudding as a luxurious dessert. After complimenting the cook and his kitchen, she contrasted the erratic service of the hospital laundry, which failed to clean the garments casualties were wearing when they arrived. As the war moved east in summer 1863, Cumming worked out of a mobile caravan ranging through Kingston, Cherokee Springs, Catoosa Springs, Tunnel Hill, Marietta, and Newnan, Georgia. On July 23, she reported on her tenuous relationship with grumpy, patriarchal male surgeons, who insisted on strict discipline for nurses and on sharing dinner with the female staff, whom one physician considered a suitable table dressing. With quick Scottish wit, Cumming labeled him a "real Pharaoh" (Cumming 1866, 78).

Cumming set up a wartime facility, Foard Hospital, in Newnan and, in August 1863, treated five hundred patients, often with the assistance of a few untrained male nurses. The shortage of women sparked her temper. On August 5, she groused: "Are the women of the South going into the hospitals? I am afraid candor will compel me to say they are not! It is not respectable and requires too constant of attention, and a hospital has none of the comforts of home!" (Cumming 1866, 88). Speaking of her own experience in an all-male environment, she could report not one offensive word or deed from male patients. With a tender, loving spirit, she assessed the dismal situation at the Burnt Shed outside Ringgold, Georgia, and treated a group of casualties from Kentucky to watered-down blackberry wine. To her delight, the Georgia Relief Committee relieved some of the burden of hunger and need, but she could not shake the urge to follow the Sisters of Charity to the front lines and treat men at field hospitals.

On October 25, 1863, Cumming recorded her impressions of Confederacy president Jefferson Davis, who arrived to take depositions from officers and men complaining about the lackluster leadership of General Braxton Bragg. The next day, mounting discontent pressed her to resign, but, as with previous depressions, the sight of men uplifted by her care renewed enthusiasm for her job. To address complaints of the sameness of the diet, which consisted of cornmeal mush, dried fruit, potatoes, rice, beef and chicken soup, and bread, she created her own invalid food out of arrowroot, eggs, wine, and preserves. As the army moved on, she and her staff packed and transported supplies and equipment to Americus, Georgia.

Cumming nourished a deep respect for Southerners, in part for their intellect and admiration for the writings of Scotland's greatest authors, Robert Burns and Sir Walter Scott. On May 24, 1864, she described her sadness at seeing sick and wounded Southern gentlemen eating with their fingers because they had no utensils. The wretchedness of their state eased somewhat in Atlanta, where she found a faithful cadre of women serving at a table set up at the depot, carrying buckets of milk, coffee, and lemonade and dressing wounds. Assisting them were elderly aristocrats too old for the army, who offered delicacies to the wounded.

After the fall of Atlanta on September 1, 1864, and later in Griffin, Georgia, in January 1865, Cumming shared the South's serious privations and worked without firewood or candles. Orders to return the mobile hospitals to Tennessee delighted her. By February, she had mixed feelings at news of an armistice and an end to the fighting. On March 9, 1865, she described the depredations of Federal marauders, who terrorized the elderly, handicapped, and vulnerable. The situation grew so fearful that the Sisters of Charity withdrew to the safety of their convent. Cumming departed from her hospital as it moved out of Sherman's reach and traveled by ambulance to view Andersonville Prison. The disastrous results of hunger, overcrowding, and widespread epidemic moved her to write, "May heaven help us all! But war is terrible" (Jones 1955, 329).

Noted as a nurse, patriot, and diarist, Cumming retired to Mobile, Alabama, then moved to her father's home in Birmingham in 1874. In 1866, she published her memoirs, *Gleaning from the Southland,* a more detailed narrative than the hospital journal. Until her death in 1909, she taught school, gave music lessons, and supported the cleaning of army graves, a project launched by the United Daughters of the Confederacy.

Sources

Cumming, Kate. *A Journal of Hospital Life in the Confederate Army of Tennessee from the Battle of Shiloh to the End of the War.* Louisville, Ky.: John P. Morton, 1866.

Cunningham, H. H. *Doctors in Gray: The Confederate Medical Service.* Baton Rouge: Louisiana State University Press, 1986.

Dodge, Bertha S. *The Story of Nursing.* Boston: Little, Brown, 1965.

Gragg, Rod, ed. *The Illustrated Confederate Reader.* New York: Harper and Row, 1989.

Jones, Katherine M. *Heroines of Dixie.* Indianapolis, Ind.: Bobbs-Merrill, 1955.

Kalisch, Philip, and Beatrice J. Kalisch. *The Advance of American Nursing.* Boston: Little, Brown, 1978.

"Kate Cumming." http://www.glue.umd.edu/~cliswp/Bios/kcbio.html.

Schroeder-Lein, Glenna R. *Confederate Hospitals on the Move: Samuel H. Stout and the Army of Tennessee.* Columbia: University of South Carolina Press, 1994.

Sherr, Lynn, and Jurate Kazickas. *Susan B. Anthony Slept Here: A Guide to American Women's Landmarks.* New York: Times Books, 1994.

Curandera

The Latino concept of *curandera,* a semiofficial shaman or community healer, derives from the Latin "to cure," meaning "to heal or restore" rather than "to mend." Surviving as an alternative to modern medicine, the *curandera,* who is typically female, is God-chosen to intercede in a medical crisis. In *The Medical Story of Early Texas* (1946), Dr. Pat Ireland Nixon recorded that, in Nacogdoches in 1810, María Benítez intervened in the case of Lorenzo Marets, a black slave so severely beaten that he required setting of a dislocated shoulder and treatment of serious contusions. A second example, María de los Reyes Martínez, a respected *curandera,* testified in a Laredo assault case in 1824 as to the nature and direction of a stab wound that she had examined. Such lay healers continue to flourish within the culture, whether in Mexico, Cuba, Houston and Los Angeles barrios, or New York's Spanish Harlem. As described by practitioner and *partera* (midwife) Juanita Sedillo, a New Mexico healer born in 1895, the *curandera* believes that God placed *remedios* on Earth to relieve human suffering. These humble folk cures include manure for setting broken bones, mud mixed with potato and vinegar for controlling fever, and herbs to speed delivery of infants.

Typically an itinerant nurse-midwife, the *curandera* may be an eccentric—a babbling

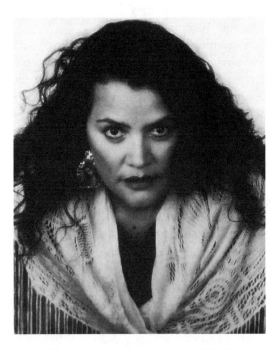

Elena Avila, curandera *and author (Jeremy P. Tarcher, Inc.)*

dispenser of love potions, Christ-crazed enchantress waving a crucifix, or suspect barbarian in a Catholic world. Sometimes called a white witch or *anciana* (old one), the practitioner accepts a divine call and sets up in the hill country or city tenement among superstitious peasants to offer a complex amalgam of herbalism, psychoanalysis, mesmerism, prayer, and magic. Her belief system, relying on the powers of faith, confession, forgiveness, and penance, may ally illness with original sin and the failings of Adam and Eve.

As God encourages balance, so does nature supply a natural cure. Thus, the *curandera*'s kit may hold ground roots; leaves of hallucinogenic plants and mushrooms; skins, fangs, and other parts of reptiles; animal bones, teeth and skulls; shells; magic stones; and the *yerba buena,* or good weed administered in teas and potions. Gregorita Rodriguez, a self-confidant *sobardora* or masseuse and acupressurist from Sante Fe, New Mexico, blends herbal cures with the laying on of hands, a time-honored method worldwide of passing positive energy into a segment of the patient's body that is blocked by negative energy.

A *curandera* survives on reputation and, consequently, must live up to community beliefs and expectations. Daily scheduling is typically informal. In the practice of Maria Sabina, a Mazatec shaman of Huautla, Oaxaca, Mexico, patients drop in as she goes about mundane home chores. A fellow practitioner in Oaxaca burns incense before pictures of the Virgin Mary and the Sacred Heart of Christ, which coexist with images derived from ancient native American folk worship.

Relying on observation, questions, and intuition, the *curandera* may summon an inborn gift for diagnosis and cleansing of body impurities. Some possess the pharmacopic knowledge bequeathed by native American forebears, who drew healing from local plants. In the late 1960s, a knowledgeable folk healer, Sabinita Herrera of Truchas, New Mexico, assisted the director of the Truchas Medical Clinic as a consultant on selecting and administering herbs.

Such folk healing, a blend of indigenous paganism with the rationalism of European medical tenets, is the central motif of Rudolfo Anaya's *Bless Me, Ultima* (1972), a classic Chicano novel. The action centers on Las Pasturas, a pastoral Indian and Spanish settlement in the post-frontier era on scrubland east of Albuquerque, New Mexico. Among *llaneros, caballeros,* and *vaqueros,* stands the vigorous, imposing figure of health—Ultima, also called "la Grande," a traditional *curandera* or folk herbalist, practical nurse, and midwife. A simply dressed peasant, Ultima carries her gunny sack and shovel up and down the riverbank in search of *la yerba del manso,* a cure for "burns, sores, piles, colic in babies, bleeding dysentery, and even rheumatism" (Anaya 1972, 37). Into a black bag tied at her waist go pinches of plant matter from oregano, a cure for coughs and fever; manzanilla, a cure for birth defects; and oshá, a panacea for contusions, coughs, colds, rheumatism, and poor digestion and a repellent for snakes. To expand her pharmacopoeia, she trades roots and herbs with patients, who pay in kind for her treatment.

In the novel, vigilantes accuse Ultima of being a *bruja* (witch). Their spite derives from a slavish adherence to Catholicism, which polarizes attitudes toward the strong, confident female healer as either a folk saint and equivalent of the Virgin of Guadalupe or a demon—the polarized clash of good against evil. The position of the *médica* (female healer) stands unevenly on a basis of superstition, folklore, and church orthodoxy as she digs healing roots, collects and dries herbs, and makes the sign of the cross over patients to lift the curse of disease. Among her other duties is a blend of witchcraft and nurse care: the formation of wax and clay dolls; burning incense and piñon wood to cleanse the air; feeding patients fresh *atole* (blue corn mush) to build strength; and bathing, purging, and sweating them with purifying concoctions to oust the death spirit. To work her spells, she sends forth an owl, the familiar who does her fearful bidding.

Because nursing in Hispanic provinces ran a close parallel to *brujería* (witchery) in colonial times, it could result in execution if practitioners breached common custom or appeared to cast the *mal ojo* (evil eye). To the question of occultism, Anaya's *curandera* explains that a wise old man gave her the owl to do good, not to thwart destiny. She proclaims her motto: "Life is never beyond hope" (Anaya 1972, 89). In a customary pagan benevolence, she blesses her grandson with goodness, strength, beauty, and a love and respect for life. In 1996, Anaya followed with *Rio Grande Fall,* a post-frontier mystery-suspense novel that reprises the motifs of witches and of the beneficent *curandera,* whose eyes look past modern-day Albuquerque to both past and future.

Unlike Anaya's Ultima, the supreme practitioner, *la curandera total,* is skilled in the whole gamut of subspecialties. According to *Nature's Healing Arts: From Folk Medicine to Modern Drugs* (1966), a publication of *National Geographic,* Tibo Chavez, an herbalist from Belen, south of Albuquerque, claims to be a descendent of Juan de Oñate, an explorer from New Spain who arrived in 1598 and was appointed first governor of New Mexico. Chavez has compiled data on his own family's specialty, particularly the manzanilla and *yerba buena* plants, and shares his stock of cures in a book on popular *remedios* and through lectures delivered at the University of New Mexico. He predicts that the era of the folk healer is coming to an end: "Our old-time *curanderos* and *curanderas*—men and women healers—are getting along in years. We've got to visit them now, and see their herbs and way of life before it's too late" (Aikman 1966, 24). To maximize his store of wisdom, he visits Mrs. Alejandro Moya, a neighboring practitioner, to swap simples and share treatments. In nearby El Cerro, Eufalia Otero dispenses decoctions of the aster family, lizard's-tail herb, and deer blood, which she recommends for heart trouble.

With the advent of modern medical practice even in remote regions, Latino populations have begun to lose their ties to *curandismo* (folk healing). Aged and discounted as relics and curiosities by the American Medical Association, these healers have fewer disciples to receive their store of folk cures and midwifery, to study the resonance between family structure and Catholicism, or to glean the woman-centered experiences of native practitioners. As personal involvement gives place to impersonal education, fewer trainees learn the patient system of neutralizing evil, which may involve a plaster likeness of Saint Gudula or Saint Teresa of Avila, palm fronds, rosaries, candles, a missal, or a small altar where the *curandera* and family members direct prayers to Jesus, Mary, or the Holy Spirit for divine intercession or a miracle.

Sources

Aikman, Lonnelle. *Nature's Healing Arts: From Folk Medicine to Modern Drugs.* Washington, D.C.: National Geographic, 1966.

Anaya, Rudolfo A. *Bless Me, Ultima.* Berkeley, Calif.: TOS Publications, 1972.

Nixon, Pat Ireland, M.D. *The Medical Story of Early Texas, 1528–1853.* Lancaster: Lancaster Press, 1946.

Pasquali, Elaine Anne. "Santeria." *Journal of Holistic Nursing* (December 1994): 380–391.

Perrone, Bobette, H. Henrietta Stockel, and Victoria Krueger. *Medicine Women, Curanderas, and Women Doctors.* Norman: University of Oklahoma Press, 1989.

Rodriguez, Raymond. "Folk Cures of My Youth Gaining Respectability." http://www.latinolink. com/opinion/opinion97/1228hi1e.htm.

Snodgrass, Mary Ellen. *Encyclopedia of Frontier Literature.* Santa Barbara, Calif.: ABC-CLIO, 1997.

Valdes, Leander J., III, Jose Luis Diaz, and Ara G. Paul. "Ethnopharmacology of Ska Maria Pastora." http://dog.net.uk/salvia.html.

Vigil, Evangelina. *Woman of Her Word: Hispanic Women Write.* Houston: Arte Publico Press, 1987.

"A Visit to the Curandera." http://www.dreamagic. com/stan/00000058.html.

"Zapata." http://ocean.st.usm.edu/~wsimkins/zapata4. html.

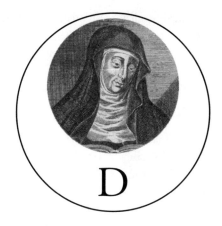

Deutsch, Naomi

A prominent nursing and social welfare activist and fellow of the American Public Health Association, Naomi Deutsch moved the East Coast public health initiatives west. Her intelligence and experience earned her a federal appointment as supervisor of the Children's Bureau, where she directed programs to preserve and bolster families in American communities and tribes. Born November 5, 1890, in Brüx, Austria, Deutsch came from a distinguished, public-spirited family that emigrated to the United States when she was a small child. She was the eldest daughter of Hermine Bacher and Dr. Gotthard Deutsch, professor of history at Hebrew Union College. Her sister, Edith Deutsch Lashmann, rose to a supervisory post of the Jewish Children's Home in Oakland, California; her brother was investigative reporter Herman Deutsch. Following training at the Cincinnati Preparatory School, Naomi Deutsch completed nurse's training in Cincinnati at the Jewish Hospital School of Nursing in 1914. Because a federal regulation denied service to nurses from hostile countries, she gave up her desire to serve in a war zone and became a public health nurse with the city's Visiting Nurse Association. Her extensive career in municipal public health took her to the Irene Kauffman

Settlement in Pittsburgh, Pennsylvania. Before tackling greater responsibilities, she completed a B.S. from Teachers' College of Columbia University.

For seven years, Deutsch joined forces with New York activist Lillian Wald as field supervisor and director at the Henry Street Visiting Nurse Service. Enlisted by the San Francisco Community Chest, in 1925 she moved to California to found and, for twelve years, direct the city's Visiting Nurse Association, a post that preceded her presidency of the California State Organization for Public Health Nursing. Simultaneous with her departmental duties, Deutsch taught public health nursing as an associate professor at the University of California at Berkeley and advised the California Department of Public Health.

Late in 1935, Catherine Lenroot, director of the federal Children's Bureau of the Department of Labor in Washington, D.C., named Deutsch director of the U.S. Public Health Department. In introducing Deutsch to the post in a letter dated October 15, Assistant Chief Martha M. Eliot stated: "I believe that such a program should be given our first attention. . . . I cannot help but believe that this pioneer work will be of greatest importance in the future of the rural nurse and that the Children's Bureau is in a strategic position to work it out with state and local health agencies and with the federal agencies that are working in the public health nursing field" (Deutsch n.d., n.p.).

Working under pediatricians Albert McCown and Robert Hood and in cooperation with Mary Irene Atkinson, director of child welfare, Deutsch managed aspects of maternal and child health and activities for crippled children. Among the agency's tasks were the study of the effects of poverty on children and publication of special health bulletins. Deutsch's office also researched infant and maternal well-being, compiled data on family income, and initiated analysis and revision of laws governing child labor, juvenile delinquency, illegitimacy, incest, foster homes, and adoption.

Sources

"Cincinnati Woman Now National Nursing Head." *Cincinnati Times Star,* January 5, 1936, 15.

Deutsch, Naomi, personal correspondence, Nursing Archives, Boston University, Massachusetts.

Dock, Lavinia, and Isabel M. Stewart. *A Short History of Nursing.* New York: G. P. Putnam's Sons, 1938.

Kalisch, Philip, and Beatrice J. Kalisch. *The Advance of American Nursing.* Boston: Little, Brown, 1978.

"Named to U.S. Post: Miss Deutsch to Head Nurses." *Oakland Chronicle,* December 15, 1935, n.p.

"Naomi Deutsch." *Pacific Coast Journal of Nursing* (September 1934): 487–488.

Disease

The history of nursing is bound to specific treatments accommodating temporal needs, which usually arise from war, natural disaster, social failing, or disease. The most devastating of diseases worldwide is smallpox, an incurable virus also known as variola. A killer of 300 million people during the twentieth century alone, smallpox accompanied wars and human migration and caused the deaths of leaders, kings, and armies. It wiped out three times the victims of war before its containment through universal vaccination.

Smallpox was a major player in the European settlement of the New World. When Spanish conquistadores carried infection to the natives of Texas, the invaders impeded European expeditions by unintentionally spreading the disease to their men. Sweeping the Atlantic coast, north to Canada, and south beyond the Amazon basin, the disease bludgeoned Amerindians, who lost some one hundred million after contact with Europeans. Brazil's Yanomami and the Iroquois of the Ohio Valley were devastated by multiple waves of infection, as were the Creek in Georgia and the Etiwan, Cherokee, and Catawba of the Carolinas; the Mandan and Assiniboin of the upper Missouri Valley were almost annihilated. Similarly doomed, the Arawak disappeared from the Caribbean, the Calusa from Cuba and Puerto Rico. The great pox killed off a third of Guatemalans and two-thirds of the Maya in Yucatan. At length, it depopulated Panama, Nicaragua, and Costa Rica. Epidemics triggered by Francisco Coronado's company in 1520 launched three centuries of devastation to Mexico; when Cabeza de Vaca settled on Galveston Island in 1528, his journals recorded treatment of subsequent infections, alternately described as smallpox and leprosy. By the nineteenth century, no tribe from the Aleutian Islands to Tierra del Fuego had been spared.

Caregivers from history are few in name and number. The work of Father Juan Larios during an epidemic at San Ildefonso south of the Rio Grande in 1674 suggests the misplaced focus of Catholic nurse care: his immediate concern was the baptism of three hundred moribund Indians. Health professionals were stymied until 1803, when an inoculation program began in Mexico. On May 20, 1804, José Antonio Cavellero, governor of Texas, issued explicit orders from the Spanish king to inoculate all: "You should set aside a hospital room in that capital, and another in each Province in your district, where the fluid will be kept fresh and communicated from arm to arm, to as many as may need it, free of charge if they are poor, the hospital staff periodically and constantly performing operations in rotation, a few at a time" (Nixon 1946, 57).

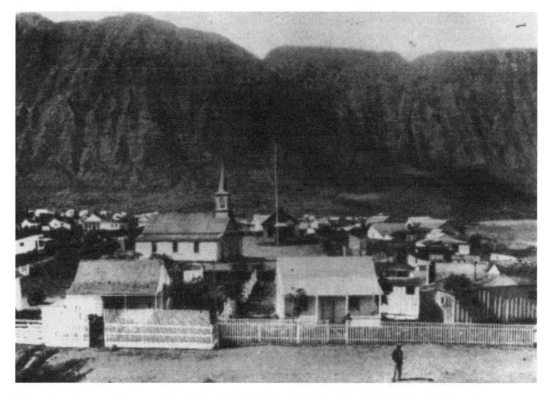

The main settlement of a leprosy colony on the island of Molokai, Hawaii, 1899 (U.S. Library of Medicine)

Within two years, the drop in cases proved the measure a godsend.

In the same year, the journal of Lewis and Clark noted the ravages of disease among tribes along the Missouri River, who lacked any method of coping with the epidemic: "The ravages of the Small Pox (which Swept off 400 men & womin & children in perpotion) has reduced this nation not exceeding 300 men. . . . I am told when this fatal malady was among them they Carried their frenzey to verry extroadinary length, not only of burning their Village, but they put their *wives* & children to *Death* with a view of their all going together to some better Countrey" (De-Voto 1953, 19). Among the Huron during the 1820s, French missionary Father Gabriel Sagard advocated quarantine, a certain containment method among those still lacking inoculation. Other tribes lessened the virulence of outbreaks by tending the sick with massage and herbs but worsened their condi-

tion with sweat baths. 15–20 percent of the unprotected died of the disease, as compared to the 2.5 percent of the inoculated who died after variolation.

A more loathsome ailment is leprosy (Hansen's disease), a virulent affliction that so filled the minds of early human ancestors that they banished the leper like a demon to some dark hole. The treatment of leprosy dates to prehistoric times in Asia, Africa, and Europe, where it decimated the populace from the eleventh to thirteenth centuries. The ancient Egyptians tended to banish victims of the "death before death" to a city of mud, a sentence less harsh than the summary execution practiced in China and India (Nikiforuk 1992, 29). Those Chinese healers who offered nostrums for leprosy suggested chaulmoogra oil, an ointment garnered from the nut of an East Indian tree. In Europe, local codes exiled the living dead with a ritual funeral mass and *separatio leprosarum* (separation of lepers). Victims had to wear long hooded gowns to conceal their lesions and avoid churches, inns and bakeries, fairs, markets, and public footpaths and drinking fountains.

The first hospital for lepers was the work of St. Basil the Great, who defied centuries of bias in 370 A.D. by founding a hospice outside Caesarea on the Mediterranean coast of Palestine. The staff, known as Knights of St. Lazarus, remained in service until 1830. A contemporary of St. Basil, Zoticus of Constantinople, was himself a victim who spent his fortune constructing a receiving center for fellow pariahs, including the daughter of the emperor Constantius. In 432 A.D., Patrick of Britain, who was revered as Ireland's patron saint, baptized sufferers and treated their lesions with his hands. St. Bridget of Ireland welcomed lepers to her hospice in Kildare. By the thirteenth century, the peak of the epidemic in Europe, most municipalities sponsored a lazer house or lazaretto, a compulsory isolation sanitarium, which offered a room and meals but little else.

Throughout Europe, the care of lepers was a long-standing charity. The first hospital, founded at York by King Aethelstan in 936, offered simple treatment. In 1101, Queen Matilda, wife of Henry I, established St. Giles's Hospital, also a standard leprosarium. In 1180, with the aid of King Henry II of England, St. Hugh of Lincoln opened his Carthusian priory in Witham, Somerset, where he personally nurtured lepers. In 1203, St. Hedwig of Bavaria built a women's convent and learning center. With her husband's help, she opened a separate hospice for female lepers at Neumarkt and supported its work until 1238. A contemporary, Fachtna of Kilcolgan, Ireland, kept a guest house for lepers until her death in 1232. About this time, the number of leprosaria in Europe had risen to nineteen thousand. In France, similar succor of lepers derived from the work of the French king, Louis IX, later called St. Louis. An educator and founder of the Sorbonne, the great Parisian university, he advocated basic nursing instruction for medical personnel and himself treated lepers with warm water, soft clothes, and healing ointments.

In 1789, John Howard, a Baptist layman, published *An Account of the Principal Lazarettos in Europe,* a summary of the rise of charity hospitals and volunteer nursing. To achieve realistic data, he sought admission at a leprosarium in Venice. Under quarantine, he noted the meager diet and abundant vermin and commented on the number of patients infected with rickettsia during their hospital stay. He deplored the low standards of hygiene at the Maltese facility, begun in the Middle Ages by the Order of St. John. From two decades of field study, Howard died in 1790 of typhus in the Ukrainian city of Kherson during the Turkish-Russian War.

In the nineteenth century, leprosy became the Christian church's cause célèbre. In San Francisco in the 1870s, church relief workers cared for Chinese immigrants, who had been left in their ghetto to die. Later in the century, Mary Reed managed a leper's colony in Chandag, India. During the reign of Kamehameha III (1825–1854), Hawaii saw its first cases of Hansen's disease, which natives called *mai pake* (Chinese disease). To stop the spread of infection among natives, lawmakers rounded up hideaways in shacks in the bush and remanded them to a receiving station at Halihi outside Honolulu. In 1873, authorities immured some eight hundred incurables and their families on a craggy peninsula on the north end of Molokai. There, Catholic missionaries and Chinese and native *kahunas* (healers) tended them using traditional herbal methods. A German nun, Barbara Cope, entered the Order of St. Francis as Mother Marianne and devoted her life to the colony. The most famous figure at the mission, Father Damien (Joseph De Veuster), fondly remembered as "the martyr of Molokai," treated exiled lepers until his death from the disease in 1889. By the mid–twentieth century, the isolation village was virtually devoid of patients because up-to-date treatments with sulfa drugs made quarantine unnecessary.

In the late twentieth century, reports from New Delhi indicated a triumph over the scourge of leprosy. India, which had more than 50 percent of the world's leprosy cases by the early 1990s, reported more than four million disfigured and suffering victims, whom the Leper Act of 1992 banned from public transportation. Since then, however, the country has applied $85 million from the World Bank and volunteer agencies to set up treatment centers and to disseminate health directives about boiling water, washing the body, and building sanitary latrines. Numbers of new cases dropped dramatically. The distribution of free antibiotics and medical care by state public health nurses, volunteers, and missionaries restored virtual pariahs to health and social acceptance.

Devastating communities throughout Asia and Europe with near instant death, the bubonic plague is unequalled as a dread stalker capable of leveling victims within hours. The Torah mentions plague in I Samuel 5–6 as a devastation of the Philistines. The disease originated with the *Yersinia pestis* (or *Pasteurella pestis*) bacterium in the Mongolian steppes and traveled on caravans to Armenia, China, and India, where natives had no immunity, then swept the Byzantine Empire in the sixth century before entering Europe and moving west to the Americas and the Pacific.

Nicknamed the "black dog" or "black death," plague is rare today and and typically strikes people who practice primitive hygiene and live in areas without basic sanitation measures. From 1346–1352, disease ravaged Europe and the eastern Mediterranean lands, costing England more than 40 percent of its population. The great European onslaught of 1348 returned as the pestis secunda in 1362 and the pestis tertia in 1369. Slow to feel the brunt of infection, Ireland was hit in 1349 and 1398.

When bubonic plague ravaged France in 1349, the Bishop of Winchester, William of Edynton, predicted the epidemic in England with a dire description: "The plague kills more viciously than a two-edged sword. Nobody dares enter any town, castle or village where it has struck. Everyone flees them in terror as they would the lair of a savage beast. There is an awful silence in such places; no merry music, no laughter. They have become dens of terror, like a wilderness" (Day 1989, 6). As soldiers returning from war infected the port of Melcombe Regis near Weymouth, early symptoms marked victims with sweating, vomiting and coughing up blood, aching limbs and head, dizziness, and sleeplessness. Diarrhea preceded delirium and hysteria, buboes or swellings of the groin and armpit, and black patches, from which derives the term "black death." In Paris in 1349, daily reports of 800 topped 500 in Pisa and 600 in Vienna. By the end of the outbreak, half of the population of Paris had died; Florence lost over 60 percent of its citizens; Venice, Hamburg, and Bremen estimated 66 percent.

The disease was so rapid in development that an attendant might sicken and die before the patient. Doctors warned the healthy: fuge cito, vade longe, rede tarde [go quickly, travel far, return slowly] (Nikiforuk 1992, 56). The profession hardest hit by mortal illness was the ministry, who remained behind to serve the sick. Monks and priests who opened monasteries to victims soon died out in record numbers, devastating both the pesthouses they visited and their own religious orders. In Montpellier, France, during the fourteenth century, 5 percent of Dominicans survived; in a Marseilles monastery, all died. England's clergy lost 50 percent; Germany's, 35 percent.

In response to panic, municipal leaders closed quarters that were hardest hit and assigned the healthy to care for the dying. Doctors treated by theory, thus keeping their distance from the hovels of the poor, who died in massive numbers. Without trained nurse care, people relied on prayer, relics, herbal concoctions, talismans, and astrology. Limited practical treatment administered by relatives or servants included lancing buboes, cauterizing wounds, purging, bleeding, and applying hot packs and mustard plasters. A few benevolent houses experienced a resurgence during the epidemic, notably the Sisterhood of the Common Life, Poor Clares, Béguines, and the Alexian Brothers, an order dating to 1348 and named for fifth-century nurse St. Alexis. Nursing nuns who moved from house to house to measure dosages and offer broth unwittingly carried contagions with them on their aprons and the sleeves and hems of voluminous habits.

The few medical workers, herbalists, and apothecaries to treat plague victims gave no thought to the real causes of disease—overcrowding, poor diet, open cesspools, or thatched roofs infested with rats. Traders continued to ply the Mediterranean and Black seas, bearing the plague to port cities in Africa, Europe, and eastern Asia. Survivors bore the brunt of a decimated populace and doubted the worth of priests and doctors. It wasn't until 1894 that French and Japanese researchers identified *Yersinia pestis* as the bacterium at fault.

Numerous Christian missions centered on plague relief, notably, St. Roch (Rock) of Montpellier, France, who focused his care on the plague victims of Piacenza, Italy, around 1368 and continued his work in Cesaria, Mantua, Parma, and Aquapendente. In the early 1500s, St. Jerome Emiliani attempted to relieve children orphaned when the plague swept Venice. Like other selfless nurses, he caught the disease, but he recovered, acquiring the immunity that multiplied his effectiveness. He remained true to the cause by establishing a hospital at Verona in 1518. St. Jerome became the rare individual reinfected by plague, which killed him in 1537. Another possible explanation is that his first infection was misdiagnosed.

The mission to comfort plague victims continued around 1538 with the charity of St. John of God, a former Portuguese mercenary. He set up treatment centers for poor plague victims in Granada, Spain, the nucleus of the Brothers Hospitallers' Order. His concepts of isolation and individualized care soon influenced treatment in Madrid, Cordova, Toledo,

Paris, and Naples and, beginning in 1602, Central and South America. St. Aloysius Gonzaga, a Jesuit healer of Castiglione, Italy, treated plague victims in the 1591 epidemic of Rome until his death from the disease. St. Martin de Porres of Lima, Peru, a Dominican friar, studied medicine with a barber-surgeon and applied his skill to the city's black and mulatto poor, who suffered alone and unattended during an epidemic around 1600. A contemporary, St. Joan de Lestonnac of Bordeaux, France, organized a cadre of young nurses to succor victims of epidemics.

In 1722, fifty-six years after the Great Plague of London, English journalist Daniel Defoe produced *A Journal of the Plague Year,* a report on the misery of poverty and sickness and the luck of those who survived. Treatment of buboes in the groin, underarms, and throat was itself a torment: "The swellings in some grew hard, and they applied violent drawing-plaisters or poultices to break them, and if these did not do they cut and scarified them in a terrible manner" (Defoe 1960, 86). Opening the buboes was a must for survival. For severely hardened tumors, cautery supplanted the lance. During painful ministrations, those patients still able to flee wrenched themselves from their caretakers and fled raving into the streets, some into rivers and wells.

Annoyed by the frenzy that sent "people in running after quacks and mountebanks, wizards, and fortune-tellers . . . even to madness," Defoe chastised physicians who offered no humane consultation and who left the suffering to the devices of mercenaries (Defoe 1960, 42). In defense of the attendants who braved contagion, he noted high numbers of nurses who died from contagion and the hardships of surviving caregivers under the Lord Mayor's stringent caution: "If any nurse-keeper shall remove herself out of any infected house before twenty-eight days after the decease of any person dying of the infection, the house to which the said nurse-keeper doth so remove herself shall be shut up until the said twenty-eight days be expired" (Defoe 1960, 47).

During sequestration, laws required attendants to air bedding and curtains and have the chamber fired or blasted with gunpowder, then sweetened with incense, rosemary, benjamin or benzoin, and rosin or purified with sulfur. No items could be sold or removed from the infected home. To ensure that the citizenry observed regulations, the constable hired watchers and searchers, who snooped into alleys and carriages and supervised the filling of a six-foot pit with the dead.

A frequent but less terrifying plague on the peoples of the Mediterranean and Asia is trachoma, a sight-threatening and disfiguring eye disease. Because it maims and blinds but does not spread from human contact, it is not listed with leprosy, favus (a contagious skin disease caused by a fungus), bubonic plague, and syphilis as universally loathsome. Under the influence of U.S. social reformer Lillian Wald, early twentieth-century school nurses and agents dispatched members of the Metropolitan Visiting Nurse bureau to counter threats to eyesight. Among New York schools, nurses found trachoma in mild to advanced stages of infection in 20 percent of students they examined. Home visits helped contain the disease and aid those already infected. Workers made inroads against suspicion by reminding parents that children who were deformed by eye inflammation or who couldn't focus on work were unemployable.

Religious workers continue to combat the disease in foreign mission fields, where granulations and scarred lids precede impaired vision and blindness. Under the auspices of Hadassah, a Jewish women's Zionist society founded by Henrietta Szold, in the mid-1900s Rose Kaplan, a reformer from Petrograd, Russia, set up a nurses' settlement in Jerusalem and carried her work in Jewish refugee camps as far south as Alexandria, Egypt, where she treated skin disease and trachoma among children.

A recurrent pestilence, yellow fever terrified medical communities in the centuries preceding an understanding of how the *Aedes aegypti* mosquito spreads the germ. In August 1793,

Philadelphia began counting deaths with 140, which rose to 1,400 in September. By the end of the epidemic, 4,044 known victims of the city's 55,000 citizens had succumbed to an agonizing course of vomiting, diarrhea, and hemorrhaging. In all, the infection struck 10 percent of the population. Because of its spread among French refugees from Haiti, Philadelphians, feeling morally superior to new arrivals from the Caribbean, charged that it was a disease of the immoral. When it claimed German immigrants, xenophobic natives dubbed it "Palatine fever" (Kraut 1994, 26). Exacerbating the treatment and care of patients was the loathsome smell that accompanied body effluvia and the immediate putrefaction of corpses, along with the burning of tar in the streets and the sprinkling of vinegar and aromatic sprigs of artemisia, commonly called wormwood.

After the wealthy deserted the city for safer climes, services to the remaining citizenry broke down at an appalling rate. The municipal coterie known as Overseers and Guardians of the Poor took charge of the almshouse on Spruce Street, hiring nurses, cooks, carters, and burial crews when workers could be found to take the jobs. The breakdown of the economy forced an increasing load of paupers on the city. A notable act of benevolence came from female convicts, who gave up their beds and linens to the sick. Most caregivers were black attendants. Under the governance of ex-slaves Absalom Jones and Richard Allen, they went from door to door checking on inhabitants, sometimes finding infants and children alone with the rotting corpses of their parents. Notables among visiting nurses were three famous blacks—Mary Scott and Sarah Bass, whom chroniclers commended for refusing to charge exorbitant rates, and Caesar Cranchal, who worked for free and died on the job. Aiding Dr. Benjamin Rush, the major medical agent of Philadelphia, were five of his pupils, who assisted with bedside care until they died from yellow fever.

Upon the failure of Ricketts's circus as a warehouse for the dying, city fathers opened a temporary lazaretto, or pest house, at Bush Hill, a prestigious address to the north of the city limits relegated to the nurse care of indigent scourge victims. Supervised by Stephen Girard and Peter Helm, the hospital staff worked under serious privation. Without water, convalescent wards, morgue, or coffins, they attended 807 patients in every space in the house, leaving none for staff residence. Carters placed new arrivals in a hole in the ground until caregivers could receive them. At a killing pace, matrons separated the dying from the sick and men from women until the house physician, Dr. Jean Devèze, could treat them. Three of the nineteen nurses were stricken; only Mary Saville, the head matron, recovered. Staff members were thereafter universally shunned as though they bore a dire infection.

Outbreaks of fever plagued other communities with sporadic menace. In Memphis, Tennessee, in late summer 1878, Annie Cook turned her sumptuous bordello, Mansion House, into a clinic. Her employees volunteered to nurse victims. After Cook died of the fever September 12, citizens lauded the unselfishness of a "Nineteenth Century Mary Magdalene" (Sherr and Kazickas 1994, 426). When yellow fever was finally defeated during the Spanish-American War, it was nurse Jane Delano, head of the Army Nurse Corps, who recognized the danger of infection by mosquito bite. A modest heroine, nurse Clara Louise Maass of East Orange, New Jersey, went to Cuba to assist in containing contagion. In March 1901, she joined nineteen human guinea pigs who volunteered to be bitten by mosquitoes. After six months of exposure and several bites on her hand, she died August 24, the only American volunteer to succumb during the project. Her body was exhumed and buried in Newark. Leopoldine Guinther located donors to a erect a pink granite monument honoring Maass's martyrdom. A stained-glass window in the United Methodist Church of Wayne, New Jersey, notes that Maass willingly sacrificed herself to quell the disease.

The spread of poliomyelitis, the virus responsible for infantile paralysis, is a more recent world terror. In 1907, when it plagued New York City, rapid infection swamped nursing referral agencies as it killed twenty-five hundred victims. By 1914, when Simon Flexner and Hideyo Noguchi identified the virus, it had spread across the country, infecting thirty thousand and killing five thousand.

In 1916, an epidemic in New York terrified people to such extremes that they nailed shut their windows and stuffed crevices with rags to prevent the virus from entering residences. People who could afford flight sent fifty thousand children from the city. As agents of the board of health, nurses persuaded parents to send infected children to hospital isolation wards, where early care might lessen crippling and death. In huge wards housing rows of iron lungs, attendants treated, fed, exercised, and encouraged victims whose breathing was affected by viral infection.

Within two years, polio again targeted children of the East Coast. Public health nurses in tenements faced a stone wall of distrust among Italian immigrants, who suffered the highest number of cases. Immigrants lumped nurses among the faceless ethnocentric authority figures who dominated their lives. Ghetto dwellers returned the slight by accusing staff nurses of marginalizing foreigners. Nurses distributing leaflets from the Department of Social Betterment of the Brooklyn Bureau of Charities and requiring quarantine in crowded tenements met with family enmity. After limiting public festivals, block parties, and public play, health agents were labeled busybodies and gossips for invoking public policy against contagion and for spreading the word that the poor were dirty and vermin-ridden.

In the South in 1944, as the rest of the nation fought World War II, residents of Hickory, North Carolina, battled polio. Ruth Council, state consultant on orthopedic nursing, alerted the Red Cross. Immediately, nurses from all parts of the country arrived and found temporary housing. Organized in shifts, they worked through the summer at such tasks as operating iron lungs by hand crank when a storm knocked out power. Nursing superintendent Ethel M. Greathouse from Louisville, Kentucky, organized a phalanx from Virginia, Mississippi, Florida, Louisiana, South Carolina, Illinois, Wisconsin, and Pennsylvania. Together, the staff created the "Miracle of Hickory," a consolidated effort of doctors, nurses, therapists, and volunteers to treat patients at a fresh air camp west of the city on the Catawba River. According to Alice E. Sink's *The Grit behind the Miracle* (1998), in nine months of operation, the camp lost only twelve of its 454 patients.

When the disease struck the western states, polio emergency volunteers (PEVs) in Ogden, Utah, relieved the strain on hospital staff by reading books to iron lung patients, feeding them to monitor proper swallowing, changing beds and diapers, and distributing comic books and toys. At St. Benedict and Dee hospitals, nurses trained helpers in hygiene to relieve the dread of contracting the poliomyelitis virus. Staff taught aides to make hot packs and apply simple therapy to atrophied limbs, the concept promoted by Sister Elizabeth Kenny, the Australian nurse who fled ridicule at home and found the first audience for her ideas in Minnesota.

When church bells rang in celebration of the Salk vaccine on April 12, 1955, thousands of volunteer workers for the March of Dimes rejoiced at the potential eradication of one of humankind's most insidious viruses. Unifying Americans as firmly as war, the fight against poliomyelitis had required the combined efforts of doctors, nurses, physical therapists, and public health workers to combat a disease that in 1952, a peak year, struck fifty-eight thousand, killing three thousand and paralyzing twenty-one thousand.

On December 6, 1998, nurse Madhu Kanta Vyas joined the World Health Organization (WHO) drive to eradicate polio from the planet by the year 2000. Among 2.6 million health workers, she carried vaccine to Salar, an isolated village in Rajasthan in north-western India, to inoculate 120 children. By the end of the campaign, WHO had treated 136 million children, topping the agency goal by ten million.

Although less spectacular than plague, polio, smallpox, and leprosy, the prime killer in Europe during the eighteenth and nineteenth centuries was tuberculosis, an ancient plague. Its telltale disfigurement is evident in Egyptian mummies; description of its wasting and shriveling of tissue colors the writings of Hippocrates in early fourth-century Greece. In the fifth century, France's King Clovis claimed to cure the scrofulous form of tuberculosis by a royal touch. The combined efforts of René Théophile Hyacinthe Laënnec, Jean-Nicolas Corvisart des Marets, and Gaspard Laurent Bayle began the long process of narrowing potential causes. Jean Antoine Villemin and Robert Koch concluded the job by 1882.

So many people fell victim to infection by tuberculosis in the nineteenth century that it earned the name "great white plague." With its long, convoluted history, it drew the consumptive artist and poet into dark rhapsodies that produced the graveyard school of art. Notable victims include poets John Keats, Percy Shelley, and Elizabeth Barrett Browning; composers Frederic Chopin and Niccolò Paganini; and writers Honoré de Balzac, the Brontë sisters, Robert Louis Stevenson, Friedrich Schiller, Anton Chekhov, and Franz Kafka. The destructive power of *Mycobacterium tuberculosis* carried off lepers, the Bantu of Africa, and victims of the Irish potato famine and reduced New Zealand's Maori by 22 percent. On the Great Plains, consumption ravaged the Sioux and Cree. Late in the twentieth century, new strains continue to decimate acquired immunodeficiency syndrome (AIDS) victims, smokers, and alcoholics.

Domestic treatment of tuberculosis in the nineteenth century followed the wrong protocols. Patients, usually cared for at home, lay among a heap of pillows in close, airtight confinement and picked at rich soups and soufflés. Europe launched the sanatorium in the early 1900s as a haven of rest, pure diet, and clean air in such welcoming climes as the Black Forest, Provence, and Swiss Alps. Pervasively understaffed, these tuberculosis hospitals thrived on the moneyed class and treated them to rigidly scrubbed cubicles devoid of wallpaper, molding, and window ledges. Although Europe made inroads against tuberculosis, it continued to thrive across Malaysia and in Hong Kong, Mexico City, and São Paulo.

Also virulent in Canada, the disease compounded the ills of immigrant populations. Toronto's first source of relief came from the House of Providence, a charitable hospice opened by the Sisters of St. Joseph in 1856. It was 1901 before Canada's municipal hospitals began receiving consumptives. In 1906, Toronto acquired the services of Christina Mitchell, a veteran of the New York City Missions and Canada's first tuberculosis nurse. With tact and skill, she allied the nursing staffs of Toronto Nursing Mission and City Mission along with the Young Men's Christian Association (YMCA), the Young Women's Christian Association (YWCA), and deaconesses of the Anglican, Methodist, and Presbyterian churches in support of city clinics.

Three early twentieth-century innovators—Dr. Edward Otis of Tufts University, Ellen La Motte, nurse-in-chief of the Tuberculosis Division for Baltimore's health department, and Jane Delano, founder of the Red Cross nursing unit—advocated hospital care as a means of control and supervision. Nurses simplified surroundings to limited furnishings, rugs, and drapes and opened rooms to sunshine and fresh air. Linens were sanitized to prevent spread of contagion to visiting family members. The nurse became the patient lifeline to quality care. A rigid schedule of temperature records, rest, moderate exercise, and tempting diet rich in eggs, milk, and meat restored patients to health. The required discipline raised the status of visiting nurses, who served as the doctor's eyes and ears. These turn-of-the-century improvements resulted in two useful texts: La Motte's *The Tuberculosis Nurse* (1915) and Delano's *American Red Cross Textbook on Home Hygiene and Care of the Sick* (1918).

No disease treatment and prevention program has so affected the spread of consumption as has the visiting nurse. After Dr. Robert Koch outlined the nature and communication of the tuberculosis bacillus in 1882, the responsibility of teaching people the value of cleanliness, pure water, fresh air, and rest fell upon visiting agents, the medical lifeline to the poor. In crowded, foul tenements, nurses combated the social problems of disease-ridden residences and large families living in few rooms. The first tuberculosis nurse was an unpaid student of Dr. William Osler of Johns Hopkins Medical School; the first paid staff position was filled in 1903 by Reiba Thelin. Extolled as a savior, she searched out Baltimore's most advanced cases, spread the doctrine of good health, and reported home conditions to relief agencies.

Supported in her work and frequently examined for signs of infection, Thelin overcame an initial discouragement and kept detailed notes of her observations. To her credit, she instilled in apathetic slum dwellers the importance of hygiene and prevention and offered the hope that others might avoid the disease that stalked their families. At the end of the first year, she resigned to join Lillian Wald's Henry Street Settlement. A replacement, Nora Holman, profited from the fervor of Osler's wife, who solicited $1 from every Baltimore citizen to fund the fight against tuberculosis. By 1910, the city's board of health took over the task of education and prophylaxis and appointed Ellen La Motte as superintendent of visiting tuberculosis nurses. With the founding of the National Association for the Study and Prevention of Tuberculosis in 1904, other cities evolved their own dispensaries.

The late twentieth century has its own "black dogs" in AIDS and Ebola. Rumors of a "gay cancer" began spreading in 1979 as a disastrous and complex disease or family of diseases struck predominantly among young male homosexuals and bisexuals. In due course, it left the New World and spread to Uganda, Japan, Brazil, Haiti, Australia, and Holland. After the Center for Disease Control in Atlanta traced infection to "Patient Zero," Gaetan Dugas, a young French-Canadian flight attendant for Air Canada linked to 150 sex partners, medical researchers sorted out a picture of infection via indiscriminate and unprotected anal intercourse. With the official naming of the virus in 1983 by Drs. Françoise Barre-Sinoussi and Luc Montagnier of the Pasteur Institute in Paris, medical theorists were still trying to explain the clues that linked medical workers in Zaire, blood transfusion, Haitians, hemophiliacs, drug use, and gays.

The misery of AIDS and the menace of its transmission to a million people under the age of fifty changed the treatment of patients in all phases of care worldwide. Along with dental hygienists, ambulance attendants, physicians, and surgeons, nurses were forced to separate themselves from their charges through the ever-present rubber glove and other artificial barriers that limit hands-on contact. According to Jeanne Parker Martin, R.N., cited in *The Person with AIDS: Nursing Perspectives,* the hospice nurse has become overall case manager who coordinates a care plan and offers housekeeping advice on disposables and impermeable containers. Diverse and complex patient needs caused by infection and neurological change require sophisticated monitoring. As the level of function declines, visiting nurses offer twenty-four-hour assistance, infection control, and bereavement counseling.

In *Borrowed Time* (1988), author and poet Paul Monette's multiple-award-winning testimony on the terror and isolation of AIDS patients, first-person accounts of treatment focus on clinical and home nursing. The quandary of collapsing human systems and exploding veins is prominent in his text, along with the high price of regular nurse visits after his family used up their insurance coverage. To ease the crisis of finding a vein that had not collapsed where an intravenous line could

be inserted, his mate, Roger Horwitz, submitted to chest catheterization. Monette recalls, "Charlene, one of our regular nurses, showed me the elaborate protocol for cleaning a port before inserting a needle. Six swabs with alcohol, six with Betadine, using a circular motion with each swab" (Monette 1988, 294). The alliance of family, neighbors, AIDS volunteers, hospice workers, and nursing staff became the life support necessary to people like Monette, who was unfamiliar with strenuous anticontagion procedures. By the end of his life, he had lost two mates to AIDS and himself died of the disease.

A contemporary heroine, Helen Miramontes, veteran critical care nurse, is a widowed mother of six, two of whom are gay men. One was diagnosed with AIDS in 1991. While working as critical care nurse at Kaiser Permanente in Santa Clara, California, she treated AIDS victims and became an activist on their behalf. As president of the California Nurses Association in the mid-1980s, she pressed for public sanitation measures and preventive education. For her work with patients with human immunodeficiency virus (HIV), mothers' groups, lobbying, and volunteering, Miramontes received the 1992 Pearl McIver Public Health Nurse Award for humanitarian involvement.

Miramontes's nursing career has covered a number of significant roles in practice, teaching, and advocacy. After entering the nursing department of the University of California at San Francisco, she served as nurse coordinator of Pacific AIDS education. In addition to a position on the Presidential Council on HIV/AIDS, Miramontes, Dr. Bernard Hirschel of Geneva, Switzerland, and activist José Zuniga are among fifty health advocates who have volunteered for the Phase III clinical trials of an HIV vaccine. Supported by President Bill Clinton and the International Association of Physicians in AIDS Care in Chicago, the experimental immunization derives from mutated virus, a product of the research of Dr. Ronald Desrosiers, a microbiologist at Harvard Medical School's New

England Primate Center. He pegs his hopes on the missing Nef gene in a dozen Australian men who have withstood infection by HIV. By replicating the conditions that have spared the few, he hopes to provide protection for the masses.

In reference to her consent to serve as a human test case, Miramontes stated, "This epidemic is very real and very personal for me. It always has been. I'm not a martyr. I'm just very, very committed to doing this work. Somebody has to take risks" (Sponselli, http://www.nurseweek,com). Although the death rate was decreasing by the late 1990s, she stressed the rise of infections among urban and minority adolescents, forty thousand of whom are infected annually. In her estimation, the development of an AIDS vaccine is the moral responsibility of the United States, even though 90 percent of infections occur in other countries.

To stem the spread of AIDS throughout the world, civil and medical authorities have engineered needle exchanges, distributed free condoms, and opened clinics for infected expectant mothers. According to Karen Codling, nutrition project officer for the United Nations International Children's Emergency Fund (UNICEF) in Bangkok, Thailand, the Thai Ministry of Health provides HIV-positive mothers with infant formula to halt breast-feeding, an intimate contact known to spread infection in 16 percent of incidence in infants. Hospital nurses are the local agents who dispense some nine hundred tins of formula mix per month to 2 percent of new mothers infected with the disease before they leave the maternity ward.

As AIDS was beginning to respond to a regular cocktail of drugs aimed at slowing its progress in the late twentieth century, a new terror burst on the scene. According to a report in *Newsweek* in May 1995, Ebola, an insidious filovirus, had struck a man in Kikwit, Zaire, in April, quickly causing blood to flow from every body orifice. Within four days, he died, his internal organs nearly liquefied. A nun and a nurse who treated him contracted the disease, spreading infection to three more nuns. The Geneva-based World Health Organization dispatched virus specialists, microbiologists, and researchers by transport planes as the military tried to curb flight from the abandoned hospital. When Ebola had run its course, it had killed 316 in southern Zaire with a mortality rate of 77 percent. The source of the disease remains a mystery.

See also: Christian Nursing; Communism, Nursing under; Kenny, Elizabeth; Medieval and Early Renaissance Nursing; Revolutionary War; Spanish-American War; Wald, Lillian D.

Sources

Amstey, Marvin S., M.D. "The Political History of Syphilis and Its Application to the AIDS Epidemic." *Women's Health Issues* (spring 1994): 16–19.

Baly, Monica E. *Nursing and Social Change.* New York: Routledge, 1995.

Bentley, James. *A Calendar of Saints.* London: Little, Brown, 1993.

Brainard, Annie M. *The Evolution of Public Health Nursing.* Philadelphia: W. B. Saunders, 1922.

Clement, J., ed. *Noble Deeds of American Women with Biographical Sketches of Some of the More Prominent.* Williamstown, Mass.: Corner House, 1975.

Cohn-Sherbok, Lavinia. *Who's Who in Christianity.* Chicago: Routledge, 1998.

Cole, Wendy. "None but the Brave." *Time,* October 6, 1997, http://www.pathfinder.com/time/magazine/1997/dom/97001/science.none_but_the_.html.

Collins, Huntly. "Mission for the Millennium: Choke Out Remains of Polio." *Charlotte Observer,* March 14, 1999, 1A, 10A.

Constable, Pamela. "India Making Big Gains in Battle against Leprosy." *Charlotte Observer,* October 4, 1998, 28A.

Day, A. Grove. *Hawaii and Its People.* New York: Duell, Sloan and Pearce, 1960.

Day, James. *The Black Death.* New York: Bookwright Press, 1989.

Defoe, Daniel. *A Journal of the Plague Year.* New York: New American Library, 1960.

DeVoto, Bernard, ed. *The Journals of Lewis and Clark.* Boston: Houghton Mifflin, 1953.

Dolan, Josephine A., R.N. *History of Nursing.* Philadelphia: W. B. Saunders, 1968.

Durham, Jerry D., and Felissa L. Cohen, eds. *The Person with AIDS: Nursing Perspectives.* New York: Springer, 1987.

Ginsburg, Ann M., M.D. "The Tuberculosis Epidemic." *Public Health* (March-April 1998).

Griffin, Gerald Joseph, and H. Joann King Griffin. *Jensen's History and Trends of Professional Nursing.* Saint Louis, Mo.: C. V. Mosby, 1965.

Grmek, Mirko D. *History of AIDS: Emergence and Origin of a Modern Pandemic.* Princeton, N.J.: Princeton University Press, 1990.

Hallam, Elizabeth, general ed. *Saints: Who They Are and How They Help You.* New York: Simon and Schuster, 1994.

Hyman, Paula, and Deborah Dash Moore. *Jewish Women in America.* New York: Routledge, Chapman and Hall, 1997.

Jamieson, Elizabeth, and Mary F. Sewall. *Trends in Nursing History.* London: W. B. Saunders, 1949.

Kraut, Alan. *Silent Travelers: Germs, Genes, and the "Immigrant Menace."* New York: Basic Books, 1994.

Kuykendall, Ralph S., and A. Grove Day. *Hawaii, a History.* Englewood Cliffs, N.J.: Prentice-Hall, 1961.

La Motte, Ellen N. *The Tuberculosis Nurse.* 1915. New York: Garland, 1985.

Lee, Gerard A. *Leper Hospitals in Medieval Ireland.* Dublin: Four Courts Press, 1996.

Lee, W. Storrs. *The Islands.* New York: Holt, Rinehart, and Winston, 1966.

McCain, Nancy L., and David F. Cella. "Correlates of Stress in HIV Disease." *Western Journal of Nursing Research* (April 1995): 141–155.

McNeill, William. *Plagues and People.* New York: Anchor Books, 1977.

Miramontes, Helen, telephone interview, June 12, 1998.

Monette, Paul. *Borrowed Time: An AIDS Memoir.* New York: Avon Books, 1988.

Murray, James P. *Galway: A Medico-Social History.* Galway: Kenny's Bookshop and Art Galleries, n.d.

Nikiforuk, Andrew. *The Fourth Horseman: A Short History of Epidemics, Plagues, Famine and Other Scourges.* Toronto: Penguin, 1992.

Nixon, Pat Ireland, M.D. *The Medical Story of Early Texas, 1528–1853.* San Antonio: Mollie Bennett Lupe Memorial Fund, 1946.

Oldstone, Michael B. A. *Viruses, Plagues, and History.* New York: Oxford University Press, 1998.

Ott, Katherine. *Fevered Lives: Tuberculosis in American Culture since 1870.* Cambridge, Mass.: Harvard University Press, 1996.

Powell, J. H. *Bring Out Your Dead: The Great Plague of Yellow Fever in Philadelphia in 1793.* New York: Time, 1965.

Royce, Marion. *Eunice Dyke, Health Care Pioneer.* Toronto: Dundurn Press, 1983.

Sherr, Lynn, and Jurate Kazickas. *Susan B. Anthony Slept Here: A Guide to American Women's Landmarks.* New York: Times Books, 1994.

Sink, Alice E. *The Grit behind the Miracle.* Lanham, Md.: University Press of America, 1998.

Sponselli, Christina. "Vaccine Volunteer." http://www.nurseweek.com/features/97-11/miramontes.html.

Thucydides. *The Peloponnesian Wars.* New York: Washington Square Press, 1963.

Tuchman, Barbara W. *A Distant Mirror: The Calamitous 14th Century.* New York: Alfred A. Knopf, 1978.

Watanabe, Myrna E. "Science, Policy Issues Put AIDS Vaccine on Slow Track." *The Scientist,* November 10, 1997, 1, 4–5.

Zinsser, Hans. *Rats, Lice and History.* New York: Black Dog and Leventhal Pubs., 1963.

Dix, Dorothea

Appointed in 1861 to superintend female nurses by Secretary of War Simon Cameron, Dorothea Lynde Dix, with the assistance of agent James E. Yeatman, headed some six thousand members of the United States Sanitary Commission (the forerunner of the American Red Cross). A determined, no-nonsense woman with a knot of hair wound neatly at the back of her head, she impressed author Louisa May Alcott as "a kind old soul, but very queer, fussy and arbitrary, no one likes her and I don't wonder" (Saxton 1977, 256). Dix recruited and interviewed, managed linens at Seminary Hospital, and, after a killing pace at her office, performed night duty dressing wounds. She later established a reputation for advancing the role of women in nursing and for upgrading prisons, almshouses, and mental asylums. A noted author, she produced diaries, memoirs, and journals of daily work directing and supplying Union hospitals and observations of prisons and mental institutions. Her work is invaluable to historians surveying nineteenth-century medical advancement.

Born into abysmal poverty in 1802 in Hampden, Maine, Dix was the child of Mary and Joseph Dix but lived with her grandmother in Boston. At age fourteen she opened a barn school for poor children. Her book *The Science of Common Things* was a popular handbook that passed through sixty editions.

As governess to the family of Dr. W. E. Channing, she first saw misery in St. Croix, Virgin Islands, where she encountered slaves working sugar plantations. Her observations preceded another influential work, *Prisons and Prison Discipline* (1845), derived from a tour of jails in the Virgin Islands, Scotland, Japan, Italy, and Sable Island, Nova Scotia.

Dix's surges of social activism ruined her health. While taking a rest cure in 1841, she kept at her mission by visiting the almshouses and jails of Massachusetts and petitioning the legislature for better care of the insane, who were incarcerated along with criminals. To arouse the public, she described similar conditions in Rhode Island, New Jersey, Pennsylvania, Indiana, Illinois, Kentucky, Tennessee, Missouri, Mississippi, Louisiana, Alabama, the Carolinas, and Maryland. In Halifax, Nova Scotia, and St. John, New Brunswick, she established up-to-date asylums but was less successful in New England after President Franklin Pierce vetoed her request for land. She learned of rescues off Sable Island after she paid for lifeboats and equipment to aid swimmers and boaters. Her petitions for social and medical reform went to notable addresses, including the English Parliament and Pope Pius IX.

The Civil War curtailed Dix's campaign to upgrade social institutions and concentrated her efforts on hospitals, nurse care, and rehabilitation. At the beginning of combat on April 12, 1861, the U.S. Medical Bureau lacked ambulance service, supply distribution channels, inspection regimens, and a nurse corps. The proposed women's nurse corps passed to President Abraham Lincoln for signature on June 1, 1861. His doubts about the efficacy of an all-female cadre of health professionals kept the concept in limbo until June 13, when he grudgingly okayed it, instituting the United States Sanitary Commission. On August 3, Congress placed nursing salaries at $12 a month, a 50 percent increase from Revolutionary War–era salaries.

Dubbed "Dragon Dix," she immediately began recruiting, publishing a circular of re-quirements, accruing recommendations, and interviewing candidates, who entered training for one hundred nurses at a time under Dr. Elizabeth Blackwell at Bellevue and New York Hospitals (Gollaher 1995, 412). Requirements for nurses included vigor, good grooming, character, sobriety, and self-discipline. Specific to the point of rudeness, Dix, who set the example of the straight-arrow, immaculate professional, announced her standards of homeliness and female submission. She declared: "All nurses are required to be plain looking women. Their dresses must be brown or black, with no bows, no curls, no jewelry, and no hoop-skirts" (Gollaher 1995, 410). For assurance of character, she required testimony of two male physicians and two clergymen. To remove the taint of promiscuity and to maintain proprieties for women in camps filled with young, lusty men, age range for nurses fell between thirty and forty-five. Two applicants whom Dix rejected as too young for the job—Cornelia Hancock and Maria Hall—found posts without authorization, Hall in several hospitals and Hancock at the battles of Wilderness and Gettysburg. Hancock privately evaluated Dix as "a self-sealing can of horror tied up with red tape" (Gollaher 1995, 413).

Under orders, Dix handpicked battlefield nurses, preferring secular staff to convent nuns. Her protégés pledged oaths of allegiance, received passes to ride government ambulances, and reported for service at commission headquarters at 14th and New York Avenues, Washington, D.C. At first, she quartered them at Columbia College Hospital in Meridian Heights. The establishment of Dix's female nurse corps unleashed the cynicism of male military and medical staff, who enjoyed opportunities for belittling and sniping. According to Jane Stuart Woolsey, author of *Hospital Days* (1870): "Was the system of women's nurses in hospitals a failure? There never was any system. That the presence of hundreds of individual women as nurses in hospitals was neither an intrusion nor a blunder, let the multitude of their unsystematized labor and achievements testify" (Austin 1971, 113). One sneering patriarch, Dr. John H. Brinton at Mound City Hospital in Illinois, chided the women for expecting room, bed, mirror, meals, and servants while they appeased their patriotic urges. In *The Personal Memoirs of John H. Brinton,* he concluded, "This female nurse business was a great trial to all the men concerned, and to me at Mound City became intolerable" (Austin 1971, 114).

Clouded by negativism, Dix's work remained unappreciated by apathetic officials until after the First Battle of Bull Run on July 21, 1861, when the initial influx of wounded from Virginia to Washington, D.C., demonstrated the seriousness of the rebellion. Immediately, she commandeered taverns, schools, churches, warehouses, and residences to receive casualties. Her flurry of telegrams and memos provoked George Templeton Strong, treasurer of the Sanitary Commission, to grouse: "Miss Dix has plagued us a little. She is energetic, benevolent, unselfish, and a mild case of monomania. Working on her own hook, she does good, but no one can cooperate with her, for she belongs to the class of comets and can be subdued into relations with no system whatever" (Gollaher 1995, 409). As newspaper accounts of the toll of wounded inspired more women to serve, Dix faced hundreds of eager volunteers—too many to examine, interview, and qualify for service.

The war was not kind to Dix. She worked from dawn until nearly 11:00 P.M., primarily corresponding with people who could benefit the war effort. Her weight dropped from 139 pounds to less than 100; her face was drawn and energy sapped by the war's mounting size and ferocity. Lacking experience in management, she lost control of her office, substituting zeal for proficiency. Gradually, ill-prepared nurses took jobs outside Dix's idealistic plan of action, filling staffs with people unfit for military rigor. After supervising the return of wounded men and nurses to their homes, she resigned on September 1, 1866, but remained at the forefront of fund-raising for an obelisk at Fortress Monroe in Hampton, Virginia, to commemorate the Union dead.

For the remainder of her career, Dix, in her mid-sixties, returned to the campaign against inhumane treatment of the insane and to the rebuilding of her own stamina. In 1870, a physician at Central Ohio Lunatic Asylum diagnosed her ailments as a combination of malaria, bronchitis, arterial disease, and rheumatic neuralgia. Undeterred, she resumed making surprise inspections on sanatoriums for the insane and sending checks and gift boxes to temperance drives, widows and orphans, and penniless young women seeking an education at Vassar College. Traveling by Pullman coach, she ranged far from home, calling in at jails and almshouses on the West Coast and touring the devastated South. Her philanthropy and political connections resulted in construction of a water fountain for Boston's dray animals, contributions to the Society for the Prevention of Cruelty to Animals (SPCA) and to the repatriation of former slaves in Liberia, and the establishment or upgrading of thirty-two institutions throughout the United States, Canada, Europe, and Japan.

After a debilitating illness in 1881, Dix, arthritic and with diminished sight and hearing, sheltered at one of her pet projects, the Trenton State Hospital in New Jersey. Until her death on July 18, 1887, she rejected laudanum for pain and continued her intense letter writing and receipt of visitors. She was buried at Mount Auburn Cemetery in Cambridge, Massachusetts. The Trenton psychiatric hospital maintains her belongings as a miniature museum. Her home is now the Dorothea Dix Memorial Park, where a marker lauds her place among the United States' medical giants.

Sources

Austin, Anne L. *The Woolsey Sisters of New York.* Philadelphia: American Philosophical Society, 1971.

"Civil War Nurses." http://www.wayne.esu1.k12.ne.us/civil/morris.html.

Denney, Robert E. *Civil War Medicine: Care and Comfort of the Wounded.* New York: Sterling Publishing, 1995.

Dolan, Josephine A., R.N. *History of Nursing.* Philadelphia: W. B. Saunders, 1968.

Felder, Deborah G. *The 100 Most Influential Women of All Time: A Ranking Past and Present.* New York: Citadel Press, 1996.

Gollaher, David. *Voice for the Mad: The Life of Dorothea Dix.* New York: Free Press, 1995.

"Gravesites of Prominent Nurses." http://users.aol. com/NsgHistory/Index.html.

"Highlights of the Army Nurse Corps." http:// www.army.mil/cmh-pg/anc/Highlights.html.

Holland, Mary A. Gardner, comp. *Our Army Nurses.* Boston: Lounsberry, Nichols and Worth, 1896.

Saxton, Martha. *Louisa May: A Modern Biography of Louisa May Alcott.* Boston: Houghton Mifflin, 1977.

Sherr, Lynn, and Jurate Kazickas. *Susan B. Anthony Slept Here: A Guide to American Women's Landmarks.* New York: Times Books, 1994.

Sterne, Capt. Doris M. *In and Out of Harm's Way: A History of the Navy Nurse Corps.* Seattle, Wash.: Peanut Butter Publishing, 1996.

du Coudray, Angélique

On October 19, 1759, King Louis XV honored Madame Angélique Marguerite le Boursier du Coudray with a formal title—the French nation's first and only itinerant specialist in midwifery. Formerly known as Madame le Boursier, she had established an admirable record of teaching and inspiring women to become *accoucheuses,* or midwives. At age forty-four, she began training a corps of peasant practitioners as well as local surgeons to advance obstetrics as a means of ensuring a healthy citizenry free of birthing injuries. The fact that male medical practitioners accepted her tutelage suggests an intelligence, skill, and sterling reputation unassailable by sexists.

For thirty years, du Coudray traveled the back country on itineraries laid out by the king, his court physicians, ministers, and royal advisers. An anomaly among the midwives of the eighteenth century, she maintained a written record of her journeys that disclosed an unusual autonomy for a woman of any station. To show students the numerous possibilities of birth complications, she invented a life-size movable pelvis and fetus model of pliant padded leather, real bone,

wicker, and linen, all mimicking the colors of human tissue. In a letter dated May 13, 1756, she described her invention, which presented a model pelvis with uterus, vagina, bladder, rectum, placenta, amnion, chorion, umbilical cord with arteries and veins, and extractable fetuses, both stillborn and viable. In the mid-1760s, Madame du Coudray augmented her obstetrical mannequin with sponges and sacs that exuded clear and red fluids to emulate amniotic fluids and blood. The only extant model is housed at the Musée Flaubert in Rouen.

An outspoken voice for professionalism, du Coudray trained in Paris through apprenticeship and hands-on pedagogy and established a lifelong motto, *Ad Operam* (To Work). In 1745, she practiced in Paris under le Boursier, her maiden name, and functioned as the unofficial head of forty city midwives. To upgrade standards, the group petitioned the Faculté de Médecine to improve their skills with anatomy course work. Because Parisian surgeons had ceased performing dissections for the edification of apprentices and failed to supervise the third-year licensing examination, midwives lacked proper preparation. Another problem for professionals was competition from quacks, who violated the integrity of midwifery by practicing without licenses.

A spirited professional, du Coudray valued her training and influence. For a three-year practicum in enlightened obstetrics, she charged beginners 300 livres, which was 50–100 percent more than her peers earned per pupil, and forced them to seek room, board, and laundry from their own purses. In 1751, she abandoned her Paris training sessions and, on court recommendation, traveled to Auvergne to instruct hundreds of apprentices from Thiers free of charge. The dismal record of rural births prefaced her concern for high mortality rates and infertility. A patriot above all, she intended to stem the abysmal loss of life by improving birthing techniques among mothers who lived too far from city centers to demand quality maternal care.

Du Coudray assembled individual lessons and published them as a birthing text, *Abrégé de l'Art des Accouchements* (A Summary of the Art of Midwifery) (1759), which offered practical advice, such as recommendations on neonatal care and breast-feeding. Based on her admirable record, the "widow du Coudray," an unmarried, childless nomad, savored her freedom to travel and teach where she chose. She may have invented a noble married name as a status booster and necessary cover for her lack of experience as wife and mother, a standard requirement for centuries among laywomen who practiced the art of birthing.

Beginning field work in Moulins and covering the heart of France, du Coudray typically accepted pupils recruited by village priests. A team of two surgeons and an apprentice, her niece, Marguerite Guillaumanche, plus a maid and menial facilitated morning and afternoon classes of as many as one hundred students, extending from Monday to Saturday for eight to twelve weeks. Students dramatized anatomy lessons using her teaching mannequin. Upon completing the course, they received certification to assure local women of their training in the royal program. Du Coudray's skill so delighted Le Nain, Moulins's local magistrate, that he published a *Mémoire,* a brochure intended to facilitate her work under fellow authorities in other regions. She broadened the project's outreach by selling male surgeons copies of her model, with which they could provide ongoing courses in midwifery. Also, each town hall displayed a silk model of the device as a substitute for other mannequins while they were repaired or replaced.

Although du Coudray began her revolution in birthing techniques under royal aegis, the immediate result of her creation of an elite cadre of modern midwives was grumbling among established practitioners and the usual intransigence of village surgeons. Mothers, too, reverted to traditional methods and rejected the new. Nonetheless, she continued to Bourgogne in 1763 to teach peasant trainees from Autun, Bourg-en-Bresse, and Chalon-sur-Saône. Her self-introduction to a third magistrate, Boutin of Bordeaux, insulted him by implying that his district was in particular need of her instruction. Unaccustomed to bold, aggressive self-starters, he rejected her offer, thus refusing the king's handpicked instructor. This debacle forced Boutin to humble himself and beg du Coudray's services for his region.

The next year, du Coudray taught in Limoges with the full cooperation of Turgot, an open-minded magistrate who welcomed an opportunity to modernize. Seeking political advancement, he ushered the king's midwife into succeeding posts, warning magistrates that du Coudray had a high opinion of her talents and brooked no interference at the local level with a task she perceived as crucial to the realm. Soon, these doubters realized the validity and worth of her teaching and endorsed her courses with genuine praise and gratitude. In Poitiers in 1765, her courses were the source of regular features for the province newspaper, *Affiches de Poitou.* The itinerary carried her to the coastal cities of Niort, Les Sables d'Olonnes, La Rochelle, and Rochefort, where she gave naval surgeons detailed demonstrations of advanced medical equipment and techniques of cesarean sections. By August 18, 1767, King Louis XV chose to award her a yearly stipend of 8,000 livres and 3,000 more as a pension.

The tour of France continued to the north with stints in Orleans, Blois, Chartres, and Montargis, concluding in winter 1768 at Bourges, where her mission bogged down from the ill treatment of an uncooperative magistrate. A bright spot on this one blot on her record was the standout student, Mme. Jouhannet, who established a lying-in clinic. Du Coudray demonstrated faith in her own efforts by investing heavily in color prints for a new edition of her printed text. With the aid of Frère Côme, who superintended her itinerary and treasury, she set out for Issoudun, Châteauroux, Périgueux, and Agen and relented toward Boutin by backtracking to Bordeaux in 1770, the final stop in her tour of the French interior.

Following a downturn in her career in 1771–1772 from rejections in Toulouse, Montpellier, Narbonne, and Marseilles, du Coudray was welcomed to Grenoble and Châlons-sur-Marne and toasted in Neuchâteau. While teaching in Flanders, she received the praise of the Comte de Nery, who passed along her credentials to Empress Maria Thérèse of Austria, mother of Queen Marie Antoinette. Du Coudray served an out-of-country assignment in Ypres, Belgium, then returned to her tour to an oversized class of 130 in Le Mans, whom the local magistrate paid to take the course, and a subsequent class of 140 in Angers. Wearied by years of dynamic classroom performance, she pushed on, accepting an appointment to the Royal Veterinary School at Alfort and other posts before her retirement in 1783. Pleased that her niece, now Marguerite Coutanceau, had established a maternal clinic in Bordeaux, written a rival handbook, and begun her own teaching cycle, du Coudray was in the process of supporting her understudy when the French Revolution altered the situation. In the war's aftermath, the Coutanceaus set up a hospice in Bordeaux. Du Coudray was reduced to penury after the national upheaval curtailed her retirement funds. At her death on April 17, 1794, she received no accolades but died with the admiration and esteem of the hundreds she had introduced to modern obstetrics.

Sources

Gelbart, Nina. *King's Midwife: A History and Mystery of Madame du Coudray.* Berkeley: University of California Press, 1998.

Hufton, Olwen. *The Prospect Before Her: A History of Women in Western Europe, 1500–1800.* New York: Vintage Books, 1995.

Marland, Hilary, ed. *The Art of Midwifery: Early Modern Midwives in Europe.* London: Routledge, 1993.

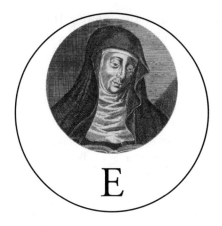

E

Etheridge, Anna Blair

Dubbed "Annie B." for her spunk, Anna Blair Etheridge was famous for rendering battlefield first aid and for galloping along with the troops to treat them as they fell. Of her, Red Cross chief Mabel Boardman wrote in *Under the Red Cross Flag at Home and Abroad* (1915, 70): "Another type of woman was Annie Etheridge, a *vivandière*, or *fille du régiment*. Like an amazon, she rode in the midst of the shot and shell, with utter disregard of danger, that she might find and aid the wounded; she encouraged the men in the trenches and led back many a straggling deserter to the battle line."

A volunteer nurse from Detroit, Michigan, Etheridge was five feet tall and only seventeen years old when she enlisted in the Union army with seventeen other nurses. Her group reported with the 2nd Michigan Regiment to Fort Wayne and left for Washington, D.C., on June 6, 1861. After the others fled and left her to nurse casualties alone, Etheridge continued as the "Daughter of the Regiment," armed with pistols and mounted sidesaddle for the trek to Alexandria, Virginia. Refusing separate accommodation for ladies, she slept on the ground rolled in an army blanket. Her first experience with battle came at Blackburn's Ford, where men fell from cannon fire.

While advancing with the troops and treating their wounds at the First Battle of Bull Run in Manassas, Virginia, on July 21, she offered her horse to a wounded Confederate soldier and continued on foot. In combat, she distinguished herself for performing first aid under fire, sewing up wounds on the battlefield, and ferrying bandages in saddlebags as she accompanied litters to aid stations. Her most famous encounter involved a wounded soldier who was blown to pieces in the field as she cradled him.

After General George McClellan took over the regiment, Etheridge was stationed at Mansion House Hospital in Alexandria, Virginia, where staff worked from reveille at 5:00 A.M. until 9:00 P.M. When the regiment returned to battle in March 1862, she traveled by boat up the Chesapeake Bay and, as a member of the Hospital Transport Service, loaded wounded aboard the *Wissahickon*, where an overload of sick men doubled up on straw mattresses. To ease their homesickness and fear, she sang "Auld Lang Syne" and "Home, Sweet Home."

Transferred to the *Wilson Small*, which received wounded from the Second Battle of Bull Run, Etheridge, nicknamed "Gentle Annie," earned the rank of sergeant major and wore the red diamond insignia of General

Philip Kearney's troops. At the Battle of Chancellorsville, Virginia, fought May 1–4, 1863, she was wounded by a minié ball to the left hand but continued at her post through the Battle of Gettysburg in early July. After a brief retreat to Cape Cod, Etheridge served aboard the *Knickerbocker,* a 450-bed transport ship that stopped at the Pamunkey River terminus to receive casualties bound for Washington, D.C., Philadelphia, and New York. Following her capture by rebels, General Philip Sheridan dispatched volunteers to return her and other Union prisoners to camp. She joined the 5th Army under General Ulysses S. Grant in spring 1864. At Petersburg, Virginia, in April 1865, a charge struck her horse Jessie, a veteran of the battles of Antietam and Spotsylvania. The mount survived to carry her mistress in a Washington, D.C., victory parade in May. For valor and length of service, Etheridge earned the Kearney Cross.

Sources

Boardman, Mabel. *Under the Red Cross Flag at Home and Abroad.* London: J. B. Lippincott, 1915.

Shura, Mary Frances. *Gentle Annie: The True Story of a Civil War Nurse.* New York: Scholastic, 1991.

Stuber, Irene. "Women of Achievement and Herstory Calendar," http://www.city-net.com/~lmann/women/history/cal4.html.

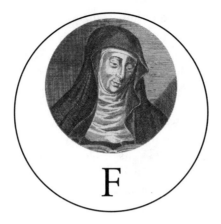

F

Farmborough, Florence

Florence Farmborough served as the Red Cross's eyes and ears on the World War I Russo-Polish front. Using a plate camera and 400,000-word diary, she recorded civil upheaval and the chaos and devastation of battle in what became a best-selling reflection on war nursing, later published as *With the Armies of the Tsar: A Nurse at the Russian Front, 1914–1918* (1974). In 1908, at the age of twenty-one, English governess and companion Farmborough left Buckinghamshire for Kiev to tutor Asya and Nadya, the two daughters of Dr. Pavel Sergeyevich Usov, a noted cardiac surgeon. When war began in 1914, she, Asya, and Nadya volunteered for the Red Cross at a Moscow hospital, staffed under the patronage of Princess Golitsin. The facility was the first to receive war wounded from field stations.

As a *krestovaya sestra* (Red Cross Sister), Farmborough learned to silence her fears and doubts and to render first aid while taking a brief medical history. Of necessity, she expanded her command of Russian. She received training at a Moscow hospital and continued studying anatomy and attending three-hour lectures each evening. After Dr. Usov's intervention, she was posted among Russian forces with the 10th Field Surgical Otryad. Dressed in nurse's uniform, apron, and veil, she journeyed to the front in the Carpathian Mountains, where the flying column was equipped with two automobiles, two horse-drawn drays, and a two-wheeled Red Cross cart topped with a canvas hood. She recalled a night of feverish work at a monastery: "Hearing, yet as with deafness, we listened to the entreaties of those agonised souls. 'Give me something to ease my pain; for the love of God, give me something, *Sestritsa.*' With cheering words we strove to comfort them, but pain is a hard master; and the wounds were such as to set one's heart beating with wonder that a man could be so mutilated in body and yet live, speak and understand" (Farmborough 1974, 41). She struggled to perform triage, dispatching patients suffering from smallpox, typhoid, cholera, and spotted fever to the contagious ward and turning away from silent moribund men who could entreat only with their eyes. Her descriptions were filled with shock at the tender age of recruits and wounds that compromised their bodily functions. Long nights of washing and bandaging were punctuated with explosions of huge German artillery shells, which rattled the hospital.

Farmborough witnessed heavy demands on the Red Cross and watched the heaving sides of agency dray horses dying of overexertion. As peasant refugees lined up for meals, feeding station attendants stretched cabbage soup and groats to accommodate them. At a railroad station, she observed the attractive hospital train sponsored by the czarina, Alexandra Feodorovna, whose name was inscribed on the side. Speaking like a war correspondent, she summarized: "The retreat was at its height. I studied the many faces in our immediate vicinity: courageous, dignified, defiant, resigned—all were there. And, as I looked, I knew that this picture of Russia in an hour of distress would never fade completely from my mind" (Farmborough 1974, 144).

Critical demand at the Polish front kept Farmborough in a constant state of readiness, snatching sleep whenever possible and abandoning film before it could be developed. On rare occasions, she found time to attend the unending funerals. Her detailed diary recounts rumors of retreats and advances, bodies strewn over the plains, the smell of decay, and pits filled with the remains of carnage.

After her unit moved south, Farmborough fled the Romanian front and trekked to Moscow, across Siberia to the Pacific port of Vladivostok and thence to the United States. Upon her return to England in 1918, she was named a Fellow of the Royal Geographical Society. She continued to follow harm's way by lecturing in Spain during the Spanish Civil War and returning home in time for the Battle of Britain during World War II.

Sources

Farmborough, Florence. *With the Armies of the Tsar: A Nurse at the Russian Front, 1914–1918.* New York: Stein and Day, 1974.

Tylee, Claire M. "The Spectacle of War: Photographs of the Russian Front by Florence Farmborough." *Women: A Cultural Review,* 8 (1997): 65–80.

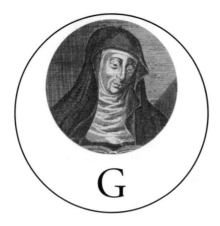

G

Galard, Geneviève de

The heroine of Dien Bien Phu, flight nurse and former prisoner of war Geneviève de Galard earned the Air Medal, Air Medical Service Silver Medal, French Legion of Honor, honorary membership in the French Foreign Legion, and a ride in a motorcade up New York City's Broadway. The U.S. Congress invited her to visit Washington, D.C., the first such gesture to a woman and the first to a French hero in over a century. The press, in ecstatic tribute to the only female at the fifty-six-day siege, dubbed her the "Angel of Dien Bien Phu."

A native of Paris, Galard was born on April 13, 1925, to a privileged family whose ancestry dates to the Crusades and the forces of Joan of Arc. Her father, Vicomte Oger de Galard-Terraube, was killed in 1934. Galard attended private school and summered at the family's chateau in Terraube. During World War II, the women of her family fled occupied Paris to Toulouse, where she continued her education under Dominican nuns. After the war, she completed additional training in home economics and fine arts and did postgraduate work at the Sorbonne in Paris. She studied nursing with the Red Cross and graduated first in her class before entering the Infirmières Pilotes et Secouristes de l'Air (IPSA),

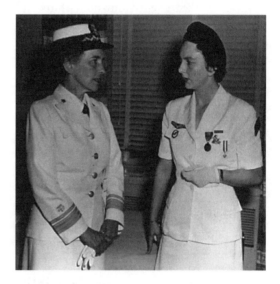

Lucile Petry (left) and Lt. Geneviève de Galard-Terraube (known as "the Angel of Dien Bien Phu"), 1954 (U.S. Library of Medicine)

an airborne nursing corps and rescue service that aided the French military in the Indochinese war.

In 1953, guided by her devout Catholicism and a family tradition of military excellence, Galard joined a Hanoi-based air rescue company to evacuate the wounded from combat sites to Saigon and ferry families from the Sahara and Morocco to Paris. On her second tour of duty in 1954, she returned to Vietnam, where nationalists had been fighting for eight years. At Dien Bien Phu, an underground fortress, where she readied critical cases for the flight to Hanoi, she found surprisingly modern hospital equipment, with refrigeration, X-ray, a surgical suite, and a dental lab, but with bunks overcrowded with wounded. Under heavy fire on March 28, her helicopter returned to the fort, where it was demolished by incoming shells from the Vietminh. The only female nurse in the fort among twelve hundred wounded, she was grounded until the French could silence enemy artillery.

At a shelter, Galard aided the fort's nineteen doctors in dressing serious abdominal wounds and attended twenty-five operations a day. She worked twenty-four-hour shifts and slept on a litter between patients. On her second day, she hopped trenches and shell craters and crawled under barbed wire to visit groups of Algerian, French, and Moroccan wounded from the 2nd Airborne, Thai Battalion, Airborne Commandos, and 8th Assault Unit. Supplied with camouflage overalls like the rest of the troop, she earned the trust of the men, who built her a private shelter concealed behind parachute silk. She collected cheese, crackers, and jam from the officers' mess to feed the Vietnamese prisoners of war, who served the hospital as spare labor.

As the siege worsened, Galard, dressed in cut-down paratrooper's uniform, worked three days and nights by lantern in the dark operating theater, and steadied the terrified men awaiting surgery. At dinner on April 29, 1954, General Christian de Castries presented her a battered Croix de Guerre with palms and Knight's Cross Legion of Honor for courage under attack. De Castries had scrounged the medal, a white enamel cross topped by a red ribbon, from his own footlocker. The next evening, Galard sewed the shield of the French Foreign Legion to her sleeve. The situation worsened after monsoon season brought damp, mold, and maggots. Snipers killed water bearers on the nightly run to the Nan-youn River. Galard continued to lift spirits with small gifts of tobacco, cookies, or fruit juice.

On May 7, after the struggle ended with the French surrender, the Vietminh allowed the medical staff to continue its humanitarian work and safely to house patients above ground in tents. Galard refused to be airlifted to safety and remained in service to patients. On May 19, she sent a personal letter on the occasion of Ho Chi Minh's sixty-fourth birthday to thank him for showing mercy toward casualties and to promise to initiate peace between the French and Vietnamese. In a second letter, she stressed: "While my joy to return home is great, it would be very imperfect if I were to leave alone, leaving behind me the other medical personnel, doctors as well as attendants" (Fall 1966, 430). She begged for clemency for all.

Ho Chi Minh personally liberated her and wished her bon voyage. For ten days, she had refused to leave her post until ordered home by the French high command. In Hanoi on May 25, she was hailed as a hero, yet she declined offers for exclusive interviews. Still aiding the wounded, she left Vietnam only after the last of the casualties were airlifted. Lauded by the U.S. Congress, she accepted honoraria from the American Red Cross, American Nurses Association, National League for Nursing, and Columbia University. New York mayor John Wagner gave her a scroll of honor; President Dwight D. Eisenhower conferred on her the Medal of Freedom, noting her service to comrades and unsurpassed courage.

Back at work as a flight nurse, Galard resumed missions to North Africa and spent off hours with veterans at Les Invalides in Paris. Some remembered her from Dien Bien Phu; others admired her reputation for kindness and modesty. A colleague, Dr. Paul Grauwin, commented on her courage and work in *Doctor at Dienbienphu* (1955), as did W. P. Holland, author of *Geneviève de Galard-Terraube*, published that same year. After training in the United States in 1955, she married Captain Jean de Heaulme in 1957 and returned to Les Invalides as a rehabilitation nurse. The couple lived in Madagascar, then returned to France in the mid-1960s. In 1963, while driving through Paris, she recognized Legionnaire Lemeunier, who had decorated her for bravery. She embraced him and made good on her famous promise, "If we ever get out of this alive, I'll pay you a bottle of champagne no matter where we meet" (Fall 1966, 348).

Sources
Current Biography. New York: H. W. Wilson, 1954.
"Dien Bien Phu." http://www.ecr.mu.oz.au/~npl/vn5.htm.
Dolan, Josephine A., R.N. *History of Nursing.* Philadelphia: W. B. Saunders, 1968.
Fall, Bernard B. *Hell in a Very Small Place: The Siege of Dien Bien Phu.* New York: Vintage Books, 1966.
McKown, Robin. *Heroic Nurses.* New York: G. P. Putnam's Sons, 1966.

Gender Issues in Nursing

The domination of nursing opportunities by either sex has fluctuated over time, depending on public, governmental, military, and religious attitudes toward sex discrimination and nursing as a profession. From early times, both men and women have held positions in nurse care and midwifery, as demonstrated by Native American healing traditions, which are open to male and female alike; by the Latino role of *curandera/curandero;* and by a roster of early Christian nurses—Fabiola, Flavia Helena, St. Cosmas, St. Damian, Flacilla, St. Marcella, St. Paula, Eustochium, St. Zoticus, St. Basil and his sister Macrina, and St. John Chrysostom. Some of these religious forerunners deliberately chose to work in single-gender companies, as did Mother Elizabeth Ann Seton's Sisters of Charity, the Order of Antonines, the Misericordia, the Ursulines of New Orleans, Quebec's Sisters of the Hôtel Dieu, and the Daughters of Charity, founded by St. Vincent de Paul and St. Louise de Marillac. In each example, society profited from the devotion and skill of medical personnel who sought opportunities to serve.

The logic of gender in nursing is often confounded by peripheral issues. One example derives from the Philadelphia yellow fever epidemic of 1793, when the unwanted job of nursing fell to those on society's bottom rung, former slaves Absalom Jones, Richard Allen, Mary Scott, Sarah Bass, and Caesar Cranchal, all of whom distinguished themselves for mercy and selflessness. Some nurses have operated outside organizations by establishing one-person outreaches devoid of gender typing, as is the case with the hospice initiatives of Father Francisco Xavier Ortiz and St. Vincent de Paul; Elizabeth Haddon Estaugh, Quaker nurse to the Indians of New Jersey; Sister Dulce in Salvador de Bahía; Father Damien, caretaker of Hawaii's lepers; masseuse and herbalist Gregorita Rodriguez of Santa Fe, New Mexico; Russian reformer Rose Kaplan's battle against trachoma in Jewish refugee camps in Alexandria, Egypt; Cuban nurse-detainee, Reynaldo Soto Hernández, whose defiant humanitarianism placed him at

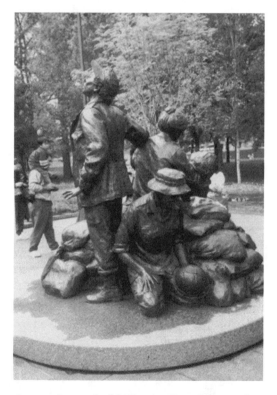

A recent photograph of the Vietnam Women's Memorial in Washington, D.C. (courtesy of the Vietnam Women's Memorial)

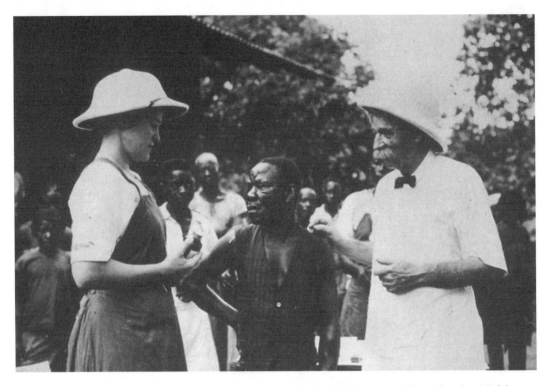

Dr. Albert Schweitzer supervises inoculations at his jungle hospital in Lambaréné, Gabon, Africa. Though most of the credit traditionally goes to Dr. Schweitzer, his wife, Hélène Bresslan Schweitzer, and daughter, Rhena Eckert, were essential to the operation of the hospital. (Agence France Presse/Archive)

odds with Castro's regime; and Helen Mira-montes, a critical care nurse from Santa Clara, California, who has volunteered to test the first acquired immunodeficiency syndrome (AIDS) vaccine. Others, like Naomi Deutsch, director of the U.S. Public Health Department, have made their way up the civil service ladder in direct competition with the dominant gender.

Typically, nursing tasks have been divided by gender. For example, in most tribes, the shaman was a man, the midwife a woman. At the healing temple of Apollo in ancient Delphi, the resident priest was male; the *pythia* (seer) and her attendants were female. When the first European missionaries arrived in South Africa in the late nineteenth century, they usually consisted of a company of Catholic priests and nuns or Protestant married couples, with the man serving as evangelist and leader and the woman as subservient nurse, facilitator, or teacher. The man-as-

dominator arrangement flourished in Brazil's Amazon Basin in 1921, where Nebraskans Leo and Jessie Halliwell carried their Seventh-Day Adventist mission, and at Lambaréné, where Dr. Albert Schweitzer, his wife, Hélène Bresslau Schweitzer, and their married daughter, Rhena Eckert, shared responsibilities for black Africans. Despite the Schweitzers' partnership, the wife's and daughter's contributions were generally ignored while the world showered honors on Dr. Schweitzer.

Another aspect of gender in nursing is the specialization that falls to men and women. In ancient times, men like King Zoser of Egypt, Maimonides of Spain, Caliph al-Muktadir, Avicenna, Rhazes of Baghdad, Hippocrates of Kos, and the Emperor Shen Nung, Chang Chung-ching, and Hua T'O of China excelled at innovation, decisionmaking, and administration, whereas women like Agnodice, founder of midwifery in the Western world, and nameless Roman slave-nurses have flourished in the nurturing, hands-on caregiving associated with wet-nursing, herbalism, ward nursing, public health, pediatrics, and family care. The Indian text *Charaka* set standards of decency and skill for anonymous female underlings. The Greek founding father of medicine, Aesculapius, demonstrated how men could confer authority on female handmaidens by sharing duties with two daughters, Hygieia and Panacea; thus, the Western concept of male hierarchy was established. It continued into the twentieth century, when innovator Elizabeth Kenny clashed with a royal commission that issued a three-hundred-page report solely to squelch the upstart Australian nurse on the issue of massaging and exercising limbs paralyzed by polio.

Two forerunners to modern nursing, the jobs of midwifery and community nurse, were traditionally relegated by default to women because male healers disdained the jobs as low-paying or insignificant woman's work. One example, the career of Elizabeth Cellier, establishes that an altruistic midwife at an English women's prison had little competition from men. In her account from the American colonial period, Martha Ballard illustrates in semiliterate diary entries the mundane, wearying nature of her chores as herbalist, healer, nurse, and midwife. Similarly, Mother Francesca Cabrini took an assignment among Italian slum-dwellers, a post previously ignored by the male medical establishment. Another charitable volunteer, Rose Hawthorne Lathrop, ministered to cancer patients in New York City, choosing the most pathetic, hopeless cases as her focus. There were few women practitioners, for example, the sixteenth-century midwife Louyse Bourgeois of St. Germain, midwife to Marie de Medici; Louyse's disciple, Marguérite du Tertre de La Marche; Luisa Rosado; and textbook authors Teresa Ployant and Valentine Seaman, who achieved notoriety as medical authorities in a male-dominated milieu.

In the Middle Ages, the promise of education and choice of career in Christian service led men and women to commit themselves as nuns, priests, or monks. Both sexes practiced nursing, although on differing bases of authority. Women, who were prohibited from the ministry, thrived as settlement workers, birthing experts, or general practitioners, as demonstrated by Margaret of Metola, Italy, who led her Mantellates into prisons to console the downtrodden. Notables of the era include St. Attracta (or Athracht) of Donegal, St. Bridget, St. Scholastica, Julia Anicia, Clothilde (or Clotilda) and Radegonde (or Radegunda), St. Bathilde (or Batilda), St. Dympna, St. Walpurga (or Walburga) of Wessex, St. Margaret of Scotland, Herrade of Landsburg, St. Clare and her Poor Clares, St. Catherine of Siena and the Caterinati, and St. Angela Merici and the Company of St. Ursula, or the Ursulines. Prominent men—namely, the Alexian Brothers, St. Columba of Gartan, St. Giles (or St. Aegidius) of Athens, St. Godric, St. Francis, and St. Hugh of Lincoln—made their niche as hospice workers and founders of orders. The Crusades brought together pilgrims, warriors, and support personnel for two centuries, producing a need for hostels, shelters, infirmaries, and hospitals and attendant monk-warriors, the first military medical corpsmen. Respected monasteries produced the Teutonic Knights of Jerusalem, Order of Trinitarians, Knights Hospitallers of St. John, and others to journey to battlefields in the Holy Lands. In their absence, nursing sisterhoods like the Sisters of the Order of St. John of Jerusalem, organized by Agnes of Rome, maintained basic womanly ward chores, tended the laundry, and cooked. On one expedition in the Seventh Crusade of 1249, the rare females, Hersend and Guillamette de Luys, accompanied Louis IX as birthing attendants to his wife, Berenger.

Outstanding female nurses of the Middle Ages were not necessarily models of feminism. The creation of the Béguines in the seventh century was a Belgian innovation—a society of unmarried laywomen led by Father Lambert le Bégue of Liège. Although free of cloistering, women such as Mary of Oignies, Juliana of Liège, Mechthild of Magdeburg,

Beatrice of Nazareth, Hadewijch of Brabant, and Marguerite Porete still functioned under male authority, as did the Gilbertines under Gilbert of Sempringham and Gerhard Groote's Sisters of the Common Life. For certain royal wives—St. Margaret, St. Elizabeth of Hungary, and St. Catherine of Genoa—aiding beggars and prisoners was the sort of dabbling in social work that relieved boredom and cleared a path to heaven. In similar fashion, St. Elizabeth of Portugal and St. Bridget of Uppland chose service more as a retreat in widowhood than a cherished career.

More public and outspoken champions of women's place in the profession flourished as abbesses, notably the Empress Cunegund of Kaufungen, Abbess Euphemia of England, Anna Comnena of Byzantium, and Frances of Rome and her Oblates of Mary, later called the Oblates of Tor de' Specchi, the first uncloistered Italian nuns. Still viable as leader, health adviser, and spokeswoman to the current age, the revered scholar, hymn writer, and textbook author, St. Hildegard of Bingen, impressed on the world the need for women's colleges and nurse training early in the twelfth century. Others succeeded in the medical realm usually dominated by males: Novella d'Andrea, lecturer to medical students, doctors Stephanie de Montaneis of Lyons, France, Jehanne of Paris, and Sarre of Paris and her daughter Florian. Likewise memorable were midwife Elysabeth Keston and the Jewish practitioners Jacoba Felicie and Sarah of St. Gilles, France.

Additional names surface as persistent, uncompromising feminists. Author and healer Trotula, a graduate of the School of Salerno, earned the title of "wise woman" and rose to chair of medicine and authority on cesarean sections. In 1771, Luisa Rosado obtained a license in a trial by ordeal: she successfully delivered the heir to the Spanish throne. In Scotland in the nineteenth century, Sophia Jex-Blake led female nurses against the Edinburgh medical establishment to demand better pay and liberation from male domination and social degradation. In 1848, English pioneer nurse-educator Mary Agnes Jones,

founder of St. Mary's Convent and Nursing Home, studied a new form of hospital administration, which did not require Christian nurses to join religious orders or commit to poverty, monastic obedience, celibacy, or enforced seclusion. Her stand against religious patriarchy freed her disciples to devote themselves fully to Christian charity and professionalism. A half-century later, in Canada in 1898, after the government beefed up military command in the Yukon, Lady Ishbel Marjoribanks Aberdeen, an aristocratic feminist, launched the Victorian Order of Nurses (VON) to honor Queen Victoria's Diamond Jubilee. The combination of Aberdeen's money and the Queen's authority overwhelmed objections from male critics.

Not all champions have triumphed against the patriarchy of government and church. A colonial martyr to midwifery, herbalist and community nurse Anne Marbury Hutchinson was exiled to Rhode Island for countering Puritan justice. Her trial demonstrated the stern male dominance of American colonial midwives and the ominous misogyny that powered subsequent witch hunts. Likewise, in the years preceding Joseph Lister's advocacy of asepsis in the second half of the nineteenth century, Mary Agnes Jones surmised that an outbreak of puerperal fever was connected with the location of a postmortem room alongside the maternity ward. While infection threatened the lives of new mothers and infants, Jones was unable to convince male doctors that hand and instrument washing was a simple solution to a deadly fever.

Some twentieth-century American women have also lost ground to male reactionaries. In 1915, birth control champion Margaret Sanger was jailed while battling the congressional Puritanism and misogyny embodied in the Comstock Act, which prohibited mailing contraceptives and birth control pamphlets. Sanger's contemporary, Dr. Marie Stopes, inventor of the cervical cap and pioneer of women's health, fought similar misogyny in England while establishing the nation's first contraception clinics.

In the struggle for supremacy in medicine, midwifery was a contested field. On the one hand, it offered an unusual opportunity to men and women to compile birthing texts, a task accomplished by seventeenth-century writers Percival Willughby and J. Sharp; Spanish authors Damián Carbón and Juan Alonso de Loy Ruyzes; Anne Horenburg of Braunschweig; and Justine Dittrichin Siege-mundin of Rohnstock, Silesia, midwife to the royal Prussian family at Brandenburg. The first major challenge to women's traditional dominance as birthing experts derived from the work of Peter Chamberlen, who invented forceps around 1630, and François Mau-riceau, author of an obstetrical text that intro-duced a method of puncturing the amnion to speed labor. By increasing efficiency, these in-novators secured the attention of male sur-geons, who realized that there was profit to be made in fast deliveries. By the eighteenth cen-tury, medical men had commandeered the birthing process, altering it from a normal, nonmedical event superintended by women to a lucrative form of surgery, a field closed to women.

In simple terms, men overran the subspe-cialty of midwifery. To ensure power, male surgeons in Navarre, Spain, usurped licensing procedures and required written examinations that were administered and graded by parish priests and municipal physicians. Obviously, the illiterate practitioner had no chance of passing. In a short time, Europe's community-based birthings had passed out of fashion, to be replaced by male-controlled medical proce-dures. Bureaucracy entangled the issue in gov-ernmental and academic red tape. In 1723, Johan von Hoorn became Sweden's first state-paid birthing instructor. Seven years later, Eu-rope's male midwives, especially in metropoli-tan areas, systematically displaced their female competitors by superintending labor and de-livery. In 1733, Thomas White licensed only male practitioners at the Royal College of Physicians in Manchester. In 1757, the province of Braunschweig legislated a birthing ordinance requiring formal course work in fe-male anatomy and physiology taught by a male professor at Das Anatomisch-Chirurgis-che Institut (the Anatomical-Surgical Insti-tute). By 1795, Barcelona College of Surgery intentionally excluded women by requiring Latin, logic, algebra, and physics, subjects taught at universities that admitted only male students.

Throughout the mid–eighteenth century, a campaign for accountability in autopsy and investigation of infanticide and the imple-mentation of forceps served male midwives in a blatant turf war. Female midwives retaliated, charging that the clamping device upped the men's year's earnings by shortening labor and increasing the number of patients each user could serve. The women complained that ex-erting force on a baby's head during pro-tracted delivery endangered mother and child. For all their protest, their grassroots revolts soon lapsed. By the end of the century, the only female midwives still in the majority were those who served the poor and outcast. The rare accepted female authority, Angélique du Coudray, became France's first and only itinerant specialist in midwifery solely by grit, persistence, and experience. Even King Louis XV had to acknowledge that she was the ex-pert of the times.

In the nineteenth century, practical mid-wifery was a lesser choice for middle- and upper-class women as the trend toward med-icalizing and institutionalizing normal births continued. In 1800, one intellectual midwife, Marie Gillain Boivin of Montreuil, France, founded L'Hospice de la Maternité for prosti-tutes, a subclass of women male surgeons re-jected. Snubbed by the Royal Academy of Medicine, she worked independently to find solutions to uterine hemorrhage and pio-neered the study of fetal heartbeat and ure-thral cancer, earning a *Doctor Honoris Causa* (honorary M.D.) from the University of Mar-burg. Her partner, Marie-Louise Lachapelle, *sage femme in chef* (chief midwife) of the Hôtel Dieu and founder of the Children's Hospital at Port Royal, authored the three-volume *Pratique des Accouchements ou Mé-*

moirs et Observations Choisies (The Practice of Midwifery or Memoirs and Selected Observations) and opened a family-centered practice. Lachapelle perpetuated the traditional regimen of massage, manipulation, oil, and herbs during natural childbirth rather than the rapid forceps deliveries preferred by men. One traditionalist, Dame Mary Rosalind Paget, a feminist spokeswoman for nursing professionalism, taught nonintervention at the Midwives' Institute, later called the Royal College of Midwives. Despite these efforts, birthing continued to move toward male-driven mechanization in the twentieth century with the lock-step use of sonograms, amniocentesis, fetal monitoring, drugs and general anesthesia, mechanical intervention, and episiotomy and other surgeries.

Unlike midwifery, which was claimed by both sexes, until the mid–nineteenth century, battlefield nursing remained the most complete and long-standing area of male medical hegemony. As a means to usurping lands, seizing treasuries, and dominating peoples, war was central to masculinity and power. From ancient times, soldiers tended their own casualties. One example in the Roman army of the Emperor Nero was the healer Pedanius Dioscorides, who traveled with the troops. Similarly, Charlemagne and Napoleon enlisted military doctors for the duration of field maneuvers. During the American Revolution, inspector-general Baron Friedrich von Steuben stated in *Regulations for the Order and Discipline of the Troops of the United States* (1778–1779) that care of sick soldiers was an essential to an officer's performance of duty.

Against such male-centered authority, a few women made themselves useful to the military. In Julius Caesar's *Gallic Commentaries,* he marveled at German women, who followed soldiers into battle and tended their wounds on the scene. Near the end of the fifteenth century, a true innovator, Queen Isabella of Castile, commandeered dressing stations and ambulances for her troops at the front, where she worked as a battlefield nurse in the world's first mobile army hospital. During the American Revolution, the danger of epidemic forced the male medical corps to value the nurse care of herbalist Margaret Vliet Warne, Martha Washington, Lucy Knox, Anna Elliott, and Kerenhappuch Turner. Outstanding among the many volunteers was Esther Gaston Walker, who served at the battles of Rocky Mount and Hanging Rock, South Carolina.

On the American frontier, individual women cited for combat duty continued the tradition. Among them are Elizabeth Black and Eleanor Felton, two nurses present at the fall of the Alamo in San Antonio, Texas, on March 6, 1836. Their compatriot, innkeeper Andrea Candelaria, nursed Jim Bowie and shielded his body from a Spanish soldier, who pierced her arm and face with a bayonet. Her colleague, Suzanna Dickerson, took casualties into the compound chapel and survived to carry the news of defeat to Governor Sam Houston. Another rare battlefield nurse, Fanny Wiggins Kelly, a captive of Chief Ottawa of the Oglala Sioux of Fort Laramie, Wyoming, wrote a memoir in 1864 about her service to the tribe during Indian raids. That same year, the Sisters of Charity treated cholera victims at Fort Harker, Kansas.

The most successful woman to overturn male domination was Florence Nightingale, whose name remains at the forefront of nineteenth-century feminists. After the Battle of Inkerman on November 5, 1854, she shamed male medical staff by asserting that she could immediately slash hospital mortality by instituting simple efficiency and cleanliness. Against the scoffing of the Royal Commission on the Health of the Army, she proved her point by setting up the landmark Scutari hospital near Istanbul, Turkey. The model, known worldwide as the Nightingale method, forced smug generals to admit that nine thousand soldiers had died needlessly, exceeding the statistics for the Great Plague of London. Within months of her return to London, poems and encomiums were lauding her example. Statues and plaques appeared on the grounds of hospitals and nursing schools bearing her name.

Americans, too, began to turn to women to staff military hospitals. In the United States, the first nurses aboard ship entered service in 1813 under a carefully controlled situation: Captain Stephen Decatur employed navy wives Mary Allen and Mary Marshall as nurses. Civil War nurses and nuns successfully staffed hospital ships, but as of 1873, the navy intentionally altered the title of nurse to bayman to indicate a preference for males. In the twentieth century, women slowly entered battlefield nursing. By July 3, 1942, Congress acknowledged their worth by conferring ranks on nurses equivalent to those for military officers.

Women who dared breach the male-only sanctum of military medicine have been tough, career-driven women who either disdained male authority or worked alone. Outstanding examples include Mary Jane Seacole, determined nurse at the Crimean front, Jane Delano, head of the Army Nurse Corps, and nurse volunteer Clara Louise Maass, hero of the military battle against yellow fever following heavy losses in the Spanish-American War. A quiet diarist, Red Cross nurse Florence Farmborough, published her observations from the Russian front during World War I; another from the era, known only as "Mademoiselle Miss," issued her daybook anonymously. Unforeseen heroism during World War I was derived from nursing English instructor Edith Cavell, whose contribution to the search for allied survivors aided Phillippe Baucq and Prince Reginald de Croy in rescuing soldiers from German territory.

American nursing history honors the most outspoken pioneers, particularly the Civil War leaders Dr. Elizabeth Blackwell, Dorothea Dix, Mary Ann Bickerdyke, and Clara Barton. Blackwell, an admirer of Florence Nightingale, stayed out of the gender fray at her New York–based training facility, forerunner of the Women's Medical College. Dix, the tough, no-nonsense organizer of frontline nursing teams, earned civil and military ridicule and backbiting from both sexes as a result of her high standards. Bickerdyke, for all her chutzpah in manipulating helpers and patients to do her will, relied on a pass signed by her protector, General William Tecumseh Sherman. In 1865, President Abraham Lincoln appeared to tiptoe into the issue of women in seats of power with his polite note stating that Clara Barton headed the national department of missing soldiers. In the South, nursing leaders Kate Cumming and Sally Louisa Tompkins reported the hardships of nursing for the losing side. Their writings attested that problems such as lack of supplies and foodstuffs were exacerbated by daily sniping from egotistical male surgeons. The same complaint permeated diaries and eyewitness accounts of northern nurses Mary Phinney, outspoken New York diarist Georgeanna M. Woolsey, and famed surgical nurse and transdresser Dr. Mary Edwards Walker, all of whom had to prove themselves repeatedly to doubting, hostile men.

Twentieth-century military nursing history continued the tradition of male decisionmaking and female dray labor. Chief of the U.S. Navy Nurse Corps Esther Voorhees Hasson was an early victim. In 1911, she resigned to end harassment and insults from her male superior, the surgeon general. As with Adolf Hitler's Nazis, military-minded communists in Cuba, China, and the Soviet bloc perpetuated the male hierarchy by organizing a medical system that functioned like an army medical corps. Under similar patriarchal mandate, Irish nurse Annie Smithson worked for Sinn Fein in 1918 and nursed wounded volunteers during Ireland's battle against British control. Her contemporary, Linda Kearns of Dromard, served as nurse and arms smuggler while operating a Red Cross field hospital during the 1916 uprising. A later venture into this hierarchy occurred in 1943 with the establishment of the Cadet Nurse Corps, which placed Lucile Petry, dean of Cornell University, as nursing director under Surgeon General Thomas Parran. When the mobile army surgical hospital (MASH) was first put to use in the Korean War in November 1953, staffing still placed men at the top and women as underlings.

As nursing standards rose in the United States, so did distaste for gender-based bias. At the height of World War II, male nurses began the push for equal opportunities for both sexes within the profession. Researcher and educator Dr. Luther P. Christman objected to the taboo against men in the military nurse corps and petitioned legislators with copies of a snide letter from a U.S. surgeon general disdaining the use of male nurses in battle zones, which were off-limits to women. A facile spokesperson, Christman carried his crusade into other venues, teaching at Cooper Hospital School of Nursing in Philadelphia, establishing nurse-physician teams at State Hospital in Yankton, South Dakota, and participating in the first national committee on postgraduate training. Active in the American Nurses Association, he completed a doctorate, taught at the University of Michigan, and served Vanderbilt University as dean of nursing. He was founder and dean emeritus of the College of Nursing at Rush University in Chicago, was named a distinguished alumnus of Temple University, and earned a lifetime achievement award from Sigma Theta Tau for achievement in nursing practice, research, education, creativity, leadership, and professional standards. In his honor, the American Association for Men in Nursing, which he founded to serve all nurses, presents an annual Luther Christman Award.

The issue of homosexuality in the military entered nursing history with the case of career soldier Colonel Margarethe Cammermeyer, a native of Norway who holds a Ph.D. in nursing and operated a successful seizure clinic. For patriotic reasons, she joined the U.S. Army Nurse Corps, served in Vietnam, earned the Bronze Star, and was named Veterans Administration Nurse of the Year. Her unblemished record ended in ignominy on April 28, 1989, when she replied candidly to a question about her relationship with artist Diane Divelbess. After lengthy investigation, the army discharged Cammermeyer on June 12, 1992; she filed suit for the unexpected slight on a spotless twenty-three-year service record. Her successful fight against discrimination won her reinstatement in July 1994. She resumed her career as chief nurse of the Washington National Guard and currently supports gay rights in the Seattle area. Barbara Streisand produced an Emmy-winning film, *Serving in Silence: The Margarethe Cammermeyer Story* (1994), based on Cammermeyer's autobiography. The screen version starred Glenn Close and Judy Davis as the much-debated lesbian couple. In April 1998, Cammermeyer, forcibly retired at age 55, launched a congressional campaign for a seat on the Washington state delegation.

Essential to a study of these gender issues is the recognition of synergy in medical history. Examples abound of men and women working cohesively, as with the influence of Jean-Henri Dunant's Red Cross on Clara Barton, founder of the American Red Cross, and the selflessness of Ethiopia's Princess Tsahaí Haíle Selassíe, who died while upgrading her father's realm by extending nurse care to poor peasants. United efforts remain the hope of those who support gender parity in the twentieth century. One heroine of American midwives, Mary Breckinridge, established the Frontier Nursing Service in Kentucky after studying Sir Leslie McKenzie's highlands and islands district midwifery practice in Scotland's Outer Hebrides. Thus, her adaptation of a man's system produced a triumph of women's nursing history.

During twentieth-century wars, women's opinions earned respect. At the beginning of the Spanish-American War, Isabel Hampton Robb offered to assist the government as agent for nurses. She led the Nurses' Associated Alumni of the United States and Canada in wartime recruitment of nurses. Dr. Anita Newcomb McGee, the nursing organizer of the era, convinced U.S. surgeon general George M. Sternberg to convene a Hospital Corps Committee, sponsored by the Daughters of the American Revolution, to augment the services of Mabel Boardman and the Red Cross. Still, antifemale feeling persisted; for example, in her writings, Spanish-American War nurse Estelle Hine identified the attitudes of corpsmen and ward masters as deterrents to quality nurse care. In the war's aftermath, one sign of women's progress was the creation of an all-female Army Nurse Corps with Dita H. Kinney as supervisor. During the Vietnam War, the equalization of nursing roles for men and women thrust home to Americans after nurses Eleanor Grace Alexander, Jeremy Olmstead, Hedwig Diane Orlowski, and Kenneth Shoemaker died in a plane crash November 30, 1967, outside Qui Nhon. By 1993, Diane Carlson Evants had evened out honor to female nurses by soliciting donations for the Vietnam Women's Memorial, sculpted by Glenna Goodacre and placed in Washington, D.C., alongside the famed "Wall," the soldiers' name for the first Vietnam memorial, designed by Maya Lin.

Peacetime brought men and women together in the search for answers to pervasive problems. In the 1970s, as feminism gained strength, Ruth Lubic made a courageous stand for childbirth centers as an alternative to male-centered hospital maternity wards and delivery rooms in the United States. By enlarging the role of fathers, children, and midwives, she reintroduced community-based parturient experiences and a normalization of childbirth. In the 1980s, Mother Clara Hale quietly worked her way into the governmental and philanthropic establishment through the media. As word of her one-woman battle to help babies addicted to drugs and infected with AIDS spread in interviews and eyewitness accounts, purse strings loosened. After President Ronald Reagan publicly proclaimed her devotion to nurse care, she channeled national attention to extend her model of child care to a string of children's homes.

Other individuals have pooled wisdom and creativity in the hospice movement. The work of William Hoare, Dr. Cicely Saunders, Quaker philanthropist Elizabeth Gurney Fry, Catherine McPardan, Ida M. Martinson, Dr. Elisabeth Kübler-Ross, Dr. Melvin Krant, Mother Teresa, Sister Frances Dominica, Ann Armstrong Dailey, Dr. Jean Quint Benoliel, Florence Wald, and Collin Murray Parkes has furthered an international concern for the dying, including suffering children and prisoners.

See also: Midwifery; Navy Nurse Corps; Sanger, Margaret; Spanish-American War; Stopes, Marie; Twentieth-Century Nursing

Sources

Allen, Lisa. "Lesbian Congressional Candidate Visits Indy." http://www.starnews.com/news/election/98/104/0417SN_cammermeyer.html.

"Alumni Information." http://www.temple.edu/education/alumni/REDLT.HTM.

"American Assembly for Men in Nursing." http://www.nursingcenter.com/people/nrsorgs/aamn.

Baker, Nina Brown. "Cyclone in Calico." *Reader's Digest* (December 1952): 141–162.

Brooks, Diane. "Cammermeyer Says She's Ready to Run." http://www.seattletimes.com/extra/browse/html97/camm_111197.html.

Byerly, Dr. W. Grimes, personal interview, August 18, 1998.

"Civil War Nurses." http://www.wayne.esu1.k12.ne.us/civil/morris.html.

Denney, Robert E. *Civil War Medicine: Care and Comfort of the Wounded.* New York: Sterling Publishing, 1995.

Dolan, Josephine A., R.N. *History of Nursing.* Philadelphia: W. B. Saunders, 1968.

Farmborough, Florence. *With the Armies of the Tsar: A Nurse at the Russian Front, 1914–1918.* New York: Stein and Day, 1974.

Gelbart, Nina. *King's Midwife: A History and Mystery of Madame du Coudray.* Berkeley: University of California Press, 1998.

"Histories of the School of Nursing." http://www.rush.edu/Departments/Archives/Nursing/index.html.

"A History of Helping Others." http://www.redcross.org/pa/lancaste/history.htm.

Holland, Mary A. Gardner, comp. *Our Army Nurses.* Boston: Lounsberry, Nichols and Worth, 1896.

Hufton, Olwen. *The Prospect before Her: A History of Women in Western Europe, 1500–1800.* New York: Vintage Books, 1995.

Kenny, Elizabeth. *And They Shall Walk.* North Stratford, N.H.: Ayer, 1980.

Kidder, Nicole. "'Serving in Silence' Author Margarethe Cammermeyer Shares Her Life Story." http://www.seattleu.edu/student/spec/02–20–97/news01.html.

Laurence, Leslie, and Beth Weinhouse. *Outrageous Practices: How Gender Bias Threatens Women's Health.* New Brunswick, N.J.: Rutgers University Press, 1997.

Lyons, Albert S., M.D., and R. Joseph Petrucelli, M.D. *Medicine: An Illustrated History.* New York: Abrams, 1987.

Marks, Geoffrey, and William K. Beatty. *Women in White.* New York: Charles Scribner's Sons, 1972.

Marland, Hilary, ed. *The Art of Midwifery: Early Modern Midwives in Europe.* London: Routledge, 1993.

McClain, Carol Shepherd. *Women as Healers: Cross-Cultural Perspectives.* New Brunswick, N.J.: University of Rutgers Press, 1989.

McGregor, Deborah Kuhn. "'Childbirth-Travells' and 'Spiritual Estates': Anne Hutchinson and Colonial Boston, 1634–1638." *Caduceus* (1989): 1–33.

McKown, Robin. *Heroic Nurses.* New York: G. P. Putnam's Sons, 1966.

Meier, Louis A. *Healing of an Army, 1777–1778.* Norristown, Pa.: Historical Society of Montgomery County, 1991.

Moore, Frank. *Women of the War: Their Heroism and Self-Sacrifice.* Hartford, Conn.: S. S. Scranton, 1866.

Mor, V. *Hospice Care Systems.* New York: Springer, 1987.

Mor, V., D. S. Gree, and Robert Kastenbaum. *The Hospice Experiment.* Baltimore: Johns Hopkins University Press, 1988.

Mosley, Leonard. *Haile Selassie: The Conquering Lion.* Englewood Cliffs, N.J.: Prentice-Hall, 1964.

"Naomi Deutsch." *Pacific Coast Journal of Nursing* (September 1934): 487–488.

Perrone, Bobette, H. Henrietta Stockel, and Victoria Krueger. *Medicine Women, Curanderas, and Women Doctors.* Norman: University of Oklahoma Press, 1989.

Pryor, Elizabeth Brown. *Clara Barton: Professional Angel.* Philadelphia: University of Pennsylvania Press, 1987.

Rose, June. *Marie Stopes and the Sexual Revolution.* London: Faber and Faber, 1993.

Ross, Ishbel. *Angel of the Battlefield.* New York: Harper and Brothers Publishers, 1956.

"Ruth Watson Lubic." *Current Biography Yearbook.* New York: Bowker, 1996, 328–332.

Saywell, John T., ed. *The Canadian Journal of Lady Aberdeen, 1893–1898.* Toronto: Champlain Society, 1960.

Sherr, Lynn, and Jurate Kazickas. *Susan B. Anthony Slept Here: A Guide to American Women's Landmarks.* New York: Times Books, 1994.

Snodgrass, Mary Ellen. *Late Achievers: Famous People Who Succeeded Late in Life.* Englewood, Colo.: Libraries Unlimited, 1992.

Sponselli, Christina. "Vaccine Volunteer." http://www.nurseweek.com/features/97–11/miramontes.html.

Spruill, Julia. *Women's Life and Work in the Southern Colonies.* New York: W. W. Norton, 1972.

Sterne, Capt. Doris M. *In and Out of Harm's Way: A History of the Navy Nurse Corps.* Seattle, Wash.: Peanut Butter Publishing, 1996.

Ward, Geoffrey C. "Queen Barton." *American Heritage* (April 1988): 14–15.

Wilbur, C. Keith, M.D. *Revolutionary Medicine, 1700–1800.* Old Saybrook, Conn.: Globe Pequot Press, 1997.

Gillespie, Mother Angela

The first staff administrator of a navy nurse corps, Mother Angela Gillespie served aboard the steamer *Red Rover* in 1862 at the height of the Civil War, supervising four nuns, five black nurse's aides, and an unspecified number of former slaves in flight from the South. Born Eliza Maria Gillespie on February 21, 1824, outside Brownsville, Pennsylvania, she attended a nearby girls academy, then boarding school in Somerset, Ohio, from 1836 to 1838. At age sixteen, she entered Visitation Academy in Georgetown, a suburb of Washington, D.C. Later she trained in administration at the Holy Cross School of Nursing at Saint Mary's College of the University of Notre Dame in South Bend, Indiana.

Primarily an educator and writer in the first two decades of her career, Gillespie worked in her hometown and taught parish grade school until age twenty-seven. After two years on the faculty at St. Mary's Seminary, a nondenominational state school in St. Mary's City, Maryland, she entered the Sisters of Mercy, a Chicago order dedicated to service. While visiting her brother at the Notre Dame seminary, she came under the influence of the institution's founder, Father Edward F. Sorin, who persuaded her to transfer to a French order, the Sisters of the Holy Cross. Under the formal title Sister Mary of St. Angela, she took the veil in April of her twenty-ninth year, when she entered a novitiate in Caen, France, preparatory to a post as director of St. Mary's Academy in Bertrand, Michigan, two years later.

A strong advocate of equal education for women, Mother Angela established course work in philosophy, mathematics, science, modern foreign languages, theology, art, and music. Her mission influenced the order's work in Chicago and Morris, Illinois. In 1860, she published *Metropolitan Readers,* an original series for primary, elementary, and advanced classes. She began editing the Catholic journal *Ave Maria* in 1866.

During this productive period of teaching and textbook authorship, Mother Angela, like other nuns and laywomen during the Civil War, offered her services to the military. Beginning in 1861 under the sponsorship of General Ulysses S. Grant, she supplied an emergency corps of nurses to the wounded and disabled wherever the need arose and administered a trained, highly disciplined nurse corps in army hospitals in Paducah and Louisville, Kentucky; Cairo, Illinois; Memphis, Tennessee; and Washington, D.C. Part of her contribution in 1862 was the establishment of a navy nurse corps aboard the *Red Rover,* a Confederate steamer confiscated and equipped as the Union's first naval hospital ship.

An admirable example of Mother Angela's volunteer management was the reclamation of storage buildings on the waterfront of Mound City, Illinois, which she converted into a fifteen-hundred-bed military hospital. Spurned by male surgeons as weak females, she and her dozen aides commandeered the wards and supervised apathetic corpsmen. The introduction of eggs, milk, rice, and chicken to the patient diet raised spirits and established that female nurses had much to offer the military. By writing hundreds of letters begging for clothing, canned fruits, jelly, wine, and provisions, she obtained the supplies to create a convalescent haven. Once more uprooted in 1862, she administered Overton Hospital in an old hotel in Memphis, Tennessee. Under fire, she traveled the river for the United States Sanitary Commission to ferry wounded and sick men and supplies to their destination. When marauders attempted to climb ladders and shoot Colonel Fry through the hospital window, Mother Angela stood in the way and refused to give ground. Fortunately, her challengers were not prepared to murder a nun and departed without firing a shot.

Mother Angela was the impetus to the expansion of her order and the establishment of an independent American branch after 1869. Between 1855 and 1882, she founded forty-five institutions. In a span of four years, she commissioned educational facilities in Austin, Texas; Baltimore, Maryland; Salt Lake City, Utah; and Washington, D.C. At her death at St. Mary's Convent in South Bend, Indiana, on March 4, 1887, after a vigorous life of service to the convent, education, and military nursing, she was honored as a war hero and the founder of the American Sisters of the Holy Cross.

Sources

Denney, Robert E. *Civil War Medicine: Care and Comfort of the Wounded.* New York: Sterling Publishing, 1995.

"First!" http://www.bluejacket.com/first.htm.

Holland, Mary A. Gardner, comp. *Our Army Nurses.* Boston: Lounsberry, Nichols and Worth, 1896.

"Mother Angela Gillespie." http://women.eb.com/women/articles/Gillespie_Mother_Angela.html.

Sterne, Capt. Doris M. *In and Out of Harm's Way: A History of the Navy Nurse Corps.* Seattle, Wash.: Peanut Butter Publishing, 1996.

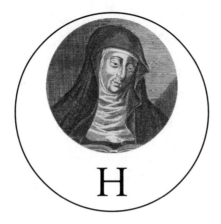

H

Hale, Clara

Returning to the earliest model of nursing, altruist and child guardian Clara Hale, called the "Mother Teresa of New York," spent her retirement years mothering and nursing a total of one thousand unwanted youngsters and special-needs babies from the East Coast drug corridor (Hine, Brown, and Terborg-Penn 1993, 513). Within Harlem's underworld misery of crack houses and death-in-life addiction, Hale House offered hope to infants born with the craving for controlled substances. Hale herself fostered infants for mothers who were forced by law to wean themselves from drugs before claiming their children.

An uneducated caregiver, Hale treated sick children instinctively. Anchored in her bentwood rocker, she nestled and soothed, petted and sang to retrieve the smallest addicts from a hellish undertow of detoxification, which causes gagging, vomiting, itching, runny noses, spasms, diarrhea, and self-mutilation. Her love of handicapped, neglected, and HIV-positive children won national acclaim. The media reported her simple one-on-one methods of treating the sick with patience and acceptance and murmurs that God loves them. In her words, "They love you to tell them how great they are, how good they are.

Somehow, even at a young age, they understand that" (Edmonds 1992, 2A).

Clara Hale learned from her own mother the importance of hands-on tenderness and a ready forgiveness of human error. A Philadelphia native born on April 1, 1905, Hale and her brother Nathan were two of the ten children her mother reared. A high school dropout, Hale married Thomas "Sam" Hale, owner of a successful floor-waxing and window-washing service. She augmented their income by cleaning theaters. In 1932, she weathered his death from cancer and nurtured sons Nathan and Kenneth and daughter Lorraine as she had promised. To supervise them in a slum environment, she ended work as a domestic and opened a child-care service in her Harlem apartment. Describing the new career, she admitted, "I didn't make a whole lot, but I wasn't starving. And the kids must've liked it because once they got there, they didn't want to go home. So what started as day care ended up being full-time" (*Current Biography* 1985, 165). In the first forty foster children she received from the Department of Social Services, she instilled a desire for education and a determination to live drug-free.

After retiring in 1968, Hale accepted a new challenge from her daughter, child specialist

Dr. Lorraine Hale, who retrieved a toddler from an addicted mother she found slumped on a park bench. The first placement grew to many more as the drug underground spread the news that Clara Hale would receive their children without hassle, charge, or lectures on morality until the mothers were able to form a stable home. Her only requirement was a weekly visit from each mother to sustain the tenuous parent-child link. Although her facility was licensed for twenty children, baby beds filled the tiny flat for the first year as Hale cared for thirty to forty abandoned children on her own funds and those of her three children. Gradually, she guided sick babies through the crying and withdrawal pain and passivity to normal behaviors.

As the drug scene raged out of control in the 1970s and early 1980s, New York City authorities attempted to stem the 10–12 percent death rate from postnatal addiction in offspring of heroin users. The multiple woes of low birth weight, respiratory irregularities, poor concentration, and learning disabilities doomed the survivors to a dependent life. To Percy Sutton, a Manhattan official seeking respite for the city's youngest citizens, Mother Hale was a godsend. He augmented her slender means by locating private funding as well as city, state, and federal allocations. Two admirers, singer-composer John Lennon and his wife, artist Yoko Ono, offered $20,000 annually, which enabled Hale to train staff in her personal nursing style.

At age seventy, Hale moved to 154 West 122nd Street, a five-story brownstone known as Hale House. In addition to dining room, kitchen, playroom, and nursery, she added hall mirrors as positive reinforcement so children could learn to identify themselves and to acknowledge personal strengths and weaknesses. On the third floor, she created a private room intended for her reception of each troubled newcomer, whose initial treatment lasted for two weeks. She refused Phenobarbital, paregoric, and methadone as she guided each addicted child through a cold turkey separation from drugs. In cribs alongside her own bed and in lengthy bouts of rocking and walking the floor, she withstood the terrors of weaning the system from its unseen torment. She said of her regimen: "The children here know that someone loves them and they're happy. I make sure that they're always clean and well fed and comfortable. I tell them how pretty they are; and what they can accomplish if they get an education. And I tell them to be proud of their Blackness, to be proud of one another, and to pull together" (Johnson 1986, 58). The day-and-night battle built trust that slowly relaxed twisted bodies and halted jerking limbs and bursts of sobs. With Hale's arms about them, they settled into contentment.

On her own, Hale accepted the challenge of changing diapers, filling bottles with formula, spooning in fruit and cereal, and mopping up drool. An adjacent medical and dental clinic provided critical care, but her steady nursing was the real source of emotional control and stronger bodies to fight infections prevalent among addicted babies. Of her first five hundred, only twelve were offered for adoption and eleven placed with foster families. As crack cocaine supplanted heroin in Harlem, sicker babies proved less predictable and more susceptible to a host of physical weaknesses and aberrant behaviors. For the first time, Hale experienced the deaths of three infants too diminished to survive.

Hale persevered in her mission, drawing referrals from the police, churches, emergency rooms, and mothers snared by addiction. Her budget mounted to $3.5 million, which underwrote programs to rehabilitate mothers and lodge those too sick with AIDS to earn a living. Seventeen years into her work, Hale came to the attention of President Ronald Reagan, who extolled her goodness on February 16, 1985, in his State of the Union speech to Congress. He cited her nightly attention to tormented children as proof that "anything is possible in America if we have the faith, the will and the heart" (Hacker 1986, n.p.). Proclaimed an American hero, she violated doctor's orders and tentatively visited the White House to shake hands with the nation's dignitaries. The experience brought a deluge of donors who enabled her to expand the receiving home at a new address, where mothers could spend time with their children and perpetuate a family bond.

As Clara Hale grew too frail to continue the pace, her daughter Lorraine began the administrative work that broadened Hale House to a chain of facilities around the country. Hale continued working with the sickest infants, whom she could barely lift. Her glass shelf of memorabilia displayed snapshots of youngsters in caps and gowns, reunited families, an autographed photo of Yoko Ono, one of Nancy and Ronald Reagan, and another of the president shaking hands with Hale. She was interviewed on "Amen" and "The Phil Donahue Show," assisted in a filmed study of her methods, and accepted two citations from the Salvation Army, including the Booth Community Service Award, Truman Award for Public Service, Leonard H. Carter Humanitarian Award, an honorary degree from the John Jay College of Criminal Justice, and a mother of the year award from the National Mother's Day Committee. Her daughter drew up plans for a larger child-care complex and a hospice for dying babies. Shortly after earning a high school equivalency diploma, Hale died on December 18, 1992, of complications from a stroke. The success of her common-sense child care brought the nation's thanks and the love of grown men and women who survived addiction because of her love.

Sources

Bidel, Susan. "When Mom's a Hard Act to Follow." *Woman's Day,* May 22, 1990, 88.

Carcaterra, Lorenzo. "Mother Hale of Harlem Has Saved 487 Drug-Addicted Babies with an Old Miracle Cure: Love." *People,* March 5, 1984, 211–214.

"Clara Hale to Get Truman Award for Public Service." *Jet,* March 20, 1989, 23.

Current Biography. New York: H. W. Wilson, 1985.

Edmonds, Patricia. "Harlem's 'Mother Hale' Dies; Took in 1,000 Babies." *USA Today,* December 21, 1992, 2A.

"$50,000 Rehab House for Cocaine-Addicted Babies." *Jet,* January 25, 1988, 23.

Hacker, Kathy. "Mother Hale: A Savior and Her Growing Mission." *Philadelphia Inquirer,* May 7, 1986.

"Hale Receives $1.1 Million to Expand Home for Babies." *Jet,* May 19, 1986, 26.

Hine, Darlene Clark, Elsa Barkley Brown, and Rosalyn Terborg-Penn, eds. *Black Women in America: An Historical Encyclopedia.* Bloomington: Indiana University Press, 1993.

Johnson, Herschel. "Clara (Mother) Hale: Healing Baby 'Junkies' with Love." *Ebony* (May 1986): 58–61.

Lanker, Brian, and Maya Angelou. "I Dream a World." *National Geographic,* August 1989, 206–226.

"Mother Hale Appears on NBC-TV's 'Amen' Series." *Jet,* February 19, 1990.

"Mother Hale Honored." *Jet,* July 10, 1989, 22.

"Mother Hale's Help." *Jet,* May 25, 1987, 36.

Nimmons, David. "The Santa Claus Awards." *Ladies' Home Journal* (December 1986): 122–129, 168.

"Ordinary Women of Grace: Subjects of the 'I Dream a World' Photography Exhibit." *U.S. News and World Report,* February 13, 1989, 54.

"Reagan Cites Clara Hale as a 'Hero' in Union Address." *Jet,* February 25, 1985, 6.

Safran, Claire. "Mama Hale and Her Little Angels." *Reader's Digest* (September 1984): 49–54.

Smith, Jesse Carney. *Notable Black American Women.* Detroit: Gale, 1992.

Snodgrass, Mary Ellen. *Late Achievers: Famous People Who Succeeded Late in Life.* Englewood, Colo.: Libraries Unlimited, 1992.

Winter, Annette. "Spotlight." *Modern Maturity* (October-November 1988): 18.

Hasson, Esther

The first chief of the U.S. Navy Nurse Corps, Esther Voorhees Hasson came to the post with war experience. Born in Baltimore, Maryland, she was the daughter of an army surgeon and veteran of the Civil War; her brother was an Annapolis graduate and naval officer until his death in 1903. Hasson attended private schools in Washington, D.C., and Germantown, Pennsylvania, before entering the Connecticut Training School for Nurses in New Haven and enlisting in the Army Nurse Corps.

During the Spanish-American War, Dr. Anita Newcomb McGee selected Hasson to serve the navy as a contract surgical nurse aboard the USS *Relief.* She wrote, "Therefore, with youth and enthusiasm sufficient to counteract the rather depressing prospect of $30 per month and one ration in kind, I started out on the Great Adventure" (Kalisch and Kalisch 1978, 205). Spiffy in a new coat of white paint girdled in green and flying the Red Cross banner alongside the Stars and Stripes, the steamer, recommissioned on May 18, 1898, was transformed into a hospital ship to evacuate the sick and wounded. In the three small rooms allotted as nurse's quarters, Hasson and her staff made do with minuscule stow holes and two drawers each for personal possessions.

Following the Battle of Santiago Bay, the USS *Relief* departed Tampa for the steamy harbor at Siboney, Cuba, on July 3. According to Hasson's unpublished manuscript, now housed in the National Archives, she and five other nurses admired the x-ray room, surgical suite, and four wards, three for enlisted men and a smaller one for officers. The influx of casualties included one with a gunshot wound and the rest ill with yellow fever, malaria, typhoid, and dysentery. In its first two months of service, the vessel received 1,485 patients, of whom sixty-five died, for a mortality rate of 4.3 percent.

After questioning by a board of examiners in first aid, therapeutics, and drugs and medical equipment, on August 18, 1908, Hasson accepted the post of superintendent of the U.S. Navy Nurse Corps. Written proofs of proficiency included a biography, an outline of military nursing duties, and a description of military organization. A demanding, idealistic public relations agent, Hasson welcomed her duties and roomed at leased housing in Washington, D.C., where she and other nurses provided their own cooking and laundry. Among her tasks was standardizing expectations and regulations for nurses at eighteen general hospitals and standardizing training procedures for hospital corpsmen, who were often the only medical personnel on board ship. In her first month, she also oversaw the appointment of chief nurses Victoria White and Martha E. Pringle. By October, the full corps rose to twenty members, called

the "Sacred Twenty" both in admiration and mocking good humor. Treated like officers, Hasson and her fellow nurses were neither enlisted nor commissioned personnel and endured the sneers of misogynists both in the military and among civilians.

Hasson published a definitive article on the Navy Nurse Corps in the March 1909 issue of *American Journal of Nursing.* Proclaiming the first navy nurses "pioneers," she added, "It rests with us to make the traditions and to set the pace for those who are to follow" (Sterne 1996, 21). Her service ended in resignation in 1911 after a series of insults and pressures from the surgeon general, Walter Wyman.

Sources

Dolan, Josephine A., R.N. *History of Nursing.* Philadelphia: W. B. Saunders, 1968.

Kalisch, Philip, and Beatrice J. Kalisch. *The Advance of American Nursing.* Boston: Little, Brown, 1978.

Sterne, Capt. Doris M. *In and Out of Harm's Way: A History of the Navy Nurse Corps.* Seattle, Wash.: Peanut Butter Publishing, 1996.

Hildegard of Bingen

In the twelfth century, St. Hildegard of Bingen, an exorcist, preacher, and prophet, was the first female in the Western world acknowledged as a church savant. As abbess of the Rupertsberg convent in the Rhineland, she pioneered natural and mystical *physica* (healing methods for application to body and mind). To Hippocrates' emphasis on the anamnesis (medical history), diagnosis in the present, and prognosis of future health of impairment, she added new meaning to wellness, a prognostic factor that became her focus. She lauded examination of the eyes as a study of the patient's physical and mental state. Consulting the Bible as well as intuition, she composed medical texts in Latin, drawing on botany for her unique description of the body's *viriditas* (greening power).

Born in 1098 of noble parentage on a country estate in Bückelhein on the Nahe River near Sponheim, from age eight Hildegard, the family's tenth child, displayed clair-

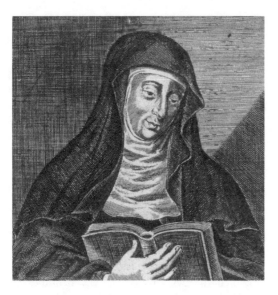

Hildegard of Bingen (Wellcome Institute Library, London)

voyance. Naturally pious and observant, she studied at the Disibodenberg cloister under the tutelage of her aunt, Abbess Yutta (or Jutta) von Sponheim, a reclusive Benedictine nun who taught her reading, composition, music and psalm singing, and needlework. At age sixteen, Hildegard made her vows; in 1136, she succeeded Yutta. A blend of seer and mystic and the chief medical writer of the time, she explained the source of her wisdom: "I see these things not with my external eyes, nor do I hear them with my external ears. I see them rather only in my soul with my bodily eyes wide open, so that I am never overcome by ecstatic unconsciousness, but see these things when I am awake during the day and during the night" (Strehlow and Herzka 1988, 140). To elucidate her visions in physical terms, she claimed to see a light within a light, the *lux vivens* (living light) that stripped away sadness and fear and returned her faculties to those of a young girl.

Relying on inner powers, herbs, and scrupulous cleanliness, Hildegard directed the care of parturient mothers. To enlarge her understanding of the circulatory and nervous systems, she concealed from the outside world her dissection of animal and possibly human carcasses. As a standardization of folk healing for nuns in monasteries, she compiled a reference book of simples, *Liber Simplicis Medicinae* (Book of Healing Herbs), and composed a two-stage medical text, *Liber Compositae Medicinae et Causae et Curae* (Book of Medical Treatment and Causes and Cures). In the latter, she recommended licorice for eye disease and lily roots for leprosy. An adjunct text, *Liber Vitae Meritorum* (Book of Life's Merits), written in 1163, is a psychotherapy handbook and study of the subconscious that notes the effects of spirituality on the body and the workings of thirty-five toxic emotions, notably anger, lust, greed, despair, and religious doubt. Her idiosyncratic methods were so intriguing that the archbishop of Mainz dispatched a monk to record her visions, which appeared in *Scivias* (That You May Know), an eleven-year project completed in 1152.

In 1147, Hildegard superintended the building of a convent at Rupertsberg, where patients thronged for counseling. During this fertile period of outreach, she corresponded with a list of rulers, bishops, popes, and commoners and composed a hymnal, *Symphonia Harmonia Coelestium Revolutionum* (The Harmonic Symphony of Heavenly Revolutions). She kept a journal, *Aphorism* (Sayings), and compiled a medieval curiosity, *Lingua Ignota* (The Unknown Language), a nine-hundred-word text in an unidentified code. She established a second priory at Eibingen in 1165.

Into her late seventies, Hildegard rode horseback and traveled by boat along the Rhine, Main, and Mosel rivers, leading a troop of nuns and medical students to patients in distant villages. By the time of her death on September 17, 1180 (alternately given as 1179 and 1181), her work had established the need for women's colleges. When her collected writings, published in nine volumes in the sixteenth century as *Physica St. Hildegardis*, were reclaimed by twentieth-century feminists, new students of her health and diet advice rediscovered the importance to digestive health of water and fiber from whole grains.

Sources

Bentley, James. *A Calendar of Saints.* London: Little, Brown, 1993.

Dock, Lavinia, and Isabel M. Stewart. *A Short History of Nursing.* New York: G. P. Putnam's Sons, 1938.

Dolan, Josephine A., R.N. *History of Nursing.* Philadelphia: W. B. Saunders, 1968.

Fischer-Kamel, Doris Sofie. "The Midwife in History with Special Emphasis on Practice in Medieval Europe and in the Islamic World." University of Arizona, 1987. Monograph.

Hallam, Elizabeth, general ed. *Saints: Who They Are and How They Help You.* New York: Simon and Schuster, 1994.

Jamieson, Elizabeth, and Mary F. Sewall. *Trends in Nursing History.* London: W. B. Saunders, 1949.

Magic and Medicine of Plants. Pleasantville, N.Y.: Reader's Digest, 1986.

Marks, Geoffrey, and William K. Beatty. *Women in White.* New York: Charles Scribner's Sons, 1972.

Ranft, Patricia. *Women and the Religious Life in Premodern Europe.* New York: St. Martin's Press, 1996.

Strehlow, Dr. Wighard, and Gottfried Herzka, M.D. *Hildegard of Bingen's Medicine.* Santa Fe: Bear and Company, 1988.

Williams, Marty Newman, and Anne Echols. *Between Pit and Pedestal: Women in the Middle Ages.* Princeton, N.J.: Markus Wiener Publishers, 1994.

Hospice

From early times, religious and secular societies have created separate housing for the sick or bereft, as demonstrated by St. Fiacre of Ireland, who opened a hospice in France and treated dying patients around 650 A.D. Archeological evidence pinpoints religious shelters in the worship centers of Greece, India, Egypt, Rome, and China. Nurse care was the task of healers or lay workers drawn to the needs of the acutely and terminally ill. In 1134 B.C., Greek plague victims were received in quarantine huts. In subsequent eras, foreigners came under the protection of the guest code, a pervasive Mediterranean code of conduct that mandated the humane and ethical treatment of strangers and visitors. By 600 B.C., Aesculapius, the father of medicine in the Western world, was elevated to a god for his care of the poor and sick. In his honor, hospices were called *aesculapia.* In India in 225 B.C., the emperor Asoka opened a similar hospice for religious pilgrims journeying to the sacred Ganges River, where they committed their bodies to be burned and the ashes scattered on the waters.

The term "hospice" derives from the Roman *hospes,* a term that is the parent of hospice, hospital, hostel, and hotel. The Romans themselves preferred the Greek term, *xenodochium,* a reception area for wanderers, pilgrims, and refugees who needed lodging and short-term care. After the establishment of Christianity in the first century, moral duty outlined by Christ impelled the devout to "love thy neighbor as thyself," a binding command that translated into the reception and nurturance of the abandoned waif, handicapped, sick, aged, mentally infirm, and injured. The value of Christian nursing and sacrifice relieved suffering on earth and elevated caregivers in heaven, a concept shared by Buddhists and Hindus.

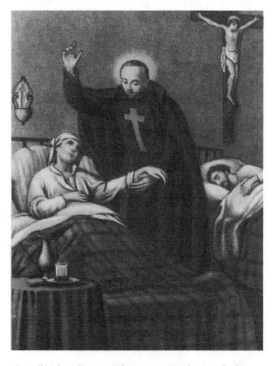

Camillus de Lellis, named patron saint of nurses for his innovative work in treating plague victims in the sixteenth century (Mary Evans Picture Library)

In 325 A.D., the Council of Nicaea sent decrees to Christian bishops to create hospices for palliative care as adjuncts to worship centers. Constantine, the first Christian emperor of Rome, expanded the church's mission by converting *aesculapia* to *xenodocia*, thus broadening the care of weary travelers. Monastery attendants and volunteers oversaw male and female inmates in separate facilities for healing, feeding, bandaging, rehabilitating, and supporting those in need. Late in the fourth century, Fabiola, a Roman aristocrat and nurse converted by St. Jerome, imported the nurturing concepts of the monasteries in the Holy Land by opening an unbiased reception center free to all comers at Ostia, Rome's seaport. Another late Byzantine hospice is credited to St. Bridget in Ireland in 500 A.D., and other establishments included one at Mount Cenis in 825 A.D. and St. Bernard's Augustinian hospices, the Great and Little St. Bernard passes in Valle d'Aosta, Italy, in 962 A.D., a facility made famous by his great shaggy dogs, who sniffed out lost travelers beneath the snow and revived them with draughts of brandy and the warmth of their fur. Muslim hospices grew out of a parallel ethos in the Islamic world. Sharing the knowledge of Aesculapius and Hippocrates, Arab caregivers evolved their own procedures and treatments that reentered the Western world during the Renaissance, when learned teachers added the works of Maimonides and Avicenna to the liberal arts and sciences.

In the Middle Ages, wanderers to and from the Crusades of the late eleventh century required wayside hospices, which sprang up where the demand was heaviest. Within two centuries, Europe boasted 820 facilities—thirty in Florence, forty in Paris, and 750 in England. Grounded in Christian dogma, these reception centers featured biblical symbols and lore in tapestries, murals, and stained glass windows. Simple but clean and inviting accommodations awaited wayfarers in wards where monks treated body and soul together in a peaceful, comforting atmosphere. Atria treated ambulatory patients and

their caregivers to fragrant oleander, palm, geranium, and citrus trees. All devout caregivers, in accordance with Catholic dictates, adhered to a strict lifestyle of poverty, chastity, and obedience. Warriors themselves supported this move toward hospices. The Knights Hospitallers of St. John built facilities on the route southeast from Europe to Syria. The Order of St. John constructed additional sites on the islands of Malta and Rhodes. The preponderance of patients were male, but a few, such as the St. Mary Magdalene Hospice, accepted females.

Folco Portinari, a banker, civic leader, and philanthropist, in Florence, Italy, founded the city's oldest hospital, Santa Maria Nuova, beyond the city walls. A charity hospice for the destitute and dying, it opened in 1288 with twelve beds. In 1296, it expanded with wards for male and female patients and welcomed plague victims.

The Renaissance made its own inroads against neglect or inhumane treatment of the dying, particularly in north and central Italy. In the mid–fifteenth century, St. Catherine of Bologna taught the Poor Clares to nurse, diagnose, and succor the dying. In Milan, St. Charles of Borromeo set up a hospice for plague victims. Guided by St. Philip Neri, in 1584, St. Camillus de Lellis of Naples, Italy, a Capuchin monk, established his ministry in a Venetian hospital and founded the Society of Servants of the Sick or Camillians, who treated victims of the plague in wards, on board ships in the harbor, and in combat in Hungary and Croatia. For his innovative regimens of fresh air, improved diet, and isolation for plague victims, he was named patron saint of nurses.

In the seventeenth century, the Catholic concept of succor for the dying survived in the century-old hospitals of the French Catholics in Quebec, the 1747 building plan of Father Francisco Xavier Ortiz in San Antonio, Texas, and St. Vincent de Paul's hospices for the orphaned, poor, sick, and dying in Paris. Staffed by Daughters of Charity, Vincentian organizations produced good works that influenced the Kaiserwerth Hospice in Prussia, staffed by Protestant sisters. Still in existence in the 1850s, these orders assisted Florence Nightingale's work at Scutari, Turkey, during the Crimean War. Civilian hospices, staffed by barber-surgeons, midwives, apothecaries, lay healers, and physicians, provided services for society's poorest, who could not afford home visits or private duty caregivers. Among the needy were the victims of the Industrial Revolution, when tuberculosis, typhoid fever, and industrial accidents and pollution shortened the lives of miners and workers clustered in unhealthy, unsanitary industrial centers.

As the medical profession evolved in dignity and value, physicians sought a reputation for success and tended to reject chronic or incurable patients, who often resorted to almshouses and workhouses during their final hours. Satirized and lambasted by Charles Dickens's novels, these facilities deserved their horrific reputation as warehouses for the unwanted. A peak in death houses occurred during the Irish potato famine, when religious caregivers claimed rejects from city hospitals. In 1879, Sister Mary Aikenhead of the Irish Sisters of Charity, a follower of Florence Nightingale, spearheaded Our Lady's Hospice and first applied the word hospice to a reception center and final home for the dying. Two decades after her death, a facility she had designed opened in Harold Cross, Dublin.

England deserves the credit for establishing the model of a national hospice network. In 1891, William Hoare opened a privately funded facility, the Hostel of God, staffed by Anglican nurses. Two years later, St. Luke's Hospice, a Methodist project, opened in the Bayswater section of London. In 1967 it became the headquarters of Dr. Cicely Saunders, founder of the contemporary hospice movement, which demedicalized the death process to free patients from the tyranny of technology and authoritarian treatment. A precedent for Saunders's work was the nineteenth-century prison reform advocacy of Elizabeth Gur-

ney Fry, a Quaker philanthropist and founder of a secular group, the Society of Protestant Sisters of Charity, who set up religious reception centers, including St. Joseph's Hospice in London.

In the 1890s, an American advocate of care for the dying, Rose Hawthorne Lathrop, daughter of author Nathaniel Hawthorne, supported centers for cancer patients. Her organization, Servants of Relief for Incurable Cancer, evolved from a volunteer effort to a religious house, Sisters of Hawthorne, an alternative to traditional medical clinics and hospitals staffed by Dominican nurses. Lathrop, working under the title Mother Alphonsa, departed from contemporary hospice programs by limiting family involvement. At the height of her advocacy, she opened St. Rose's Hospice in Manhattan, which preceded six additional free hospices in New York, Denver, Philadelphia, and St. Paul.

In this same period, Catherine McPardan provided in-home support for the terminally ill on Manhattan's Lower East Side. Her group of Irish Catholic volunteer nurses founded Calvary Hospital in New York City, one of the few U.S. facilities offering minimal forms of traditional medical treatment augmented by the two key features of a hospice— pain control and spiritual solace. Additional centers opened in the Featherbed Lane section of the Bronx, staffed by three orders of Catholic nuns—the Little Company of Mary, Dominicans of Bleauvelt, and Sisters of the Sick Poor.

The international hospice concept, a social movement embracing the normalization of the dying process, grew out of the research and work of Saunders and Dr. Elisabeth Kübler-Ross, a Swiss psychiatrist and author of On Death and Dying (1969). Both sought to reduce the trauma of terminal illness by altering traditional medical care to suit the needs of the patient. From a psychological point of view, Kübler-Ross gained broad-based public support by objecting to the isolation of the dying from normal human affairs and insisting that everyone has a stake in the public's attitude toward death. From a nursing perspective, Saunders proposed centers where holistic, nonintrusive treatment would prioritize patient concerns over medical protocols.

During the height of the AIDS epidemic in the 1980s, additional support by nurses and physicians brought hospices into the public domain as a charity worth supporting for the good of all. The combined creativity of notable caregivers evolved the idea of dying with dignity into a widespread issue, which people added to their wills and discussed with their families. Among the developers of hospice were these innovators:

- In the 1970s, Ida M. Martinson, professor and chair of the Department of Family Health Care Nursing at the University of California, completed a national model on home care for a dying child. Funded by the National Cancer Institute, the concept influenced other national programs. Martinson presided over Children's Hospice International, a global clearinghouse that encourages family-centered care for terminally ill youngsters.

- In 1974, a similar effort evolved from the work of Dr. Melvin Krant at Tufts University in Boston with support from the National Cancer Institute. The resulting Psychosocial Cancer Unit aided families and patients in coping with suffering and grief. Additional centers around the globe include Mother Teresa's ninety-eight hospices among the poor of India and Bishop Francis Chanlay's Mount Miriam Hospital in Malaysia, where Franciscan Sisters of Divine Motherhood minister to the poor.

- In 1978, Sister Frances Dominica, a pediatric nurse and superior general of the Anglican Society of All Saints, pressed for home treatment of dying children, who were ill at ease in the clangor of modern, hyperscheduled hospitals. In November 1982, her solicitation led to the opening of Helen House in Oxford, England, a pleasing eight-room facility that housed patient and parent. Adjunct amenities include a hydrotherapy pool, play and study rooms, garden, and hobby labs. Sister Dominica's model launched a series of children's hospice programs to reduce the distress of families and children, so that they can die peacefully and without pain in the arms of their parents.

- In 1983, Ann Armstrong Dailey founded Children's Hospice International, which promised shelter and care for critically ill children. In addition to nurse care, her worldwide mission offers grief support groups and nurse training programs.

- Dr. Jean Quint Benoliel, a nurse-educator and veteran of World War II, implemented psychological advancement in thanatology by training transitional nurses to ease communication between patients and caregivers. By clarifying for patients the effects of disease on their bodies, these nurses alleviated fears and provided data to make choices easier.

- Sister Florence of Les Filles de la Charité (The Daughters of Charity) in Canada countered community resistance to an AIDS hospice by opening a facility on inherited land in Martinville, Quebec. With the assistance of social worker Louise Lalonde, Sister Florence provided services to two patients whom others rejected. Because the backlash of fearful locals resulted in telephone threats and public dissension, she ended her mission to AIDS patients and converted the nuns' hospice into a battered women's shelter.

The right of dying patients to choose the amount of intervention in their final treatment—a parallel concern to hospices—provoked controversy in the 1950s. A study consortium, the International Work Group on Death, Dying, and Bereavement (IWG), coordinated the energies of several social reformers. Florence Wald, dean of Yale's nursing school, profited from the breakthroughs of Dr. Cicely Saunders, Collin Murray Parkes, and Elisabeth Kübler-Ross, noted researcher in the field of thanatology. Subsequent IWG sessions in China, England, Norway, and the United States continued to examine standards of care for the dying. By the 1960s, group interest extended from hospices to nursing schools, church and mission groups, city planners, universities, social service departments, and volunteer agencies.

Feminism added its impetus to the treatment of catastrophic illness. The rise of the women's movement empowered nurses to influence areas of patient care that had previously been reserved for the attending physician. More licensed practical nurses and registered nurses received B.S. and M.S. degrees in nursing. Their leadership ranged beyond ancillary roles to control of nurse-practitioners, Women, Infants, and Children (WIC) programs, nursing homes, birthing clinics, and home health care agencies.

First proposed in Connecticut by Florence Wald and a Yale study group in 1967, the American concept of hospice care for the dying came into popular use in 1971, when Hospice, Inc. became the first twentieth-century home care service for the terminally ill. By 1975, an international committee was establishing the parameters for hospice care. The group's four central precepts ally treatment dynamics with compassion:

- control by the terminally ill over their care
- merger of personal goals and preferences with style of treatment
- alliance of health professionals with family and friends
- assistance to health professionals who cope with the dying

Rapidly, the project grew from two hundred programs in 1980 to fifteen hundred in 1985. With the support of insurance reimbursement from Medicare, Medicaid, and private firms, the creation of local hospice initiatives rapidly introduced across the United States the long-lived European model that religious orders had begun during the Crusades.

The first American program, Hospice, Inc., of New Haven, Connecticut, launched a home care initiative in 1971. The following year, Connecticut Hospice, Inc., opened in Branford as a model of the community-based initiative. The staff trained other interdisciplinary teams through National Hospice Symposia, begun in 1975. The second venture into care of the dying began at McGill Medical Hospital in Montreal, Canada. It was followed by St. Luke's Hospice in New York City, a teaching facility founded by Chaplain Carlton Sweetser to dispatch a hospice team to home-bound patients. Inspired by Dr. Cicely Saunders's lecture tour, he disseminated the hospice concept at thanatology conferences. After leaving Sloan Kettering Hospital, he headed the chaplaincy of St. Luke's, where the hospice board coordinated staff outreach. With a grant of $60,000 from the Episcopal Society of Women, he hired a full-time nurse and part-time director to initiate the program, which started simply with a nine-to-five scatter-bed model. Because the acute care staff rejected the idea of a separate ward, teams visited patients' bedsides throughout the hospital. Expansion of the original team added a social worker, radiologist, physician, and administrator.

From these pioneering programs have come a set of national standards that offer a liberal approach to death with dignity. By 1978, the U.S. Department of Health, Education, and Welfare (HEW) published a report that labeled the concept a viable method for providing humane care for the terminally ill at a reduced cost. HEW advised Congress to fund hospices. In 1979, the Health Care Financing Administration set up twenty-six model programs nationwide to determine cost effectiveness and purpose. The W. K. Kellogg Foundation furthered national studies with a grant to the Joint Commission on Accreditation of Hospitals. By 1982, lawmakers were convinced that the hospice movement was working and offered Medicare benefits to cover patient expenses.

In subsequent years, Congress upped per diem benefits and added hospice care to CHAMPUS, the medical program covering military families, as well as the Indian Health Service and prison hospice units. In 1992, Clara McBride Hale, a public hero and child care champion of babies infected with AIDS or addicted to alcohol and drugs, died before she could achieve her dream—a hospice for dying children. Nonetheless, with the creative know-how of her daughter, Dr. Lorraine Hale, the stalled plan gained the support of New York Mayor David Dinkins. As a result of grassroots and legislative support, from 1989 to 1998 the numbers of hospices grew from thirty-one to more than two thousand.

Each participating hospice complies with the law to offer health options to patients and their families. Care integrates round-the-clock service in institutions and at home according to the patient's wishes and needs or, in the case of infants and children, the parents' wishes. Trainers educate staff and volunteers to aid those who have no family support. Caregivers respect privacy and personal beliefs while providing palliative therapy and ongoing assessment of quality of life. Follow-up support provides grief counseling to survivors for a year after a death. One specialist in terminal illness, nurse Joy K. Ufema, was the subject of "A Matter of Life and Death" (1981), a television movie about hospice nursing starring Linda Lavin. Ufema summed up her belief in the hospice creed with simple grace: "I know that death is not the enemy; inhumanity is. I will die well, knowing that whenever I had doubt, I risked it!" (Schorr and Zimmerman 1988, 363).

See also: Disease; Hale, Clara; Medieval and Early Renaissance Nursing; Saunders, Dr. Cicely; Teresa, Mother; Wald, Florence

Sources

Cohn-Sherbok, Lavinia. *Who's Who in Christianity.* Chicago: Routledge, 1998.

Corr, C. A., and D. M. Corr. *Hospice Approaches to Pediatric Care.* Annapolis, Md.: Springer, 1985.

"Elisabeth Kübler-Ross." http://www.wic.org/bio/eross.htm.

Hallam, Elizabeth, general ed. *Saints: Who They Are and How They Help You.* New York: Simon and Schuster, 1994.

"The History of Hospice." http://www.cptel.net/pamnorth/history.htm.

Humphry, Derek. "Films Dealing with Dying and Euthanasia." http://www.rights.org/~deathnet/ergo_films.html, 1995.

"Interview with Florence Wald." http://www.npha.org/intjwald.html.

Kastenbaum, Robert. *Death, Society, and Human Experience.* New York: Charles E. Merrill, 1986.

———, and Beatrice Kastenbaum, eds. *Encyclopedia of Death.* New York: Avon, 1989.

Kübler-Ross, Elisabeth. *On Death and Dying.* New York: Macmillan, 1969.

Levy, M. H. "Pain Control Research in the Terminally Ill." *Omega* (1987–1988): 265–280.

Marks, Geoffrey, and William K. Beatty. *Women in White.* New York: Charles Scribner's Sons, 1972.

Mor, V. *Hospice Care Systems.* New York: Springer, 1987.

Mor, V., D. S. Gree, and Robert Kastenbaum. *The Hospice Experiment.* Baltimore: Johns Hopkins University Press, 1988.

Mother Frances Domina. "Reflections on Death in Childhood." *British Medical Journal,* no. 294: 108–110.

Nixon, Pat Ireland, M.D. *The Medical Story of Early Texas, 1528–1853.* San Antonio: Mollie Bennett Lupe Memorial Fund, 1946.

"A Prison Hospice Model for the Future." http://www.npha.org/ftworth.html.

Saunders, Cicely. *The Management of Terminal Disease.* Hospital Medical Publications, 1967.

Schorr, Thelma M., R.N., and Anne Zimmerman, R.N., eds. *Making Choices, Taking Chances: Nurse Leaders Tell Their Stories.* St. Louis: C. V. Mosby, 1988.

Sebba, Anne. *Mother Teresa: Beyond the Image.* New York: Doubleday, 1997.

Sherr, Lynn, and Jurate Kazickas. *Susan B. Anthony Slept Here: A Guide to American Women's Landmarks.* New York: Times Books, 1994.

Siebold, Cathy. *The Hospice Movement: Easing Death's Pains.* New York: Twayne, 1992.

Twycross, R. G. *Pain Relief and Cancer.* Philadelphia: Saunders, 1984.

Zimmerman, J. *Hospice: Complete Care for the Terminally Ill.* Baltimore: Urban and Schwarzenberg, 1981.

Hutchinson, Anne

Perhaps the first New England colonist to serve the dual role of nurse and evangelist was Anne Marbury Hutchinson. Her fearful encounter with Puritan justice resulted from the stern accountability required of colonial midwives and the ominous misogyny that powered subsequent witch hunts. Throughout her travail in religious courts, she maintained her innocence and claimed that she served Boston's parturient women for humanitarian reasons. Twentieth-century feminists acclaimed her a martyr to women's rights.

A devout Puritan and native of Alford, Lincolnshire, Hutchinson was reared in a rigorous faith and developed a strong spirituality. Although her talents tended toward theology, she studied medical books. Self-confident and steady of hand, she practiced herbal healing and focused on gynecology. She emigrated from England in summer 1634 with her husband and ten children to the Massachusetts Bay Colony, where her oldest son Edward had built a house in Boston. Like other colonial nurse-midwives, she made her own potions and salves from fresh herbs, dried roots in a stillroom, and mastered Indian cures for fever.

According to Hutchinson's mentor, Reverend John Cotton of Boston, an eminent theologian, she had thrust herself into colonial life upon arrival from England and carried faith and midwifery to local women: "She did much good in our Town, in womans meeting at Childbirth-Travells, wherein shee was not onely skilfull and helpfull, but readily fell into good discourse with the women about their spiritual estates. . . . So as these private conferences did well tend to water the seeds publikely sowen. Whereupon all the faithfull embraced her conference, and blessed God for her fruitfull discourses" (Hall 1968, 412). Governor John Winthrop's *A Short Story of the Rise, Reign and Ruine of the Antinomians, Familists & Libertarians* (1644) records a parallel acknowledgment of her assistance "in the times of child-birth and other occasions of bodily infirmities" (Hall 1968, 263). She offered her simples and services to neighbors as a supplement to the medications prescribed by three area doctors.

On October 17, 1637, Hutchinson and assistant Jane Hawkins, an established birthing coach, attended the lying-in of Mary Dyer, the only fully documented medical case attached to Hutchinson's medical practice. Only weeks before she faced public interrogation by Governor Winthrop's court at Newton, she delivered Dyer of a badly deformed stillborn female, born two months early. Its birth shook the bed and produced a foul odor, which caused onlookers to vomit and children to twitch and hurry out of the room. Rumor declared that the child was headless, scaly, and equipped with claws; to superstitious Puritans, its horrific appearance suggested a manifestation of the devil. John Cotton advised Hutchinson to bury the corpse quietly and to conceal its birth from authorities.

A bold freethinker and magnetic speaker, Hutchinson, who led a splinter group of women twice a week in open discussion, was already under investigation and had developed a disquieting reputation for innovative worship and egalitarian thought. Growing antipathy toward her women's circle derived from Puritan leaders' fear of heresy and resultant social disorder. Three years after the delivery of Dyer's monstrous stillborn daughter, the established male clergy forced a trial, followed by excommunication of both midwives and exile of Jane Hawkins from the Massachusetts Bay Colony. Part of the case against Hutchinson involved Dyer's anomalous infant. The court exhumed the corpse and noted evidence of horns and talons. In addition to these portents, a physician testified that Hutchinson had produced large uterine tumors, which prosecutors determined were signs of her intercourse with Satan.

In a scathing denunciation, Governor Winthrop accused her of using midwifery as a means of insinuating her unorthodox beliefs into Boston via its female citizens. In a bold strike against her, he maligned her potions as spiritual poisons and labeled her philosophy antinomian, a quasi-sacrilegious stance against

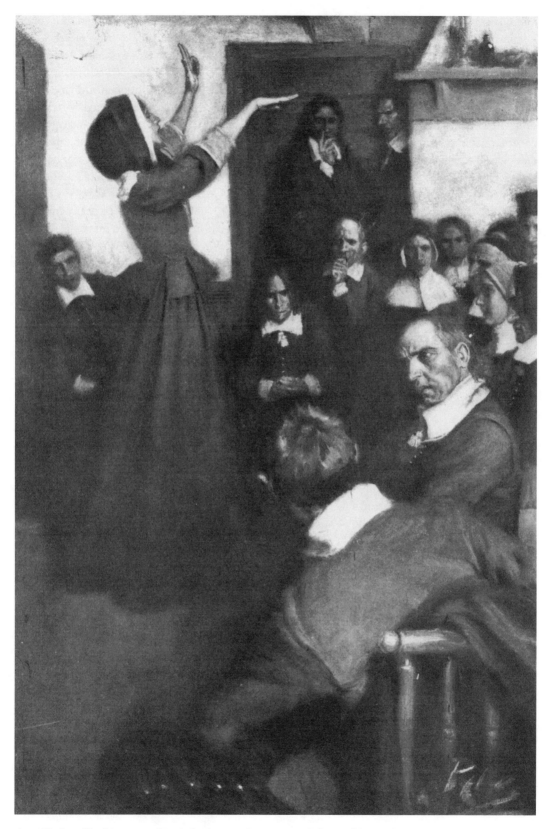

Anne Marbury Hutchinson preaching in her house in Boston, 1901 (Library of Congress)

moral law. His judgment, imputing evil in her role in Dyer's delivery, blamed "monstrous errours" (Hall 1968, 281). Implicit in his accusation was the Puritan abhorrence of witchcraft and demonology, which created a pervasive suspicion of the midwife's profession. Reverend John Wilson supported the governor's summation by declaring her philosophy "to be dayngerous and damnable and to be no lesse than Sudducisme and Athiisme" (Hall 1968, 358). Another Puritan, the Reverend Peter Bulkeley, defamed her female followers as familists, freethinking women who turned from the nuclear family to live apart from holy matrimony and practice free love. The Reverend Hugh Peters added his own thoughts on women who presumed to think for themselves: "You have rather bine a Husband than a Wife and a preacher than a Hearer; a Magistrate than a subject" (Hall 1968, 383). Winthrop banished her, calling her haughty and bolder than a man. The accusation suggested the narrow confines of the midwife's authority and the frail egos of colonial males, who did not hesitate to trounce a powerful woman in their midst.

Reestablished in Aquidneck south of Providence, Rhode Island, Hutchinson shared with neighboring tribes her considerable medical knowledge. Adding to the weight of trial and public humiliation was the birth of her child, a fetus more monstrous than Mary Dyer's. Governor Winthrop took the opportunity to affirm his opinion that Hutchinson suffered God's vengeance for forming a heretical band of women. Following Hutchinson's husband's death, in 1642 she, six of her children, and other settlers moved to Long Island, but found the Indians less amenable to their presence. Resettled in the Dutch colony of New Amsterdam at Pelham Bay, she continued her work for six years until Siwanoy tribesmen kidnapped her daughter Susanna and slaughtered Hutchinson and the rest of her household in August 1643. The Hutchinson River and nearby parkway carry her name. An imposing statue of her with Bible in hand stands in the Massachusetts State House. The Newport Historical Society erected a bronze plaque dedicated "To the memory of Anne Marbury Hutchinson from the women who won't forget" (Rau 1999, 4).

Sources

Augur, Helen. *An American Jezebel: The Life of Anne Hutchinson.* New York: Brentano's, 1930.

Battis, Emery. *Saints and Sectaries: Anne Hutchinson and the Antinomian Controversy in the Massachusetts Bay Colony.* Chapel Hill: University of North Carolina Press, 1962.

Burgess, Barbara. "The Puritan Exiles the Separatists." http://www.naccc.org/congregationalist/Volume157/Number4/exile.html.

Curtis, Edith. *Anne Hutchinson.* Cambridge, Mass.: Washburn and Thomas, 1930.

Faber, Doris. *Anne Hutchinson.* Champaign, Ill.: Gerrard Publishing, 1970.

Hall, David D., ed. *The Antinomian Controversy, 1636–1638: A Documentary History.* Middletown, Conn.: Wesleyan University Press, 1968.

McGregor, Deborah Kuhn. "'Childbirth-Travells' and 'Spiritual Estates': Anne Hutchinson and Colonial Boston, 1634–1638." *Caduceus* (1989): 1–33.

Rau, Elizabeth. "Anne Hutchinson: Courage Ahead of Her Time." http://www.projo.com/horizons/elect96/229spr1.htm.

Rogers, Jay. "America's Christian Leaders: Anne Hutchinson." http://www.forerunner.com/forerunner/X0193_Anne_Hutchinson.html.

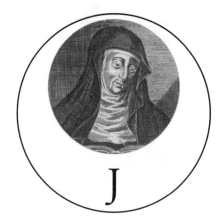

Jones, Mary Agnes

Mary Agnes Jones, founder of St. Mary's Convent and Nursing Home and an influence on the work of Florence Nightingale, studied hospital administration at the Community of the Nursing Sisters of St. John the Divine, or St. John's House, which set the example for training staff to aid the poor. Born in Tamworth, Staffordshire, in 1812, she was the daughter of a cabinet maker, whose earnings paid for minimal schooling. Largely self-educated, she displayed the qualities associated with professional success, including intelligence, ability, character, and fluency in French. Jones was thirty-five years old when she requested that the Bishop of London place her in a religious community. A devout Christian, she lacked funds for classes and worked as a sister-housekeeper to cover the annual tuition of £50.

On March 21, 1856, Jones joined sixteen other pioneers—three sisters, nine nurses, and four probationary nurses—in staffing King's College Hospital, a London center for the destitute. The organization set up the ward system, which provided food, housekeeping, and obstetrical and medical treatment. In addition to scrubbing floors, sanitizing bedding, and upgrading patient diet, Jones's group rid the halls of intrusive visitors and halted public consumption of alcohol. Nurse rotation introduced each worker to trauma, surgical, contagious disease, and midwifery.

In an era when women had little control over the medical establishment, Jones became an advocate for the professional nurse. In exchange for loyalty to patient care and the hospital, she demanded respect for staff along with private sleeping quarters, washrooms, and an off-duty lounge. More lenient scheduling and amenities guaranteed a daily allotment of fresh dairy products, tea, sugar, and ale and regular meals in a private dining area, where Jones delivered pep talks to elevate character. As the King's College Hospital nursing program drew visitors from Prussia, Poland, France, and Russia, her philosophy established the norm by which other systems were judged. Within a few years, both St. Thomas's Hospital in London and the Royal Liverpool Infirmary offered similar lounges and dormitories for staff.

The problem of complete care for the sick forced Jones to reach beyond hospital grounds to tenements and homes where destitute invalids suffered alone and women gave birth untended. With funds from philanthropist William Rathbone, in 1859, she established district nurses and advised him on the best way to upgrade the Liverpool Workhouse Infirmary. The success of the nursing program in the early 1860s encouraged her to open an orphanage and convalescent home. She dispatched a sister to oversee the Galignani Hospital for the English outside Paris. Within a year, Jones took the post of nursing administrator at London's Charing Cross Hospital.

A nadir in Jones's career came in 1867, with an outbreak of puerperal, or childbed, fever. In a letter to Florence Nightingale, Jones expressed her concern that the post-mortem room was too close to the maternity ward. She regretted the doctors' refusal to wash their hands upon entering the lying-in ward, a situation that rapidly spread infection, threatening the lives of new mothers and infants. The connection between clean hands and instruments and improved recovery rates for mothers remained unclear until hospital acceptance of Joseph Lister's proposals for carbolic acid antisepsis, which remained in contention as late as the 1880s.

Overall, the responsibilities that Jones undertook are impressive. Her staff provided four thousand meals daily to outpatients, regular home visits, and supervision of the London docks during the cholera epidemic and the Staffordshire collieries during a typhoid fever outbreak. Two of her staff died from treating scarlet fever in Surrey and Buckinghamshire. In the midst of an overwhelming workload and shortage of trained staff, she supervised the Hospital for Sick Children in Nottingham. At age fifty-three, she wrote to Florence Nightingale, "I cannot say that my work is quite easy to me, for some months past I have not felt quite well—yet I fear more of laziness than real illness—for I do so long really for rest very often now though I would fain not be weary or laggard till my work is done but each month the necessity for constant unflagging work seems to increase" (Myers 1996, 11). In 1866, concerned friends donated French books, fresh country produce, and a bed to relieve Jones's back strain. She retreated to Lea Hurst, the Nightingale family's Derbyshire home, and used the time to draft institutional regulations for St. John's House.

During this segment of her career, Jones clashed with Archibald Campbell Tait, Bishop of London, over the issue of religious commitment and its influence on nursing. On October 12, 1867, she seceded from St. John's House by severing relations with the religious council. In January 1868, to Nightingale's dismay, Jones and seven others established the Community of St. Mary and St. John Evangelist, an independent Augustinian sisterhood outside Church of England authority. The order remained on precarious ground, depending entirely on donations. In 1873, Jones became mother superior of St. Mary's Convent and Nursing Home in Kensington, her newly created day nursery and refuge for incurables. Tubercular and arthritic patients ineligible for the workhouse infirmary sought care from the staff, consisting of seven sisters, two probationary nurses, and three female servants.

Because no records survive of Jones's last years of service, history relies on surmise and anecdote. On March 29, 1887, at age seventy-five, she and Sister Laura Girdlestone suffered typhoid fever, which weakened them for three months. Florence Nightingale inquired daily and dispatched jelly, meat puree, soup, brandy, and champagne along with encouraging messages until Jones's death on June 2.

Sources

Goodnow, Minnie. *Nursing History.* London: W. B. Saunders, 1942.

Griffin, Gerald Joseph, and H. Joann King Griffin. *Jensen's History and Trends of Professional Nursing.* Saint Louis, Mo.: C. V. Mosby, 1965.

Jamieson, Elizabeth, and Mary F. Sewall. *Trends in Nursing History.* London: W. B. Saunders, 1949.

Kalisch, Philip, and Beatrice J. Kalisch. *The Advance of American Nursing.* Boston: Little, Brown, 1978.

Myers, Pamela. *Building for the Future: A Nursing History 1896–1996.* Chiswick, London: St. Mary's Convent, 1996.

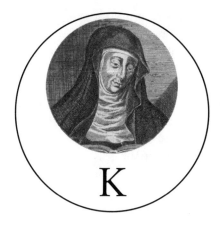

Kenny, Elizabeth

An Australian nurse who developed a treatment for polio victims, Sister Elizabeth Kenny initiated her career in the backcountry with isolated polio victims. Far from orthopedic centers, she fought creeping paralysis with stimulation and hot packs, the only weapons she had against advancing muscular atrophy. The concept, similar to that of Juan Castro, a Tolcha Indian from Texas, relaxes the muscles and restores vitality. When her system began increasing motility and halting tissue deterioration, she published anecdotal findings to the jeers of the medical establishment. Only when the Mayo Clinic and the University of Minnesota accepted her method did it begin to influence treatment of polio worldwide. Vindication proved a mixed blessing. Throughout the Minnesota epidemic of 1946, she challenged her limits, endangering her health. At her death from Parkinson's disease on November 30, 1952, in Toowoomba, Queensland, the media recognized her as a pragmatic healer of the polio era—an innovator and reformer who nursed patients by instinct rather than protocol.

A native of Warialda, New South Wales, Kenny, born September 20, 1886, was one of the nine children of an Irish veterinarian and the granddaughter of a Scottish sea captain. She was a twenty-three-year-old bush nurse in 1910 when she encountered her first case of infantile paralysis—a toddler lying awkwardly twisted on a cot in a tenant shack of a cattle station in North Queensland. Traveling miles by buggy to a telegraph office, Kenny wired her mentor, Dr. Aeneas John McDonnell, for instructions. He relayed the world's blank on polio: no research center had solved the virus puzzle. The only treatment must be directed at symptoms.

Challenged by the unknown, Kenny returned to the child to apply the layperson's first aid. She heated salt in a skillet, filled a bag, and applied the warm grains to the aching leg, then tried the standard linseed poultice. Neither method helped. As a third regimen, she boiled blanket strips, wrung them out, and used them to massage and stroke the wry limbs until spasms yielded and the patient could sleep. The simplicity of the method worked on the next five victims, yet McDonnell opposed the treatment as the opposite of standard practice, which required immediate splinting of affected limbs.

Kenny opened a cottage polio clinic in 1913 in Clifton, where parents brought sick children. A volunteer during World War I, she was serving at the front in France when she suffered shrapnel wounds to the knee and calf.

After three weeks of recuperation, she accompanied wounded soldiers home to Australia and continued as ship nurse on subsequent round trips. Aboard the *Marathon* out of Liverpool in October 1918, she survived a shipboard epidemic of influenza and, with one other nurse, tended five hundred patients before the armistice returned her to Australia. She was appointed temporary matron at the Enoggera Military Hospital when she collapsed from a heart attack.

Following treatment in Stuttgart, Germany, Kenny resumed caring for polio victims and was again victorious in reeducating a young girl's limbs that had been encased in splints. While caring for paralytics in her family's home, she defrayed expenses by patenting a litter known as the Sylvia Stretcher, an invention she named for a little girl she transported from farm to hospital. In the backyard of a residence in Townsville, Queensland, in 1933, she established a clinic to rehabilitate seventeen intractable cases of polio. Her successes impressed pediatricians, orthopedic surgeons, and health officials, but at a lecture in Brisbane, her description of spasm brought laughter and gibes. Despite the combative atmosphere, the government health authorities acceded to popular pressure and, in 1934, sponsored the Kenny Clinic and Training School. The next year, a royal commission went to great lengths to refute Kenny's claims about paralytic muscle spasms and published a three-hundred-page report to silence the upstart nurse, yet the stinging retorts carried no weight with parents. To honor Sister Kenny, they built the Elizabeth Kenny Park and Children's Playground.

Kenny's influence spread to England, where she supervised a ward at Queen Mary's Hospital at Carshalton and treated children from France, China, and Poland. Gradually, she made converts and triumphed in Australia in 1939 when the government offered the Kenny treatment as an alternative to orthodox splinting of rigid limbs. In 1940, accompanied by her namesake and aide, Mary Stewart Kenny, Sister Kenny demonstrated the efficacy of the wet-pack treatment on muscle spasms at the Minneapolis General Hospital for the staff of the University of Minnesota School of Public Health and the National Foundation for Infantile Paralysis (NFIP). Approved by the American Medical Association and the NFIP in December 1941, the method was the focus of the Sister Kenny Institute of Minneapolis, her first training center for physiotherapists and nurses, established in 1942.

In record time, as Kenny centers spread, the reformed view of creeping paralysis revolutionized treatment. She received a gold key from the American Congress of Physical Therapy and an invitation to lunch with President Franklin D. Roosevelt, a chair-bound polio victim. Rosalind Russell starred in the film *Sister Kenny* (1946), adapted from Kenny's autobiography, *And They Shall Walk* (1943). After a tour of Europe and South America, Kenny aided Centralia, Illinois, in establishing a Kenny clinic. In 1950, the U.S. Congress granted her diplomatic status so that she could cross borders without a visa or passport. Crippled in her mid-fifties, she died on November 20, 1952, in the midst of the 1950–1954 series of polio epidemics, three years before Jonas Salk answered her prayers for a polio vaccine.

Sources

Fessler, Diane Burke. *No Time for Fear: Voices of American Military Nurses in World War II.* East Lansing: Michigan State University Press, 1996.

The Grolier Library of Women's Biographies. Danbury, Conn.: Grolier Educational, 1998.

Kenny, Elizabeth. *And They Shall Walk.* North Stratford, N.H.: Ayer, 1980.

McKown, Robin. *Heroic Nurses.* New York: G. P. Putnam's Sons, 1966.

Sherr, Lynn, and Jurate Kazickas. *Susan B. Anthony Slept Here: A Guide to American Women's Landmarks.* New York: Times Books, 1994.

"The Stubborn Sister." *Time,* December 8, 1952, 80–81.

"Transition." *Newsweek,* December 8, 1952, 67.

Korean War

Beginning in June 1950, the police action known as the Korean War halted the benign

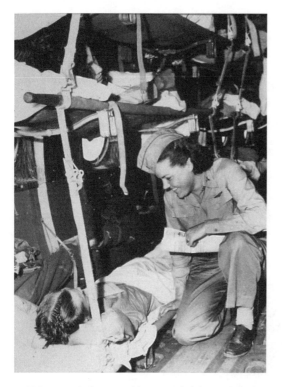

A U.S. nurse checks on a soldier wounded during fighting in the Korean War. (Archive Photos)

political and economic glow that followed World War II. As soon as President Harry Truman legitimized combat following the North Korean communists' breach of the 38th parallel, the U.S. Army Nurse Corps left for the front, where war continued until July 27, 1953. In all, demand for medical services drew 260 army nurses to serve ten hospitals in addition to forward units, field stations, and the first mobile army surgical hospital (MASH) units. The Navy Nurse Corps rose to 3,238 members and staffed three hospital ships, the *Consolation, Repose,* and *Haven.* The newcomers, the Air Force Nurse Corps, officially launched in July 1950, assigned two hundred flight nurses to evacuate the wounded. The famed "limited war" cost more than fifty thousand American lives and employed nurses to treat the wounded in-country and to rehabilitate casualties at support units in Japan and other countries of the Pacific Rim. Overall, 3,081 active duty and 1,704 reserve navy nurses served in the con-

flict, in which none were killed. Of the 540 army nurses involved in the action, Genevieve Smith was the only death, which occurred en route to her post aboard a C-54, which left Kimpo Air Base and crashed in the Sea of Japan.

One of the most decorated female soldiers in U.S. military history, Californian Lillian Kinkela-Keil, a captain in the Air Force Nurse Corps, flew two hundred evacuation missions and twenty-five transatlantic crossings in World War II and returned to duty from civilian work to fly hundreds more in Korea. She served as technical adviser for a film about her wartime adventures, *Flight Nurse* (1953), starring Joan Leslie and Forrest Tucker. Overall, Kinkela-Keil earned eleven battle stars, the Air Medal with oak leaf clusters, Presidential Unit Citation, Korean Service Medal, American Campaign Medal, United Defense Medal, and Republic of Korea Presidential Citation.

Thirty nurses served at the 4th Field Hospital, a large installation set up in a converted teacher's college after the Inchon invasion on September 15, 1950. Working twelve hours daily, seven days a week, staff managed an operating theater, anesthesia, and surgical and medical wards. Among the challenges of the war was the task of examining and interviewing Chinese and Korean combatants as well as Japanese, Turkish, British, Filipino, and Australian participants in the international task force. For questioning people speaking unfamiliar languages, staff resorted to sign language or summoned interpreters.

On the second floor of the hospital, primitive housing with crumbling doors and windows, kerosene stoves, and five-gallon cans of water greeted the nurses in their off hours. Amenities consisted of folding canvas buckets, foot lockers, cots, and rice straw mats. Despite the squalor, Californian Margaret Feil spoke for her compatriots when she remarked to an interviewer: "I don't feel that I'm making a great sacrifice there. I wouldn't be doing anything else in the world. I know that if they offered to let me go home, I wouldn't go. I'd want to finish this first—and stay as long as

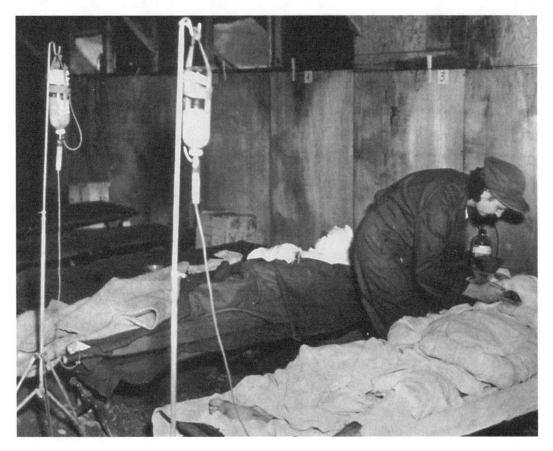

Blood transfusions at a forward base in Korea, distributed by Captain Dot I. Dodd (Archive Photos)

everyone else does" (Samuels 1951, 33). This spirit of involvement sparked rage in volunteers after stateside nurses ignored the call for three thousand more nurses.

One of the surprises of the so-called forgotten war was Richard Hooker's satiric novel, *MASH* (1968), a fictional representation of the mobile army surgical hospital, an innovation in expert field treatment that placed a sixty-bed facility in service to a single division as close to combat as 8 miles. Devised in 1944 as a means of landing aid stations with amphibious units fighting in the Pacific, this innovative treatment package was a departure from the traditional protocol of treating casualties within a two-hundred-soldier company and then transporting more serious cases to a battalion aid station only 5–10 miles from the front and on to a field hospital and general

hospital 25–100 miles away for more sophisticated care, such as ophthalmic or maxillofacial surgery. The MASH unit limited care to surgery, general debridement, resuscitation, x-ray, and stabilization before the patient was airlifted by helicopter to a complete care facility. The typical MASH outfit required sixteen medical officers, sixteen nurses, and one hundred enlisted men to staff preoperative and postoperative wards, the operating suite, and anesthesiology for general, thoracic, and orthopedic surgery (Figure 1).

First tested in Korea at Iwon in November 1950, the initial MASH unit received 171 surgical cases in its first month of operation, and according to Captain John M. McGuire, all patients survived. When moved near Kyungju, the mission expanded to a two-hundred-bed field hospital because of a lack of

Figure 1: The organization of MASH units during the Korean War

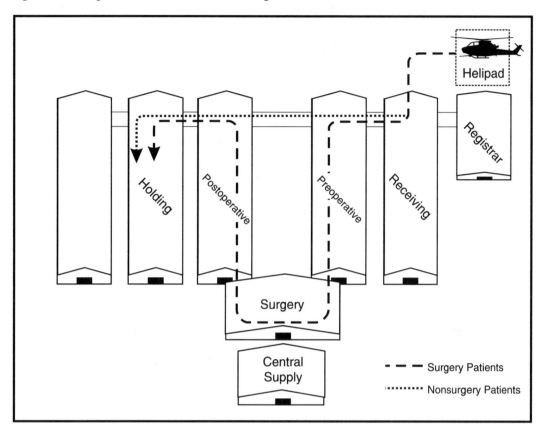

evacuation sites in Korea. For this alteration in the original plan, the more complex unit required an upgrade of staff to twenty medical officers, twenty nurses, and 120 enlisted men. Its increase in sophistication and mission greatly altered the original concept of mobility as it received surgical and medical cases from the 1st Marine Division, 2nd and 7th Infantry Divisions, and 187th Regimental Combat Team.

The MASH concept established one of the principles expounded by Florence Nightingale during the Crimean War—the sooner treatment begins, the more lives saved and the higher the morale of frontline warriors. As described by Lieutenant Colonel John L. Mothershead and Captain Samuel L. Crook of the 8076th MASH, its primary function was to perform emergency, life-saving surgery and to stabilize patients to be transported to rear medical installations. The arrangement of tents consisted of a U-shaped passage of patients from reception to the preoperative, surgery, and postoperative areas and out to two holding tents on the far wing. MASH units also included annexes to distribute supplies. The experiment proved valuable during the Korean action by reducing the mortality rate to half that of World War II.

Hooker's book became an Oscar-winning 1970 film, spelled *M*A*S*H,* Hollywood-style, starring Sally Kellerman as Nurse "Hot Lips" Houlihan, also known as the "goose girl." The movie spawned an irreverent, antimilitary television phenomenon running from 1971 to 1981, starring Alan Alda as chief surgeon and Loretta Swit as Head Nurse Houlihan and demonstrating the exigencies and hazards of frontline nursing. Derived from the 8055th MASH unit, the comic episodes convey the insanity of war and the muck, gore, and shot-up bodies of patients who shuttle in and out of preoperative, surgery, and postoperative areas with their host of physical and emotional problems. For all its satire on the ongoing Vietnam debacle, the series mirrored an international conflict that was safely past and easily mocked.

Sources

Byerly, Dr. W. Grimes, personal interview, August 18, 1998.

"18th Medcom Nursing." http://www.seoul.amedd.army.mil/nursing/18121dnm.htm.

Kalisch, Philip, and Beatrice J. Kalisch. *The Advance of American Nursing.* Boston: Little, Brown, 1978.

"Medical Corps." http://www.army.mil/cmh-pg/books/korea/22_1_5.htm.

"Post WWII and Korea." http://userpages.aug.com/captbarb/femvets6.html.

Samuels, Gertrude. "With Army Nurses Somewhere in Korea." *New York Times Magazine,* April 15, 1951, 14, 33–34.

Snodgrass, Mary Ellen. *Encyclopedia of Satirical Literature.* Santa Barbara, Calif.: ABC-CLIO, 1996.

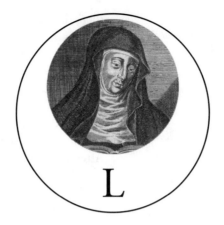

L

La Flesche Picotte, Susan

In the last years of the nineteenth century, Susan La Flesche Picotte became the first female Indian healer trained in the white world. She was the daughter of Mary "The One Woman" Gale La Flesche, of mixed Iowa blood, and French-Omaha chief Joseph "Iron Eyes" La Flesche, a pragmatic native spokesman who believed that the best course of action for Indians was to acclimate to white society. Born in Nebraska in 1865, La Flesche Picotte completed the early stages of her education at the Elizabeth Institute for Young Ladies in New Jersey. On return to the reservation, she assisted a white reservation doctor as volunteer nurse and began to question the unequal treatment of her people.

Influenced by the volunteer nursing among the Poncas of her sister Susette "Bright Eyes" La Flesche Tibbles, La Flesche Picotte entered the Hampton Institute in Virginia and profited from the example of Dr. Martha M. Waldron, a strong feminist. La Flesche Picotte studied healing with Presbyterian and Quaker missionaries and, with a grant from the Women's National Indian Association, completed training at the Women's Medical College in Philadelphia, Pennsylvania, graduated valedictorian of her class, and interned at the nearby Woman's Hospital. As reservation doctor and medical missionary on the Omaha reservation in northeastern Nebraska, she traveled on horseback and by buggy from 1889 to 1893 in extremes of weather to treat chronic alcoholism, cholera, typhoid, dysentery, tuberculosis, influenza, and conjunctivitis. She is said to have examined or treated all thirteen hundred of the widely scattered Omaha nation and served as healer, nurse, and public health educator in matters of sanitation, nutrition, and infant care.

In her late twenties and thirties, La Flesche Picotte moved from healing to activism. Under the auspices of the Women's National Indian Association, she launched a temperance drive in 1891. After marrying Henri Picotte, of French-Sioux descent, she set up a community practice in Bancroft, Nebraska, and regularly lighted a lamp at dusk as a beacon to patients arriving at night. Widowed in 1905, she allied with the mission of the Blackbird Hills Presbyterian Church and settled in Walthill, Nebraska, where she opened a hospital in 1913. Her intervention in tribal difficulties in 1910 took her to Washington, D.C., as a lobbyist. Among her accomplishments was a covenant to end the sale or possession of alcohol on Omaha land. At her death in 1915 from a mastoid infection, she was buried in Bancroft.

Sources

Bataille, Gretchen M., ed. *Native American Women: A Biographical Dictionary.* New York: Garland, 1993.

Gridley, Marion E. *American Indian Women.* New York: Hawthorn Books, 1974.

Kent, Jacqueline C. *Women in Medicine.* Minneapolis, Minn.: Oliver Press, 1998.

Sherr, Lynn, and Jurate Kazickas. *Susan B. Anthony Slept Here: A Guide to American Women's Landmarks.* New York: Times Books, 1994.

Waldman, Carl. *Who Was Who in Native American History: Indians and Non-Indians from Early Contacts through 1900.* New York: Facts on File, 1990.

Webster's Dictionary of American Women. New York: Merriam-Webster, 1996.

White, Julia. "Susan La Flesche, Omaha." http://www.powersource.com/powersource/gallery/womansp/omaha.html.

Lubic, Ruth

In the late twentieth century, nurse-educator and anthropologist Dr. Ruth Watson Lubic, winner of the MacArthur Foundation award and March of Dimes nurse of 1985, single-handedly bolstered the nurse-midwife program in the United States. The general director of New York's Maternity Center Association from 1970 to 1995, Lubic superintended the nation's first freestanding birthing facility and oversaw a model nursing program during a quarter-century of phenomenal growth fueled in part by the women's movement. Following the centuries-old example of midwives, she advocated hands-on care with a minimum of instruments and machinery. A low-cost method of normal delivery, this time-honored concept of midwifery prefaced a transformation of birthing from brightly lit delivery suites back to the calmer, less intrusive birthing room of the past that welcomed whole families. As Lubic announced, "We're demonstrating that maternity care can be safe, satisfying and economical" ("For 'New Nurse'" 1980, n.p.).

Native to Bristol, Pennsylvania, Lubic, the daughter of pharmacist John "Doc" Russell Watson and office manager Lillian Kraft Watson, was born January 18, 1927. After her fa-

ther's death, fifteen-year-old Lubic assisted her mother in stocking and running the family drugstore. In the company of a local physician, she began going on calls and considering a nursing career. Integral to her preference for natural nursing were the techniques of her aunt Alice, who taught a system of body mechanics that used rhythm to lessen stress. After high school, Lubic ran the drugstore and earned tuition to nursing school.

In 1952, Lubic began a three-year program at Philadelphia's School of Nursing at the University of Pennsylvania. At her graduation, she earned the Florence Nightingale Medal for nursing practice and the Letitia White Award for academic excellence. Lubic's first post took her to the forerunner of the Sloan-Kettering Center in New York. She achieved a bachelor's degree from Hunter College and advanced to head nurse before completing course work at Teachers College of Columbia University in 1959. Her experience with motherhood influenced work toward an M.S. degree in medical-surgical nursing and midwifery, a specialty then in disfavor with the American College of Obstetricians and Gynecologists. After clinical certification from Kings County Hospital, she taught nursing for a year at New York Medical College and midwifery at the Maternity Center Association (MCA). On a 1973 visit to China, she joined an American medical delegation as the only nurse.

Lubic's advancement to the head of the Maternity Center Association preceded its development of an experimental program of home care for low-risk mothers. To enable families to perceive birth as a natural experience, midwives from MCA opened a Childbearing Center in 1975 in a townhouse on New York's Upper East Side. After selecting expectant mothers free of heart disease, diabetes, or past delivery problems, the center coached them through safe, pain-reduced births and mastered conditions demanding acute care. To combat the possessiveness and objections of obstetricians and neonatologists, Lubic and others at the center spoke out against gender oppression, also the subject of her dissertation, entitled "Barriers and Conflict in Maternity Care Innovation." Within a few years, Lubic's courageous stand for women and homey childbirth centers began a growing trend to liberalize delivery and free it of male domination. By enlarging the role of fathers, children, and midwives, Lubic revived interest in home delivery and influenced hospitals to lessen dependence on electronic monitoring devices and anesthetics, to put mothers and newborns in the same room, and to encourage early bonding and breast-feeding. In 1983, thirty states reported home birthing plans at 103 centers. In fifteen years, the number was about 245.

In 1988, following the publication of *Childbearing: A Book of Choices,* which she wrote with Gene R. Hawes, Lubic was instrumental in establishing a parallel center in the Bronx, which served the opposite end of the economic scale. Her creation of a specialized midwifery course assisted the Community-Based Nurse-Midwifery Education Program, which embraced her holistic birthing model by including fathers and older children. Her service to the World Health Organization, American College of Nurse-Midwives, American Public Health Association, and Institute of Medicine of the National Academy of Sciences broadened her influence across the medical spectrum. To raise the infant survival rate in the nation's capital and developing nations, she has expanded MCA's outreach to Washington, D.C., and eastern Europe. For her work, she was named one of *Ladies Home Journal's* 100 most important women and has earned the Rockefeller Public Service award, the Lillian D. Wald Spirit of Nursing award, and five honorary degrees.

Sources

"A. J. Wright." http://eja.anes.hscyr.edu/anes/anest–1/1992/92_01.txt.

"For 'New Nurse': Bigger Role in Health Care." *U.S. News and World Report,* January 14, 1980.

"On the Frequency Distribution of Recent Time Cost Studies." http://www.lib.ncsu.edu/stacks.

"Ruth Watson Lubic." *Current Biography Yearbook.* New York: Bowker, 1996, 328–332.

Schorr, Thelma M., R.N., and Anne Zimmerman, R. N., eds. *Making Choices, Taking Chances: Nurse Leaders Tell Their Stories.* St. Louis: C. V. Mosby, 1988.

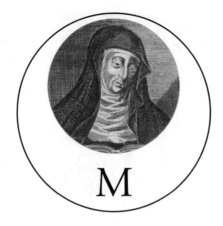

M

Medieval and Early Renaissance Nursing

In the Middle Ages, both sexes practiced nursing, although on differing bases of authority. In lieu of the ministry, which was closed to females, the task of healer became a standard role for active, liberated women interested in altruistic medicine, whether as midwives, herbalists, or *empirics,* the folk healers or general practitioners common to rural areas. From Ireland and across continental Europe to the Mediterranean, the late fifth to early sixth centuries produced nurses and nurse companies among royalty and aristocrats who professed a joy in attending the sick.

Details of medieval healers and their practice are sketchy and padded with legend. Their inflated biographies establish an overall dedication to humane comfort of sufferers:

- Around 400 A.D., St. Alexis, only son of a Roman senator, renounced marriage on his wedding day and journeyed to Syria to live as a hermit. He returned to his home in disguise to serve among the suffering. In the image of Alexis's tender care of the dying, in 1348, Tobias of Mechelen, Belgium, founded the Alexian Brothers, or Cellites, a conservative beggar house that aided poor sufferers of

the bubonic plague and buried the abandoned dead.

- Half a century after Alexis, St. Attracta (or Athracht) of Donegal, Ireland, followed the example of St. Patrick and opened an abbey in Lough Gara, Sligo, that welcomed ailing beggars. She erected a simi-

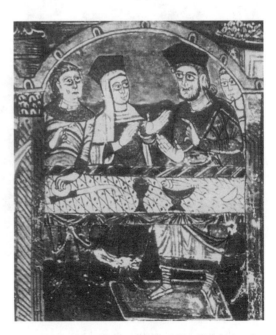

Saint Radegonde, here seated at the table of her husband, King Clothaire, founded a convent-hospital and leper sanctuary in France. (North Wind Picture Archive)

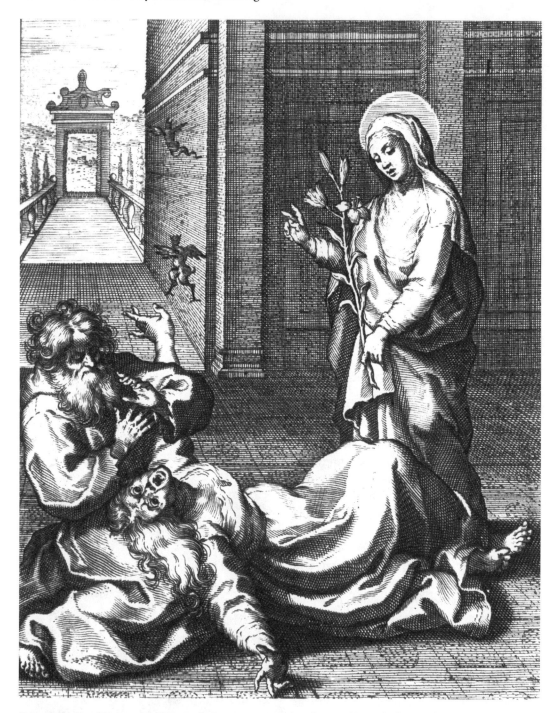

Saint Catherine of Siena was well known for her passionate work with incurables in the fourteenth century. (Lauros-Giraudon/Art Resource, NY)

lar hostel at Killaraght that remained in use until its destruction in 1539.

- Celtic women of late sixth-century Kildare depended on the nurse-midwife St. Bridget (also Bride or Brigid), Ireland's patron saint and the patron of healers. At her double monastery, which accommodated men and women in separate lodgings, she welcomed outcast lepers. In this same period, an obscure contemporary, St. Scholastica, twin sister of St. Benedict, fought plague at her convent near Monte Cassino, Italy, and taught her skill to others.

- A sixth-century Irish charismatic, St. Columba of Gartan, also a disciple of St. Patrick, founded religious houses at Kell, Derry, and Durrow. After he was exiled in 565 to the Scottish island of Iona, he introduced Christianity to Scotland and built a hospice for lepers, where he relied on *aquavit* and *usque-beatha,* the original Irish whisky, as stimulants.

- In Constantinople, the wife of Emperor Olybrios, Julia Anicia, born in 472 A.D., studied medicine and supported the work of hospitals.

- In Gaul two women pioneered modern nursing—Clothilde (or Clotilda) of Burgundy, consort of Clovis I, a Frankish king and Christian convert who ruled from 481 to 511 A.D., and their daughter-in-law, Radegonde (or Radegunda) of Thuringia, consort of King Clothaire, a Frankish monarch. The matriarch of a saintly family, Clothilde was canonized for her volunteerism. She is best remembered tending patients at a hospice and at the monastery of St. Martin's at Tours, where she retired at age thirty-seven following her husband's death. She was beloved as the Queen Widow and patroness of the lame. By the mid–sixth century, Queen Radegonde had become an unassuming royal who devoted her ministrations to beggars, lepers, and local handicapped peasants. As abbess of Holy Cross Monastery at Poitiers, she erected a modern hospital heated and plumbed by the Roman underfloor system. In comfort, she educated two hundred nurses to care for indigent patients.

- In the seventh century, Radegonde's kinswoman, St. Bathilde (or Batilda), a former Anglo-Saxon slave and consort of King Clovis II, founded religious houses at Corbie and Chelles north of Paris. Revered as a patroness of children, she retired to nurse the poor.

- In the late 600s, an Irish caretaker of the insane, St. Dympna, was martyred at Gheel, Belgium, where she was honored as the patron of the mentally ill. At a hospital built in her honor in 1286, patients thronged for treatment, turning the town into a center for psychiatric care. Villagers established a tradition of opening their homes to recovering patients and tenderly introducing them to normal lives.

- An obscure nursing brother, St. Giles (or St. Aegidius) of Athens settled near Nimes, France, on the Rhone River around 683. He earned respect for aiding lepers, cripples, and nursing mothers and for founding twenty-four hospitals, 162 churches, and an abbey, Saint Gilles of Provence. In 1117, Matilda, wife of Henry I, honored St. Giles with a leprosarium near London.

The seventh century saw the establishment of an influential order, the Béguines, an amorphous, free-ranging Belgian society of unmarried north European laywomen who renounced a secular life to become medical missionaries and nurture the poor under the name of Father Lambert le Bégue of Liège. His first convert, Mary of Oignies, chose care of lepers as her specialty. In 1184, subsequent medical missionaries took the name Béguines. Among them were Mechtilde of Magdeburg (ca. 1212–ca. 1282), Beatrice of Nazareth (ca. 1200–1268), Hadewijch of Brabant (fl. 1221–1240), and Marguerite Porete (?–1310), who was burned at the stake for heresy. Unhampered by cloistering, Béguines flourished in hostels in France, Belgium, Germany, Holland, and Switzerland under the patronage of such generous supporters as Jeanne of Flanders and her sister Margaret. During a period of religious ferment, these Christian workers ventured beyond the restricted life and powerlessness of medieval womanhood to pioneer socially approved alternatives to the roles of wife or cloistered sister. Their medical villages, called Béguinages, consisted of huts, convent, chapel, infirmary or hospital, and cemetery. Though unfettered by church rule, Béguines suffered persecution, denunciation, and excommunication by refusing the coercion of religious hierarchy. Their independence produced a public display of growing disdain for Catholic patriarchy. By 1350, their ranks grew to 200,000.

Throughout the late Middle Ages, names and deeds of additional religious and lay nurses dotted manuscripts and history books:

- In the eighth century, St. Walpurga (or Walburga), a Wessex princess and volunteer evangelizer of the Swabians, went to Germany to teach pagans modern medical techniques. As abbess of Hildersheim, she founded a double monastery and hospice that received plague victims. Her innovation parallels that of St. Gall's Benedictine monastery and medical school in Switzerland, established in 720. According to the priorities of St. Benedict, the facility took nurse care as the highest charge because it was commanded by Christ. Within the first century of operation, St. Gall's expanded to a six-bed wing, physician's quarters, pharmacy, and herb garden.

- An eleventh-century healer, the Empress Cunegund, wife of Holy Roman Emperor Henry II, compensated for childlessness by joining her husband in charitable deeds. She built a Benedictine abbey at Kaufungen and spent her retirement years as a nurse.

- In the twelfth century, a German Benedictine nurse, St. Hildegard of Bingen, composed medical handbooks as instruction for her visiting nurse staff. Some of her treatments concentrated on a cure for leprosy, the most loathsome

disease of the age. The great thinkers of the era consulted with her and sent ailing and handicapped people to her for observation and diagnosis. Her contemporaries, St. Margaret of Scotland and Herrade of Landsburg, set up receiving centers for the sick. St. Margaret, a royal wife, washed and treated the sick and aided wandering beggars and prisoners. In the late twelfth century, Herrade served as abbess of Hohenburg, an abbey and hospice on Mt. St. Odelia in the Vosges Mountains in Alsace.

- An unusual Christian convert, St. Godric of Walpole, Norfolk, was a peddler in Lincolnshire before entering the trade of sea merchant and sailing to Scotland, Flanders, and Denmark. In 1105, under the influence of St. Cuthbert of Innisfarne, he changed his life by giving up merchandising and returned to Palestine to nurse in a hospital.

- Queen Matilda, wife of Holy Roman Emperor Henry V, established the Hospital of St. Katharine in London in 1148 and dispatched health workers to visit poor communities.

- The founder of the Gilbertines, England's only indigenous religious order, was Gilbert of Sempringham, who took holy orders in 1122. He established the Rule of St. Benedict for local *conversae* (laywomen) in the mid–twelfth century. He is credited with building leprosariums, orphanages, and thirteen additional houses for monks and nuns.

- A popular figure from La Grande Chartreuse monastery, St. Hugh, Bishop of Lincoln, opened a Carthusian priory in Witham, Somerset, in 1180. He fed and tended lepers and sheltered the homeless. While repairing earthquake damage to his cathedral, he carried bags of lime and stone like a common mason. His shrines in England, France, Flanders, German, Italy, and Spain remain a favorite stopping place of religious pilgrims.

Perhaps the most famous altruist of the Middle Ages, St. Francis of Assisi left a life of luxury among the privileged of Umbria to work at the Church of San Damiano. Content as a mendicant, he repaired churches, nurtured the poor, and treated lepers. An outstanding influence on twelfth-century religious missions, Clare (or Clarissa) dei Sciffi, from a wealthy house in Assisi, Italy, followed the example of poverty and service set by St. Francis, whom she heard preach in her teens. Dressed in the ash-colored robe and hemp belt of the Benedictines, she departed from a comfortable home for Sant'Angelo di Panzo to serve suffering humanity as the "Little Flower of St. Francis." With sisters Agnes and Beatrice, she founded an austere order of Franciscan nuns familiarly known as the Poor Ladies of San Damiano, or Poor Clares. Francis named Agnes abbess of the convent of Monticelli outside Florence. Bolstered by newcomers that included Agnes of Bohemia, the movement expanded with branches in Rome, Venice, Siena, Pisa, and Mantua as well as Prague, Germany, England, and France. At San Damiano, disciples constructed huts of wattle and daub, where they treated the chronically ill whom Francis remanded to their convent. He, too, sought their ministrations after he was afflicted by blindness.

During the first half of the thirteenth century, a number of lesser holy healers served England and France, establishing in small increments the standards and practices of charity that endure to the present day.

- From 1226 to 1257, Abbess Euphemia of England superintended Wherwell Priory, a Benedictine house in Hampshire founded by Queen Alfrida in the tenth century. As a *medica* (female physician), Euphemia built a modern infirmary above a stream as a method of ridding the building of sewage and of decontaminating the premises.
- In her short life, St. Elizabeth of Hungary, wife of Louis (Ludwig) of Thu-

ringia, craved an austere, penitential milieu. With her husband's permission, she spent her dowry on the poor. During the famine of 1226, she took grain from the royal storehouse to bake bread for the hungry. In 1227, she was widowed. Influenced by the Poor Clares, she joined the Franciscan Tertiary Order at Marburg, Hesse, as nurse to lepers and the elderly. Her good works included catching fish to supply meat for the poor, teaching new parents to care for infants, and spinning wool and sewing clothing for the homeless. She established more than a dozen hospitals, each named St. Elizabeth. For her goodness, she was named patron of the homeless, nurses, and widows.

- In 1265, Stephanie de Montaneis of Lyons, France, practiced medicine that she learned from her father, Dr. Étienne Montaneis. Another healer of the era, Sarre of Paris, took her own daughter Florian as apprentice, an act common to families of healers who typically passed the tradition from father to son. An obscure healer, Jehanne of Paris, is affirmed by a listing on the Paris tax rolls in 1292 as a *sage femme* (midwife).
- Contemporaneous with the work of Stephanie de Montaneis, Margaret of Cortona founded Spedale di Santa Maria della Misericordia in Lavinio, Italy, and trained a corps of nurse-nuns known as *le poverelle* (the poor little ones).

In addition to these hallmarks of nursing were the thousands of nameless but essential wet nurses who lived with families, assisted at births, and assumed the role of nurturer and helpmate. For the poor, the post of wet nurse was reassuring to working-class women who had lost children and still had milk available. It was the job of the supervising midwife to match the gentrified or aristocratic mother with a suitable candidate. For at least eighteen months, the wet nurse was assured kind treatment, quality nutrition, shelter, and rest. Cash proceeds were valuable to smallholders and sharecroppers, who had few alternatives but to farm out their wives as nursery maids when crops were bad.

Not all female accomplishments were so unassuming and modest. In the late eleventh century, author and healer Trotula of Salerno in southern Italy, possibly the wife of Dr. Johannes Platearius, was accorded the title of *sapiens matrona* (wise woman) (Marks and Beatty 1972, 44). Publishing under the pseudonym Eros or Erotian, she produced *Passionibus Mulierum Curandorum* (Curing Women's Diseases), also called *Trotula Major,* the first European handbook on diet, exercise, menstruation, contraception, obstetrics, and sexual dysfunction. By way of preface, she explained: "Wherefore I, Trotula, pitying the calamities of women, and at the urgent request of certain ones, began to write this book on the diseases which affect [women]" (Williams and Echols 1994, 47). Among her innovations was quilling, the practice of puffing an irritant such as pepper or euphorbia into the mother's nostrils to induce sneezing as a means of expelling the placenta. Trotula's writings stayed in circulation for five centuries.

A graduate of the liberal, pro-woman School of Salerno, which Constantinus Africanus founded in 1075, Trotula was not accorded the full title of M.D., yet she accepted the post of chair of medicine and performed cesarean sections. Among her practices were the use of opiates during labor and her theory that both men and women could be infertile. The former violated Church dictates that women should suffer as did the biblical Eve; the second innovative concept shocked a patriarchal society that blamed women for being childless. Trotula and her son John compiled a medical encyclopedia *Practica Brevia* (A Short Practical Handbook). Her later writing, *De Aegritudinum Curatione* (Concerning the Cure of Diseases), also known as *Trotula Minor,* remained in print throughout the era and influenced scholars and physicians. So powerful was her reputation that male medical scholars proposed that she was either a misidentified male named Trottus or else a legend.

The twelfth century brought a flurry of hospital building and improvement. In Bruges, Belgium, St. John's Hospital, operated by an Augustinian staff, opened its doors in 1118; London acquired St. Bartholomew's Hospital in 1123. In 1148, Queen Maud (or Matilda) of Scotland founded the Hospital of St. Katharine in London and dispatched health nurses to attend the poor at home. One nurse of the period, Princess Anna Comnena, biographer of her father, Alexis I, did more than the pious, who merely garbed themselves in tatters, sprinkled dust on their heads, and walked among the suffering as a means of readying themselves for the Christian afterlife. Anna went beyond a show of piety to manage the Panocrator Hospital, teach classes, and publish medical texts.

Altruism in the thirteenth century sparked a renaissance of social outreach and more construction of hospitals. In London, St. Thomas's Hospital opened in 1213; in Paris, the Hôtel Dieu, home of *la Grand Chambre des pouvres* (the great room of the poor), the oldest ward in continuous use, set aside a women's ward as a birthing chamber attended by *la dame des accouchées* (the mistress of births). Individuals made their mark in patient care:

- The era is epitomized by Margaret of Metola, Italy, a deformed waif who led a band of followers known as Mantellates into prisons to treat hunger, despair, and "jail fever."
- In 1222, the Grey Sisters, or Sisters of Mercy, evolved a hospice like the Béguinages and launched a public nursing practice among the poor. Other Béguines of this period include the Brethren of the Misericordia in Florence, Italy, begun in 1244 by Pier Bossi, and the Sisters of the Common Life, instituted by Gerhard Groote (or

Geert de Groote) of Deventer around 1375. The brethren chose black robes and masks to conceal their identity while they offered first aid to wayfarers and transported corpses for burial. Bearing a "zane" or basket litter, they staffed a 24-hour rescue operation that remains in service.

In the fourteenth century, the life span of women was compromised by childbearing and attendant complications. From the ages of twenty to forty, they were more likely to die than men. After forty, women's chances of survival soared above men's. Some put their later years to good use in nursing:

- In 1320, a Jewish nurse, Jacoba Felicie, appeared before the Paris magistrate to ask for female practitioners to protect the modesty of female patients. Her crimes consisted of visiting the sick, prescribing medicine, and accepting only what fees patients could pay. Among her arguments in favor of nurse care and midwifery is the reminder that men were not allowed to ask about, observe, or examine the breasts, abdomen, and pudenda of women.
- St. Elizabeth of Coimbra, Portugal, also called Isabel, withdrew from her husband's worldly milieu to rear her children. In 1325, she joined the Franciscan Poor Clares to open a hospital for abandoned infants, aid the poor, and reclaim prostitutes.
- In the 1360s, the University of Bologna hired a female lecturer, Novella d'Andrea, although nothing is said of her expertise.

In general, healers applied pharmacopoeia dating to ancient times, notably, opium, mandrake, and hemlock as anesthesia. Scientifically based treatments called for herbs, purgatives, hot plasters, rare spices and powdered jewels, and earthenware bowls and lancets for cupping and bleeding. Practitioners, like their Babylonian and Egyptian forebears, studied charts and analyses of the planets for assurance that treatment would benefit rather than harm.

One of the most controversial establishments of the era, the Hospital of St. Mary of Bethlehem, opened in London on land donated by Simon Fitzmary and became England's first treatment center for the insane. Badly managed, in 1377 it attempted public service by warehousing lunatics, chaining them to walls, and immuring them in cages with little more than straw for comfort. Attendants did little more than feed them and remove their corpses when they were mercifully relieved of their torment. The ravings of wretched mental patients produced the term "bedlam," a condensation of Bethlehem, a descriptive term that equated with ravings and chaos. Renovated in the early nineteenth century, the upgraded hospital offered more up-to-date treatment and humane care.

A notable medieval failure was the series of military and political expeditions lumped together as the Crusades. Europe's attempt to colonize the Middle East from 1100 to 1300, ostensibly to spread Christianity among Muslims, cost many lives as well as the wealth of nations. Although military might made no significant dent in the Islamic power base, the era opened western Asia to Europeans, broadened world trade, intermingled elements of culture from East and West, and initiated medical innovations. The astonishing stream of pilgrims, warriors, and support personnel during two centuries of conflict called for the establishment of hostels, shelters, infirmaries, and hospitals along the route where volunteer nurse staff treated diseases from the Mediterranean world as well as wounds, malnutrition, and exhaustion. Staffing these way stations was the work of the Catholic Church. Teams of monk-warriors were the first military medical corpsmen. They provided resource information on disease and wellness as well as nursing home care and hospices. Their infirmaries, herbariums, and pharmacies welcomed the needy from all points, made no demands on allegiance, and asked no payment. Among their standard pharmacopoeia were plants valued by ancient Mediterranean healers: thyme as an antispasmodic, alchemilla (lady's mantle) as a restorative for the elderly, mint and fennel to soothe dyspepsia, poppy and mandrake for pain, valerian for rest, and St. John's wort to hasten healing.

Military nursing orders of monks, nuns, and lay volunteers combined religious and medical services for the sake of wanderers far from home:

- In 1050, a nursing order called the Knights Hospitallers of St. John opened St. John of Jerusalem, a one-thousand-bed hospital managed by Peter Gerhard. Attendants dressed in armor topped by black vestments marked by a white Maltese cross and served in an emergency capacity wherever needed, building additional shelters and receiving centers at busy metropolitan centers in Rhodes, Cyprus, Malta, and England. Innovations in their hospitals include written patient charts and scribes to record doctors' prescriptions. In the absence of the knights from headquarters, a nursing sisterhood, Sisters of the Order of St. John of Jerusalem, organized by Agnes of Rome, staffed the wards, tended the laundry, and maintained food supplies. Their uniform consisted of a red habit topped by a white Maltese cross. Later, the base color altered to black. Resettled on Malta after the capture of Jerusalem, the nuns set international standards for professional nursing.
- The Teutonic Knights of Jerusalem, a German order founded in 1100, created the first portable tent emergency rooms staffed by men who doubled as warriors and corpsmen, identified by their white tunics marked with a gold-edged black Maltese cross. Female members wore the same uniform as the men, shared a cloister, and ranged about the neighborhood tending the sick. These forerunners of visiting public nurses were often members of healing families who passed cures and treatments to their children and to apprenticed nieces and nephews.
- A pious brotherhood, the Order of Trinitarians, established in Paris by St. John of Math and Felix of Valois in 1197, carried first aid to casualties of war and domestic outbreaks of plague. Traveling on humble mounts rather than horses, they were simple almoners eventually called "Friars of the Ass." Throughout France and Spain, they were identified by a distinctive uniform—a white tunic marked on the front with a cross formed of a red upright and blue crossbar. A particular service, the ransoming and succor of Christian captives held in Muslim jails, earned them high regard in the military community.
- When Louis IX of France journeyed to the Holy Land in 1249, he added to his staff Hersend and Guillamette de Luys, both midwives who tended the queen at the birth of a fourth son and treated and delivered the children of soldiers' wives. In 1293, Louis's sister, Marguerite of Bourgogne, built an attractive stone hospital in Tounerre, France, which featured stained glass panels, artistic fretwork, and Romanesque detailing capturing the spirit and service of the Crusades.

Preceding the Renaissance, the energy of wise and compassionate women supported less mercenary healing ministries. Listed among practitioners are these:

- In 1326, Sarah of St. Gilles, a Jewish healer in Marseilles, France, received royal permission to train an apprentice.
- A Scandinavian Cistercian nun and visionary, St. Bridget of Upland, patron saint of Sweden, managed two careers in her long life. She was married and bore eight children, one of whom became St.

Catherine of Sweden. Simultaneously, she served Queen Blanche of Namur as lady-in-waiting. Widowed in 1344, Bridget joined the Cistercians and composed *Revelationes Caelestes* (Heavenly Revelations). At her urging, King Magnus II donated to the poor funds he might have spent on luxuries. In 1346, Bridget founded the Bridgettine order at Vadstena, a mixed house of nuns and monks that spawned seventy monasteries. She left the mission network to local management and migrated to Rome, where she founded a hospice, treated the sick, and supported local healers until her death in 1373.

- Around 1367, Caterina Benincasa, later called St. Catherine of Siena, patron saint of Italy, treated victims of epidemics. Allied with the Order of St. Dominic, her outreach was the beginning of the Caterinati, who focused on lepers, plague victims, and other incurables. Her work in 1372 during an outbreak of plague demonstrated piety and Catholic zeal to help those near death. As a result of her compassion for victims of catastrophic illness, Siena was the location chosen for the Hospital of Santa Maria della Scala.

- At the beginning of the fifteenth century, Frances of Rome and her sister-in-law, Vannozza, conducted social work and served the community as visiting nurses. In addition to offering public prayers for the needy, they worked in the wards of the Ospedale di San Spirito (Hospital of the Holy Spirit). Frances formed an order of gentlewomen or lay nuns attached to the local Benedictine house, officially recognized in 1425 as Oblates of Mary, later as the Oblates of Tor de' Specchi, the first uncloistered Italian nuns. Their work continues in Switzerland and the United States.

- Some fifteenth-century nurses found work in monastery infirmaries or as retainers of a wealthy household, as is the case with Elysabeth Keston, respected practitioner in the household of Isabelle Despenser, Countess of Warwick. In 1439, the countess recognized Keston's work with a stipend.

- In the late fifteenth century, St. Catherine of Genoa, member of the influential Fieschi family of Liguria, and author of *Dialogues on the Soul and the Body*, treated plague at St. Laurence Hospital in Genoa, Italy. In Brescia, the company of Divine Love, an outreach to victims of syphilis, organized an auxiliary of nurses to tend female victims, most of whom were prostitutes and social outcasts. Led by St. Angela Merici, the sisterhood provided halfway houses for women, offering education and help in reestablishing their lives. The corps were the beginnings of the Ursulines.

- In this same period, Queen Isabella of Castile, Spain, became a forerunner of Florence Nightingale by turning her attention to battlefield nursing. Isabella stocked tent dressing stations and ambulances for her troops to take to the front and invented the first movable hospitals, where she personally dressed wounds. She is best known for dispatching Christopher Columbus to the New World and for establishing the mission of Bartolomé de Las Casas, Apostle to the Indies, to evangelize and succor American Indians in Mexico.

See also: Christian Nursing; Disease; Gender Issues in Nursing; Hildegard of Bingen; Hospice; Midwifery

Sources

Baugh, Albert C., ed. *A Literary History of England.* New York: Appleton-Century-Crofts, 1948.

Bean, William B., M.D. "Medicine's Forgotten Man—the Patient." *Nursing Forum* (1963): 46–69.

Bois, Danuta. "Trotula of Salerno. "http://www.net-srq.com/~dbois/trotula.html.

Bradley, S. A. J., ed. *Anglo-Saxon Poetry.* London: J. M. Dent, 1995.

Brainard, Annie M. *The Evolution of Public Health Nursing.* Philadelphia: W. B. Saunders, 1922.

Bryant, Arthur. *The Medieval Foundation of England.* Garden City, N.Y.: Doubleday, 1967.

Butler, Alban. *Lives of the Saints.* New York: Barnes and Noble, 1997.

"The Catholic Encyclopedia." http://www.knight.org/advent/cathen.html.

"Catholic Online Saints." http://www.catholiconline.com/saints.html.

Cavendish, Richard, ed. *May, Myth and Magic.* New York: Marshall Cavendish, 1970.

Cohn-Sherbok, Lavinia. *Who's Who in Christianity.* Chicago: Routledge, 1998.

Crystal, David, ed. *The Cambridge Biographical Dictionary.* Cambridge: University of Cambridge, 1996.

Deen, Edith. *Great Women of the Christian Faith.* Westwood, N.J.: Barbour, 1959.

Delehaye, Hippolyte. *The Legends of the Saints.* Dublin: Four Courts Press, 1955.

Dobson, R. B. "Gilbert of Sempringham and the Gilbertine Order: ca. 130–ca. 1300." *English Historical Review* (February 1998): 147–149.

Dolan, Josephine A., R.N. *History of Nursing.* Philadelphia: W. B. Saunders, 1968.

Duby, Georges, and Michelle Perrot, general eds. *A History of Women in the West.* Cambridge, Mass.: Belknap Press, 1992.

"Famous Belgians: Lambert le Bégue." http://ourworld.compuserve.com/homepages/tielemans/hp67marc.htm.

Farmer, David Hugh. *The Oxford Dictionary of Saints.* Oxford: Oxford University Press, 1992.

Fischer-Kamel, Doris Sofie. "The Midwife in History with Special Emphasis on Practice in Medieval Europe and in the Islamic World." University of Arizona, 1987. Monograph.

Franck, Irene M., and David M. Brownstone. *Women's World: A Timeline of Women in History.* New York: HarperPerennial, 1995.

Griffin, Gerald Joseph, and H. Joann King Griffin. *Jensen's History and Trends of Professional Nursing.* Saint Louis, Mo.: C. V. Mosby, 1965.

Hallam, Elizabeth, general ed. *Saints: Who They Are and How They Help You.* New York: Simon and Schuster, 1994.

Hastings, James, ed. *Encyclopedia of Religion and Ethics.* New York: Charles Scribner's Sons, 1951.

"The History of St. Giles." http://www.oxford.anglican.org/Parishes/stgilesoxford/history.htm.

Hollister, C. Warren. *Medieval Europe: A Short History.* New York: McGraw-Hill, 1994.

Kalisch, Philip, and Beatrice J. Kalisch. *The Advance of American Nursing.* Boston: Little, Brown, 1978.

Kauffman, Christopher J. *Tamers of Death: The History of the Alexian Brothers.* New York: Seabury Press, 1976.

Kent, Jacqueline C. *Women in Medicine.* Minneapolis, Minn.: Oliver Press, 1998.

Kirsch, J. P. "St. Dymphna." http://www.madnation.org/Heroine.htm, 1999.

Knuth, Elizabeth T. "The Beguines." http://www.users.csbsju.edu/~eknuth/xpxx/beguines.html, December 1992.

Lee, Gerard A. *Leper Hospitals in Medieval Ireland.* Dublin: Four Courts Press, 1996.

Lewis, Lionel Smithett. "The Celtic Church." In *St. Joseph of Arimathaea at Glastonbury.* London: James Clarke, 1955.

Lopez, Robert S. *The Birth of Europe.* New York: M. Evans, 1967.

Magnusson, Magnus, general ed. *Cambridge Biographical Dictionary.* Cambridge: University of Cambridge, 1990.

Mantinband, James H. *Dictionary of Latin Literature.* New York: Philosophical Library, 1956.

Marks, Geoffrey, and William K. Beatty. *Women in White.* New York: Charles Scribner's Sons, 1972.

McCall, Andrew. *The Medieval Underworld.* New York: Dorset Press, 1979.

McKown, Robin. *Heroic Nurses.* New York: G. P. Putnam's Sons, 1966.

McSkimming, Sammy. "The Coming of Saint Columba." http://www.dalriada.co.uk/Archives.columba.htm, 1992.

"Medieval Sourcebook: Life of St. Goderic." http://www.fordham.edu/halsall/source/goderic.html, 1996.

Murray, James P. *Galway: A Medico-Social History.* Galway: Kenny's Bookshop and Art Galleries Ltd., n.d.

O'Ceirin, Kit, and Cyril O'Ceirin. *Women of Ireland: A Biographical Dictionary.* Galway: Tir Eolas Newtownlynch, 1996.

O'Croinin, Daibhi. *Early Medieval Ireland, 400–1200.* London: Longman, 1995.

"The Order of Trinitarians." http://www.knight.org/advent/cathen/15045d.htm.

Paor, Liam de. *Saint Patrick's World.* Dublin: Four Courts Press, 1996.

Parry, Melanie, ed. *Larousse Dictionary of Women.* New York: Larousse Kingfisher Chambers, 1994.

"Psautier de 'Lambert le Bégue.'" http://www.ulg.ac.be/libnet/enlumin/en10302.htm.

Raby, F. J. E., ed. *A History of Christian-Latin Poetry.* Oxford: Clarendon Press, 1953.

Ranft, Patricia. *Women and the Religious Life in Premodern Europe.* New York: St. Martin's Press, 1996.

Rawcliffe, Carole. *Medicine and Society in Later Medieval England.* Gloucestershire: Alan Sutton Publishing, 1995.

Rice, David Talbot, ed. *The Dawn of European Civilization: The Dark Ages.* New York: McGraw-Hill, 1965.

"St. Columba." http://www.heritagehouse.uk.com/columba.thm.

———. http://www.reformation.org/vol2ch20.html.

"St. Gilbert." http://www.hullp.demon.co.uk/SacredHeart/saint/StGilbertS.htm.

Smaridge, Norah. *Hands of Mercy: The Story of Sister-Nurses in the Civil War*. New York: Benziger Brothers, 1960.

Steinberg, S. H., ed. *Cassell's Encyclopaedia of World Literature*. New York: Funk and Wagnalls, 1953.

Thornhill, Gill. "Trotula of Salerno." http://www.amazoncity.com/technology/museum/trotula.html.

Trager, James. *The Women's Chronology*. New York: Henry Holt, 1994.

Tuchman, Barbara W. *A Distant Mirror: The Calamitous 14th Century*. New York: Alfred A. Knopf, 1978.

"Wherwell." http://www.hants.org.uk/localpages/north_west/andover/wherwell/about.html.

Williams, Marty Newman, and Anne Echols. *Between Pit and Pedestal: Women in the Middle Ages*. Princeton, N.J.: Markus Wiener Publishers, 1994.

Midwifery

Although midwifery has varied widely over time, the universal place of the midwife in family health establishes the birthing practice as a folk art. Descriptions of birthing in Mamluk, Egypt, from 1250 to 1517 A.D., describe collective drama—a festive gathering of seven days, concluding with the midwife displaying the newborn, followed by the mother, who tossed salt and cumin throughout the house.

Anthropologists surmise that, among early peoples who developed strong trunk muscles and squatted by firesides with their knees spread wide, giving birth was less arduous than for modern women. Attendant midwives tended to work with partners. When they assisted women in labor, the junior or apprentice partner steadied the mother from behind and at each side and massaged and kneaded the abdomen to comfort and en-

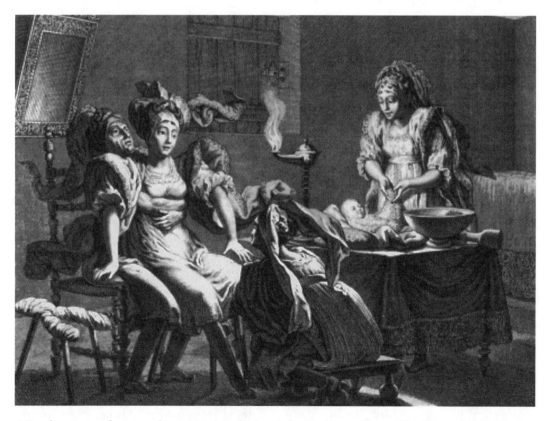

A French engraving of an upper-class woman giving birth with the aid of three midwives (U.S. Library of Medicine)

courage normal contractions. The senior partner commanded the front view and reached into the birth canal to turn the infant and to ease its delivery. This vertical style of birthing altered over time. As described in colonial New England, social or community birthing teams, called gossips, bonded neighboring goodwives in a woman-centered bedside ritual of love and support. Amid lighted candles in a darkened room, they sipped their caudle, a ceremonial drink brewed from beneficial botanicals for the occasion. The tone of the ceremony was pious and fearful in anticipation of physical danger to both mother and child. The midwife's role required uncomplicated services to the mother: a single birthing coach guided the infant from the birth canal, severed the umbilical cord, removed the afterbirth, and tended to the nurturance and washing of the infant until the mother was ready to breast-feed. The event concluded with the upsitting, arrangement of the mother and child on pillows to receive male kin and wellwishers.

Early examples of women's cycles and parturition procedures come from cave drawings, bas-reliefs, statues, and papyri. According to the women of India and Afghanistan, Sanskrit *samhitas* or religious handbooks, describe the work of the *dai*, the traditional midwife. Clad in a white sari that suggests the uniform of Mother Teresa's order, she supervised prenatal and postnatal care, labor, and delivery. As named in the Farsi language, the *mommah* is the traditional source of herbal remedies, massage, and folk treatments for impaired lactation, swelling, backache, and morning nausea; today in Sri Lanka, the *marthuvichi* continues the tradition of family health care by vaccinating infants and distributing formula. The Tunisian *qabileh* practices ancient methods of pain relief and healing.

In the Far East, midwifery allies with deeply ingrained moral and social values. The *chu san wan* of Korea perpetuates a tradition of unifying families to support the mother and witness the birth. In Mandarin China, where birthing practices of the *tu tan se* (midwife) earned mention in scripture, the thrust of birthing philosophy is summarized in the *Tao Te Ching* of Lao-tzu (sixth century B.C.), which offers surprisingly modern advice: "You are a midwife: you are assisting at someone else's birth. Do good without show or fuss. Facilitate what is happening rather than what you think ought to be happening. If you must take the lead, lead so that the mother is helped, yet still free and in charge" (Shroff 1997, 34). The text concludes with a reminder that midwifery is a time-honored act of enabling. When the child is born, the midwife should stand in the background so the mother can experience a sense of accomplishment.

The *daya*, the Arabic midwife of Sudan and Egypt, could join doctors in the study of gynecology and obstetrics at the temple of Sais near the Nile River's Rosetta estuary. Women practiced medicine from 2730 B.C. and, according to the Kahun Papyrus of 2160 B.C., performed cesarean section. As stated in the Westcar Papyrus, Egyptian midwives of 1700 B.C. preferred birthing chairs as a means of support for the parturient woman. Beginning in 1500 B.C., midwives studied at Heliopolis, a coeducational priestly institution that may have included Moses and his wife Zipporah among its alumni. Egyptian healers included two queens: Hatshepsut around 1500 B.C. and Cleopatra around 60 B.C. Bas-reliefs from Luxor's palace birth chambers depict midwives assisting women of the royal family and picture Isis, goddess and patron of women, surveying the event. By the fifth century B.C., attitudes had changed: women were brought up in seclusion by a repressive patriarchy and shamed because of the shape, odor, and function of their bodies. Midwives crept into birthing chambers to conduct their work out of the public eye.

These bits and pieces of birthing history testify to the importance of midwives to a healthy, ordered society. The book of Genesis in the Pentateuch, the Ebers Papyrus, and the Talmud refer to the midwife, including the Jewish attendant on the last delivery of

Rachel, Jacob's favorite, around 1800 B.C. In Exodus, the Egyptian pharaoh enlists Hebrew midwives to help him exterminate all Hebrew males at birth, thus limiting the immigrant population in his realm. During the Hebrews' travails in the first chapter of Exodus, Egypt's king instructed Hebrew midwives Shiprah and Puah to kill male infants. When the women disobeyed, they made up a lie that Hebrew women deliver so fast that the boy babies were already received into the family when the attendants arrived. The fact that a king would consult with birthing specialists indicates that they were respected (although manipulated) medical professionals in the time of Moses. From the tenth century B.C., a graphic passage about Tamar, David's daughter, describes the birth of her twins, Perez and Zerah, and the midwife's attempt to mark the firstborn with a scarlet cord, an oriental sign of blessing. To her surprise, the second son managed to be born first.

The Greeks and Babylonians concurred on the tradition of respect for those who attended women in childbirth. In Athens during the fifth century B.C., Socrates' mother is named as a practitioner. In the second century, Aspasia, a Milesian intellectual who became Pericles' consort, served as obstetrician and surgeon. Soranus, the Ephesian scholar educated at Alexandria, lectured and practiced obstetrics in Rome during the early second century A.D. He wrote *De Morbis Mulierum* (Concerning Women's Disease), the first identified text on midwifery. Devoid of the usual arrogance toward midwives, he treasured their secret arts and set the standards for the *obstetrix* in a treatise known as "The Hygiene of a Midwife." His outline did not require that the midwife herself be a mother; rather, Soranus called for literacy, good sight and hearing, robust health, and intelligence. He expected the midwife to make keen observations, keep secrets of the examining room and birthing chamber, and to avoid the superstitions that impeded empiricism. As to fees, he stressed: "She must not be greedy for money, lest she give an abortive wickedly for payment" (Lefkowitz 1992, 266).

Of particular influence in ancient Greece and Rome were those folk practitioners who had themselves experienced healthy pregnancies and easy births and older midwives, who suffered less control by males. Such assistants to parturition the Greeks called *maia*, followers of the semilegendary Agnodice, a transdressing gynecologist whom Greek women revered as the first midwife. A funerary stela from the fourth century B.C. pictures the midwife Phanostrate; a bas-relief from first-century Ostia, Rome's seaport, shows a two-woman team, one supporting the mother in a birthing chair and the other seated at the mother's knees and gripping the fetus as it emerges from the womb.

The world's midwives maintained esteem primarily from the people who most needed their services—women of childbearing age and men anxious over their lack of a thriving male heir. Although 25–40 percent of parturient mothers died in childbirth during the Renaissance, female patients avoided the misogyny of male doctors by seeking gynecological and obstetrical advice and care from other women, who guarded their privacy and the secrecy of the lying-in chamber. Derived from the Middle English for "with woman," the term "midwife" parallels the Latin *uxor obstetrix*, Arabic *muwallida*, French *sage femme*, Dutch *stadsvroedvrouw*, Italian *comadre*, Yiddish *vartsfroy*, Hawaiian *pale keiki*, and the Appalachian "granny woman." The field worldwide comprises compassionate local woman known for their commitment to fellow citizens, advocacy of women, accessibility in time of labor and delivery, or, less logically, for having the most successful pregnancies and live births among community women. In Casablanca, Morocco, the midwife is a respected family associate on a par with a godmother. The association of delivery nurse and family members continues until the child is betrothed and married. The midwife holds an honored position at circumcision and naming rituals and washes the corpses of the family's dead.

From early in the twentieth century, "Aunt Ella" Ingenthron Dunn, author of *The Granny*

Woman of the Hills, traveled by mule, horse, buggy, farm wagon, and car to treat the women of Walnut Shade, an Ozark village in Missouri. The impetus for her job came from her mother, who had been a midwife and homesteader before her. To Aunt Ella, "Being a granny woman was more like an angel-of-mercy business than a job." She worked long hours for five or ten dollars, and occasionally for "only a 'thank you'" (Aikman 1966, 21). Her simples, carried in a little black bag, consisted of goldenseal, catnip leaves, watermelon seeds, and the basics—cotton, muslin, scales, scissors, camphor, cornstarch, and goose grease.

The protocols of "handywomen," or lay midwives, preserved a blend of natural traditions that couple barnyard observations with herbalism, chants, religious ritual, and phases of the moon. A particularly versatile wise woman, the South African *ou tantes,* even expanded the practice of midwifery to the care and delivery of farm animals. In general, early midwives were greathearted and hospitable caregivers who welcomed parturient women to their homes, which served as temporary lying-in clinics, or stayed unspecified amounts of time with patients, who could remain in labor for days. When unwed mothers fled their home communities to seek discreet midwives, they typically left their infants in the midwife's care for placement in foundling homes and orphanages. In the case of abortions, it was the midwife who buried or discarded the evidence. When the mother delivered a freak too frail or handicapped to survive, the midwife might seek temporary lodging for the newborn or quietly strangle it and inter its remains. If the mother expired while giving birth, the midwife was skilled at performing a cesarean delivery to save the imperiled babe and at laying out the mother's corpse for burial.

Worldwide, the standard midwife's kit included compresses; the birthing stool, chair, or tub; and such additions as magic stones. Georgian granny women of the plantation era augmented the basics with black string to tie around the waist, cobwebs to coagulate blood, a blue bottle to blow into, and chicken feathers to dispatch evil. Each professional bundle contained twine for pulling the infant in cases of difficult presentation and knives for embryotomy, the dissection of a stillborn infant practiced in pre-Christian Hawaii. Handled with care were vials of linseed or olive oil, ale and spirits, pinches of lady's mantle to stanch bleeding, hops as a palliative, birthwort, smut rye, and belladonna, an antispasmodic for regulating contractions. For analgesics, they carried wormwood, henbane, poppy, and mandragora (mandrake). If the birth were delayed, it could be hurried with pennyroyal, savin, coriander, or ergot, specifics that the midwife shared with prostitutes, who used them as abortifacients. For imminent miscarriage, Spanish midwives might administer a poultice of vinegar, plantain, and the juice of nightshade, a common pasture weed; the black plantation granny preferred black haw root tea. The frontier American practitioner applied oil and wine to the newborn, spoon-fed brandy or wild cherry bark tea to stimulate mother and child and poppy tea to quiet a crying infant, and administered tansy tea to bring on a miscarriage or cure irregular menstrual cycles, hasten menstrual extraction, relieve clotting, and prevent or cure venereal disease.

Native American healers favored masks and ceremonial chants and prayers to treat women and ease delivery. They selected their pharmacopoeia from indigenous plants: aromatic pennyroyal or wild ginger to cure an erratic monthly cycle; allspice for menstrual flooding; croton tea or soapweed to induce abortion; blue cohosh to bring on labor; golden ragwort, spikenard, and juniper to hasten slow labor; and nightshade, highbush cranberry, or red alder bark for painful labor. The Navaho prescribed broom snakeroot to expel the placenta. The Penobscot trusted a decoction of white ash to cleanse the womb. For problems of lactation, they used ginseng and slippery elm for breast pain and saguaro or snow-on-the-mountain to start the flow of milk. North American Indian birthing attendants chose pine for swelling; agrimony, willow bark, and angelica for fever; alumroot and cherry for hemorrhage; bearberry and burdock for venereal disease; Mormon tea or *yerba-mansa* for syphilis; buckeye for infection; quinine for malaise; and mugwort for menopause. For infants there was arrowhead tea for fretfulness, smartweed to halt thumb sucking, and nettle for teething. Louise Plenty Holes, a Lakota elder and *pejuta win* (medicine woman) of the Pine Ridge Agency in the Dakotas, speaks of a white puffball found on the prairie that contains brown powder suitable for coagulating the umbilicus.

Because midwives and their clients are traditionally female and thus linked biblically to evil and the fall of man, they have historically suffered the denigration that attaches to the sex. In the thirteenth century, female healers were suppressed and excluded from universities. During the witch hunts from the fourteenth to the seventeenth centuries, male doctors sought a medical monopoly. They allied with church courts to link midwifery and sorcery in the minds of zealots. These superstitious know-nothings turned to doctors to identify witches and then tormented and burned at the stake thousands of health workers who came under suspicion of complicity with dark forces or outright carnality with Satan, in a wave of killing tantamount to cultural genocide.

In 1484, Dominicans Heinrich Kraemer and Jacob Sprenger, under the auspices of Pope Innocent VIII, published *Malleus Maleficarum* (Hammer of Witches), a handbook for witch hunters. The text targeted midwives for practicing the black arts and harming or murdering mothers and eating unbaptized newborns, usually the offspring of peasants. Fraught with patriarchy and misogyny, the text warns of old women, midwives, and powerful females, all threatening the superiority of men. Chosen punishments included starving, beating, ducking, shaving, applying thumbscrews, using spikes, and stretching on the rack.

Usually a mature, trustworthy figure, either married or widowed, the midwife named in histories was typically uneducated in medicine and anatomy but probably apprenticed to a senior midwife or surgeon. One notable practitioner, Louyse Bourgeois of St. Germain, outside Paris, was an anomaly, a midwife not of the laboring class. She married a physician, Martin Boursier, and assisted a master surgeon and retired midwife, Ambroise Paré, who had practiced at the Hôtel Dieu in the 1530s. Although she lacked the license of the *matrone jurée* (sworn midwife), which required the testimony of a medical doctor, two surgeons, and two midwives, she treated the poor and published an obstetrical textbook in 1609, the first scientific handbook published by a woman. The work, which describes how to revive a moribund fetus, stayed in print for a century, passing through six upgrades.

Bourgeois's skill brought her into the service of aristocrats, whom she charged 1,000 ducats for delivering a male infant and 600 for a girl. She was the attendant of Marie de Medici, wife of Henry IV, to whom the textbook was dedicated. Seven times, she treated Marie and delivered the child later crowned as Louis XIII. After a patient, the Duchesse d'Orléans, died of puerperal fever in 1627, Bourgeois's reputation declined, but she established a practice for a successor, her daughter. Another student, Marguérite du Tertre de La Marche, excelled at obstetrics, supervised the birthing clinic of the Hôtel Dieu, and published a textbook for her own classroom use.

The well-read midwife may have owned one of several handbooks about midwifery, such as the work of two male practitioners— Percival Willughby, inventor of a forerunner of forceps, who wrote *Observations in Midwifery* (ca. 1670), or J. Sharp, author of *The Midwives Book, or the Whole Art of Midwifery Discovered, Directing Childbearing Women How to Behave Themselves in Their Conception, Bearing and Nursing of Children* (1671), both written in vernacular English rather than the more scholarly Latin. In the late seventeenth century, Spanish authors Damián Carbón and Juan Alonso de loy Ruyzes published birthing handbooks in Castilian vernacular specifically worded for use by midwives. A text issued by Anne Horenburg of Braunschweig in 1700 employed the artful rhetorical device of a conversation between two sisters. A popular German work published illustrations and observations by Justine Dittrichin Siegemundin of Rohnstock, Silesia, and was reissued in Dutch. In practice in Liegnitz, Poland, she served the royal Prussian family at Brandenburg as a practitioner of natural childbirth.

In contrast to the stereotype of the crabbed hag, the midwife was typically bright, energetic, and innovative, like Peter Chamberlen, the inventor of forceps whose grandson, Hugh Chamberlen, tried to unionize English midwives in 1634, and François Mauriceau, author of an obstetrical text that pioneered a method of puncturing the amnion to speed labor. The female practitioner was often married to a prosperous burgher and trained as deputy midwife for up to seven years under a relative or *maestra* (senior practitioner) before developing a group or private practice.

Parish women's groups superintended midwifery, as demonstrated by a remonstrance in Swarthmore, England, dated October 12, 1675, upbraiding a careless midwife and limiting her service to assistance of other professionals. A letter dated September 12, 1677, from a Dublin parish concerning supervision of sisters and midwives asked that female parishioners "looke into & consider whether there be amongst you any women who profess truth [that] take upon them [the] office of a midwife, nurse or nurse-keepers . . . whether they keep truth cleare and keep up their testimonys for [the] Lord in faithfullness" (Marland 1993, 62–63). By the seventeenth century, the College of Physicians in Zaragoza, Spain, required four years of apprenticeship of its recognized *parteras* and *matronas;* the London diocese licensed practitioners and kept records of their deliveries. An example from St. Andrew Holborn names Debora Bromfield and the six respectable women who supported her petition for registry in 1663. All

told, she had successfully delivered them of thirty-two healthy children.

Challenges to midwives and midwifery abound in nursing history. A personal attack against Jane Creighton of Charleston forced her to advertise in the *South Carolina Gazette* on April 28, 1759, that she had been maliciously accused by a patient and was ready to answer all allegations. In Posen, Poland, in 1677, anti-Semitic laws required Jews to treat only their own ethnic group. In 1729, a similar dictum from Hamburg officials forbade Jewish midwives from attending Gentile parturient women. Regional regulation usually broadened circumstances where and when licensed midwives could practice and under what conditions. Out of civic, religious, and moral obligation, midwives served poor women gratis. For those treating women too poor to afford their services or for practical or visiting nurses who only chanced on women in labor, some municipalities waived licensing fees or allowed practitioners to work outside regulations. Other services expected of midwives included a form of in-house spying to report to authorities on contagious disease, lewd behavior, marital or child abuse, or sex crimes, such as, in 1677, the rebuke of Margaret Treadway, a respected Quaker midwife, to a Buckinghamshire girl accused of incest.

Excellence of service could be judged by word-of-mouth quality control (the numbers of recommendations versus the number of deaths) and by the size of repeat business from satisfied clients, including first and second generations of patients in a single family. Another factor was the rank of patients, which was indicated by the honorifics "mistress," "madam," "gentlewoman," or "lady." Clients often included physicians' and ministers' wives and nurses, whose patronage attested to the midwife's skill, sobriety, integrity, and discretion, such as Mrs. Abraham Colfe, an English country parson's wife who attended the sick in the 1640s, and Catharina Schrader of Dokkum, Holland, widow of a surgeon. Her diaries, published as *Mother and Child Saved: The Memoirs of the Frisian Midwife Catharina*

Schrader, 1693–1745, tell of intense emotions at the loss of a new mother. An American practitioner, Temperance Worthington, wife of the Reverend Cotton Mather Smith, in 1784 performed the nursing and midwifery chores expected of minister's wives as a means of saving parishioners from smallpox and adding members to the church roll.

The number of midwives who gave signed testimony in ecclesiastical courts about virginity, rapes, premature births, stillbirths, post-quickening abortions, infanticide, and deaths in childbirth proves both their educational attainments and the community's respect. Common examples derive from Hispanic communities in eighteenth- and nineteenth-century California, where mestizo midwives attended Indian women. Acting as lay ministers, they baptized stillborn infants and performed last rites for moribund women and infants, whom the parish church reported as converts to Catholicism. A dramatic example from a trial in San Antonio records the 1795 court appearance of midwife Manuela Matiana de Lara concerning the rape of a thirteen-year-old girl by her father. A second-hand report states: "Asked if, in the inspection she has made of María Antonio-Manzola, [Manuela] noticed that she had been violated, she replied that she had not been completely raped, but that she had certainly had her virginity offended" (Nixon 1946, 83). Other services of respected nurse-attendants included the witnessing of birth records and naming ceremonies and emergency baptisms. These tasks placed some practitioners under church control, which recognized that midwives rivaled priests for the job of baptizing infants. In Italy, the midwife, the only female admitted to the baptism, supervised female morality. Another church-centered service resulted from witch hunts, when midwives applied their knowledge of anatomy to searches for marks of the devil, who allegedly left identifiable proof of copulation with female witches.

In most areas, birthing was a neighborly task and a form of female bonding and networking, as displayed by Catherine Blakley, respected deliverer of three thousand children in the colonial capital of Williamsburg, Virginia. The job of a normal delivery and after-birth care required no assistance from a physician. If obstetrical anomalies such as eclampsia, ectopic pregnancy, or premature labor proved beyond the practitioner's talents and equipment, she was obliged to summon a surgeon, who possessed the requisite knives, tongs, and griffin's feet and crochets, two types of hooked needles. However, for isolated women, no such backup existed. Among mountain and rural folk, the resulting higher death rate for mother and child attests to the need for reliable laypersons.

Earnings varied, depending on where midwives practiced and the status of their clients. Fees for *Weise Frauen* in fifteenth-century Germany ranged from 2 to 8 gulden annually, or about 20 percent of the earnings of a barber-surgeon, plus a pittance for the *Kindbetthelferinnen* (childbed helpers); in England during the seventeenth century fees ranged from two shillings six pence to ten shillings and were often augmented with tips. In Jewish ghettos, an annual salary assured the services of a midwife, perhaps as an inducement for families to remain and as an assurance that the poor were not neglected. In Posen, Poland, in 1675, the community's Jewish midwife earned 12 florins annually; by the end of the eighteenth century, the stipend had risen to 600–900 florins per year. In 1763, Sara van der Wegh, a Dutch midwife in Delf-shaven, earned 60 guilders a year. A pious Yiddish midwife, Hanna Sandusky of Pittsburgh, Pennsylvania, immigrated to the United States around 1860. Along with matchmaking and sewing shrouds, she attended 3,571 births, for which she charged no fee. Others in the immigrant community, who called her "Bobba," accorded their respect and admiration for her kindheartedness. Where the demand was great, a midwife might make a career of a single service and set up a fee scale that accepted coins, goods, or services, such as a load of firewood, a milk cow, or plowing. In some rural situations or parishes where practitioners competed for trade, a midwife might work at farming, looming, and other tasks or as a visiting nurse and caregiver to the terminally ill.

The work of birthing fluctuated with the vicissitudes of war, epidemics, natural catastrophes, a failing economy, or social and moral castigation of select groups such as Jews, Quakers, Catholics, Huguenots, Gypsies, or immigrants in general. Around 1649, Quaker sisters were expelled from Anglican hospitals; in 1662, an ecclesiastical court in Stockport, England, harassed Ann Shield and her daughter Constance, Quaker midwives who practiced in a parish of the Church of England. What seem to be traditionally negative comments about midwives and their practice may be open to reinterpretation when considered by medical historians from the twentieth century. A case in point is Elizabeth Cellier, dubbed the "Popish Midwife" and castigated by political enemies in the early 1680s, when political unrest among London Protestants victimized Catholics.

The eighteenth century saw multiple crises in midwifery. The cause of conflict was the intrusion of male medical figures in the birthing process, which women had previously considered a normal, nonmedical phase of their lives. In Navarre, Spain, licensed midwifery depended on written examinations administered and graded by parish priests and municipal physicians. In 1723, Johan von Hoorn, author of a midwives' handbook, became Sweden's first state-paid teacher of midwifery. In France in 1728, Louis XVI demanded that his wife, Queen Maria, deliver on her back so he could observe the process. Because of the royal example, French women abandoned the birthing stool and more comfortable birthing positions that used gravity to assist their labors. Around 1730, Europe's male midwives began acquiring advanced training and assuming more responsibility for labor and delivery, especially in metropolitan areas. In 1733, Thomas White licensed only male practitioners at the Royal College of Physicians in Manchester. In 1757, Matthew Turner offered

formal midwife training in London, the same year that Braunschweig legislated a midwifery ordinance that ousted illiterate practitioners by requiring formal course work in female anatomy and physiology taught by a male professor at Das Anatomisch-Chirurgische Institut (the Anatomical-Surgical Institute).

Throughout the mid–eighteenth century, surgeons began ousting midwives from the task of autopsy and investigation of infanticide. By 1766, male physicians and barber-surgeons encouraged the use of forceps, a tool rarely found in a midwife's kit. Midwives charged that the device shortened labor to the detriment of mother and child, primarily to increase the deliverer's patient load and earnings. An impassioned letter in an issue of the *Virginia Gazette* dated February 11, 1766, decried the notion of male midwives, declaring, "It is a notorious fact that more children have been lost since Women were so scandalously indecent as to employ Men than for Ages before that Practice became so general" (Spruill 1972, 275). Such outbursts did little to promote the cause of all-female midwives as the trend toward male attendants continued. In 1773, a municipal action against Isabel Cortés, a midwife of Archidona, Spain, stripped her of authority to administer compounds to combat sterility and postpartum complications. In 1795, Barcelona College of Surgery offered courses in midwifery that deliberately excluded women by requiring proficiency in Latin, logic, algebra, and physics. By the end of the century, the switch from midwifery to male-dominated hospital care had altered the trend toward midwifery for all but the poorest families.

The eighteenth century also produced notable institutional and official ferment on the subject of birthing. The Madrid College of Surgery created a *cátedra de partos* (chair of childbirth) in 1787. That same year, Teresa Ployant, a French midwife at the Naples hospital for incurables, published *Breve Compandio dell' Arte Ostetricia* (A Short Handbook on the Obstetrical Art), a manual for midwives that recommended assiduous study of medical principles to prevent male doctors from subsuming women's role in childbirth. In 1798 at New York Hospital, Valentine Seaman organized a nursing and midwifery training program, an educational forerunner of curricula in the next decade at Woman's Hospital in Philadelphia, New England Female College of Boston, New England Hospital for Women and Children, and the Philadelphia Dispensary, where Quakers began upgrading standards and procedures.

Throughout Europe and the United States, the nineteenth century continued the trend toward medicalizing and institutionalizing the normal birth process and denigrating the practice of midwifery within the medical hierarchy. Although midwifery gained from Ignaz Semmelweis's training of nurses in sanitary procedures to control puerperal fever, other losses to medicine were considerable. One scholarly midwife, Marie Anne Victoire Gillain Boivin of Montreuil, France, studied under nuns at Etampes. She set up L'Hospice de la Maternité in 1800 and focused on the treatment of prostitutes, whom doctors tended to reject. Refused admission to the Royal Academy of Medicine, which accepted no female students, she turned her energies to translating studies on uterine hemorrhage and became one of the first practitioners to study fetal heartbeat. For her skill, she earned a *Doctor Honoris Causa* (honorary M.D.) from the University of Marburg. Working with Marie-Louise Lachapelle, *sage femme in chef* (chief midwife) of the Hôtel Dieu and founder of the Children's Hospital at Port Royal, Boivin produced a text on female organs, the first to record urethral cancer. Lachapelle, author of the three-volume *Pratique des Accouchements ou Mémoirs et Observations Choisies* (The Practice of Midwifery or Memoirs and Selected Observations), treated charity cases and followed a family-centered tradition of midwifery. She organized a maternity department and taught apprentices her science. Out of some forty thousand cases, she relied on natural childbirth and performed only one cesarean section. Like most midwives, she waited patiently for the delivery and used no instruments when slow presentation inconvenienced her.

Other innovators improved the lot of mothers across Europe. In Venice in 1800, Benedetta Trevisan upgraded the profession with scientific principles that overrode superstition, a challenge also undertaken by Maddalena de Marinis of Naples in 1838. In London in 1828, midwives lost clients because of the move toward male dominance of birthing at University College, which appointed its first professor of midwifery. The difference in practice lay in the male midwife's use of forceps as opposed to the time-honored regimen of massage, manipulation, oil, and herbs preferred by the female midwife. Thus, midwifery stood out as a natural, traditional, and somewhat old-fashioned method, as opposed to hospital-based delivery that required episiotomy, drugs and general anesthesia, mechanical intervention, fetal monitoring, or surgery. A champion of the natural method, Dame Mary Rosalind Paget protected infants and mothers from technical intervention by founding the Midwives' Institute, later called the Royal College of Midwives.

In Spain, a move toward community education centers opened doors of liberal education to peasant midwives both under and outside the control of universities, thereby elevating the status of female practitioners. The birthing profession began preserving traditional methods as midwives themselves began teaching in-depth courses. At Madrid University, Francisca Iracheta set up a training regimen for midwives. Under the supervision of her husband, surgeon José López de Morelle, she taught beginners from her own illustrated handbook, *Examen de Matronas* (Instruction of Midwives), published in 1870, the first medical textbook issued by a Spanish woman. Her syllabus, composed in question-and-answer form, covered a standard field. Appended to the manual was a pattern for making a practice pelvis and a pronouncing glossary of medical terms. The following year, the University of Cordoba issued its own obstetrical text. Another author, Pilar Jáuregui, published articles in the 1870s in *El anfiteatro Médico Español* (The Spanish Medical Amphitheater) advocating training for midwives and prosecution of unlicensed laywomen. An outspoken contemporary, Eloisa Vílchez, was appointed resident midwife at Granada's maternity home, a salaried post that advanced from 912 pesetas in 1886 to 1,250 two years later. In 1895, Pilar Ortiz Grimaud and Cristina Martín served the *Casa de Socorro* (Assistance House) as *matronas titulares* (official midwives). Grimaud rose in rank to specialist in diseases of the womb and served as consultant to the resident gynecologist. A sister specialist, María Morales, served the University of Madrid as consultant in cases of sterility.

Beyond more advanced countries lay the job of midwifery in developing nations, immigrant communities, and mission fronts. According to New York City's records for 1891, 48 percent of births were attended by midwives, primarily at the demand of immigrant women. A parallel dependence on midwives persisted on the frontier. In Utah, Brigham Young preferred females for attending births and supported training and herbology for practitioners. At a time when Mormons led the nation in number of women studying medicine, in 1842, Emma Smith, wife of Prophet Joseph Smith, founded the Mormon Relief Society, which extended compassionate service to white and Indian women and their families. Mormon midwife Patty Bartlett Sessions kept track of deliveries in *Mormon Midwife,* which covers her frontier experiences from 1846–1888. Nurse-midwives like Eliza Cook of Mottsville, Nevada, a practitioner who traveled Carvon Valley in a horse and buggy, continued until mid-century in the traditional style of European caregivers by spending weeks with a family, tending to mother and infant, and cooking and washing for other small children. In Red Willow, Nebraska, for example, the mother of Dr. Mary Canaga Rowland performed the neighborly act of helping women in confinement. The

pay was small, as Rowland reported in *As Long as Life: The Memoirs of a Frontier Woman Doctor* (1994, 4–5): "She delivered the baby, took care of mother and baby, and in addition did the housework and cooked for the rest of the family for up to two weeks, all for five dollars a week."

In Africa, a valiant masseuse and midwife from Leipzig, Germany, Emmy Krigar Suren studied with the Red Cross before accepting assignment in 1898 as the first trained midwife in South Africa. At the height of World War I, she opened a practice among German soldiers' wives in Windhoek, Namibia, and traveled by oxcart and on horseback. Although she was expelled from the country from 1916 to 1921, she returned and delivered more than nine hundred babies. Her high standards of cleanliness, competence, and devotion to duty earned her the title of "the Florence Nightingale of South Africa" and a commendation from Prince Louis Ferdinand of Prussia. A colleague, Sister Franzeska, a German nun of the Order of the Sacred Heart of Jesus, established standards for training midwives and thrived as a nursing educator.

The second wave of midwives included some firsts for Africa. Miss E. S. E. Perala of Helsinki, Finland, who arrived in 1924, was the first midwife qualified in instrument deliveries; Sister Zoe Maneli became the first black registered nurse from South Africa. Manela trained Hulda Ngatjiekare Shipanga, the first Herero nurse, who practiced midwifery at the King Edward VIII Hospital in Durban before specializing in orthopedics. With the opening of the Onandjokwe Midwifery School in 1965, local trainees studied an illustrated text in the Owambo language. Written by matron Magrieta Airaksinen, a nun from the Finnish Mission Society, the work demonstrated the focus of the Namibian outreach: "We regard midwifery as the spearhead of our health services and if we cannot train midwives, the midwifery work now being done must collapse and the witch doctors take over again. We are confident that we can train [local women] to be competent registered midwives" (van Dyk 1997, 109).

One Namibian graduate, Ester Iimene Hango, completed training in the Afrikaans language and became the first pupil to qualify both in midwifery and general nursing and to operate one of the missionary clinics. Although political unrest and skirmishes exiled some of the local staff to the north, the program quickly recovered and evolved a multicultural workforce of black Africans and white Europeans. Ultimately, the establishment of modern obstetrics reduced Namibia's child mortality rate and elevated life expectancy in one of Africa's poorest evolving nations.

Similarly primitive was the medical network among the Blasket Isles off southwestern Ireland at the beginning of the twentieth century. Villagers selected Méiní O'Shea Dunlevy, daughter of Irish parents, who was a native of Massachusetts and a veteran of her own births and stillbirths. At the parish priest's request, she took over the work of Nell Mhicil Mitchell, the revered midwife long past her prime, and settled among locals to nurse and deliver babies. Isolated offshore where infant mortality was high, Méiní set up practice after a mainland doctor issued certification for a fee of 12.5 pence, wedge of tobacco, and a stiff drop of whiskey in his coffee mug. She became a household name among those who needed tending. Patients served as an audience for her avocation, bilingual storytelling. She remained in practice until 1933, when she moved to the mainland to tend her aged mother.

After medical science absorbed the midwife's task in industrialized countries, except for isolated examples, particularly Holland and Ireland, the role diminished as the job of *accoucheur* (midwife) and general practitioner took prominence. To stem the infant mortality rate and lessen the trauma of labor and birth with soporific drugs and general anesthesia, more women went to hospitals for male-controlled birthing. Fewer expected the services of a female practical nurse on return home. Instead, they set up a series of appointments with doctors, whose numbers had increased along with their cultivation of pre- and postnatal visits.

Additional competition from *visiteuses* (visiting nurses), maternity nurses, and welfare and public health agents plus the decline in the birth rate lessened the role of the midwife, costing some their livelihood. Throughout Europe, new questions arose concerning the suitability of midwifery. In Germany, medical protocol directed midwives to defer to male doctors. The Danes, led by Dr. N. Salomon, directed the *jordemoder* (midwife) to control septic conditions through harsh sterilization techniques calling for carbolic acid, bleach, lye, and sulfurous fumes. The Spanish required current practitioners to take additional course work. Swedish midwives introduced instrument deliveries and broadened their field to include general health care and home hygiene.

For the certified U.S. midwife, registration became the norm for trainees in the twentieth century. The first to be licensed was Carolyn C. Van Blarcom, a graduate of Johns Hopkins Training School for Nurses and author of *The Midwife in England* (1913). In 1918, the nonprofit Maternity Center Association, the first nurse-midwife school and family education facility, opened in New York City. Run by an all-female staff, the facility challenged a disturbing high point in mortality rate for mothers. To improve care for women, it was the first in the area to arrange classes for expectant parents and rapidly justified its existence by lowering the mortality rate for both mother and child. In a similar program, the Dutch concentrated on service to impoverished mothers. In 1919, Mademoiselle Marie Perneel worked toward a formal Belgian affiliation, the International Midwives' Union (IMU), which evolved into the International Confederation of Midwives (ICM).

Throughout the Western Hemisphere, the medical community remained ambivalent toward traditional midwifery. In 1912, Clara D. Noyes, R.N., superintendent of training schools for Bellevue Hospital and its satellites, addressed the International Congress of Hygiene and Demography, calling for advanced obstetrical nurses to replace midwives to "provide better teaching, better nursing and eventually better medical assistance to the less highly favored classes" (Shoemaker 1984, 8). With the institutionalization of obstetrics, birthing specialists declined in Georgia in 1925, when the State Board of Health began licensing the nine thousand rural granny women. By 1944, their number had declined to twenty-two hundred, as the state sent the dwindling number of apprentices to New York's Maternity Center Association; Frontier Graduate School in Midwifery in Wendover, Kentucky; and Alabama's Tuskegee School for Training Nurses in Midwifery, which opened in 1941.

One candidate, although lacking in literacy, drafted a compelling request to a Georgia public health nurse: "Pleas i want you to make me out a Lison Blank for grannie doctor. Thay is a tight cornder out here. Need us right now. Say thay ant noBody clost anuff. Want me. i want you to fix me up. i Bee up just as soon as i can get a way to come. it 10 miles out here an no way to get to town now tell i can catch a way" (Campbell 1946, 12). The petitioner had already undergone training and had collected money to pay for the maternity pamphlet and booklet on regulations issued by the state board. Visiting nurses followed up on preliminary training by supervising deliveries, stressing standards of cleanliness and requisite supplies, and ruling out the candidate's use of talismans, roots, herbs, homemade salve, and patent medicines.

A major breakthrough in the midwifery quandary was the nurse-midwifery program begun in 1925 by the Frontier Nursing Service, established by Mary Breckinridge in Leslie County, Kentucky. Initiated as the Kentucky Committee for Mothers and Babies, the project began as a means of reducing infant and maternal deaths in rural areas. Breckinridge and a staff of two nurses opened their clinic at Wendover. For four decades, she re-cruited courier assistants to visit families in remote coves by horseback. In 1932, her assistant, Rose McNaught, opened the first U.S. nurse-midwifery training program at the Maternity Center Association Lobenstine Clinic in New York City. In 1939, Breckinridge began training local women at the Frontier Graduate School of Midwifery. The demand for the Breckinridge model increased into the 1990s, when there were about five thousand certified practitioners, but not enough to staff remote clinics.

Today midwives continue their work among certain ethnic populations and augment their service by fitting contraceptives and conducting well-baby clinics. In Las Vegas, New Mexico, *partera* and *curandera* Jesusita Aragon claims to have attended twenty thousand deliveries from the beginning of her practice in 1923 until 1984. She apprenticed under her grandmother after learning to birth calves on the farm and mastered methods countenanced by the American Medical Association. In practice, she relies more on intuition than Western regimen and, in difficult situations, calls on a kindly spirit, Santo Niño de Atocha. For the Amish, midwifery holds an honored place among a people who reject technology. A heroine in Mount Eaton, Ohio, for four decades, Barb Hostetler entered the profession in the time-honored fashion. After producing her own six children, she became a trusted birthing specialist. Disdaining the electrical gadgetry of modern obstetrics, she timed labor by kerosene lantern in her own farmhouse before helping to establish Ohio's first birthing center. Constructed with Amish donations rather than government funds, the center features both electric and kerosene lamps and hand-built Amish cribs.

In the 1960s, during the rise of feminism and of such grassroots initiatives as the Lamaze movement and La Leche League, the social context of midwifery shifted from indigent or rural mothers to suburban women. To avoid the domination of male obstetricians and hospitals, educated metropolitan parents resumed the ancient tradition of midwifery and home-centered care as a means of ensuring normal, family-centered deliveries. In the words of Sharon Robinson, daughter of baseball great Jackie Robinson, midwifery succeeds because it is "holistic in approach . . . We get involved with a woman's spiritual, emotional and physical well-being. We often become just another member of the family during the pregnancy" ("Another" 1982, 107). Practicing in South Boston and Danville, Virginia, in 1982, she looked forward to strengthening rural clinical experience for partners in birthing.

A parallel drive in Canada brought feminist midwives into a gynocentric coalition with participants from a variety of cultures as well as with disabled, imprisoned, teenage, and lesbian mothers. One alliance of Iman Al-Jazairi, an Iraqi immigrant, with Sapna Patel, a writer from Lusaka, Zambia, produced a blended world vision of fundamental women's rights. A different slant from Ontarian Mennonites is the "Jesus-way," a nonviolent approach that chooses a serene home birth to welcome children into a worshipful community (Shroff 1997, 282). Another view comes from Jocelyne Maxwell, a francophone Canadian from the Manitoulin-Sudbury district in northern Ontario, who champions using practitioners with the same linguistic background as the expectant mothers they serve.

Unlike the Swedish model of state-run midwifery, the Canadian view calls for harmonious relationships between parents and birthing assistants and for reproductive autonomy free from cold, sterile hospital suites, intrusive instruments and monitoring devices, and hurry-up, male-dominated birthing. Central to the disdain for patriarchy is a belief that Western medicine is primarily destructive to the birthing process and culturally inappropriate. After midwifery was legalized and covered under the Ontario Health Insurance Plan, Patel and Al-Jazairi supported women of color from Sri Lanka, Pakistan, India, Sudan, Tunisia, Korea, Iran, Egypt, and China in seeking the uninhibited, holistic care their cultures had depended on from ancient times.

With similar fervor, Mennonite and aboriginal parents returned to the sacred paradigm that was once the norm in preindustrial Canada.

By 1998, Canada saw its first registered midwives in practice in British Columbia. Preceding the overhaul were a number of confrontations between the medical and traditional communities. One 1983 court case charged Linda Wheeldon and Charlene MacLellen, midwives in rural Nova Scotia, with criminal negligence causing death following the loss of an infant born in respiratory distress. After nine months of legal struggle, the case was dismissed and $14,000 raised to defray the defendants' expenses. MacLellen recalls that, on arrival at the courtroom, she heard a female news photographer echo the sentiments of many supporters, "God bless you midwives" (Shroff 1997, 336).

After a lengthy restructuring of services, Canadian authorities replaced a folk system that countenanced the untrained practice of aboriginal and immigrant midwives, particularly the Gulf Islanders and West Kootenai Indians. Maintaining the spirit of midwifery, the Medical Practitioners Act called for an end to amateurism and a licensed practice under the supervision of the College of Physicians and Surgeons. The purpose of regulation was to reduce dangers to mothers and infants while maximizing choice. As a compromise measure, mothers selecting home birth began consulting a sympathetic physician who would partner with a midwife.

The strength of the pro-midwife force is felt in the United States as well. By 1970, there were twelve hundred nurse-midwives, a national body of medical workers recognized by the American College of Obstetricians and Gynecologists as members of the maternal care team. By late 1997, the number had risen to six thousand. As educators of parents in family planning, breast-feeding, vaccination, and prenatal and postnatal care, nurse-practitioners continue to serve outback and immigrant families. A testament to their value is found in the record of deliveries and healthy mothers aided by Maude Callen, country nurse-midwife traveling the rutted back roads of Pinesville, South Carolina. She and other certified nurse-midwives answer questions during pregnancy and screen mothers for such life-threatening situations as obesity, hypertension, diabetes, and the tendency to deliver prematurely. During labor, practitioners can enlarge the mouth of the vagina by episiotomy but cannot perform forceps or cesarean delivery. In emergencies, they summon medical assistance and monitor mother and child until help arrives.

Where salaried midwives work with a team of women's health providers, they attend women in clinic or hospital settings; perform pelvic examinations; keep records; and wash, weigh, and swaddle newborns. Registered nurse-midwives augment their basic education with one- or two-year programs plus a practicum at major medical schools and obtain certification from the American College of Nurse-Midwives, assisting at 5 percent of births nationwide, totaling 185,000 in 1992. The rate of cesarean births for midwives is less than half that of obstetricians, who now perform surgery on one in four mothers. Other benefits are the lessening of labor complications and dependence on drugs. An added bonus, according to the *Journal of the Nurse-Midwifery,* home births in 1999 cost $1,500 compared to $5,000 for a hospital birth. Overall, Ruth Freeman, professor emeritus of Johns Hopkins University, sees midwifery as a boost to the concept of wellness. In her words, "Midwifery focuses on health rather than illness, on helping families to deal with their own problems rather than to rely on artificial outside support" ("Return" 1972, 56).

In U.S. maternity wards and lying-in clinics, doulas (or doules) serve as labor coaches and assisted with birth but lacked the knowledge of a professional midwife. The program involving these birthing supporters thrives in Guatemala, South Africa, Canada, and Finland and officially began in the United States in 1992 with the work of Penny Simkin, a Seattle, Washington, physical therapist and childbirth educator. The nonprofit Doulas of North America (DONA) evolved into a program of training and certification and introduced such equipment as the gymnastic ball, on which women in labor rest and distribute the pressure of contractions. By 1996, one hundred U.S. doulas were in service. According to nurse and doula overseer Cindy Hopkins at Presbyterian Hospital in Charlotte, North Carolina, staff hoped that providing additional support for parturient women would reduce the number of cesarean sections. The program cut surgeries by half and stemmed requests for epidural anesthesia by 60 percent and labor-inducing drugs by 40 percent. In addition, doula supervision shortened labor by 25 percent and lessened the need for forceps deliveries by 40 percent.

A controversial act by doctors, nurses, and midwives brought to light in June 1998 was the sterilization of Third World women with quinacrine, an inexpensive compound linked to risks of cancer. According to Catherine Olian on CBS-TV's *60 Minutes* on October 18, 1998, the drug, distributed as pellets, was first used as a sterilization agent in Santiago, Chile, in 1973. It is forced into the uterus with an intrauterine device (IUD) inserter. The simple procedure produces transient symptoms: short-term pain, bleeding, backache, fever, and headache. Within an hour, the drug dissolves and scarifies the fallopian tubes, blocking the passage of ova and preventing pregnancy. The use of quinacrine produces a quick, nonsurgical sterilization, a dramatically cheap and uncomplicated answer to overpopulation in India, Bangladesh, Pakistan, Malaysia, the Philippines, Vietnam, Morocco, Egypt, Iran, Croatia, Romania, China, Colombia, Chile, Venezuela, and Costa Rica. In these countries, the risks of pregnancy compromise the life expectancy of women, raising the likelihood of death during pregnancy to eighteen times the rate for women in industrialized countries. However, laboratory studies in the United States indicated that quinacrine has carcinogenic properties. The World Health Organization (WHO) and women's rights advocates condemned use of the toxic compound and lambasted health workers who indoctrinate women into submitting to treatment without understanding the irreversible effects of the drug. With the backing of the World Health Organization, health officials in India and six other countries banned quinacrine clinics in 1998. In October of that year the U.S. Food and Drug Administration ordered a halt to sale of the drug.

A more pressing problem is the prevalence of female genital mutilation, a patriarchal initiation rite common to animists of twenty-six African nations and among some Islamic, Christian, and Jewish women worldwide. Often the work of tribal midwives, the ritual scarification and removal of female genitalia exists in three forms:

- Most common in Africa is type 1 clitoridectomy, the ritual surgery performed on 85 percent of young women undergoing genital mutilation, which removes all or part of the clitoris.
- Type 2 clitoridectomy involves removal of the clitoris and parts of the labia minora.
- Type 3 and type 4 infibulation (or pharaonic circumcision), which accounts for 15 percent of African mutilations of women, is the drastic excision of the clitoris, the center of female sexual sensation, as well as the labia minora and labia majora. The degree of damage depends on the choice of practitioners, who stitch or pin the raw edges to narrow the vaginal opening as an inducement to sexual purity before marriage. The small aperture that remains allows the voiding of urine and menstrual flow. First intercourse and deliveries require additional rupture of tissue and restitching. Nurse Meserak Ramsey of Ethiopia described her own genital mutilation as a sexual death.

Armed with such crude instruments as knives, glass shards, and razor blades, midwives may prepare the subject with ice or local anesthesia and an encouragement to be brave or may commandeer village women to hold the unsuspecting child while performing the operation. Other methods involve piercing, stretching, cauterization, and scraping. Only the wealthy can afford to pay a surgeon to perform the operation under general anesthesia. Among those receiving no anesthesia, death can result from immediate organ damage, hemorrhage, pain, shock, gangrene, abscess, tetanus, septicemia, transmission of AIDS, and urinary or pelvic infection.

After visiting midwives, American novelist and activist Alice Walker reported to *Ms.* magazine in December 1993 on the prevailing impersonal, callous point of view: "Interviewing the circumcisor, I asked what she felt when the children cried and screamed. She didn't hear them, she said . . . Interviewing her was very difficult. I glanced at her hands—extremely dirty, with black gunk under the nails—and thought of their coarse hardness against the tenderest parts of these girls" ("Female Genital Mutilation," http://www.albany.net, 1). Walker quoted midwives who justify their work as a tradition expected of the community's women.

In the 1990s, this practice, performed worldwide on 135 million children ages 4–8 and as young as newborn, is the subject of study for the World Health Organization, the United Nations International Children's Emergency Fund (UNICEF), and the U.S. Immigration and Naturalization Service, which weighs the requests for political asylum from terrified women seeking to avoid unnecessary surgery to their genitals. Feminists warn that, unless the world community halts the practice, six thousand girls daily continue to suffer irreversible damage. Activists call for laws throughout Africa and the Middle East to end the age-old tradition and demand investigation of the practice among immigrants in industrialized nations.

See also: Ballard, Martha; Cellier, Elizabeth; Christian Nursing; *Curandera;* du Coudray, Angélique; Hutchinson, Anne; Lubic, Ruth; Native American Nursing; Nazi Nurses; Paget, Dame Mary

Rosalind; Public Health Nursing; Rosado, Luisa; Twentieth-Century Nursing

Sources

Abrams, Lynn, and Elizabeth Harvey, eds. *Gender Relations in German History: Power, Agency and Experience from the Sixteenth to the Twentieth Century.* Durham, N.C.: Duke University Press, 1997.

Adamson, Peter. "Commentary: A Failure of Imagination." http://www.unicef.org/pon96/womfail. htm.

Aikman, Lonnelle. *Nature's Healing Arts: From Folk Medicine to Modern Drugs.* Washington, D.C.: National Geographic, 1966.

Ailinger, Rita L., and Maria Elena Causey. "Health Concept of Older Hispanic Immigrants." *Western Journal of Nursing Research* (December 1995): 605–613.

"Another Robinson Pioneer." *Ebony* (December 1982): 106–107.

Apple, Rima D., ed. *Women's Health, Health and Medicine in America: A Historical Handbook.* New Brunswick, N.J.: Rutgers University Press, 1992.

Bing, Elisabeth. "Lamaze Childbirth: Then and Now." http://www.lamaze-childbirth.com/bingart. html.

Brainard, Annie M. *The Evolution of Public Health Nursing.* Philadelphia: W. B. Saunders, 1922.

Bushman, Claudia Lauper, and Richard Lyman Bushman. *Mormons in America.* New York: Oxford Press, 1998.

Campbell, Marie. *Folks Do Get Born.* New York: Rinehart, 1946.

Crichton, Jennifer. *Delivery: A Nurse-Midwife's Story.* New York: Warner Books, 1986.

Cushman, Karen. *The Midwife's Apprentice.* New York: HarperTrophy, 1995.

Dempsey, Patricia, and Theresa Gesse. "Beliefs, Values, and Practices of Navajo Childbearing Women." *Western Journal of Nursing Research* (December 1995): 591–604.

Dictionary of National Biography, 1942–1950. New York: Oxford University Press, 1959.

Ehrenreich, Barbara, and Deirdre English. *Witches, Midwives, and Nurses: A History of Women Healers.* New York: Feminist Press, 1995.

"Female Genital Mutilation." http://www.albany. net/~crystal/GG1/Naturopath/FGM.html.

———. http://www.amnesty.org/ailib/intcam/femgen/fgm1.htm.

———. http://www.int/inf-fs/en/fact153.html.

Fischer-Kamel, Doris Sofie. "The Midwife in History with Special Emphasis on Practice in Medieval Europe and in the Islamic World." University of Arizona, 1987. Monograph.

Fraser, Gertrude. *African American Midwives in the South.* New York: Cambridge University Press, 1998.

Freedman, Alix M. "Disputed Third World Sterilization Drug Rooted in N.C." *Charlotte Observer,* June 20, 1998, 1A, 19A.

Freudenheim, Milt. "As Nurses Take on Primary Care, Physicians Are Sounding Alarms." *New York Times,* September 30, 1997.

"The Frontier Nursing Service." http://www. achiever.com/freehmpg/kynurses/fns.html.

"Frontier School History." http://www.midwives. org/history.htm.

Garloch, Karen. "Lean on Me." *Charlotte Observer,* December 7, 1998, 1E, 4E.

Hall, David D., ed. *The Antinomian Controversy, 1636–1638: A Documentary History.* Middletown, Conn.: Wesleyan University Press, 1968.

Hanson, Jillian. "Choosing a Childbirth Educator." http://pregnancytoday.com/reference/articles/simkin-choose.htm.

"History of Nurse-Midwifery in the U.S." http:// www.acnm.org/educ/fenmhist.htm.

"The History of the Frontier Nursing Service." http://www.barefoot.com/fns/fns.html.

Hufton, Olwen. *The Prospect Before Her: A History of Women in Western Europe, 1500–1800.* New York: Vintage Books, 1995.

Hurd-Mead, Kate Campbell. *A History of Women in Medicine: From the Earliest Times to the Beginning of the Nineteenth Century.* Haddam, Conn.: Haddam Press, 1938.

Hyginus. *Hygini Fabulae.* Leyden, Holland: A. W. Sythoff, 1933.

Hyman, Paula, and Deborah Dash Moore. *Jewish Women in America.* New York: Routledge, Chapman and Hall, 1997.

Kelly, Katy. "Doc Lehman Is a Bridge to Divergent Worlds." *USA Today,* June 9, 1998.

Kraut, Alan. *Silent Travelers: Germs, Genes, and the "Immigrant Menace."* New York: Basic Books, 1994.

Leavitt, Judith Walzer. *Brought to Bed: Childbearing in America 1750–1950.* Cambridge, Mass.: Oxford University Press, 1986.

Lefkowitz, Mary. *Women's Life in Greece and Rome,* Baltimore: Johns Hopkins University Press, 1992.

Lepper, Elisabeth. "Midwifery Services in Holland." *Nursing Times,* November 29, 1979, 2084–2087.

Light, Luise. "Health Watch." *New Age,* March/April 1999, 30.

Lyons, Albert S., M.D., and R. Joseph Petrucelli, M.D. *Medicine: An Illustrated History.* New York: Abrams, 1987.

Magic and Medicine of Plants. Pleasantville, N.Y.: Reader's Digest, 1986.

Marcus, Jacob R. *Communal Sick-Care in the German Ghetto.* Cincinnati, Ohio: Hebrew Union College Press, 1947.

Marks, Geoffrey, and William K. Beatty. *Women in White.* New York: Charles Scribner's Sons, 1972.

Marland, Hilary, ed. *The Art of Midwifery: Early Modern Midwives in Europe.* London: Routledge, 1993.

Marland, Hilary, and Anne Marie Rafferty. *Midwives, Society and Childbirth: Debates and Controversies in the Modern Period.* London: Routledge, 1997.

"Mary Breckinridge, 1881–1965." http://www.ana.org/hof/brecmx.htm.

Matson, Leslie. *Méiní the Blasket Nurse.* Dublin: Mercier Press, 1996.

Nixon, Pat Ireland, M.D. *The Medical Story of Early Texas, 1528–1853.* San Antonio: Mollie Bennett Lupe Memorial Fund, 1946.

"Notes on Advanced Nursing." http://www.search.com/Infoseek/1,135,0,0200.html.

Patterson, Lotsee, and Mary Ellen Snodgrass. *Indian Terms of the Americas.* Englewood, Colo.: Libraries Unlimited, 1994.

Read, Phyllis J., and Bernard L. Witlieb. *The Book of Women's Firsts.* New York: Random House, 1992.

"Rebirth for Midwifery." *Time,* August 29, 1977, 66.

"Return of the Midwife." *Time,* November 20, 1972, 56–57.

Rogers, Nicole. "Wimmenspeak on Midwifery Lore." http://www.murdoch.edu.au/elaw/issues/v2n3/rogers.txt.

Rowland, Mary Canaga. *As Long as Life: The Memoirs of a Frontier Woman Doctor.* Seattle, Wash.: Storm Peak Press, 1994.

"Ruth Watson Lubic." *Current Biography Yearbook.* New York: Bowker, 1996, 328–332.

St. Pierre, Mark, and Tilda Long Soldier. *Walking in the Sacred Manner: Healers, Dreamers and Pipe Carriers—Medicine Women of the Plains Indians.* New York: Simon and Schuster, 1995.

Schlissel, Lillian, Vicki L. Ruiz, and Janice Monk, eds. *Western Women: Their Land, Their Lives.* Albuquerque: University of New Mexico Press, 1988.

Shearer, Benjamin F., and Barbara S. Shearer. *Notable Women in the Life Sciences.* Westport, Conn.: Greenwood Press, 1996.

Sherr, Lynn, and Jurate Kazickas. *Susan B. Anthony Slept Here: A Guide to American Women's Landmarks.* New York: Times Books, 1994.

Shoemaker, Sister M. Theophane. *History of Nurse-Midwifery in the United States.* New York: Garland Publishing, 1984.

Shroff, Farah. *The New Midwifery.* Toronto: Women's Press, 1997.

Spruill, Julia. *Women's Life and Work in the Southern Colonies.* New York: W. W. Norton, 1972.

Stoddard, Marthe. "Program Delivers Birth Support." *Lincoln Star,* June 23, 1995, 1, 8.

Ulrich, Laurel Thatcher. *A Midwife's Tale: The Life of Martha Ballard, Based on Her Diary, 1785–1812.* New York: Alfred A. Knopf, 1990.

van Dyk, Agnes. *A History of Nursing in Namibia.* Windhoek: Gamsbert Macmillan, 1997.

Van Olphen-Fehr, Juliana. *The Diary of a Midwife.* Westport, Conn.: Greenwood Press, 1998.

Weiner, Lynn Y. "Reconstructing Motherhood; The La Leche League." *Journal of American History* (March 1994): 1–12.

Wigginton, Eliot, ed. *Foxfire 2.* Garden City, N.Y.: Anchor Books, 1973.

Williams, Marty Newman, and Anne Echols. *Between Pit and Pedestal: Women in the Middle Ages.* Princeton, N.J.: Markus Wiener Publishers, 1994.

"Women in Medicine." http://www.med.virginia.edu/hs-library/historical/antigua/stext.htm.

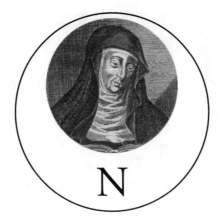

N

Native American Nursing

Dating to prehistory, Native American nurse care is a sacred profession. It deviates so completely from European tradition in style and methodology that the word "nurse" falls short. Imbued with respect for religious, psychological, and physical laws, valid native medical therapy by a shaman, herbalist, or medicine man or woman allies body and spirit after some imbalance has thrown overall health off-kilter. According to the introduction to *Medicine Women, Curanderas, and Women Doctors* by Bobette Perrone, Henrietta Stockel, and Victoria Krueger (1989, 11): "It is assumed that the spiritual being has definite relationships with the earth, with other spirits (living and dead), and with powers both animate and inanimate. These powers take the forms of animals, deities, elements of nature, objects, one's relatives, and one's relationship to all of these entities."

To harmonize elements, the Navajo may perform a medicine sing; a loving Sioux caretaker may summon a prayer circle; the Cherokee prefer to smudge by burning a twist of sweetgrass and inhaling the fumes. The Micmac offer the mother a trillium root to chew to initiate labor. The Nishnawe of Canada purify with sage and rely on the squawvine or partridge berry to ease birthing and sage tea to suppress lactation. Postpartum ceremonies may link the burial of the afterbirth and umbilical cord with a naming ritual. To restore a symmetry between mind, body, and heart, officiating medicine women may sing, chant, wave eagle feathers, apply porcupine quills in a form of acupuncture, or perform a ritual that draws on the power in sand painting, a feather fan, rattles, animal hides, teeth, or claws. Overall, the patient's trust in a blend of charms, spells, plant lore, and psychotherapy enhances effectiveness, but no single element is identifiable as a cure.

Models of Native American caregiving are unassuming yet sustaining members of the community. A Pueblo nurse-midwife, Gia Khuun (Mother Corn) of Santa Clara Pueblo, served her community in the late nineteenth century as central contributor to tribal continuity. A nurturing medicine woman, herbalist, and obstetrician, she delivered the children of her extended family and neighbors and treated their illnesses. As demonstrated by her practice, the *gia* (maternal qualities) foster caring, sharing, and interdependence, the hallmarks of tribal life. According to Ruthbeth Finerman in *Women as Healers: Cross-Cultural Perspectives,* Saraguro Indians of Ecuador expect healing to be the natural work of married women. Without fanfare, Saraguro

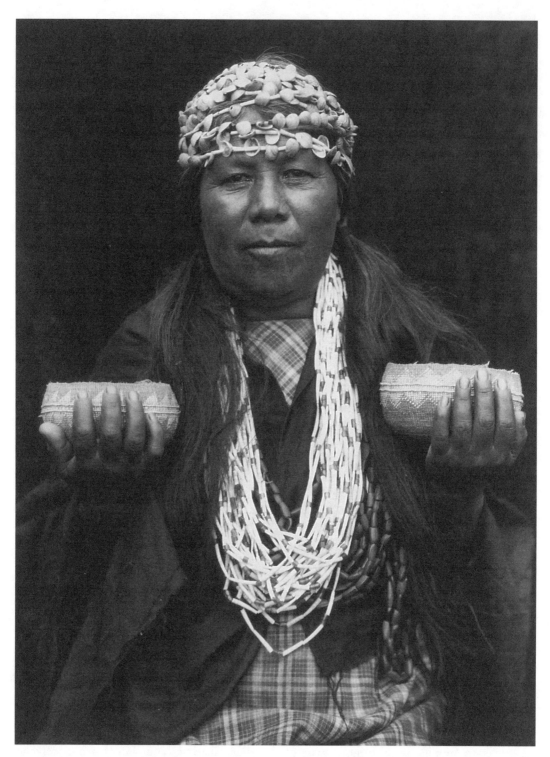

An Edward Curtis photograph of an Athapaskan Hupa shaman of Northwest California taken in 1923 (Library of Congress)

mothers treat 86 percent of family illness and 75 percent of tribal cases. In the 1980s, the use of informal, empathetic cures devised by untrained Saraguro women contrasts with the intervention of two *curanderos* to treat alcoholism, chronic and emotional ills, and sterility; six herbalists to treat diet and personal problems; midwives to manage contraception, birth, and fertility problems; and eight nurse-practitioners to vaccinate and teach hygiene.

Native plants are essential to Indian treatments. In the Lukachukai Mountains of Arizona, Navajo medicine man Ray Winnie maintains a stock of seven basic herbs and advises the Navajo Community College on oral tradition and herb collection. Outside Branson, Missouri, Chick Allen, of Delaware and Cherokee ancestry, reported to an interviewer from *National Geographic* that white settlers learned to use roots and herbs from native healers. In his estimation, "Many a life in the early frontier days was saved with these remedies" (Aikman 1966, 19–20). Among the Tewa of the Isleta Pueblo in New Mexico, the combined knowledge of native healers and Anglo and Hispanic settlers has produced a complex of simples and treatments for a list of human ills. Alice Norris, a Papago health worker in Sells, Arizona, attests to the logic of tribal medicine, which involves a three-person team—the diagnostician, the singer, and the herbalist. Her associate, Papago medicine man Sam Angelo, works in conjunction with the U.S. Public Health Service to offer traditional cures along with modern treatment.

Native healing is intrinsically pragmatic. It accords the right of practice to male and female and typically calls for payment up-front, whether in quartz, a rabbit, or coins. Within the Indian pharmacopoeia of North, Central, and South America and the Caribbean isles lie elements valued worldwide—hemlock spruce, an antiscorbutic; willow bark, the forerunner of aspirin; the painkiller coca or cocaine; foxglove, also known as digitalis; oshá root for cough suppressant; and stoneseed, a contraceptive. Medical equipment invented from nature includes the obsidian lancet for bloodletting and the drainage and irrigation syringe, composed of sheep belly or animal bladder bulb attached to a length of duodenum with a hollow quill or bone at the end. Ancient treatments ranged from extracting teeth to rubbing, pressing, setting bones, cutting, cauterizing, douching, fumigating, making poultices, drawing out abscesses and snake venom, countering irritation, scarifying, suctioning out disease through a reed, smoking sacred tobacco, and sweating in a vapor bath. Of the latter, the attendant helped the patient into a small oven-shaped structure, where the embers of a fire maintained heat. Stripped naked, the patient perspired and then was plunged into a cold stream. It is notable that the native understanding of wounds and healing produced fewer amputees and cripples than did the more sophisticated European systems of the mid–sixteenth to nineteenth centuries.

First-person accounts of healing methods abound in pioneer and missionary journals, for example, the experience of Juan Ortiz, a nobleman from Seville, Spain, who was tortured by an unidentified Indian tribe in Florida. After the cacique ordered him stretched over a grill, Ortiz dangled above hot coals and cried piteously for aid. Native women unbound him and bathed his hurts in extracts of fresh herbs, thus saving his life. Such abbreviated examples are the only written record of native treatments and of the decimation of tribes from initial contact with European diseases, especially smallpox, measles, typhus, typhoid, scarlet fever, whooping cough, dysentery, plague, tuberculosis, and cholera.

European explorers who expected to teach native healers were often receivers of medical expertise, as was the case with Dr. Diego Alvarez Chanca, a late fifteenth-century professor from the University of Salamanca and fleet surgeon on Christopher Columbus's second voyage. While touring the Caribbean, he collected and studied quinine, cascara sagrada, and balsam, all of which he introduced to the Spanish medical establishment on his return.

- In 1519, Hernán Cortés, conqueror of Mexico, reported to Emperor Charles V on the tamarind purgatives, narcotics, and indigenous drugs used by Aztecs, who divided health professionals into specialties. The Apaches recommended sarsaparilla, jalap, coca, castor oil, moxa, and datura as medicaments. They dispatched midwives to perform abortions and treat obstetrical needs, which were less frequent than in white society because native mothers preferred to give birth unaided in the wild. As a contribution to the welfare of Mexico City and a gesture of atonement for his cruelties to Indians, in 1524 Cortés established the Hospital of the Immaculate Conception, the first European hospital in the Americas.

- In 1528, Álvar Núñez Cabeza de Vaca began ministering to natives of Texas, applying European methods and learning from native healers. In his firsthand report, *Castaways,* he reports on observations while visiting Malhado, the Isle of Misfortune: "They tried to make us into medicine men, without examining us or asking for credentials, for they cure illnesses by blowing on the sick person, and by blowing and using their hands they cast the illness out of him; and they ordered us to do the same and to be of some use" (Cabeza de Vaca 1993, 49). This unusual regimen for treating internal disease brought laughter from the Spaniards, who saw no use in passing hot stones over the aching stomach, making small cuts over the painful body part and sucking out the pain, or applying beneficial cautery. In a humorous ethnic turnabout, Cabeza de Vaca preferred his own form of ritual healing, "by making the sign of the cross over them and blowing on them and reciting a Pater Noster and an Ave Maria."

- Nicolás Monardes collected in his *Joyfull Newes out of the Newe Founde Worlde* (1545) an assortment of treatments and medicinal "Trees, Plantes, Herbes, Rootes, Joices, Gummes, Fruites" from the Americas (Aikman 1966, 114). On an Apache guaiacum treatment he reported: "A Spanyarde that did suffer great paines of the Poxe [syphilis], whiche he had by the companie of an Indian woman, but his servaunte beyng one of the Phisitions of that countrie, gave unto hym the water of Guaiacan, wherewith not onely his greevous paines were taken awaie that he did suffer; but healed verie well of the evill" (Nixon 1946, 20). Other derivatives Monardes praised include the Peruvian coca; the Aztec copal, a sweet gum used to cure toothache; and sassafras, a panacea valued by Florida Indians.

- As recorded by Pedro de Castaneda, historian of Francisco Coronado's expedition of 1540–1542, Spanish military surgeons learned herbal techniques from the Indians of Kansas, such as the healing properties of quince. The guide Ysopete, a Wichita, introduced fresh mushrooms, dock, mustard, sorrel, wild onion, elm bark paste, and lamb's quarter to military diets to prevent scurvy and demonstrated the use of meal poultices for skin lesions, coffee bean root and slippery elm bark as laxatives, milkweed and dock root for diarrhea and dysentery, and foxglove for chills and fever.

- A priceless Aztec herbal, the Badianus Manuscript (1552), housed in the Vatican library in Rome, contains translations of botanical formulae. Compiled by two Catholic-educated Aztecs, Martin de la Cruz and Juannes Badianus, at the College of Santa Cruz at Tlaltelco, Mexico City, the text is written in Latin and Aztec. The eight chapters group ailments by type or location from head to foot and append illustrations of 204 healing herbs and trees valued by native healers. Viceroy Don Francisco de Mendoza brought the manuscript to King Charles V as a gift.

- In 1633, Calancha of Peru, an Augustinian prelate, was the first to describe how an extract made from the bitter cinchona bark immediately relieved pain and fever. By 1640, missionary priests were shipping the valuable bark to Europe to cure malaria. Named quinine in 1820, it was synthesized a century later.
- A giant step into native lore, Fernando Hernández's *Rerum Medicorum Novae Hispaniae Thesarus, seu Plantarum, Animalium, Mineralium Mexicanorum Historia* (1651) (A Treasury of Medicine of New Spain, or a History of Mexican Plants, Animals, and Minerals), referred to 1,200 medical plants in the native pharmacopoeia.

Additional details of Native American medical treatment consist essentially of anecdotal fragments. The Comanche stanched blood by plugging wounds with wads of rotted wood and treated snakebite with alder bark and peyote poultices. The Tejas cured amebic dysentery with chaparro amargosa. The Oglala Sioux employed refined cottonwood bark in powder form to break up cataracts. The Choctaw taught a white doctor to use lye and tobacco juice on hemorrhoids and wild sage plasters on tumors. The Karankawa prized ipecac to control dysentery. Natchez healers treated fever with magnolia seed and toothache with acacia. In a dramatic example of euthanasia, a Comanche chief slit his wife's throat to end her suffering from a debilitating illness. Nearly all tribes possessed some nostrums for indigestion, intestinal parasites, and arthritis, the diseases that had troubled them most before European settlement. To these native remedies, missionaries added lime bark, blister plasters, nutmeg, peppermint, calomel, magnesia, epsom salts, and opium, the standard pharmacopoeia of the early nineteenth century, and introduced smallpox vaccination.

A remarkably detailed account of the meeting of Native Americans and frontiersmen occurs in the *Journals of Lewis and Clark,* a faithful daybook describing visits to ailing tribe members along the exploring party's trek up the Missouri River, west to Washington state and the Pacific Ocean, and back to St. Louis. Lewis records the native use of venom from rattlesnakes, administered to his Shoshone guide and translator Sacagawea, to hasten childbirth. Father Felix Espinosa marveled at a native form of quarantine, which required the tribe to abandon smallpox victims in a thorny spot to die alone and be eaten by animals and birds, thus ridding the village of infection.

On May 19, 1806, Lewis, a cheerful dispenser of frontier remedies, treated villagers with laudanum, cathartic, eye ointment, and liniment. Four days later, as Sacagawea's son, Jean Baptiste Charbonneau, grew ill with swollen neck glands, Lewis made a poultice of wild onion, followed two weeks later with a salve of pine resin, beeswax, and bear grease. Explorer John Sheilds treated a sick chief with a method of sweating and cooling that he had applied to explorer William Bratton. Similar to an ancient Mayan method, alternating temperature required a hole 3 feet in diameter and 4 feet deep, in which he built a fire and placed a board near the embers for the patient to rest his feet while sitting under willow poles arched overhead and covered in a thick awning of blankets. While sprinkling water on the embers, the patient breathed steam as long as he could stand it, then plunged into cold water before returning to the sweat hut and sipping tea made from horsemint or snakeroot. Lewis seemed pleased to report on June 8 that his patients were recovering.

Indian healers derived ingenious methods from nature. A detailed treatment recorded in 1836 concerning a throat ailment of William Bent, an Indian agent on the Arkansas River, credits a Cheyenne healer named Lawyer with a unique device. He connected strands of sinew to tiny burs and maneuvered them into Bent's obstructed throat to remove mucus and prevent choking. A century before Sister Kenny evolved a hot pack therapy for polio, the Tolcha were treating paralysis with a vigorous application of hot sand, soaks in hot goat's milk, massage, poultices, and salve of goat marrow and pungent herbs. Patient diet consisted of corn and goat meat, fat, cheese, and milk, followed by decoctions of herbs and mescal, a powerful antispasmodic. Other eyewitness accounts laud the work of Blue Earring Woman, a Minneconjou Lakota born around 1850 on the Cheyenne River Reservation, and Isabel Ten Fingers, an Oglala healer born in 1905 who treated tuberculosis, arthritis, and diabetes. In Smith Point, Texas, in 1850, a Cherokee healer, Sarah "Sallie" Ridge Paschal, transformed her two-story residence into a yellow fever clinic and brewed teas to control fever. A respected late nineteenth-century Assiniboin healer, Iron Woman, impressed her grandchildren by the simplicity of herbs and treatments for humans and animals and the use of a digging stick, the world's most primitive agricultural tool, to locate beneficial roots.

White society's respect for native cures followed an erratic course. In 1891, the U.S. government classified as civil service workers the nurses of the Indian Health Service, thereby bringing native health outreach into alliance with invasive surgery, x-ray and laboratory testing, and chemical drugs. The steady erosion of Native American reliance on natural cures stabilized in the 1970s, with a renewed interest in native healing. From hippie-era books, movies, and television arose a glorified vision of the native healer. In place of a confident, low-key caretaker, the media hyped the image of a wonder worker and wielder of supernatural power, a perception far removed from reality.

Among the caregivers of the twentieth century are sensitive, spiritual healers in the old tradition along with modern nurse-midwives and medical educators who support programs that bolster maternal and fetal health and tribal wellness:

Isabelle Cobb, a Cherokee physician and health educator from Morgantown, Tennessee, treated patients at the Nursery and Children's Hospital in West New Brighton, New York. In the early 1900s, while serving in Wagoner, Oklahoma, she tended the sick in their homes in lieu of taking them to the hospital.

A Catholic project, the *Catholic Maternity Institute and School for Nurse-Midwifery,* opened in 1943 in Santa Fe, New Mexico. Headed by sisters M. Helen Herb and M. Theophane Shoemaker, the program augmented the work of native birthing experts. Nurse-midwives received parturient women living in a 30-mile radius of the center and supervised deliveries in the home. Funding for the program derives from the Society of Catholic Medical Missionaries, Federal Children's Bureau, and New Mexico State Department of Health.

Inspirational health activist *Annie Dodge Wauneka,* daughter of Chee Dodge, a Navajo chief from Sawmill, Arizona, has been the conduit for both the traditional Blessing Way and modern health methods. While attending a government school at Fort Defiance, she was only eight years old when she aided nurse Domatilda Showalter in treating classmates during the 1918 flu epidemic. In adulthood, Dodge became the first woman elected to the Navajo Tribal Council. By visiting hogans to disseminate facts about hygiene and inoculation and compiling a medical handbook in Navajo for the use of doctors and nurses, she removed some of the suspicion and misunderstanding that inhibited patients from seeking preventive and medical care. Because of her influence, two thousand consumptive Indians agreed to hospital care, and families replaced dirt floors in their hogans with planks. In 1960, she broadcast health advice through twice-weekly radio programs from Gallup's station KGAK. Her service to the National Tuberculosis Association and Surgeon General's Advisory Board and a television documentary by Walter Cronkite helped to earn her a 1963 Presidential Medal of Freedom, conferred by President John F. Kennedy. In 1976, *Ladies' Home Journal* named her Woman of the Year.

Ruth Muskrat Bronson, native to the Delaware District of the Cherokee nation, campaigned for better health care from her office at the Washington bureau of the National Congress of American Indians. As health educator at the San Carlos Apache Indian Reservation in 1957, she upgraded native lifestyles. Her work earned her the 1962 Department of Health, Education, and Welfare Superior Service and Oveta Cult Hobby awards.

In the mid-1960s, *Dr. Connie Redbird Pinkerman-Uri,* a Choctaw-Cherokee from Wheatland, California, established Los Angeles's first Indian Free Clinic. She has campaigned to turn Fort McArthur into an Indian hospital, end forced sterilization of native women, and improve health at Chino State Prison. Her contemporary, Lois Fister Steele, is an Assiniboin health activist who has sponsored an innovative traveling medicine show and standardization of health systems for the Pascua Yaqui of Tucson, Arizona.

Named Top Indian Woman in 1970, Seminole nurse *Betty Mae Jumper* worked at the Kiowa Indian Hospital in Oklahoma before entering public health nursing. Her study of pervasive problems on the Seminole Reservation in Florida led to political activism that affected the health, welfare, and economic self-sufficiency of the Seminole.

The official religious dreamer for the Kashaya Pomo Reservation, California nurse *Essie Parrish,* was a traditionalist. She served local people as a healer and compiled a Kashaya dictionary and anthology of legends. At her death in 1979, she was ranked "the most important California Indian of the twentieth century" (Bataille 1993, 198).

Annie "Flower That Speaks in a Pollen Way" Kahn, a Navajo herder of the Water Clan in Lukachukai, Arizona, who teaches and heals from her hogan, values *hozhooji,* a blend of harmony and otherworldliness that respects nature's flora and fauna. She maintains that she was chosen a healer at a Blessing Way ceremony before she was born. Before each patient interview, she steadies her spirit. Her method consists of a six-stage therapy: consciousness raising, ordering, obedience to law, spiritual power, preparation for ceremony, and ritual.

On a ridge outside Santa Fe, New Mexico, Apache basket weaver *Tu Moonwalker,* a descendent of Cochise and Mangas Coloradas, follows a heritage of healing as distinguished teacher and medicine woman. She learned herbalism from her grandmother, Dorothy Naiche. Moonwalker conquered polio in childhood and readied herself for a vision quest that required her to remain alone on the desert for a week. As a therapist, she alerts the suffering to healing energies in baskets and in medicine herb pouches.

Dhyani Ywahoo, a spiritualist, teacher, and keeper of the priest craft of the Ani Gadoah Clan of the Cherokee nation, is a healer at the Sunray Meditation Society in Vermont. She reveres meditation and resonation as healing forces. A proponent of good humor and wellness, she applies nonintrusive methods to restore balance and uses sacred quartz crystals to calm and instruct.

A prominent professional nurse and health services activist from San Diego, California, *Carmella Ignacio,* a member of the Papago tribe, was elected a director of the American Indian Health Center in 1984 for her concern for the quality of native life.

A Canadian midwife, *Irene Beardy,* from Bearskin Lake, Ontario, fits new ways with old traditions. In her words: "We had our own way. It was suited to the lifestyle of the past. Now we have new ways which need to include modern medicine" (Shroff 1997, 275). Her task may be to encourage young mothers to exercise more and eat better, as opposed to past midwifery that treated active women working on traplines and eating traditional foods.

In Povungnituk, Quebec, a birthing center combines the work of midwives with First Nations practitioners. One Hotanoshoni leader, *Katsi Cook,* founding member of the College of Midwives of Ontario, actively researches and writes about traditional methods as well as cultural and ecological issues. She influenced Carol Couchie, a Scots-Ojibway practitioner of midwifery and primary health care under the name Healing Cedar Woman. Based in

Toronto, Couchie offers training sessions under Canada's Aboriginal Health Professions program and extols the Six Nations birthing center, where patients receive holistic care.

A contemporary of Couchie, *Herbert Nabigon,* is a pipe carrier and traditional instructor in Cree healing traditions and coordinator of the Native Human Service Program at Laurentian University.

Sarah Ellen Albertson, a Delaware/Seneca from Denver, Colorado, who specializes in Indian health, serves the Red Cross and the affirmative action commission of the Colorado Nurses' association.

Much of Native American nursing centers on reducing infant mortality and facilitating early childhood survival. Among current nurse caregivers in the area of family health are these:

- Staff nurse at the Puyallup Indian Clinic and women's advocate for education and family planning Ruth Wallis Backup, an Athabascan from Fort Yukon, Alaska, specializes in Indian health services and chairs the Commission on Nursing Practice and Education.
- Donna Blair Beckstrom, a Minnesota Chippewa from Philadelphia, supports family wellness as women's advocate from the Native American Breastfeeding Association and researcher on maternal and newborn health. Belma T. Colter, a Shoshone/Bannock from Fort Hall, Idaho, supports family planning, women, infants, and children (WIC) care, prenatal care, and child advocacy projects.
- Narcissus Gayton, a Mescalero Apache from Mescalero, New Mexico, is a Save the Children committeewoman and women's advocate on such health issues as cancer screening and maternal health.
- Darlene Monteaux Herndon, a Sioux healer from Rosebud, South Dakota, specializes in health workshops and family nurse practice in women's health.

- Carol Matte Lipscomb, a Salish/Kootenai from St. Ignatius, Montana, focuses a tribal health nursing program on family planning, prenatal care, and child care programs.
- Manuella Real Bird Mesteth, a Crow from Crow Agency, Montana, works toward maternal and child health at prenatal, family planning, and cancer detection clinics.
- Women's advocate Betty Owl Nephew, a Seneca/Cayuga/Cherokee from Rochester, New York, supports temperance, health delivery, and WIC prenatal programs.
- A lay midwife, Katsitsiakwa Cook, an Akwesasne Mohawk from Akwesasne Reservation, New York, is a women's health specialist with expertise in reproductive choice, sterilization, WIC and prenatal care, and rural women's advocacy.
- Sharron K. Johnson, a Comanche from Lawton, Oklahoma, teaches parenting and directs a child abuse outreach and family crisis program.

Other nursing specialties center professional energies on adult problems:

- In the treatment and prevention of alcoholism, three women focus on native abusers. Sonja R. Dana, a Passamaquoddy from Perry, Maine, develops community health plans for family counseling and drug and alcohol abuse. Cecilia Marden Gallerito, a Mescalero Apache from Los Angeles, counsels alcoholic Indian women. Grace Elizabeth Lincoln, an Inuit from Kotzebue, Alaska, treats alcohol abuse.
- Psychiatric nurse-consultant Virginia Knoki-June, a Navajo from Fort Defiance, Arizona, serves as instructor, consultant, and speaker on the whole spectrum of native health issues.
- Geriatrics is another concern to native caregivers. A proponent of nutrition

programs for the elderly, Loretta M. Bad Heart Bull, a Standing Rock Sioux from Fort Yates, North Dakota, serves the Medex program of the University of North Dakota, which employs nurses in primary care for communities, and the National Indian Council on Aging. Michelle Margaret Jenson, an Omaha/Winnebago from Omaha, Nebraska, supports the elderly, helps families cope with crisis, and promotes women's health.

- Involved in home health care delivery systems are Frances Sylestine Battise, an Alabama-Coushatta from Livingston, Texas, and Cherry Maynor Beasley, a Lumbee from Pembroke, North Carolina, who has aided national and state task forces on family planning and mental health and works to educate Native Americans about the dangers of high blood pressure.

See also: Disease; La Flesche Picotte, Susan; Midwifery; Twentieth-Century Nursing

Sources

Aikman, Lonnelle. *Nature's Healing Arts: From Folk Medicine to Modern Drugs.* Washington, D.C.: National Geographic, 1966.

Anderson, Owannah. *Ohoyo One Thousand: A Resource Guide of American Indian/Alaska Native Women.* Washington, D.C.: U.S. Department of Education, 1982.

Bataille, Gretchen M., ed. *Native American Women: A Biographical Dictionary.* New York: Garland, 1993.

Cabeza de Vaca, Álvar Núñez. *Castaways.* 1528. Berkeley: University of California Press, 1993.

Clement, J., ed. *Noble Deeds of American Women with Biographical Sketches of Some of the More Prominent.* Williamstown, Mass.: Corner House, 1975.

Clores, Suzanne. *Native American Women.* New York: Chelsea House, 1995.

DeVoto, Bernard, ed. *The Journals of Lewis and Clark.* Boston: Houghton Mifflin, 1953.

Dock, Lavinia, and Isabel M. Stewart. *A Short History of Nursing.* New York: G. P. Putnam's Sons, 1938.

Dolan, Josephine A., R.N. *History of Nursing.* Philadelphia: W. B. Saunders, 1968.

Gridley, Marion E. *American Indian Women.* New York: Hawthorn Books, 1974.

Kraut, Alan. *Silent Travelers: Germs, Genes, and the "Immigrant Menace."* New York: Basic Books, 1994.

Lamps on the Prairie: A History of Nursing in Kansas. Emporia.: Kansas State Nurses' Association, 1942.

Lewis, Dale. "Woman Is Medicine: An Interview with CheQweesh Auh-Ho-Oh." *Woman of Power* (winter 1987).

McClain, Carol Shepherd. *Women as Healers: Cross-Cultural Perspectives.* New Brunswick, N.J.: University of Rutgers Press, 1989.

"Medicine Women." http://www.powersource.com/ powersource/gallery/womansp/medwomen.html.

Muina, Natalia. "To Make Whole." *Woman of Power* (winter 1987).

Native American Women. New York: American Indian Treaty Council Information Center, 1975.

Nelson, Mary Carroll. *Annie Wauneka.* Minneapolis, Minn.: Dillon Press, 1972.

Nixon, Pat Ireland, M.D. *The Medical Story of Early Texas, 1528–1853.* San Antonio: Mollie Bennett Lupe Memorial Fund, 1946.

Perrone, Bobette, H. Henrietta Stockel, and Victoria Krueger. *Medicine Women, Curanderas, and Women Doctors.* Norman: University of Oklahoma Press, 1989.

"Prehistory." http://www.geocities.com/Athens/Forum/6011/sld003.htm.

"Return of the Midwife." *Time,* November 20, 1972, 56–57.

St. Pierre, Mark, and Tilda Long Soldier. *Walking in the Sacred Manner: Healers, Dreamers and Pipe Carriers—Medicine Women of the Plains Indians.* New York: Simon and Schuster, 1995.

Schlissel, Lillian, Vicki L. Ruiz, and Janice Monk, eds. *Western Women: Their Land, Their Lives.* Albuquerque: University of New Mexico Press, 1988.

Sherr, Lynn, and Jurate Kazickas. *Susan B. Anthony Slept Here: A Guide to American Women's Landmarks.* New York: Times Books, 1994.

Shoemaker, Sister M. Theophane. *History of Nurse-Midwifery in the United States.* New York: Garland Publishing, 1984.

Shroff, Farah. *The New Midwifery.* Toronto: Women's Press, 1997.

Steer, Diana. *Native American Women.* New York: Barnes and Noble, 1996.

Steiner, Stan. *The New Indians.* New York: Delta Books, 1968.

Sterne, Capt. Doris M. *In and Out of Harm's Way: A History of the Navy Nurse Corps.* Seattle, Wash.: Peanut Butter Publishing, 1996.

Wilson, Amy V., R.N. *A Nurse in the Yukon.* New York: Dodd, Mead, 1965.

Navy Nurse Corps

Nurse care aboard ship is a unique area of military medicine. In a bold experiment in 1813, Captain Stephen Decatur, a naval commodore aboard the frigate *United States* and commander of a squadron of three ships during the War of 1812, employed nurses Mary Allen and Mary Marshall, wives of his sailors, on board his ship during combat. Until Decatur's unconventional mixing of the sexes at sea, navy nurse care was a haphazard arrangement calling for shipboard appointment of helpers or corpsmen dubbed "loblolly boys." John Wall, the first naval loblolly boy on record, enlisted in June 1798. A famous nurse-sailor, English novelist Tobias Smollett, claimed the title of loblolly boy over a half century earlier for his post as surgeon's mate on H.M.S. *Chichester* in the West Indies during the War of Austrian Succession, which began in 1739 (Kemp 1988). As an aide to the surgeon and the surgeon's mate, the loblolly boy removed amputated limbs, tidied the deck with sand and seawater, and stoked charcoal braziers to heat tar, which the surgeon applied to the hemorrhaging stumps. The name, derived from loblolly, a thin gruel or porridge made of cereal or meal thickened with boiling milk or water and spoon-fed to invalids, stayed in use until 1861, when navy corpsmen earned the full status of nurse.

In 1814, navy physician Dr. William Paul Crillon Barton published "A Treatise Containing a plan for the Internal Organization and Government of Marine Hospitals in the United States together with a scheme for Amending and Systematizing the Medical Department of the Navy," a dissertation calling for nurses to staff, manage, and administer military hospitals. He specifically requested females of good disposition, compassion, vigorous health, neatness, and strong character. To maintain the traditional chain of command, he recommended: "They should obey

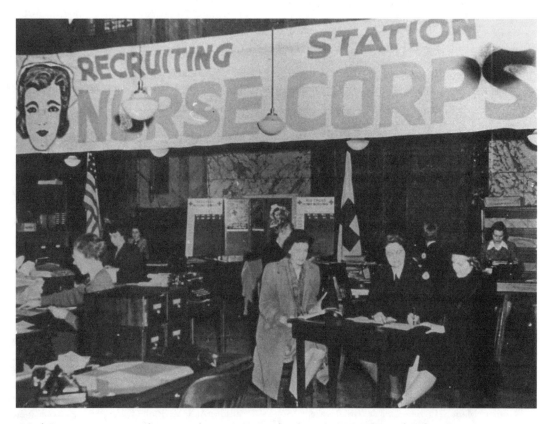

A Red Cross recruiting station for army and navy nurses, Pittsburgh, 1943 (U.S. Library of Medicine)

punctually all orders from their superiors; and should exact a ready acquiescence in their commands, from the attendants under them" (Sterne 1996, 2).

Simultaneous with Barton's unheard-of call for women in administrative positions, the navy issued stiffer regulations for corpsmen. Selected from a ship's crew, these orderlies aided the ship's surgeon by washing, shaving, and feeding inmates, assisting at recruitment examinations, and hauling tubs of sand to absorb body fluids from surgical procedures to prevent them from contaminating wooden decking. A subsequent navy regulation established a company of six landsmen to serve each hospital ship as nurses. When Barton was named senior medical officer of the naval hospital at Portsmouth, Virginia, naval authorities overruled his intent to hire female nursing superintendents or matrons for military hospital wards.

During the Civil War, the Union navy formed a medical fleet from six mismatched vessels—the *Ben Morgan, Home, A. Houghton, Mohawk, New Hampshire,* and the navy's first official hospital ship, *Red Rover,* a luxury Mississippi steamer. A Confederate paddle-wheeler seized in combat in 1862 and converted at a cost of $3,500, the *Red Rover* offered bathrooms, icebox, laundry, elevator, kitchens, amputation theater, gauze blinds, and a full corps of surgical nurses. An adjunct of the fleet was the *Valparaiso,* a lazaretto, or quarantine, ship. Augmenting the staff in emergencies were Catholic nuns from the Sisters of the Holy Cross, supervised by Mother Superior Angela Gillespie. That same year, the *Red Rover* acquired its own staff of nuns, the navy's first official nurse corps, consisting of Sister Adela, Sister Callista, Sister St. John, and Sister Veronica, nurses from the Holy Cross School of Nursing, a division of Saint Mary's College at Notre Dame University in South Bend, Indiana. Aiding the sisters were five black volunteer nurses—Alice Kennedy, Sarah Kinno, Ellen Campbell, Betsy Young, and Dennis Downs—plus a few unnamed black nurses who assisted unofficially while

fleeing slavery. Each staff member earned 50 cents per day in wages as compared to the army salary of 40 cents daily. When the navy established a military hospital in a Memphis hotel in September 1863, Sister St. John headed the nursing staff, which included Sister de Sales O'Neill, later the Sister Superior of a Catholic hospital in Ohio. After the *Red Rover* was decommissioned in November 1865, ward logs record the sisters' patient load as 2,947, an average of one thousand per year.

In the wake of a respectable war record, public acclamation and pride furthered the growth of the Navy Nurse Corps. With the support of the American Medical Association, in 1869, a demand for nursing schools arose in most states. As a result, the navy led the nation with its first nursing hospital in Mare Island, California, followed by the New England Hospital's school in 1872, and Bellevue Hospital in New York, the country's first Nightingale facility. The navy pursued better care for wounded in 1870 with the commissioning of the *Pawnee* in Norfolk, Virginia, and the *Idaho* at sea off Japan. As of 1873, alteration of the title of nurse to bayman indicated the separation of sexes, with men rather than nuns performing the job. A sheaf of job descriptions dated 1887 required each staff nurse to care for fifty patients over a seventy-five-hour work week in addition to stoking the ward stove with coal; trimming wicks, cleaning lamp chimneys, and filling wells with kerosene; and keeping detailed patient records. As a matter of naval pride, shipboard nurses, like their civilian equivalents, were expected to maintain standards of integrity, sobriety, and professionalism. By 1897, to supplant volunteer and contract nurses, the U.S. Navy Hospital Corps became the official nursing arm of the navy for trained male graduates seeking a career in the military.

The corps's intransigence on the matter of female nurses lasted until the Spanish-American War. With the sinking of the battleship *Maine* in Havana Harbor on January 25, 1898, a new impetus required a larger medical staff, which included the navy's first degreed nurses. Ten female nurses joined the staff of the naval hospital in Brooklyn, New York, along with five nuns from the Sisters of Charity. Four more nurses held a post in Key West, Florida; eight staffed the navy's first Red Cross hospital ship, the *Solace,* which patrolled the blockade off the Cuban coast, collected the wounded and fever victims from Guantánamo Bay, Cuba, and ferried them to the New York Naval hospital or installations in Boston, Norfolk, and Fort Monroe, Virginia. A sister ship, the *Relief,* carried Esther V. Hasson, on loan from the army, for trips from the Caribbean to the army's Montauk Point hospital in Long Island, New York. Hasson later served the *Sherman,* a navy transport vessel in the Philippines. In a wartime climate, Sophia Palmer, an advocate of a nursing union and editor of the *American Journal of Nursing,* advocated examining boards and state licensing boards to ensure high standards.

It was 1902 before the female navy nurse sought a formal organization. On the advice of the surgeon general of the navy, a congressional bill proposed establishing a navy nursing corps, to consist of a superintendent, eight head nurses, and forty staff members, comprising sixteen first-class and twenty-four second-class nurses. Limited to the ages of twenty-six to forty, female nurses would be allowed a fifteen-year career and additional service in the Navy Reserves. For all its appeal, the bill failed in 1902 and again in 1904. It was February 6, 1908, before the U.S. Navy Nurse Corps became a reality.

Headed by Esther Hasson, the first twenty members organized the corps in Washington, D.C., before being parceled out to the eighteen navy hospitals. As of 1913, the uniform acquired the gold oak-leaf pin, adorned with shield and anchor. That fall, instructors Mary H. Humphrey and Corinne Anderson set up a training academy for native girls in Tutuila, Samoa, like the one on Guam. There Nellie M. Scherzinger, a victim of tuberculosis, became the first navy nurse to die in service. By the end of World War I, two of Hasson's "Sacred Twenty" had earned letters of commendation: chief nurses Elizabeth Leonardt and Martha E. Pringle. Two on loan to the army, Mary Elderkin and Jeannette McClellan, achieved the same award.

A month before the United States declared war on Germany in 1917, navy nurses from the Brooklyn Hospital and Philadelphia Methodist Hospital, monitored by Chief Nurse Frances Ban Ingen, sailed aboard the *Henderson* with a convoy bound for Brest, France. By the end of the war, Ingen had earned army certification for meritorious service for field work. She and other uniformed nurses displayed corps pride in velour hats, blue capes lined in red with acorn-and-leaf collar insignia, ankle-length skirts, gloves, and sturdy lace-up shoes. Only Ingen's cape bore the distinctive gold band marking a supervisor. Chief Nurse Alice M. Garrett and her staff of forty nurses followed in the second wave aboard the *St. Louis.* They landed at Southampton, England, and crossed the English Channel in rough seas for the naval installation at Brest, set up in an abandoned Catholic convent. Immediately, the staff began treating wounds, burns, and poison gas injuries. At a crude field hospital set up in France, nurse-anesthetist Elizabeth Dewey, recipient of a frontline commendation, reported the squalor of the makeshift arrangement and treatment of gangrenous wounds overrun by maggots. Between July 18 and 26, 1918, her unit treated thirty-five hundred wounded. She reported one stretch of fourteen hours at the operating table without a break. In her off-hours, she visited patients. Similar reports came from Chief Nurses Elizabeth Hogue in Strathpeffer, Scotland, and Alice Garrett in Brest.

Doubling the patient load were cases of Spanish influenza, the war's surprise killer, which raged from September 1918 to August 1919. Incidence of flu rose to a devastating sixty thousand cases a week and didn't slacken until June 1919. Decades before aspirin and viral studies increased the survival rate, nurses relied on palliative care—sponging faces and extremities, spoon-feeding liquids, and combating chills with heated blankets. The navy's famous designer of its nursing uniform, Esther Nelson Behr Hunter, wrote: "God have mercy on the boys who suffered so severely. The U.S.A. never will know the long sorrow list until months have passed" (Sterne 1996, 46).

The eyewitness accounts attest to the hardships and losses of the epidemic. At the base hospital in Whitepoint, Ireland, was Chief Nurse Grace MacIntyre, who described sailing aboard the *Briton.* Her letters reported dodging three submarines, a minor inconvenience compared to an outbreak of influenza, which boosted the sick bay population from six to 160 within two days. Among reports from the stateside hospital in Portsmouth, navy nurse Ada McGrath detailed the deluge of patients evacuated from France and the hasty hammering together of bungalows and contagion wards to accommodate meningitis, diphtheria, measles, and scarlet fever. One troop ship brought seven hundred medical cases requiring quarantine, which sidelined some nurses until the contagion passed. The Great Lakes Hospital alone treated twenty-eight hundred patients. Additional military clinics accommodated civilians as well. A nearby camp took the overflow of one thousand more. On the difficulty of meeting both military and civilian needs, Chief Nurse Beatrice Bowman reported: "And oh, we needed nurses. My nurses didn't stop to get orders to do double duty . . . They were wonderful women" (Sterne 1996, 50). The first navy nurse buried in Arlington National Cemetery, Maude Coleman, died of flu on September 22, 1918, in the first few weeks of the outbreak. Two nurses who died at the Brooklyn Naval Hospital received full military funerals.

Throughout Europe, the nursing staff remained on duty for two months after the armistice was signed on November 11, 1918. Of the 1,551 who served their country, none died of enemy fire: nineteen died of disease, one in Leith, Scotland; after the war's end, seventeen more expired. Four of the corps earned the Navy Cross—Marie Louise Hidell, Lillian Mary Murphy, Edna Elizabeth Place,

and Lenah S. Higbee, the first nurse for whom the navy named a destroyer.

The postwar period brought new challenges in military medical care, in part from suggestions and observations made during the conflict. By December 1918, Chief Nurse Sophia V. Kiel was readying the first transport home, the *George Washington,* the ship that had carried Woodrow Wilson to the Paris Peace Conference. An outward-bound contingent embarked for the Caribbean to set up training schools in the Virgin Islands. Chief Nurse Alice M. Garrett and Eva R. Dunlap were among the first to arrive. One pair— Chief Nurse Lucia D. Jordan and Josephine Y. Raymond—aided Catholic nuns in launching a two-year French-language nursing course in nearby Port au Prince, Haiti. For work among lepers and the insane in the Caribbean, Elsie Jarvis earned a commendation.

With Beatrice Bowman heading the corps, navy nurses entered the between-the-wars calm with plenty to do. Chief Nurse Sophia Kiel, along with Ada Chew and Viola M. Visel, compiled the nursing segment of the *Hospital Corps Handbook.* The lull in nursing activity altered to a decided stir in 1940, as the American military anticipated involvement in World War II. On the morning of December 7, 1941, Ruth Erickson, later director of the Navy Nurse Corps, reported hurrying to work and immediately receiving wounded and burn victims from gas fires in the dock area of Pearl Harbor. Aboard the *Solace,* Chief Nurse Grace Lally witnessed the first explosions and fires on oily waters. With a staff of twelve, she began treating victims retrieved from the wreckage of the battleship *Arizona,* which Japanese bombers sank. Over the next weeks, nurses worked eight-hour shifts with four-hour breaks. For her staff's efficiency, Admiral Chester William Nimitz awarded Lally a citation of meritorious achievement, lauding "the successful care of all casualties and the saving of many lives" (Sterne 1996, 109).

The Pacific war jeopardized navy nurses as never before. The Japanese imprisoned Mary

Chapman, Dorothy Still Danner, Helen Gorzelanski Hunter, Goldie O'Haver Merrill, Margaret Nash, Mary Rose Harrington Nelson, Eldene Paige, Susie Josephine Pitcher, Bertha Evans St. Pierre, C. Edwina Todd, and Chief Nurse Laura Maye Cobb. At the end of 1941, captors transported them to Japan along with corpsmen and patients. Many suffered bayonet wounds in the back. Others serving in the Philippines battled malnutrition, beriberi, scurvy, kidney infection, dysentery, tuberculosis, and fever as internment spanned into months.

The war brought significant change. The navy's medical units were dispensing synthetic quinine and vaccines against tetanus and yellow fever and introducing penicillin and blood plasma, the medical breakthroughs of the age. Insect containment squads sprayed areas with DDT, a new insecticide. On January 5, 1942, Alberta Rose Krape appeared on the front cover of *Life* magazine in white uniform and cap above a caption calling for fifty thousand nurse volunteers, which, for the first time in military history, included married women. Visits by First Lady Eleanor Roosevelt lifted the spirits in numerous clinics and wards. By July 3, 1942, Congress authorized ranks for nurses equivalent to those for military officers and established a blue double-breasted coat and serviceable blue-and-white cap and dress as the new uniform. In December, Lieutenant Commander Sue Sophia Dauser, a veteran of World War I as well as of Guam and the Philippines during World War II, headed the corps as the navy's highest-ranking female officer.

By 1943, navy nurses were stationed in the Virgin Islands, Puerto Rico, Trinidad, Cuba, Samoa, Alaska, Newfoundland, Hawaii, New Zealand, Panama, the Philippines, and New Hebrides plus the hospital ships *Solace* and *Relief.* Within the year, additional postings dispatched staff to the Aleutian Islands, Bermuda, Australia, Guam, New Guinea, Oran, Algiers, Tunisia, Naples, Palermo, Sicily, the Solomon Islands, the Russell Islands, and Curaçao and aboard the hospital ships *Bountiful, Refuge,* and *Samaritan.* The need for professional nurse care encouraged a landmark in gender equality—the enrollment of male nursing students in four schools by 1943. Still, Congress chose to widen the gap between the sexes by rejecting the commissioning of male nurses, thereby placing female officers over noncommissioned male aides.

In an unprecedented shift in standards, the army allowed its nurses to marry, but, despite exigencies of war, the Navy Nurse Corps held fast to its traditional standards. By the end of 1943, two navy nurses, Lieutenant Stephany J. Kozak and Lieutenant Dymphna M. Van Gorp, entered training as flight nurses. As staff members of the first in-air evacuation school, they reported to Rio de Janeiro to train Brazilian Air Force nurses in the use of life rafts and swimming and in outfitting planes with straps and brackets to secure stretchers and medical equipment. For their competence, the two flight nurses and a third, Lieutenant Catherine M. Kain, earned the Navy Commendation Ribbon.

On January 6, 1945, President Franklin D. Roosevelt asked Congress for a Selective Service act to draft nurses into the military. Nurses' organizations backed his request, which included a call for full integration, but the bill came too late in the war for legislative action. Another evidence of end-of-war nurse shortages was the establishment of the Cadet Nurse Corps. To fill gaps, Lucile Petry Leone recruited 135,000 volunteers by the end of 1945.

As though imprisoned in a time warp, the eleven captive nurses, still alive with 2,147 other prisoners, remained stalwart during the final months of combat. In a hostile, potentially deadly atmosphere, they became experts at making do. To assist in caring for internees, Laura Cobb welcomed volunteer Filipino and British nurses at the internment camp at Los Baños in the Philippines, where Japanese guards had transported eight hundred internees. Under a cover of hibiscus leis, she concealed service records in her bodice to preserve details of captivity. Goldie O'Haver Merrill constructed replacement uniforms out of denim. Margaret Nash informed an Australian man of the difficulty of cleansing instruments and described a sterilizer, which he improvised from scrap metal.

Reduced to eating rice laced with vermin, the survivors supplemented limited meals with pig grass, banana tree roots, and slugs. Trembling, they often lurched and fell; their quaking hands made treatment difficult and surgery chancy. The situation was desperate in the final days as General Douglas MacArthur's forces penetrated enemy territory to raid the camp on February 23, 1945. After thirty-seven months of captivity, nurse-internee Edwina Todd wrote of her tears when she saw planes painted on the side with the word "RESCUE." Within hours of liberation, navy nurses helped army personnel set up reception clinics. On the return flight to the United States, the eleven heroines were back in uniform and enjoying their new rank by the time their plane made the final hop from Johnston Island to Pearl Harbor. Susie Pitcher had acquired a heart problem; Laura Cobb had to be hospitalized. One internee, Margaret Nash, remained in a New York navy hospital, receiving treatment for tuberculosis, pellagra, and beriberi until 1946. All eleven survivors earned the army's Bronze Star and Distinguished Unit Badge, the American Defense Service Ribbon and Star, Pacific and Asiatic Service Ribbon with two stars, Philippine Defense Ribbon, Philippine Liberation Ribbon with one star, and the Navy Gold Star. Their example illustrated to recalcitrant brass that female nurses, like their male counterparts, displayed the "right stuff."

See also: Civil War; Gillespie, Mother Angela; Hasson, Esther; Spanish-American War; World War I; World War II.

Sources

"First!" http://www.bluejacket.com/first.htm.

Griffin, Gerald Joseph, and H. Joann King Griffin. *Jensen's History and Trends of Professional Nursing.* Saint Louis, Mo.: C. V. Mosby, 1965.

Kalisch, Philip, and Beatrice J. Kalisch. *The Advance of American Nursing.* Boston: Little, Brown, 1978.

Kemp, Peter. *The Oxford Companion to Ships and the Sea.* Oxford: Oxford University Press, 1988.

McHenry, Robert, ed. *Liberty's Women.* Springfield, Mass.: G. C. Merriam, 1980.

Sterne, Capt. Doris M. *In and Out of Harm's Way: A History of the Navy Nurse Corps.* Seattle, Wash.: Peanut Butter Publishing, 1996.

"Voices from the Past . . . Visions of the Future." http://www.ana.org/centenn.htm.

Nazi Nurses

The situation that confronted German nurses during the Nazi rise to power drew the definitive line in the sand: patriotic medical workers had to demonstrate that they were prepared to perform the eugenic cleansing that the Führer outlined for the Fatherland. At the beginning of Adolf Hitler's attempt to rid the Aryan race of impurities, he assigned Dr. Leonardo Conti as Nazi Party of the Reich Health Chief. In 1935, Conti set up the Nazi Women's Bureau to report on undesirables, notably hereditary deaf-mutes, schizophrenics, the developmentally disabled, epileptics, dwarves, prostitutes, and victims of venereal disease, all of whom were marked for extermination. A parallel group, the League of German Girls, initiated young women into the mindset of the master race so as to indoctrinate the next generation. Eager for an immediate return on his planning, Hitler wearied of delays caused by Conti's insistence on refining Germany's laws. In secret, Hitler issued an aggressive fiat—a monstrous plan to exterminate undesirables.

On September 15, 1935, Hermann Goering announced the Nuremberg Laws, a classification system that reduced chosen groups to second-class status. A high-sounding action, the Law for the Protection of German Blood and Honor, prevented genetically deficient people from procreating. Although Goering's instructions named mostly doctors, it is clear that, from 1933 to 1937, nurses, their aides, and orderlies forcibly sterilized 200,000 young people, some without their knowledge. In six death camps, these loyal professionals initiated the unthinkable—the eradication of some six million unwanted citizens. In hospital settings, Nazi nurses informed German mothers that seriously ill children could be mercifully euthanatized and guided parents toward a choice in keeping with Hitler's idealized plan for a blemish-free race. In nursing homes and mental institutions, so-called mercy killings rid the state of the infirm and mental defectives. The blood-soaked era produced an unprecedented blot on nursing history.

At war's end in 1945, evidence presented at the Nuremberg trials established that the mandated separation of people into desirable and undesirable hinged on a systematic annihilation of subjects suffering from mental defects, schizophrenia, manic depression, and hereditary epilepsy, Huntington's chorea, blindness, deafness, and other severe genetic abnormalities. In four death camps the totals reached nearly two million:

- Belzec, nearly 600,000
- Chelmno, nearly 300,000
- Sobibor, more than 250,000
- Treblinka, 700,000–800,000

Coupled with suicides, disease, starvation, and malnutrition, the total staggered the civilized world with the immensity of Hitler's war crimes.

In addition to outright murder, state-run army medical facilities, civil clinics, and the SS, the security police of the Nazi state, medical service conducted inhumane experimentation on additional undesirables, including Jews, Gypsies, Freemasons, Jehovah's Witnesses, homosexuals, and political prisoners. The majority of victims were women, many of whom died outright or were permanently maimed. The grisly work began July 10, 1942, on one hundred women transported to Auschwitz. Protocols tested new drugs and treatments such as lethal injections of anthrax and typhus, exposure to phosgene gas and gangrene bacilli, and phosphorus burns, which provided data to determine Germany's ability to survive biological and chemical warfare. Extending German surgeons' mastery of battlefield procedures were amputations and bone and muscle transplants. To enhance

their knowledge of reproduction, doctors destroyed uterine linings and sterilized the innocent with radiation to determine survivable dosages. An ingenious plot to isolate pairs of twins produced information on the genetic qualities of whites, Jews, and blacks.

With no compassion on their human guinea pigs, staff conducted studies of the human tolerance to cold, high altitude, ingested seawater, and pain to benefit the air force and submarine fleet. Photographs from Dachau attest to the effects of oxygen deprivation in a decompression chamber, where the subject suffered anoxia, convulsions, and subsequent unconsciousness. Under the expert supervision of Karl Brandt, chief of German medical services, and Dr. Ernst Robert Grawitz, the SS chief medical officer, some experiments produced up to 100 percent fatalities and untold suffering. Perpetrators denied their victims painkillers and offered no warning as to the nature and outcomes of the experiments. The final mortality figures will never be known, despite the German penchant for meticulous record keeping. Among the most feared and despised war criminals, Brandt was executed on June 2, 1948; Conti and Grawitz committed suicide while awaiting trial for crimes against humanity.

Postwar detective work disclosed the structure of Hitler's killer hierarchy. Conti's role in eugenics—which eroded by 1943 to a staff position under the control of Heinrich Himmler—was initially pervasive. For the sake of political expediency, he exploited Germany's zealous male-centered control of motherhood. Ostensibly to free hospital beds for German military casualties, he stepped up the use of holistic or organic medicine, euthanasia for defective infants, and government-sanctioned natural childbirth. His prime agent was Nanna Conti, his mother, a reputable midwife who had a significant influence on his career. As chief midwife for the Reich, she sponsored recruitment and training of practitioners and raised the retirement age to keep more state-licensed midwives in service. In addition, she supported breast-feeding and the donation of breast milk, a sanitary measure that ensured nourishment from pure sources.

Conti's work meshed with other insidious assaults on traditional loyalties, including the saturation of public radio with military music, pro-Nazi rallies, and the manipulation of the revered Reichsverband Deutscher Hausfrauen-vereine (National Union of German Housewives' Associations). On Mother's Day in 1934, the Reichsmütterdienst (State Mothers' Service), a conduit for German values, began training mothers in child care as a means of promoting the Nazi ideal of racial purity. The success of the total eugenics program is verifiable:

- In 1909, there were thirty-eight hundred German midwives in service. By the end of the Weimar period, there were twenty thousand, an increase of 426 percent.
- In 1933, midwives performed 29 percent of deliveries in Germany. According to *Ärztin,* a journal for women doctors, the number rose conservatively to 39 percent in 1935, then burgeoned to 75 percent by 1937. As of 1939, salaries rose to 1,400 Reichmarks annually. Regulations required that all German babies be delivered by registered midwives, who were members of the Reichsfactscraft Deutscher Hebammen, a professional union charged with ridding Germany of substandard citizens. The stepped-up infant delivery machine faltered, however, from a lack of training facilities to manage the huge influx of farm girls and village women seeking salaried careers in midwifery.

A heavy patina of patriotism overlaid the dirty work. Stalwart members of each staff could anticipate an Iron Cross—the traditional Maltese cross and ribbon the Prussians issued for valor in combat. According to a chapter by Susanne Hahn in *Medicine, Ethics and the Third Reich* (Michalczyk 1994), in 1933, a schism developed over professional roles in the discipline and control of racial purification. In 1934, only 9.2 percent of German nurses joined the National Socialist Nurses Organization, nicknamed the "Red Swastika nurses." Christian hospitals abstained from the master plan; Catholic nuns took no part in abortion, sterilization, and euthanasia. Those who refused lost jobs to the Nazi Order of Nurses, known as "brown sisters," a description of their state uniforms. By 1937, the rise of fanatic nationalism stoked prejudice against Catholic Charities nurses and midwives, who deliberately concealed genetically damaged children whom Hitler had marked for slaughter. On behalf of German Catholics, in July 1941, Clemens August Count von Galen, Roman Catholic bishop of Munster, rebuked Hitler for his heinous euthanasia program.

In the legal actions that followed the war, stark statements of medical malfeasance accompanied testimony. In the words of the chief prosecutor at the Nuremberg trials: "The defendants in this case are charged with murders, tortures, and other atrocities committed in the name of medical science. The victims of these crimes are numbered in the hundreds of thousands. A handful only are still alive; a few of the survivors will appear in this courtroom. But most of these miserable victims were slaughtered outright or died in the course of the tortures to which they were subjected. For the most part they are nameless dead" ("Opening Statement. 9 December 1946," 1). Into the last decade of the twentieth century, zealous stalkers of war criminals pursued fleeing Nazi medical staff into obscure corners of the world and applied evolving computer and chemical technology to the scraps of evidence that linked Germany's medical elite to the war crimes of the century.

See also: World War II

Sources

Abrams, Lynn, and Elizabeth Harvey, eds. *Gender Relations in German History: Power, Agency and Experience from the Sixteenth to the Twentieth Century.* Durham, N.C.: Duke University Press, 1997.

Annas, George J., and Michael A. Grodin. *The Nazi Doctors and the Nuremberg Code.* New York: Oxford University Press, 1992.

Burleigh, Michael. *Death and Deliverance: Euthanasia in Germany, 1900–1945.* Cambridge: Cambridge University Press, 1994.

Gilbert, Martin. *Atlas of the Holocaust.* New York: William Morrow, 1993.

Gutman, Israel, editor in chief. *Encyclopedia of the Holocaust.* Vol. 3. New York: Macmillan, 1990.

Kater, Michael H. *Doctors under Hitler.* Chapel Hill: University of North Carolina Press, 1989.

Koonz, Claudia. *Mothers in the Fatherland.* New York: St. Martin's Press, 1981.

Loftin, Robert Jay. *The Nazi Doctors.* New York: Basic Books, 1986.

Michalczyk, John H., ed. *Medicine, Ethics and the Third Reich.* Kansas City, Mo.: Sheed and Ward, 1994.

Ofer, Dalia, and Lenore J. Weitzman. *Women in the Holocaust.* New Haven, Conn.: Yale University Press, 1998.

"The Opening Statement of the Prosecution of Brigadier General Telford Taylor, 9 December 1946." http://www.ushmm.org/research/doctors/telfptx.htm.

Proctor, Robert N. *Racial Hygiene: Medicine under the Nazis.* Cambridge, Mass.: Harvard University Press, 1988.

Schreiber, Bernhard. *The Men behind Hitler: A German Warning to the World.* http://homepages.enterprise.net/toolan/hitler/htm.

Thornton, Fr. James. "Defying the Death Ethic." http://www.execpc.com/~jfish/na/052697n1.txt.

Nightingale, Florence

Dubbed "the Star of the East" and the idealized "lady with the lamp," Florence Nightingale excelled at convincing skeptics. A model of self-confidence and organizational genius in an era of female submission to males, she elevated nursing from the level of domestic help to the modern professional concept of competent healing. She applied her concepts to military medicine and hospital design, established training hospitals, and published an enviable canon of 150 pamphlets and six books—*Notes on Matters Affecting the Health, Efficiency and Hospital Administration of the British Army* (1857), *Notes on Hospitals* (1859), *Notes on Nursing: What It Is and Is Not* (1859), *Training of Nurses* (1882), *Nursing the Sick* (1882), and *Sick Nursing and Health Nursing* (1893). The third, *Notes on Nursing,* remains a fixture in medical training and on the shelves of public libraries worldwide. More than a century after its publication, Nightingale's succinct commentary cuts to the core of the nurse's responsibilities.

Born in Florence, Italy, on May 12, 1820, to wealthy landowner William Edward Nightingale and Frances Smith Nightingale, Florence was a sickly child reared at family homes in Derbyshire, Hampshire, and London. With her father's tutoring, she achieved the rare gift to female children in Victorian England—a quality education in languages, philosophy, science, math, and history and instruction in the liberal philosophies of Plato, Jean-Jacques Rousseau, and René Descartes. She flourished in the milieu of the upper middle class yet grew apart from the focus and mores of a genteel social rank. An early clue to her leanings was her treatment of wounded animals and the generous nursing care she expended on family servants.

During an outbreak of fever in Spitalfields, Nightingale, then only seventeen, had a religious experience on February 7, 1837, when she heard a divine voice compelling her toward a selfless mission. Drawn away from debutante balls and husband hunting to a noble working-class calling, she outraged her parents, who feared that she would languish as an old maid, contract a contagious disease, or fall to social and moral ruin among the dissolute who frequented and staffed hospitals. Her mother remained adamant, but her father relented after receiving some of his daughter's tender care during his illness. In 1849, Nightingale traveled abroad in Greece, Egypt, Italy, France, and Germany to study nursing methods and administration. Significant to her career was a fortnight spent at the Institution of Protestant Deaconesses, a hospital and orphanage at Kaiserswerth, founded by Theodor Fliedner in 1833 outside Düsseldorf, Germany.

Her mind made up, Nightingale returned to Kaiserswerth in 1851 to train under

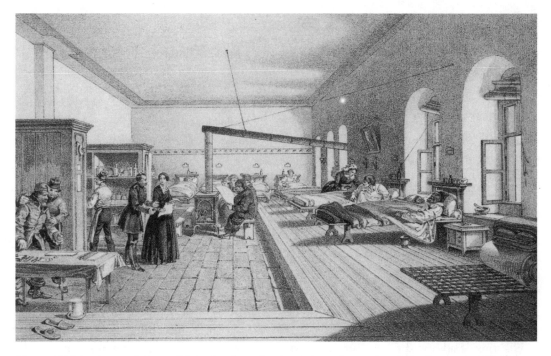

Florence Nightingale at work in a well-lighted, well-ventilated, orderly ward; copy of a painting in a hospital (Corbis-Bettmann)

Lutheran direction; in St. Germain near Paris the following year, she enlisted at a facility staffed by the Sisters of Mercy. From August 12, 1853, to October 1854, she superintended the Institute for the Care of Sick Gentlewomen in Distressed Circumstances, a hospital for invalid women on Upper Harley Street in London. An innovator and problem-solver, she upgraded its organization and efficiency and modernized the physical plant by installing patient call buttons, hot and cold water taps on each floor, and elevators to transport hot food from the cellar kitchen to patient wards. The facility was one of the first to welcome patients of all creeds and social levels.

At the outbreak of the Crimean War after England and France allied against Russia in 1854, the stirrings of nursing professionalism challenged an appalling neglect of soldiers wounded at the front. War correspondent William Howard Russell reported through the London *Times* the abysmal care and bluntly denounced indecent linens, stench, and fetid air. One of his strongly worded articles begged

for nurses: "The soldiers have to attend upon each other . . . the manner in which the sick and wounded are treated is worthy only of the savages of Dahomey—not only are surgeons not to be had, but there are no dressers or nurses to carry out the surgeon's directions. . . . Why have we no Sisters of Charity?" (Brainard 1922, 92). Calling on able-bodied and patriotic Englishwomen, the writer seemed to speak directly to Nightingale.

Obsessed with her religious calling and bankrolled by an annual stipend of £500 from her father, Nightingale heeded a second call to heal the destitute. After Turkey, England, France, and Sardinia allied against Russia, she volunteered for duty in the resulting September invasion of Sevastopol, the official beginning of the Crimean War. Prim and ladylike both in person and in correspondence, she tendered a formal offer to Sydney Herbert, British secretary of war, on October 14. Before her letter arrived, he had written his own, against the advice of the military, offering her the job of superintendent of nurses. She immediately accepted.

Under Nightingale's direction, thirty-eight nurses from Catholic, Anglican, and municipal hospitals bolstered the primitive army medical corps. After indoctrination at St. John's House on October 19, 1854, this initial wave of medical staff sailed on October 21 from England for Scutari, Turkey, a base of operations and receiving center for casualties on the Bosporus. After being ferried across the Black Sea from the combat zone, malnourished, maimed, and cholera-weakened soldiers lay in stone galleries of the Barrack Hospital, an abandoned Turkish army barracks outside Constantinople. As reported, fifty French nuns from the Sisters of Mercy were treating their nation's casualties; some four thousand British sick and wounded were dying untended at the rate of 42.7 percent (alternately reported as 50 percent and 60 percent).

Nightingale advanced to the Turkish coast of the Black Sea, shepherding her staff to Scutari on November 5 (Figure 2). Promised adequate support, the women encountered a debacle. Among the sights and smells of offal, vermin, body effluvia, and sewer gas, they witnessed patients suffering dysentery and frostbite in an overcrowded facility both filthy and unfurnished. The men lay on coarse straw under canvas sheets. The only water for bathing was unheated and impure. Rats and lice raised the mortality rate by spreading cholera and typhus. Staff requisition forms passed numerous signers in the cumbrous chain of command before acquiring the medical and surgical necessities. Deliveries of foodstuffs, medicines, and bandages were inadequate for the influx of wounded, who filled four miles of beds.

After the Battle of Inkerman that same day, Nightingale shamed the male staff by asserting that efficiency and cleanliness could immediately reduce hospital mortality. Significant to past losses were open sewer drainage, lack of laundries, substandard supplies and food, disorganized medical staff, and the absence of nurses. To attend to these multiple needs and nurse a deluge of misery, she kept a skeleton crew of the most efficient: J. Davy,

Maria Huddon, Margaret Jones, Sarah Kelly, Margaret Goodman, Mrs. Parker, Mrs. Roberts, and Elizabeth B. Turnbull. The others of her staff of thirty-eight nurses either became too sick to work, died, or failed because of incompetence, dismissal, or disinterest. With the remaining eight reliable assistants, Nightingale met the challenge of battlefield casualties and diseased patients, of whom an alarming number had previously not survived.

Mary Jane Seacole, a Jamaican colleague and healer who practiced Creole medicine and established a hostel at the Crimean front in Russia, visited Florence Nightingale at Scutari Hospital, described the efficiency of the staff, and approved of the simple kitchen and clean surroundings. Of Nightingale, she reported, "A slight figure, in nurses' dress; with a pale, gentle, and withal firm face, resting lightly in the palm of one white hand, while the other supports the elbow—a position which gives to her countenance a keen inquiring expression, which is rather marked" (Seacole 1988, 90–91). In wholehearted approval of England's heroic nurse, Seacole lauded her as "that Englishwoman whose name shall never die, but sound like music on the lips of British men until the hour of doom."

Over twenty-one months, Nightingale applied her own funds and those of private donors to upgrade combat medical aid. To improve mortality rates, she established sanitation and protocol for the barracks hospital. A laundry and hospital kitchen operated around the clock. She commandeered supplies and issued nightshirts, socks, utensils, bathtubs, linens and pillows, soap, combs, scissors, bedpans, and operating tables. As the sole female night nurse, she patrolled the wards by the light of her lamp, an image that Henry Wadsworth Longfellow immortalized in his lyric war memoir, "Santa Filomena" (1858):

Lo! in that house of misery
A lady with a lamp I see
Pass through the glimmering gloom,
And flit from room to room.
And slow, as in a dream of bliss,

Figure 2: A map of the Crimean War showing where Florence Nightingale and Mary Jane Seacole worked

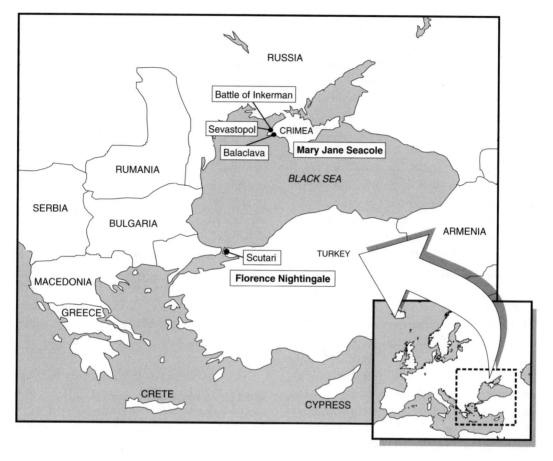

The speechless sufferer turns to kiss
Her shadow, as it falls
Upon the darkening walls. . . .
A Lady with a Lamp Shall Stand
In the great history of the land,
A noble type of good,
Heroic womanhood.

For all its idealization and Victorian sentimentality, it solidifies the image of Nightingale that has dominated medical history, art and cinema, and women's biography for 140 years.

Battling her own sufferings from Crimean (typhoid) fever, in July 1856, four months after the war ended, Nightingale returned to Lea Hurst, England, an international idol. She received a unique decoration, the Victoria Cross, consisting of three stars atop an oval containing the biblical line "Blessed are the Merciful," above the word "Crimea" and signed on the back, "To Miss Florence Nightingale, As a Mark of Esteem and Gratitude for Her Devotion Towards the Queen's Brave Soldiers. From Victoria R., 1855" (Kalisch and Kalisch 1978, 43). Queen Victoria and Prince Albert invited her to brief them and Prime Minister Henry John Temple, Viscount Palmerston, on the shortcomings of the military medical corps and accepted her advice on practical means of overcoming inadequacies.

Because authorities barred women from serving on government commissions, Nightingale informed an investigating panel, the Royal Commission on the Health of the

Army, in writing of the horrors of the Crimea. She emphasized the needless deaths of nine thousand—a number exceeding the statistics for the Great Plague of London. Deaths resulted more often from disease than trauma and could have wiped out the British force. Her extensive notes, line graphs, and color-coded wedge diagrams, which she called "coxcombs," expressed her vision of nursing. She established the worth of treating casualties as near to the front as possible and of reducing the pathetic mortality rate for soldiers in peacetime, who died at double the rate for civilian males of the same age category. A forerunner of the demographic statistician, she subsequently earned admittance to the Royal Statistical Society in 1858 and to the American Statistical Society in 1874.

Nightingale and a data consultant turned from the Crimea to India, the jewel of the British Empire. When the Sepoy Rebellion arose in India in 1857, she launched a campaign to appoint another investigating commission. At the top of her priorities was the establishment of necessary sanitary measures in India, a nation cowed by perennial waves of cholera and plague. Working from home, she completed her own report within two years to draw attention to a death rate of troops that was six times that of British civilians. The combined efforts of her statistics and military reform dropped the mortality rate from 6.9 percent to 1.8 percent. National findings not only saved the nation and its soldiers from needless loss but also established the importance of statistics to military and public health standards.

Still debilitated from illness and battle stress, Nightingale became a virtual recluse in her London quarters and lived off the royalties from her publications while directing her input into nursing education. Despite her total withdrawal from public appearances, her example, charts and graphs, monographs, consultations, and more than twelve thousand letters made their mark on society and its expectation of clean, professionally sound hospital wards. In a light moment, she remarked on the public's lack of clear definition of the profession: "No man, not even a doctor, ever gives any definition of what a nurse should be than this—'devoted and obedient.' This definition would do just as well for a porter. It might even do for a horse. It will not do [for a nurse]" (Maggio 1996, 487).

Using the Nightingale Fund of nearly £50,000, donated by admirers and veterans of the Crimean War, in 1860 she promoted the image of the career nurse by founding the Nightingale School of Nursing, a model teaching program based at St. Thomas's Hospital, a secular school in London under the supervision of Matron Sarah Wardroper, and at King's College Hospital. To modernize care, these institutions taught the curriculum that she dictated. Among her strongest injunctions to the probationer was her reminder that "Nature alone cures. . . . What nursing has to do . . . is to put the patient in the best condition for nature to act upon him" (Maggio 1996, 488).

The first ten students to study the Nightingale philosophy arrived on June 15, 1860, and donned the trainee's uniform—brown tunic topped by immaculate white apron and cap. Focusing on bedside care, they learned to splint broken bones, observe the sick and convalescent, dress sores, transport helpless patients, and replenish linens while the bed was occupied. Nightingale nurses attended lectures covering the principles of surgery, chemistry, and medication. Soon, the Nightingale nurse set the standard for St. Catherine's Hospital in Canada, Bellevue Hospital in New York City, Connecticut's New Haven Hospital, and Boston's Massachusetts General, which opened as an auxiliary the Boston Training School for Nurses under the supervision of Linda Richards, a Nightingale nurse.

In addition to nursing education, Nightingale spearheaded numerous causes: separate hospital facilities for children and the insane, quarantine for those infected with contagious diseases, public health initiatives, women's rights, education for women, and recognition of nursing as a respectable profession. Devoid of Catholic or Anglican dogma, her model of secular vocational nursing called for an amalgam of theory and practicum. In *Notes on Nursing,* her evaluation of sick people warranted a personal observation about the ideal hospital environment: "In watching disease, both in private houses and in public hospitals, the thing which strikes the experienced observer most forcibly is this, that the symptoms or the sufferings generally considered to be inevitable and incident to the disease are often not symptoms of the disease at all, but of something quite different—of the want of fresh air, or of light, or of warmth, or of quiet, or of cleanliness, or of punctuality and care in the administration of diet, of each or of all of these" (Thatcher 1984, 38). In answer to these shortcomings, she founded a pragmatic protocol known as the environmental adaptation theory: for maximum healing, the patient should receive proper dressing and remedies, ventilation, warmth, light, cleanliness of room, bedding, and person, quality diet, cheer and quiet, and suitable observation. Her demands of character were rigorous—chastity, sobriety, honesty, truth, trustworthiness, punctuality, self-control, and attention to duty. To the question of the nurse's gender, she exhorted, "Oh, leave these jargons, and go your way straight to God's work, in simplicity and singleness of heart" (van der Peet 1995, 160). In 1857, her single-minded campaign prefaced the founding of the British Army Medical School.

Nightingale's success in upgrading England's military operations brought her to the attention of the United States War Department, which, in 1861, sought her advice on setting up installations during the Civil War. Although she was deathly ill and bedfast, she replied to Simon Cameron, Secretary of War, and to Dorothea Dix, head of the United States Sanitary Commission. Subsequent social reform from her bed table writing board included lying-in hospitals, visiting nurse programs, improved ward systems for sick indigents, pediatric clinics, and barracks for married soldiers. Before a second collapse in 1867,

she targeted infant mortality rates and the necessity of putting "one female trained head" over hospital management and discipline, her most straightforward condemnation of male-centered medicine (Moore 1988, 5).

Nightingale remained at the forefront of nursing philosophy into old age. In 1893, she published the Nightingale Pledge, a standard work in nursing texts: "I solemnly pledge myself before God and in the presence of this assembly, to pass my life in purity and to practice my profession faithfully. I will abstain from whatever is deleterious and mischievous and will not take or knowingly administer any harmful drug. I will do all in my power to elevate the standard of my profession, and will hold in confidence all personal matters committed to my keeping, and all family affairs coming to my knowledge in the practice of my calling. With loyalty will I endeavor to aid the physician in his work and devote myself to the welfare of those committed to my care" (Goodnow 1942, iv). Impaired, but persistent, at age sixty-seven, she helped organize the British Nurses' Association. In 1901, she lost her sight and engaged the care of a housekeeper. Six years later, King Edward VII conferred on her the Order of Merit, making her the first female honoree. At her death on August 13, 1910, survivors rejected plans for a state funeral and burial in Westminster Abbey. They honored her wishes for a simple burial among family and a headstone marked "F. N. Born 1820. Died 1910."

The influence of Florence Nightingale remained strong throughout the twentieth century. Hospitals scrambled to hire Nightingale nurses, a designation ranking them at the top of the profession. A statue of Nightingale in London duplicates the posture and facial features of a giant of modern medicine. Her life continues to intrigue biographers. Hollywood versions of her courage cast Kay Francis in *The White Angel* (1936) and Anna Neagle in *The Lady with a Lamp* (1951); a television film, *Florence Nightingale* (1985), starred Jaclyn Smith. Nightingale's work toward army medical service reform, standardization of nurse training, and public health in India solidified the concept of the nurse's moral calling throughout the world.

Sources

Baly, Monica E. *Nursing and Social Change.* New York: Routledge, 1995.

Barritt, Evelyn R., R.N. "Florence Nightingale's Values and Modern Nursing Education." *Nursing Forum* (1973): 7–47.

Brainard, Annie M. *The Evolution of Public Health Nursing.* Philadelphia: W. B. Saunders, 1922.

Cohen, I. Bernard. "Florence Nightingale." *Scientific American* (March 1984): 128–132.

Dolan, Josephine A., R.N. *History of Nursing.* Philadelphia: W. B. Saunders, 1968.

Felder, Deborah G. *The 100 Most Influential Women of All Time: A Ranking Past and Present.* New York: Citadel Press, 1996.

"Florence Nightingale." http://www.dnai.com/~borneo/nightingale//38.htm.

Goodnow, Minnie. *Nursing History.* London: W. B. Saunders, 1942.

Griffin, Gerald Joseph, and H. Joann King Griffin. *Jensen's History and Trends of Professional Nursing.* Saint Louis, Mo.: C. V. Mosby, 1965.

The Grolier Library of Women's Biographies. Danbury, Conn.: Grolier Educational, 1998.

Kalisch, Philip, and Beatrice J. Kalisch. *The Advance of American Nursing.* Boston: Little, Brown, 1978.

Longfellow, Henry Wadsworth. "Santa Filomena." *Atlantic Monthly* (November 1857). http://www.theatlantic.com/atlantic.html.

Maggio, Rosalie, ed. *The New Beacon Book of Quotations by Women.* Boston: Beacon Press, 1996.

McKown, Robin. *Heroic Nurses.* New York: G. P. Putnam's Sons, 1966.

Moore, Judith. *A Zeal for Responsibility: The Struggle for Professional Nursing in Victorian England, 1868–1883.* Athens: University of Georgia Press, 1988.

Myers, Pamela. *Building for the Future: A Nursing History 1896–1996.* Chiswick, London: St. Mary's Convent, 1996.

Nightingale, Florence. *Notes on Nursing: What It Is and Is Not.* 1859. London: Harrison and Son, 1946.

O'Ceirin, Kit, and Cyril O'Ceirin. *Women of Ireland: A Biographical Dictionary.* Galway: Tir Eolas Newtownlynch, 1996.

Olson, Christopher G. "Historical Nursing Leader: Florence Nightingale." http://www.internurse.com/flo.htm.

Seacole, Mary. *Wonderful Adventures of Mrs. Seacole in Many Lands.* New York: Oxford University Press, 1988.

Thatcher, Virginia. *History of Anesthesia, with Emphasis on the Nurse Specialist.* New York: Garland, 1984.

van der Peet, Rob. *The Nightingale Model of Nursing.* Edinburgh: Campion Press, 1995.

Woodham-Smith, Cecil. *Florence Nightingale.* New York: McGraw-Hill, 1951.

Nineteenth-Century Nursing

In the early nineteenth century, hospitals damned themselves because of a low level of quality service and an even lower ebb of reputation. In the years preceding the century, Guy's Hospital of London regularly commandeered patients to stoke coal and assist the watch nurse or else be fined a day's food or summarily tossed out. In Bath, a formal declaration concerning pauper charity, dated April 3, 1872, noted with shame that the city was the only one of its size and means in England that had no hospice to serve the poor. The document stated local resolve to build a dispensary and staff it with physicians, an apothecary, and a matron and night nurse.

More almshouse than medical treatment center, according to nurse Louisa Twining's *Recollections of Workhouse Visiting and Management during Twenty-Five Years* (1880), facilities were custodial warehouses of mendicants and paupers. Unaccustomed to paying patients, they existed as refuges for abandoned waifs, retreats for the disabled and feebleminded, and isolation centers for plague and cholera victims. Across the board, they earned a reputation for filth, stale air, overcrowding, and foul odors. Treatments tended to the extreme, notably purging with calomel, traumatic surgeries, and dosing with soporifics—laudanum, a tincture of opium, mandragora, henbane, or water of nightshade.

Paid somewhere between six shillings and nine shillings six pence weekly, the only people willing to work under these conditions were the altruistic *matrum* (head nurse), lay nurses, nuns, or aged housekeepers, charwomen, and cooks, as well as the chronically jailed or unemployed, alcoholics, laudanum addicts, mental defectives, and wastrels, as

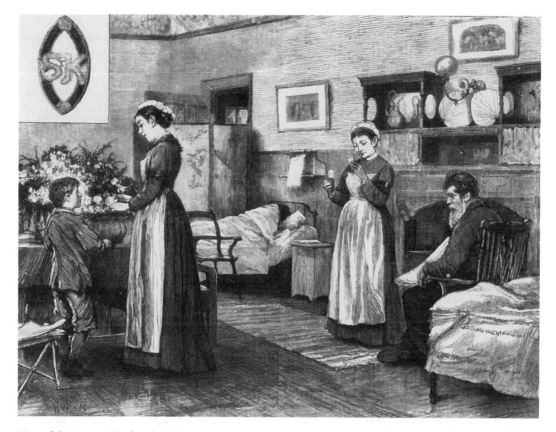

View of the Bouverie Ward in the Westminster Hospital, The New Order of St. Katherine for Nurses (U.S. Library of Medicine)

typified by Sairey Gamp, the scheming nurse-midwife in Charles Dickens's *Martin Chuzzle-wit* (1843–1844). The caricature of some seventy London workhouse nurses depicts an ungainly, overweight glutton wearing "a very rusty black gown, rather the worse for snuff" along with shawl and bonnet from a second-hand shop. Red-faced, swollen, and reeking of gin, she epitomized a pervasive lack of professionalism. In Dickens's words, "she went to a lying-in or a laying out with equal zest and relish" (Dickens 1965, 340). Her most despicable act was lining her chair with a pillow snatched from the bed of a comatose patient.

On the American frontier, nursing in the tradition of Puritan herbalist Anne Hutchinson was a blend of natural remedies and neighborly good deeds, as demonstrated by the mother of Carrie Young, author of *Nothing To Do but Stay: My Pioneer Mother*

(1991). With no medicine or knowledge of how to treat influenza, she resorted to canning jars of hot chicken soup delivered by sled over the frozen prairie to people in need. In *No Life for a Lady* (1941), Agnes Morley Cleaveland, a settler southwest of Albuquerque, New Mexico, reported the suffering of a man whose arm was blackening from frostbite. A Mexican servant applied the folk remedy of the times: "We got a large onion and peeled off the outer leaves. Then taking a few of the inner succulent leaves we put them on live coals raked from the fireplace; when they were toasted to a degree of tenderness we put a pinch of Duke's Mixture . . . into each leaf, spread these leaves on a cloth, and applied them warm" (p. 147). The course of treatment, followed every three hours over a three-week period, saved the man's arm. Cleaveland's memoirs venture into more perilous medical catastrophes—rabies, typhoid, and smallpox—as well as grave digging.

Other newcomers to the frontier made a harsh country a little less forbidding. At the fall of the Alamo in San Antonio, Texas, March 6, 1836, two women risked their lives in a doomed struggle. At Sam Houston's request, Andrea Candelaria, an innkeeper, nursed Jim Bowie through consumption and remained at his side during hand-to-hand fighting. While she shielded his body, a Spanish soldier pierced her arm and face with a bayonet. A colleague, Suzanna Dickerson, treated the fallen in the compound chapel and survived to carry the news of the slaughter to Sam Houston. Under fire at Fort Ridgely in Fairfax, Minnesota, Eliza Muller nursed refugees and soldiers after the Sioux Indian Outbreak of 1862. Agnes Freeman, a settler of Beatrice, Nebraska, in 1863, learned medicine from hands-on nursing and assisting her husband, Dr. Daniel Freeman. Fanny Wiggins Kelly, a captive of Chief Ottawa of the Oglala Sioux of Fort Laramie, Wyoming, served the tribe as nurse during Indian raids, which she described in *Narrative of My Captivity among the Sioux Indians* (1864).

Isolated figures retrieve the nursing history of the era from some of its ignominy. In Huntsville, Utah, Mary Heathman Smith, an immigrant from England, was nurse-midwife and healer for three decades to the people of Ogden Valley. Concepcion Arguello of San Francisco, California, suffered a broken heart and turned to nursing and charity work to ease her pain. In 1851, she entered the Dominican convent in Monterey as Sister Mary Dominica and remained a nun until her death in 1857. A pioneer nurse who emigrated to Arizona from Ireland in 1880, Nellie Cashman turned Russ House into an inn, where she nursed indigent wanderers and sheltered the homeless. Her good works earned her the name of "angel of Tombstone" (Sherr and Kazickas 1994, 24). Another greathearted volunteer nurse known only as Silver Heels left her work in an Alma, Colorado, dance hall to tend victims of a smallpox outbreak. She van-

ished from the community after the contagion ruined her face. For her generosity, locals named Mount Silverheels in her honor.

According to *Lamps on the Prairie: A History of Nursing in Kansas* (1942), Sara T. D. Lawrence Robinson, a doctor's wife, offered care to overnight visitors and wayfarers stranded by illness. Amy Loucks of Lakin treated a near scalping by sewing the flap in place with violin string and a dressing of carbolic acid and used a razor and embroidery scissors to amputate a railroad brakeman's three crushed fingers. A settler in Kansas City, Kansas, Mary Stewart, planted an herb garden and originated recipes for decoctions of roots, flowers, and leaves. She successfully treated cases of spotted fever with soda baths, thin soup, and purgatives. Another innovator, Lida Todd Aaron, of Wichita, chose spice or mustard plaster to sweat the patient's chest and relieve congestion. A visiting nurse in Pawnee County in the 1880s, Lucy Ann Davis Wheeler, stayed in service throughout the influenza epidemic of 1918. During a cholera epidemic at Fort Hays, volunteer lay nurses accepted as aides women from local bordellos, who took their turns on lamp-lit, tent-to-tent rounds. Late in the century, Dr. Ellis Reynolds Shipp delivered more than six thousand babies around Salt Lake City, Utah, and founded a school of nursing and obstetrics from which her daughter, Olea Shipp, graduated. In a museum display honoring the Utah Hall-of-Famer, Shipp's work garments and medical kit attest to the simplicity of her practice.

Catholic medical workers significantly affected frontier health. Mother Mary Baptist Russell, the first superior of the Sisters of Mercy, emigrated from Newry, Ireland, and established St. Mary's Hospital in San Francisco, the West Coast's first Catholic facility. Among her projects were soup kitchens for the poor, visits to death row prisoners in San Quentin, and a hospice for the aged and terminally ill. In 1868, the hospital served as a receiving center for smallpox victims. At her death in 1898, the *San Francisco Bulletin* proclaimed her the "best-known charitable worker on the Pacific Coast" (O'Ceirin and O'Ceirin 1996, 198).

Healers in Kansas made a notable beginning at offering quality health care. The Sisters of Charity, who opened Kansas's first civilian hospital in Leavenworth in 1864, fed and treated cholera victims at Fort Harker and rescued children orphaned by the outbreak. The first trained nurse in Kansas, Sister Joanna Bruner, arrived while the state was still being settled. The second and third civilian facilities—Christ's Hospital in Topeka, superintended by Sister Huberta of Olpe, Germany, and St. Mary's Hospital in Emporia, established by Ellen S. Bowman Vail and superintended by Fannie G. McKibben—opened in 1884.

Begun in a sailor's shed set up in New York by the West India Company in 1658, American hospital care, like that of industrialized Europe, made strides toward responsible administration. The nucleus of Bellevue Hospital, the shed expanded in 1816 to serve the multiple purposes of workhouse, almshouse, insane asylum, and orphanage. Overcrowded with up to two thousand patients, it was the site of outbreaks of typhus and other infectious diseases. Officials commandeered nursing staff from prisons and allotted one attendant per twenty patients. Parallel facilities in Philadelphia and Charleston offered little beyond minimal housekeeping and removal of the dead. Significant to Charleston's growth was the Ladies Benevolent Society, a band of nonsectarian lay workers who served admirably in the early nineteenth century and into the Civil War. Reorganized in 1881, the society maintained its pride in being the first official group of visiting nurses in the United States.

The status of nurse care in the era received much castigation from varied sources. An 1837 report from the Bellevue Hospital Visiting Committee commiserated with dray nurses who were treated as maids-of-all-work. In general, they were low-paid, poorly fed, and housed in barns like cattle. To account for their status, the report proposed the cause of the profession's denigration: nurses were drawn from society's dregs and were, consequently, unprincipled and untrustworthy. Services varied widely from parish to parish, usually employing no staff head or trained nurses and allowing the lowest standards of sanitation and hygiene.

Great Britain was no better off. In England, the low-end job of ward staffer fell to pauper nurses, poor women who earned extra money by prostitution, who drank and took drugs on the job, and who stole patient meals and clothing to give to their own families. Scottish nurses led by Sophia Jex-Blake stormed the Edinburgh medical establishment, demanding better pay and liberation from male domination and social degradation. In 1855, Irish nurse Mary Agnes Jones, Nightingale's prize pupil, reported on a Liverpool workhouse hospital, "A hospital is a sad place, but a Workhouse! It almost seems as if over so many of these beds NO HOPE must be written, with reference to this world" (Myers, 1996, 2). Jex-Blake's theatrics and Jones's candid estimation reflect a mounting revolt against uninhabitable infirmaries and general hospitals alike.

At this low point in nursing history, religious houses were the fount of reform. Out of love and service to fellow humans, Catholic nursing orders began setting up hospitals to elevate nurse care. Between 1845 and 1875, the Anglican Church founded forty-two religious communities, most providing nurse care. Spurred by the acute demand for higher standards of professionalism, the outreach paralleled the rise in England's population from 8.9 million to 13.9 million—a virtual flood of people swamping metropolitan areas with social and health needs as manufacturing drew more outsiders into factory communities. Thus, the social upheaval stirred by the Industrial Revolution precipitated medical modernization.

A force for change, lay church members initiated improvements. Following the example of France and Holland and of St. Mary di

Rosa of Brescia, founder of the Handmaids of Charity, England's Protestant sisterhoods set up visiting nurse programs to offer advice on health and cleanliness and to improve home care of invalids. A crusader for humane prisons, hospitals, and asylums, Elizabeth Fry organized London's Quaker Nursing Sisters in 1840 and influenced bedside care across Europe. During the Irish famine of 1844, Joanna Bridgeman, known as Mother Jane Francis, supervised the Sisters from Limerick in a mission to the sick and starving with funding from the Vatican and American Quakers. Bridgeman also worked at Scutari during the Crimean War and managed Kouali Federal Hospital in Turkey. In 1848, the Community of the Nursing Sisters of St. John the Divine, or St. John's House, set the example for training staff to aid the poor. In these classes, Mary Agnes Jones, founder of St. Mary's Convent and Nursing Home, studied hospital administration. She and others welcomed the liberal spirit of Anglican nurse training, which, unlike medieval forerunners, had "no vows, no poverty, no monastic obedience, no celibacy, no engagements, no cloistered seclusion, no tyranny exercised over the will or conscience, but a full, free and willing devotion to the cause of Christian charity" (Myers 1996, 4). Guided by the chaplain's morning and evening prayer from the Book of Common Prayer, the staff promoted high standards of behavior and character while ridding nursing of its centuries-old tie with convent sisterhoods bound by Catholic dogma.

Unlike facilities that turned out midwives and nursing home staff, St. Mary's produced medical assistants as adjuncts to the medical staff for all areas of health care. In the style of Nightingale nurses, trainees began with the rudiments of laundry and patient hygiene. Promising candidates advanced to the next level of study, which offered eighteen months of lectures and treatment of illness and trauma under the supervision of doctors from Westminster Hospital and King's College Hospital. Three years of ward practice preceded certification, the forerunner of the registered nurse

degree. Alongside the first professional nurses labored a staff of volunteer sisters, who supervised nurses and maintained standards of character. Graduates entered wards and domestic services nationwide as true professionals.

The concept of career nursing faced its first major challenge during the cholera epidemic of 1853–1854, followed the next year by the Crimean War. As a result of Nightingale's success in elevating standards of cleanliness, comfort, nutrition, and treatment, a grateful populace donated generously to nursing programs. One medical facility, the Royal Prince Alfred Hospital in Sydney, Australia, applied the Nightingale model in 1881. The staff adopted the paradigm of neatness, obedience, and scrupulous morality, the three hallmarks of the era. Housing for nurses in cubicles off the front hall kept them constantly under surveillance and in service to the wards, where they cleaned linens, earthenware, and appliances and performed mending and repairs in addition to tending patients. It was not until 1902 that the hiring of ward maids relieved nurse staff of general housekeeping. In the program's infancy, nurses earned £30 annually, with probationers making £20; ward nurses received £35, acting sisters £45, and sisters £50. In-service instruction required regular attendance at lectures, leaving little private time for rest, family visits, and relaxation.

Equipment and other necessaries were a crucial element of the success of Sydney's Royal Prince Alfred Hospital. Staff maintained a horse-drawn ambulance at the hospital stable and used the kitchen for diet and sterilizing instruments. Each nurse on night duty bore a screened hurricane lamp, cleaned and fueled nightly by the junior member of the team. It was the task of the matron, Elizabeth Lelia Murray, a graduate of London's King's College Hospital, to obtain stimulants from the local pub, which she hid in her cape until safely back at the dispensary. Strict record-keeping produced a summary of the first year's 1,069 admissions and 6,660 outpatients: 118 cases of typhoid, 141 accidents, and 147 surgeries. In 1883–1884, the hospital recorded 224 deaths and a breakdown of medical cases: 220 typhoid cases, 79 pulmonary tuberculosis, 62 rheumatism, 51 pneumonia, 40 bronchitis, 31 pleurisy, 31 heart disease, 25 kidney disease, 22 cirrhosis of the liver, 19 larval cysts, 13 abscesses, 12 hemiplegia, 7 bowel obstruction, 6 aneurysm, 5 pericarditis, and 3 anemia. Treatments consisted largely of bathing and sponging, ice packs, hot moist towels, poultices, and cough mixtures, all dispensed without drugs. More complicated nurse care called for cupping and leeches, which had been standard practice for several hundred years. Between 1882 and 1919, patients suffering consumption and typhoid fever remained in the general wards. Despite heavy reliance on carbolic acid, it is not surprising that nine nurses died, all from typhoid.

In industrialized nations, the end of the nineteenth century saw a vast, almost miraculous improvement in health care. In England, nurse Ethel Gordon Fenwick, a graduate of the Royal Infirmary and nursing supervisor at St. Bartholomew's Hospital in London, founded a nursing association as a means of raising standards and also issued the *Nursing Record,* later called the *British Journal of Nursing.* In the Western Hemisphere, an English immigrant, Alice Fisher, arrived at Philadelphia's worst hospital in 1884 and, with the aid of Edith Horner, transformed its Byzantine sanitation and service into the renowned Philadelphia General Hospital, a model of efficiency. Sister Mary Bernard, founder of the Sisters of St. Joseph of Wichita, Kansas, became a pioneering nurse-anesthetist at St. Vincent's Hospital in Erie, Pennsylvania, in 1887.

Anesthesiology developed as a duty of ordinary nurses. In 1880, sisters Aldonza Eltrich and Vanossa Woenke, Franciscan nuns at St. John's Hospital in Springfield, Illinois, learned the new science and taught others. A multitalented laborer, Lotta Frejd, served the Augustana Hospital School of Nursing in Chicago as cook, laundress, janitor, porter, and anesthetist in 1885. In 1886, Mary Cyrilla Erhard of the Sisters of St. Francis in Syracuse, New York, carried her nurse-anesthetist training to Malulani Hospital in Wailuku, Maui.

In the last decade of the century, the advent of general anesthesia added a new dimension to nursing and evolved into a nurse specialty. By 1893, Alice Magaw of St. Mary's Hospital in Rochester, Minnesota, began performing laboratory technology and established a model program of open-drop chloroform and ether anesthesia at the Mayo Clinic. In fourteen thousand surgical procedures at which she demonstrated her skill to hundreds of observers, she caused no death from overdosing. For her contribution to nurse-anesthetists, Dr. Charles Mayo named her the "mother of anesthesia" (History of Nurse Anesthesia, www.aana.com). In 1899, Ethel Baxter began dispensing anesthesia at a hospital in Yazoo City, Mississippi, becoming the first nurse-anesthetist in the South. A contemporary, Canadian practitioner Agatha Hodgins, studied the ether drop method at the Mayo Clinic and practiced her profession during World War I at Neuilly, France. Aided by Anne E. Beddow of Birmingham, Alabama, Hodgins organized nurse anesthetists in 1923. Such trained personnel became the norm in industrialized nations.

The advancement of professional health care workers is evident in figures bridging the nineteenth and twentieth centuries. Recorded by the U.S. Government Printing Office in 1949, this growth period indicates the phenomenal increase in professional nurse staff as compared to the slower addition of practical nurses and midwives to the health care labor pool:

Table 2

Year Trained	Practical Nurses	Student Nurses and Midwives
1870	1,204	10,569
1880	1,537	13,080
1890	4,589	39,987
1900	11,804	101,511
1910	83,327	123,534
1920	149,128	145,795

Source: Thatcher 1984, 38.

Unlike the prospering metropolitan regions, the outback still demanded less specialization, as demonstrated by the jack-of-all-trades work of Elizabeth Deane, head of the hospital staff of Circle City, Alaska, in 1897. The following year, after the Canadian government built a military community to serve the Yukon, Lady Ishbel Marjoribanks Aberdeen, a stalwart blend of aristocrat and feminist, launched the Victorian Order of Nurses (VON) to honor Queen Victoria's Diamond Jubilee. In her private papers, published as *The Canadian Journal of Lady Aberdeen, 1893–1898* (Saywell 1960), she countered opposition from conservatives to improved medical care among pioneers and miners. VON work filled her social calendar with fancy dress balls, garden parties, and carnivals and kept her on the move over thousands of miles of Canada as she built consensus and solicited funds. She gloried in the professional zeal of nursing probationers and remarked, "The faces of the girls in training were sufficient witness of the work being carried on, so full were they of a steadfast look of holy determination and devotion" (Saywell 1960, 435).

Late in November, Aberdeen's diary named enemies—Orangemen, rabid "temperance people," fusty medical associations, aristocrats, and the full cadre of Toronto mossbacks. Her plan of attack was simple: "The only thing to be done was to go straight ahead as if totally unconscious of the opposing hosts" (Saywell 1960, 441). At the core of her mission lay the hardships of pioneer nurse care. On December 8, 1897, she penned her concerns for those in the heartland: "The cry for help is very urgent—accidents, very many & painful cases of frostbite & inevitable fever & malaria. So our pioneers are brave women" (Saywell 1960, 446).

The Canadian far west profited from the arrival of four sourdough VON nurses—Rachel Hanna from Toronto General Hospital, Georgia Powell from New Brunswick, Margaret Payson from Nova Scotia, and Amy Scott from England—to minister to miners, suppliers, and adventurers. Much lauded in Lady Aberdeen's notes, the foursome traveled by rail from Vancouver to Fort Wrangel before joining two hundred members of the Royal Canadian Mounted Police to steam up the Stikine River to Glenora and Telegraph Creek and overland some 200 miles to their appointed places. Of their hardships, Aberdeen comments, "The worst part was the horrible swamps through which they had to wade up to their waists. And nothing to eat but hard biscuits, rancid strong bacon & black tea & this in the midst of great heat & under perpetual attack from the biggest bloodthirstiest hordes of mosquitoes" (Saywell 1960, 458). The most common complaints the foursome encountered were scurvy, frostbite, gangrene, rheumatism, and pneumonia along with the broken bones and contusions caused by falls and camp violence. The rigors of frontier nursing brought its perpetual list of complaints. Georgia Powell reported a heavy influx of diseased patients: "Such sick men! nor was the sickness all, but the filth and the vermin; and we had so little to do with" (Backhouse 1994, 134).

Amid the explosion of medical innovation in the Edwardian era, Aberdeen's brainchild was in good company. In this same period, Mrs. R. A. Edgerton, an English Red Cross nurse, opened a private facility and later superintended nursing at Dawson's Good Samaritan Hospital in the Yukon. On July 11, 1898, a religious initiative, the mission of the Sisters of St. Ann, brought three nursing missionaries—Mary of the Cross, Mary Joseph Calasanctius, and Mary John Damascene, the operating room supervisor—upriver by steamer to assist at St. Mary's Hospital, the first permanent medical facility of the gold-mining region. Situated near Dawson, the hospital drew on untrained attendants, sisters Mary Zephyrin, Pauline, and Prudentienne, who had treated the sick at Akulurak, an Inuit community on the tundra bordering the Bering Sea. The staff's first emergency was a Klondike typhoid epidemic. An influx of 140 patients overran the poorly equipped two-story log building, which lacked plumbing and housed the sick on bare sacks of sawdust, over which they furnished their own sheets.

To rid the hospital of mounting debt, the mission sisters toured the creeks on borrowed horses in May 1899. Within four weeks, they collected $10,000 dollars in donations. That winter, to boost hospital funds, Dawson women hosted a week-long Christmas charity bazaar. According to Faith Fenton, editor of the daily *Paystreak,* activities luring people out into the dark nights included a gypsy fortune-teller, wheel of fortune, bobbing in the lily pond, and buying lottery tickets and handicrafts. Pro-hospital revelers enjoyed music, dancing, café noir, and bonbons. The total—$12,000—retired much of the hospital's debt and assured Dawson a start toward quality care.

See also: African-American Nurses; Barton, Clara; Bickerdyke, Mary Anne; Blackwell, Dr. Elizabeth; Christian Nursing; Civil War; Cumming, Kate; Etheridge, Anna Blair; Gillespie, Mother Angela; Jones, Mary Agnes; La Flesche Picotte, Susan; Midwifery; Native American Nursing; Navy Nurse Corps; Nightingale, Florence; Paget, Dame Mary Rosalind; Public Health Nursing; Red Cross; Richards, Linda; Seacole, Mary Jane

Sources

Abel-Smith, Brian. *A History of the Nursing Profession.* London: Heinemann, 1960.

Armstrong, Dorothy Mary. *The First Fifty Years: A History of Nursing at the Royal Prince Alfred Hospital, Sydney, from 1882–1932.* Sydney: Royal Prince Alfred Hospital Graduate Nurses' Association, 1965.

Backhouse, Frances. *Women of the Klondike.* Vancouver: Whitecap Books, 1995.

Baly, Monica E. *Nursing and Social Change.* New York: Routledge, 1995.

Bentley, James. *A Calendar of Saints.* London: Little, Brown, 1993.

Cleaveland, Agnes Morley. *No Life for a Lady.* Lincoln: University of Nebraska Press, 1941.

Dickens, Charles. *Martin Chuzzlewit.* New York: Signet Classics, 1965.

Dictionary of National Biography, 1942–1950. New York: Oxford University Press, 1959.

Ehrenreich, Barbara, and Deirdre English. *Witches, Midwives, and Nurses: A History of Women Healers.* New York: Feminist Press, 1982.

Griffin, Gerald Joseph, and H. Joann King Griffin. *Jensen's History and Trends of Professional Nursing.* Saint Louis, Mo.: C. V. Mosby, 1965.

"History of Nurse Anesthesia Practice." http://www.aana.com/information/infohistory.htm.

Jamieson, Elizabeth, and Mary F. Sewall. *Trends in Nursing History.* London: W. B. Saunders, 1949.

Lacey, Candida Ann, ed. *Barbara Leigh Smith and the Langham Place Group.* New York: Routledge and Kegan Paul, 1987.

Lamps on the Prairie: A History of Nursing in Kansas. Emporia: Kansas State Nurses' Association, 1942.

McKown, Robin. *Heroic Nurses.* New York: G. P. Putnam's Sons, 1966.

Moore, Judith. *A Zeal for Responsibility: The Struggle for Professional Nursing in Victorian England, 1868–1883.* Athens: University of Georgia Press, 1988.

Murphy, Claire Riddle, and Jane G. Haigh. *Gold Rush Women.* Anchorage: Alaska Northwest Books, 1997.

Myers, Pamela. *Building for the Future: A Nursing History 1896–1996.* Chiswick, London: St. Mary's Convent, 1996.

Newlin, George, ed. and comp. *Everyone in Dickens.* Vol. 1. Westport, Conn.: Greenwood, 1995.

O'Ceirin, Kit and Cyril O'Ceirin. *Women of Ireland: A Biographical Dictionary.* Galway: Tir Eolas Newtownlynch, 1996.

Saywell, John T., ed. *The Canadian Journal of Lady Aberdeen, 1893–1898.* Toronto: Champlain Society, 1960.

Sherr, Lynn, and Jurate Kazickas. *Susan B. Anthony Slept Here: A Guide to American Women's Landmarks.* New York: Times Books, 1994.

Sterne, Capt. Doris M. *In and Out of Harm's Way: A History of the Navy Nurse Corps.* Seattle, Wash.: Peanut Butter Publishing, 1996.

Thatcher, Virginia. *History of Anesthesia, with Emphasis on the Nurse Specialist.* New York: Garland, 1984.

Underwood, Larry D. *Love and Glory: Women of the Old West.* Lincoln, Neb.: Media Publishing, 1991.

Young, Carrie. *Nothing To Do but Stay: My Pioneer Mother.* New York: Delta, 1991.

Nutting, Adelaide

Adelaide Nutting, a contemporary and colleague of some of the twentieth century's memorable names in nursing, was the first American nurse to become a university professor and the first nursing archivist and historian. She directed the first university department of nursing education, which was

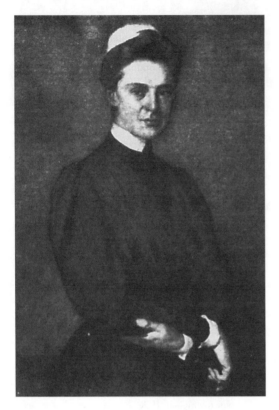

Mary Adelaide Nutting, ca. 1923 (U.S. Library of Medicine)

recognized internationally for quality performance. A cool, logical voice for excellence, she applied natural leadership to the growing pains that beset the nursing profession, which was still proving itself in the medical community. From her programs came the nation's revered faculty and deans of nursing. In 1921, Yale University conferred on her an honorary M.A. Columbia University honored her accomplishments with an archive, the Adelaide Nutting Historical Nursing Collection.

Nutting's career bore little resemblance to her girlhood preparation. The daughter of a civil service worker, she was born in Waterloo, Quebec, on November 1, 1858, and grew up in Ottawa, where she attended a small academy before entering a convent school in St. John to study French. From there, she progressed to Bute House in Montreal, demonstrating her talent for language and music.

She continued her education in Lowell, Massachusetts, where she boarded with relatives.

On her return to Ottawa, Nutting was introduced to nurse care during her mother's extended illness. Grieving over her mother's death, Nutting turned to church work, accepted private music pupils, and then taught music at the Cathedral School for Girls in Newfoundland. Still unsettled at age thirty, she read about Baltimore's Johns Hopkins Hospital Training School for Nurses, headed by a Canadian nurse, Isabel Hampton. The strain of twelve-hour stretches of duty plus classroom work compromised Nutting's health, but she refused to yield to physical limitations.

On graduation from the two-year program in 1891, Nutting entered the profession amid an explosion of nursing programs that drew eleven thousand students in the year 1900. She rose quickly in the hospital hierarchy, from head nurse and assistant superintendent to school principal as Hampton's replacement. One of Nutting's prime acts was to abolish schedules that linked classes with ward duty, a burden that had so limited her ability to study. Her purpose was a shift from hospitals exploiting probationers as cheap labor to a beneficial practicum of hands-on training. A second contribution to her alma mater was the extension of the course from two years to three to accommodate the growing number of specialties, notably anesthesia. She fought for an endowment to separate the school from the hospital budget and established a tuition system similar to the university fee structure.

To combat mediocrity in nursing schools, in 1903 Nutting led the Maryland State Nurses Association in a campaign for nursing regulations. She thrived in administrative and leadership roles and served as secretary of the American Society of Superintendents of Training Schools for Nurses and president of the American Federation of Nurses. To provide the profession with an overview, she joined feminist nurse Lavinia Dock in researching a four-volume *History of Nursing,*

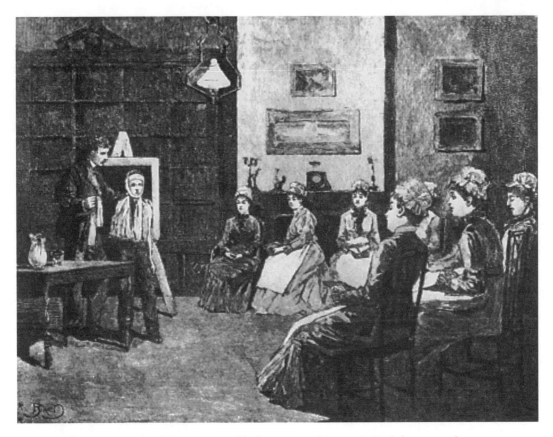

An illustration from A History of Nursing: *M. Adelaide Nutting and Lavinia L. Dock demonstrate the proper bandaging techniques of the early twentieth century. (U.S. Library of Medicine)*

drawn in part from books in Nutting's private library, which contained a first-class collection of works by Florence Nightingale.

In 1906, Nutting accepted a promotion to full professor of institutional administration at Columbia University's teachers college, which carried the responsibility for curriculum development. To round out the program, she added courses in theory and practice. With the help of Lillian Wald, nurse and social reformer at the Henry Street Settlement, Nutting acquired financing for courses in public health and, in 1910, launched the first Department of Nursing Education, which she directed. A teacher as well as administrator, she influenced the career of Isabel Maitland Stewart, a Canadian nurse from Chatham, Ontario, who joined Nutting's staff and sup-

ported the National League of Nursing Education. As one of the nation's most respected experts on nursing, Nutting continued aiding schools by strengthening their programs to produce qualified, well-rounded professionals. At her retirement in 1925, she was honored for inspiring others and for demanding the best from herself and her school.

Sources

Apple, Rima D., ed. *Women's Health, Health and Medicine in America: A Historical Handbook.* New Brunswick, N.J.: Rutgers University Press, 1992.

"The History of Nursing." http://www.lib.auburn.edu/madd/docs/unionlist/h24.html.

"Johns Hopkins Hospital Centennial." http://hopkins.med.jhu.edu/BasicFacts/hundred.html.

Yost, Edna. *American Women of Nursing.* Philadelphia: J. B. Lippincott, 1947.

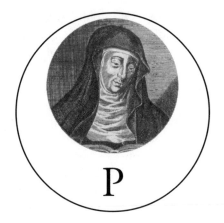

P

Paget, Dame Mary Rosalind

A skilled nurse and midwife, suffragist, and opponent of male-dominated health care for women, Dame Mary Rosalind Paget saw nursing as essential to the security of England's informed female citizenry. A champion of natural birthing methods, she protected infants and mothers by founding the Midwives' Institute, later called the Royal College of Midwives. Begun in 1881, the union buoyed professional esprit de corps into the pre–World War I era by acknowledging the value of midwives to women's health care, registering members, offering scholarships to trainees, and encouraging cooperation among lay practitioners. Uppermost in her respect for clients was a belief that all parturient women deserved the aid of a midwife, regardless of the client's moral standards or respectability.

Paget derived strength from a family devoted to social welfare. Born January 4, 1855, in Greenbank, Liverpool, to reformer Elizabeth Rathbone and attorney and police magistrate John Paget, she was a niece of William Rathbone, a Quaker member of Parliament and voice for nursing reform. Paget grew up in a household that honored feminism and the move toward enfranchisement of women. Her personal mission was the fostering of

women's suffrage and active citizenship. To facilitate her ideals, she chaired the third Conference of the Association of Queen's Superintendents in the Northern Counties and attended the Congress of Italian Midwives. From the beginning, her driving principle was the need for improved morals, character, and sobriety among England's mothers to ensure a stable, voting citizenry for the twentieth century.

Paget maintained a staunch professionalism. As Queen Victoria's personal nurse since 1891, a staff member at the London Hospital, and founder of the Charter Society of Physiotherapy, she introduced and edited *Nursing Notes,* forerunner of *Midwives Chronicle.* She valued close ties with other birthing specialists and urged lawmakers to pass a bill to register midwives. Because members of Parliament considered the act an intrusion on liberty, they voted down the bill in 1890, thus maintaining England's backward status among more progressive European nations. To assist the poor in obtaining the best obstetrical service, Paget expanded their options by fighting for registration, which was enacted in 1902.

In 1896, Paget addressed the National Union of Women Workers about promoting natural methods of childbirth and prenatal care by creating an enlightened network of midwives, especially for the working class. Of concern was the departure of middle-class women from the fundamentals of midwifery as they abandoned home-centered birthing for obstetrical clinics and male doctors. Another problem she foresaw was the muddling of issues of birthing with the mission of philanthropists, whose outreach she considered parallel but apart from the midwife's concerns. To achieve an enlightened sisterhood of women abstaining from drink and working toward stronger families, she combined the roles of nurse and political activist. In 1907, she composed a letter challenging the Council of the Queen Victoria Jubilee Institute for Nurses on the matter of unwed mothers and exhorted nurses to tend the sick poor without judging their circumstances. She emphasized that nonjudgmental treatment to mothers could rescue unwed parents and illegitimate children from ignominy.

Paget helped the midwives' union grow in membership from 240 in 1894 to 1,235 in 1914 by supporting lower-class midwives in upgrading their skills and expressing the concerns of their clients. In Liverpool in 1909, she followed the example of her cousin Eleanor Rathbone in delivering a paper on midwifery and maternity nursing at the Jubilee Congress on District Nursing. A spirited, good-natured leader and campaigner, she and her associate, Paulina Ffynes Clinton, supported the cause of lying-in services in the 1911 Insurance Bill by polling influential medical leaders, nominating likely candidates for provisional insurance committees, and drafting a letter to the media. Paget's campaign centered on informing women's groups of the social, moral, and religious value of women's welfare. Recognition of the issue of home and family versus work outside the home placed her in the minority who recommended well-paying jobs to keep mothers out of crime and prostitution. She proclaimed, "And who shall dare to be hard upon women driven by starvation? For we do not hear of state support for these mothers" (Marland and Rafferty 1997, 91). Her activism challenged

philanthropic foundations to build responsibility among the poor rather than a perpetual climate of need.

Paget proved useful in practical matters, particularly the thorny issue of pay for midwives. She joined Paulina Clinton and Amy Hughes in advocating higher fees to separate the midwives' life-sustaining careers from those of rescue workers and other volunteers and altruists. To save poor clients from having to pay more for deliveries, Paget demanded that districts supplement income for midwives. By legitimizing and ennobling the status of women's work, she advanced the cause of midwifery, thus upgrading the health and morals of women and young families. In 1935, at age eighty, she received her first national recognition of service. After her death August 19, 1948, in Bolney, Sussex, her portrait adorned the headquarters of the Royal College of Midwives.

Sources

Dictionary of National Biography, 1942–1950. New York: Oxford University Press, 1959.

Hannam, June. "Rosalind Paget: Class, Gender, and the Midwives' Institute." *History of Nursing Society Journal* 5 (1994–1995): 133–149.

Marland, Hilary, and Anne Marie Rafferty. *Midwives, Society and Childbirth: Debates and Controversies in the Modern Period.* London: Routledge, 1997.

Rivers, J. *Dame Rosalind Paget: A Short Account of Her Life Work.* London: Midwives' Chronicle, 1981.

Public Health Nursing

Visiting nurse care has its roots in the spontaneous charitable missions and neighborly kindnesses dating to ancient times and the work of Phoebe, a Christian deaconess, the Western world's first visiting nurse. Essential to house-to-house service were the needs of city dwellers. Their existence in crowded warrens surrounded by animal droppings and above-ground sewer mains bred the outbreaks of disease that terrorized and decimated communities. Added health threats from foul cisterns and public baths spread disease among people who had no knowledge of bacteria from septic air and water and no concerted plan to prevent and stop contagion.

Evolving from the ministrations of altruistic nuns and midwives during the Renaissance, the concept of home visits claims among its originators the Damsels of Charity, founded by Prince Henry de la Mark in 1560, and the Sisters of St. Charles of Nancy, a French company of lay nurses begun in 1652 to comfort and treat plague victims. The first identifiable municipal visitation system began with the social reform of the seventeenth century. The English Poor Law of 1601 diverted responsibility for indigents from families to parishes, whose concern for society's most miserable citizens aimed at bettering life for all.

In France, where duty toward the poor had not developed into a national concern, Bishop Francis de Sales of Geneva and his partner, Madame Jeanne de Chantal of Dijon, enlisted noblewomen to join the Order of the Visitation of Holy Mary and St. Jane Frances de Chantal. A coterie of the high-minded, these caregivers distributed alms and clothing, laundered linens, and called on the sick of Autun. Remaining in close touch with the terminally ill, the order provided a mortuary service that included washing and arranging corpses for burial. To characterize her professional intent, de Chantal dressed in a demure plain serge and white collar and sleeves, a forerunner of the Victorian nursing uniform. In 1606, she overtaxed herself in treating dysentery victims. Admiring villagers acknowledged her selflessness by naming her the Saint of Monthelon. In 1610, when her children were grown, she helped de Sales found a permanent congregation of women in Annecy, Savoy.

A subsequent benefactor of the ill, Father Vincent de Paul, organized teams of men and women to systematize the route of the visiting nurse. His public succor, the Society of Missioners, began in 1617 with parish priests; within a decade, the ravages of war drew his workers over much of the countryside. During the famine of 1651, the staff distributed bread to those at the point of death. Simulta-

neously, contagion distressed neighboring villages, which the Missioners visited on mules or on foot. De Paul's parallel experiment, Les Dames de Charité (Ladies or Sisters of Charity), began with one needy case and spread over much of France.

With so many volunteers at hand, de Paul suggested forming an uncloistered volunteer cadre of charity workers to call on the rural poor. He admonished the rich to lay aside jewels and fine raiment and to plunge themselves into hands-on charity. Supervised by Mlle. Louise le Gras, later known as St. Louise de Marillac, the nurses established territories to lighten the burden and consolidate efforts. De Paul enlisted assistants from the peasant class, Les Filles de Charité (Daughters of Charity), who undertook the menial jobs of housecleaning, laundry, and bathing patients.

St. Vincent de Paul's public mission inspired other communities. In this same era, Theophrastus Renardot, a Paris physician, emulated de Paul's concept and originated a band of doctors to spend two days a week diagnosing and prescribing treatments and medicaments for the poor. Likewise, Montreal, Canada, profited from the Vincentian model in the work of Marguerite d'Youville, a disillusioned widow who in 1737 organized Les Soeurs Grises (Grey Sisters), visiting nurses in gray habits and silver crosses who visited the elderly at L'Hôpital Général and treated patients in wards and at home. A separate mission rescued foundlings and housed them at La Crèche d'Youville (The Cradle of Youville) before placing them in local homes. Likewise benefited were the handicapped, prostitutes, French and English soldiers, and American Indians during a smallpox epidemic. In 1990, St. Marguerite d'Youville was the first Canadian to be canonized.

In Protestant nations, religious workers devised their own networks of nurses to treat home-bound patients; visit hospitals, workhouses, and prisons; succor orphans; shelter distressed women; and bury the dead. In 1789, Isabella Graham, a Scottish immigrant to New York, enlisted Presbyterian widows to perform charitable work for the poor. Joined by Sarah Ogden Hoffman, the Widow's Society tended the sick and dying in their cellars, garrets, and huts. In Philadelphia, Dr. Joseph Warrington organized a society of nurse-midwives in 1832, the Lying-in Charity for Attending Indigent Women in Their Homes. He launched a second group, the Nurse Society, in 1839, to provide an active mission of pious, mature private-duty nurses to live with patients and treat illnesses or handicaps of any type. The society, supervised by a doctor, offered training suited to each volunteer's level of proficiency. Veteran members of the society received certification that allowed them to freelance.

Taking his cue from Mennonite deaconesses in Holland and Elizabeth Fry's reform at London's Newgate Prison, Reverend Theodor Fliedner of Kaiserswerth, Germany, raised funds for a parish nurse system. Aided by his wife, Frederika Münster, he began a Women's Society of Visiting Nurses and opened a kindergarten and a halfway house for female prisoners. His expansive plans called for a hospital and training school, a lasting contribution to social reform. On April 20, 1836, he purchased an ample residence that became Kaiserswerth Hospital and began accepting sturdy laboring-class women of good character and maturity. Graduates, dressed in a plain blue shift, white apron, and frilled cap, went into the community to treat the sick or teach school.

Fliedner's second wife, Caroline Bertheau, a former pupil employed at a Hamburg hospital, helped him dispatch *geimeinde diakonissens* (parish deaconesses). The concept prospered and influenced similar agencies dispatching trained village nurses in England, France, and Switzerland. In London, Elizabeth Fry began a Kaiserswerth model in 1840 and enlisted Queen Adelaide as a patroness. In Paris the following year, the Institute of Protestant Deaconesses, also known as the Protestant Sisters of Charity, offered both nurses and aides to communities in need. Before mid-century, the job of nurse, buoyed by Kaiserswerth graduate Florence Nightingale and her protégés, began to take on the tone of a profession.

The creator of England's district nursing program, William Rathbone, instituted his work in Liverpool in 1859. Himself a visiting volunteer for the District Provident Society and Relief Society, patterned after the parish lay visitors of Elberfeld, Germany, he set up a model that emulated nurse Mary Robinson's nurse care of his wife during a three-month terminal illness. Using a grid system that placed one visitor in a specified area, volunteers canvassed streets, houses, and individuals to study the conditions that influenced well-being. Annoyed with the trappings of aristocratic socialites, with their self-ennobling charity balls and bazaars, Rathbone initiated a disciplined system, described in his books *Method Versus Muddle and Waste in Charitable Work* and *The History and Progress of District Nursing* (both 1890). More than a visionary, he oversaw proper nurse care and instruction in hygiene and sanitation, which he contended prevented human ills and cost less than hospitalization.

To carry out his work, Rathbone hired Mary Robinson to initiate a three-month trial of his concept. In addition to intervention in illness, she taught family members how to wash, dress, medicate, and feed the sick, elderly, and debilitated. Lessons in home cleanliness bound Rathbone's nurses to social work as well as medical treatment in the most squalid sections. The size and condition of Liverpool's slums threatened Robinson with defeat at the end of one month. After a pep talk from Rathbone, she returned to duty, becoming England's first district nurse. He praised her professionalism, noting that good deeds radiated far from one household to the health of the community and helped to rid the area of drunkenness, abuse, and crime.

To spread the job over other districts, Rathbone sought nurses from the Nightingale School of Nursing at St. Thomas's Hospital and from St. John's House. On the advice of

Florence Nightingale, he set up a nursing school at the Liverpool Royal Infirmary to educate hospital, private duty, and district nurses. The success of the project precipitated changes at the Liverpool Workhouse Infirmary, an appalling facility that ostensibly cared for paupers. School superintendent Mary Agnes Jones, a graduate of Kaiserswerth and the Nightingale School, began work on May 16, 1865, with a staff of twelve nurses, eighteen probationers, and fifty-four aides. Within two years, the women had revolutionized the workhouse system as the Brownlow Infirmary. The first casualty of the hard job was Jones herself, who died in 1887 of typhoid and fatigue.

Following the success of Liverpool's Brownlow Infirmary, London established its East London Nursing Society in 1868 to treat the poor. A subsequent community project, the Nursing Branch of the Biblewomen's Mission, opened a benevolent house of humble women dedicated to helping slum families but limited in nurse care training. The latter group, called Ranyard Nurses after their organizer, grew rapidly from five thousand volunteers in 1870 to 27,690 the following year. In 1874, Florence L. Lees-Craven, a Nightingale nurse trained at Kaiserswerth, Dresden, and Berlin, offered an alternative to the amateur Ranyard nurses by setting up a staff of trained district nurses. Instead of using one hundred visiting nurses to serve 3.5 million people in London, Lees-Craven proposed staffing 115 districts with gentlewomen, whom she trusted more than nurses of the lower classes. A subscription brought in £20,000 to underwrite the program. Nurses wore distinctive brown Holland dresses trimmed in blue linen bands and topped with an apron, a bonnet, oversleeves, and an alpaca cloak. These demure, intelligent health care volunteers set an example of propriety and order later lauded by Florence Nightingale as the height of professionalism.

In the fiftieth year of her reign, Queen Victoria, a proponent of regional health programs, set aside £70,000 from the Women's Jubilee Fund to found the Institute for the Training and Supervising of District Nurses. In 1889, she chartered the Queen Victoria Jubilee Institute for Nurses, a nonsectarian women's organization that preceded the establishment of district nursing homes throughout the British Isles. For those districts lacking funds to support a Queen's nurse, county associations trained village nurses and midwives, who had to meet the standards of Amy Hughes, the institute's superintendent-general. By 1922, the number of such rural practitioners reached 5,478.

Coinciding with the creation of public nursing networks in England, American hospitals initiated community programs, starting in 1877 with the New York City Mission. Nurse Frances Root, a graduate of the training program at Bellevue Hospital, became New York's first official visiting nurse. The following year, Dr. Felix Adler launched the New York Society for Ethical Culture, a nonsectarian system of nurse care for the poor. Employing nurse Effie Benedict, also a Bellevue graduate, he arranged for care of DeMilt Dispensary patients after they returned home. Directed by attending physicians, Benedict's staff followed posthospitalization orders in treating family members and instructing parents in cleanliness and child care.

As England's example intensified efforts in the United States, Boston profited from the altruism of Abbie Crowell Howes and Phoebe G. Adam, both members of the Women's Education Association, who instituted their own society of district nurse-educators. Allying with a local dispensary, the group, later named the Instructive District Nursing Association, hired Amelia Hodgkiss on February 8, 1886. In the first year, she and two others served the heart of the city, treating illness and demonstrating hygiene and health care. An at-large nurse joined the trio to treat patients in outlying districts. Among immigrants who were suspicious of their "help" and spoke substandard or limited English, Boston's visiting nurses won over their clients on a woman-to-woman basis. Together, they made 7,182 calls and visited 707 cases; the second year, their case load rose to 1,836 for an astounding 17,066 visits.

In the same year that Howes and Adam set up their service in Boston, Elizabeth Pratt Jenks established a visiting nurse project in Philadelphia. Inspired by a description of visiting nurses in Manchester, England, Jenks corralled several generous, public-spirited women to fund the experiment for a month. Beginning March 1, nurse Sarah G. Haydock solicited patients willing to receive a visiting nurse, an unheard-of service in the city. By 1887, the Visiting Nurse Society of Philadelphia stood on firmer ground and offered treatment at a minimal fee ranging from 50 cents to $1, depending on the time allotted per patient. The group adopted a uniform consisting of seersucker tunic, white apron, collar and cuffs, cape, and bonnet or straw hat. In 1891, Linda Richards, the United States' first trained nurse, headed the project, which treated the poor along with paying clients.

Chicago philanthropists were also inspired by English and American successes and formed their own visiting nurse association, suggested by William N. Salter, a lecturer at the Chicago Ethical Society. One of the city's most welcome practitioners, Czech immigrant Anne Prochazka, a specialist in orthopedic nursing, spoke to her elderly clients in their own language and sometimes rescued abandoned infants and the homeless from the streets. Employing nurse Mary Margaret Etter, who served the fledgling project until her death three years later, the group disbanded and reformed as the Augusta Memorial Visiting Nurses, founded by Clarissa Shumway and staffed by nurse Eleanor M. Brown and assistant nurse L. M. Seymour. A consortium of thirty physicians took over the task after Shumway resigned and nurtured it into an official municipal department, the Visiting Nurse Association of Chicago. Before century's end, similar projects sprang up in Buffalo, Kansas City, Detroit, Baltimore, Providence, and Cleveland.

The focus of visiting nurses broadened to feature specialty care for cancer patients, tuberculosis treatment and prevention, well-baby clinics, and school and industrial nursing. Among turn-of-the-century specialists were Ada Mayo Stewart, Ellen Morris Wood, Lydia Holman, Anna B. Duncan, and Dr. Sara Josephine Baker. Stewart, a graduate of Waltham Training School, worked for the Vermont Marble Company in 1895 as a company visiting nurse. Employed by company president Fletcher D. Proctor to improve employee welfare, she visited workers' families in West Rutland and Rutland Center, cared for surgical patients and mothers-to-be at no charge, and referred those with serious medical problems to a doctor. The following year, Wood instituted a rural visiting nurse program at Mt. Kisco in Westchester County, New York. In 1900, Holman established a similar project in Ledger, North Carolina, working alone for eleven years. On the staff of a mercantile company, Duncan served the John Wannamaker department store as the first company nurse in 1897.

In New York tenements and eventually to the industrialized world, Baker proved the worth of municipal visiting nurse care. She and her thirty-member team treated sick babies door-to-door in 1902 and designed baby sacks that opened down the front to prevent suffocation. To address the problem of young girls left in charge of siblings, she inaugurated Little Mothers' Leagues. Her knowledge of breast-feeding, nutrition, disease prevention, and prenatal care dropped the annual infant morality rate by twelve hundred. From 1908 to 1923, she lowered the infant death rate from 144 to sixty-six per thousand. As assistant to the commissioner of health, in 1907, she joined the successful search for "Typhoid Mary" Mallon.

A lecturer at New York University Bellevue Hospital Medical School on child hygiene for fourteen years, Baker became the first woman to receive a Ph.D. in public health. She was president of the American Child Health Association; consultant to the federal Children's

Bureau; and author of *Healthy Babies, Healthy Children* (1920), *Healthy Mothers* (1920), *The Growing Child* (1923), and *Child Hygiene* (1925). In her memoir, *Fighting for Life* (1939), she captured the essence of her profession with her comment, "Sick people need immediate help, understanding and humanity almost as much as they need highly standardized and efficient practice" (Maggio 1996, 487). In honor of Baker's devotion to humanistic public health, she became the first woman appointed to the League of Nations and served on its health committee from 1922 to 1924.

The Depression placed new demands on visiting nurses as the rate of illness among the unemployed rose 48 percent. Usually assigned to preventive and educational projects, they assumed curative roles and bedside care in desperate situations, most notably through the work of Mary Breckinridge and her frontier nurse cadre in the Kentucky hill country. Both on duty and on call, they staffed emergency hospital sections and mobilized clinics and first aid to stricken populations. The total reduction in lost lives, health, and money provided a return on municipal investments of 1,000 percent. In commendation of public health nursing, President Herbert Hoover remarked: "One good community nurse will save a dozen future policemen" ("Naomi Deutsch" 1934, 486).

A viable model from the post–World War II era was the Red Hook Experiment, a four-year program begun in 1947. According to Doris R. Schwartz, veteran of hospital ship nursing in the Pacific theater, a valuable experiment in primary nurse practice occurred at the union of New York City's Department of Health with Brooklyn's Visiting Nurse Association. The resultant mission treated the inner-city poor, an outreach she later termed "people caring for people" (Schorr and Zimmerman 1988, 320). Among the underclass, she enjoyed a rich experience that other cities adopted to improve community welfare. Supported by Cornell University's home care program, she duplicated aspects of the project on the Navajo reservation in Arizona. From her team's study of families from disparate cultures, she deduced that "respect for the personhood of patient and family makes it possible to establish and continue a relationship that permits the nurse to give effective care while continuing to search for the cause of behavior. That respect for personhood we believe to be among the patient's and the family's rights" (Schorr and Zimmerman 1988, 317).

Schwartz's admiration for the nurse-practitioner derived from her experience among Scottish geriatric patients. To provide better care to them, she applied her principles to a day hospital for rehabilitation and maintenance of the aged. In 1979, she published "Fruit, on the Tree of an Early Ambition," a poem expressing her delight in cooperative efforts. With a humanitarian glow, she concluded that through nursing, "Happiness adds and multiplies as we divide it with others" (Schorr and Zimmerman 1988, 320).

In Canada, where cholera had decimated populations in 1834, public health nursing offered a solution to municipal and back-country problems. The Public Health Act provided for the supervision of ailing citizens and looked toward control of infectious and pestilential diseases. Subsequent regulations enacted in 1835, 1839, and 1849 attempted to stanch waves of smallpox, diphtheria, scarlet fever, typhoid, and typhus, which the refugees from Ireland's potato famine brought from home. At the height of immigration and settlement, patients in isolated areas bore the brunt of a nursing shortage. A viable service, the Victorian Order of Nurses (VON), began meeting the needs of a far-flung nation in 1898.

At the urging of the National Council of Women, Lady Ishbel Marjoribanks, Lady Aberdeen, an admirer of Florence Nightingale, promoted the visiting nurse model to alleviate suffering and elevate standards of public welfare. Against the backlash of physicians and taxpayers, Aberdeen joined forces with Charlotte MacLeod, superintendent of the Waltham

Training School for Nurses, and Dr. Alfred Worcester, Waltham's founder, to woo hostile medical men. By December, Canada had its network of nurses, whom Queen Victoria honored with the royal badge already in use throughout England, Scotland, and Ireland. Beginning with sixteen nurses, the program grew to a staff of six hundred by its sixtieth anniversary and profited from the patronage of Queen Mother Elizabeth as the order's president. The service, which targeted families, the elderly, and victims of catastrophic illness, ran on endowments, donations, and patient fees, which were deposited in a community chest.

Canadian health officials also supported specialty nursing as a means of controlling contagion and epidemics. A pioneer of public health nursing, Eunice Henrietta Dyke, a native of Lockport, New York, and superintendent of the Toronto Health Department, began her career as a tuberculosis nurse in 1911. Teaming with associate Janet Neilson, a dispensary nurse, Dyke located eight hundred consumptives for treatment at St. Michael's Hospital. Upon verifying the diagnosis, the team removed the patient to a ward, fumigated the home, and initiated treatment. Her jurisdiction expanded to include public schools, mental health, and control of the 1918 epidemic of Spanish influenza. By 1921, her work earned Toronto a good health rating. In 1923, she was invited to address the Red Cross League of France. Her subsequent contributions to the department include child health centers and family health crisis management.

Among Native Americans, Canada's public health nurse Amy V. Wilson surveyed families around the Peace River and Lesser Slave Lake. During the building of the Alcan Highway through the Yukon, she opened a clinic at Whitehorse, treating victims of the 1949 diphtheria epidemic as well as cases of scabies and attending at births. In her memoir, *A Nurse in the Yukon* (1965, 17), she documented the abysmal conditions in far-flung Indian camps that made up her territory: "By daylight the sick people looked even more ghastly than they had at night. Their meager supply of thin, ragged blankets shocked me almost as much as did their cotton summer clothing, so inadequate against the freezing temperatures."

Tending the medical needs of the three thousand natives in the Yukon and northern British Columbia, she traveled by car, plane, boat, and dogsled and lived in tents and shacks to save people from the "choking sickness." By the end of her tenure, she had earned respect from the government and patients. At her death from cardiac illness in October 1965, in Olds, Alberta, she was honored with a posthumous medal. She left behind a district nurse's prayer, which concludes, "Give me good judgment, Lord, I pray,/And let my hands be steady" (Wilson 1965, 209).

The World Health Organization used the visiting public health nurse model in developing countries. Like the nurse-midwives in English and American villages, the "Missi Ubat" (medicine miss) of Malaysia made similar visits to improve community welfare, especially for mothers, infants, and preschool children. In the late 1950s, field nurse Rosina Binte Karim traveled by Land Rover, boat, and bicycle and on foot to conduct prenatal sessions and child eye, ear, nose, and throat examinations. In areas where villagers were hostile or suspicious of health clinics, Karim appealed to motherly instincts and lured children with sweets and chocolates to combat such problems as yaws, an ulcerative bone disease similar to syphilis. A lasting contribution was the cooperation of local teachers, headmen, and husbands, whose influence established the worth of getting inoculations and using powdered milk to bottle-feed at-risk infants.

See also: Ancient Times; Christian Nursing; Deutsch, Naomi; Disease; Jones, Mary Agnes; Midwifery; Red Cross; Richards, Linda; Wald, Lillian D.

Sources

Brainard, Annie M. *The Evolution of Public Health Nursing.* Philadelphia: W. B. Saunders, 1922.

Clement, J., ed. *Noble Deeds of American Women with Biographical Sketches of Some of the More Prominent.* Williamstown, Mass.: Corner House, 1975.

Dolan, Josephine A., R.N. *History of Nursing.* Philadelphia: W. B. Saunders, 1968.

"Histoire brève de Marguerite d'Youville." http://www.sgm.qc.ca/FRmmy1.htm.

Jamieson, Elizabeth, and Mary F. Sewall. *Trends in Nursing History.* London: W. B. Saunders, 1949.

Kalisch, Philip, and Beatrice J. Kalisch. *The Advance of American Nursing.* Boston: Little, Brown, 1978.

Karim, Rosina Binte Haji Abdul. "Missi Ubat—the Malayan Medicine Miss." *Nursing Outlook* (April 1959): 224–225.

Kraut, Alan. *Silent Travelers: Germs, Genes, and the "Immigrant Menace."* New York: Basic Books, 1994.

Livingston, M. Christine. "The Victorian Order of Nurses for Canada." *Nursing Outlook* (January 1958): 42–44.

Maggio, Rosalie, ed. *The New Beacon Book of Quotations by Women.* Boston: Beacon Press, 1996.

McHenry, Robert, ed. *Liberty's Women.* Springfield, Mass.: G. C. Merriam, 1980.

McKown, Robin. *Heroic Nurses.* New York: G. P. Putnam's Sons, 1966.

"Naomi Deutsch." *Pacific Coast Journal of Nursing* (September 1934): 487–488.

Royce, Marion. *Eunice Dyke, Health Care Pioneer.* Toronto: Dundurn Press, 1983.

Schorr, Thelma M., R.N., and Anne Zimmerman, R.N., eds. *Making Choices, Taking Chances: Nurse Leaders Tell Their Stories.* St. Louis: C. V. Mosby, 1988.

Sherr, Lynn, and Jurate Kazickas. *Susan B. Anthony Slept Here: A Guide to American Women's Landmarks.* New York: Times Books, 1994.

Stuber, Irene. "Women of Achievement and Herstory Calendar." http://www.city-net.com/~lmann/women/history/cal4.html.

Webster's Dictionary of American Women. New York: Merriam-Webster, 1996.

Who's Who in America, 1978–1979. New Providence, N.J.: Marquis Who's Who, 1979.

Wilson, Amy V., R.N. *A Nurse in the Yukon.* New York: Dodd, Mead, 1965.

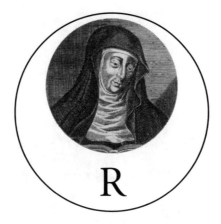

R

Red Cross

The Red Cross insignia is a global emblem of humane care. The famous red-on-white banner, designed by battlefield nurse and ambulance driver St. Camillus de Lellis, came to symbolize the work of Jean-Henri Dunant, a Genevan philanthropist, who established a temporary field hospital during the Battle of Solferino, Italy, in June 1859. Setting up in a church, he treated thousands of wounded from both sides of the conflict. In 1862, he published *A Memory of Solferino,* describing some of the forty thousand casualties he treated, and projected a network of neutral volunteer societies worldwide to care for fallen warriors. At an international conference held in October 1864, he launched the International Committee of the Red Cross (ICRC), which spread within the year to twelve nations and ultimately to 165. Expansions on the original philosophy of goodwill and kindness to the sick and wounded sought to remove unnecessary brutality from warfare. A series of Geneva Conventions led to coverage of victims on land in 1864, sailors at sea in 1906, prisoners of war in 1929, and civilians in 1949.

The idea of international crisis intervention prospered from royal support. Underwritten by Marie Louise Augusta, Queen of Prussia and Empress of Germany, an admirer who also cut and rolled bandages, the Women's Patriotic Society quickly brought Dunant's idea to national acceptance. To maximize preparedness, the society trained nurses and erected barrack hospitals reserved for emergency and combat casualties. Certain units of the society created *mutterhausen* (mother houses), patterned after the Kaiserswerth Institution. Living like denizens of a convent, nurse-trainees elevated their skills in trauma care and, by their example of competence, drew other young females into their order.

The Japanese contingent modeled its *Hakuiaisha,* the Japanese Red Cross Society, on the Austrian Patriotic Society. Dispatched by Count Tsunetami Sano, the Japanese Minister to Austria, founders toured aid society demonstrations at the Vienna World Exposition in 1873. The agency took shape in 1877 during a civil war, the Satsuma Rebellion, when nurses cared for the fallen of both armies. By 1890, *Hakuiaisha* was issuing a monthly journal. Baron Ishiguro Tadunori, Japan's surgeon general, dispatched a magic lantern show to explain the Red Cross concept in outlying villages. Preparedness proved beneficial in the 1894 Sino-Japanese War, when Lieutenant-Colonel Shimidzu led the

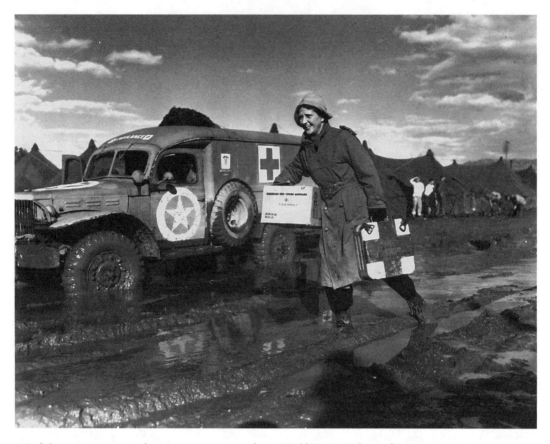

A Red Cross nurse carries supplies at a temporary camp during World War II. (Library of Congress)

Japanese Red Cross in training uniformed physicians, nurses, pharmacists, and corpsmen to aid the military in war zones. A year after skirmishes with Korea in 1894, Nagao Ariga returned to European aid societies to study emergency preparedness and to set regulations to facilitate the war ministry. During the Boxer Rebellion of 1900, Japanese nurses treated Admiral Zenovy Petrovich Rojestvensky, head of the Russian fleet, and aided the wounded of both sides after the fall of Port Arthur outside Shantung, China. By comparison to the Japanese Red Cross, czarist medical aid was less dedicated to preventing disease than the Japanese agency, which excelled at balance and sanitation control.

When peace was restored, the Japanese Red Cross became a national institution. Princess Komatsu broke tradition for noblewomen by heading the Red Cross Ladies' Volunteer Nursing Association and setting the example for conduct of nursing staff. As described in *Under the Care of the Japanese War Office* (1905) by nurse Ethel McCaul, a Royal Red Cross decoration recipient, the Japanese agency thrived on the national concept of cooperation and submission to authority, two virtues pervasive in Japanese society. When the American agency sent food during a severe famine, Baron Ozawa, vice president of the Japanese Red Cross, went to the huts of the poor to name the source of their food parcels. The Empress Haru-Ko supported other peacetime efforts with an endowment of $50,000.

Later in Red Cross history, the concept of an impartial humanitarian task force won support among Americans. The United States chartered the league in 1882 at the urging of Charles Bowles, a U.S. representative to the

1864 Geneva Convention, and of Clara Barton, founder of the American Red Cross. An editorial from the Chicago *Inter-Ocean* dated March 31, 1884, summarized the agency's humanitarian goals in compelling language: "The supplying of material wants—of food, raiment, and shelter—is only a small part of its ministry in its work among suffering humanity. When fire or flood or pestilence has caused widespread desolation, the Red Cross seeks to carry to people's hearts that message which speaks of a universal brotherhood" (Ross 1956, 281).

Bowles's vision of crisis intervention derived from the experiences of the United States Sanitary Commission, the flawed, often chaotic Union army medical department that attempted to supply staff and hospital equipment during the Civil War. As a model of disorganization, the Civil War medical service pointed up the necessity for a bureau dedicated to wartime and disaster relief. Bowles divided assignments strictly by gender: medical men were to inventory surgical instruments, arrange transportation for the wounded, and answer "all of the specialized questions that are beyond the competence of women" (Hutchinson 1996, 81). Female volunteers were to manage "women's work," which Bowles particularized as stocking linens, locating wartime nursing staff, and soliciting money and books.

Barton headed the American Red Cross until 1904, when she was replaced by Mabel Boardman, who led the organization to national renown. During Boardman's tenure, after cyclones struck in Hattiesburg, Mississippi, and Omaha, Nebraska, scattered Red Cross volunteers were on the scene. In *Under the Red Cross Flag at Home and Abroad* (1915, 133), an overview of agency organization and mission up to World War I, she captured the essence of the agency's disaster relief: "They not only nursed the sick, but they proved of incalculable value to the health authorities in the prevention of epidemics by their inspection and their instructions to the people. Promptly in the field, they donned rubber boots, waded through mud and climbed over debris to reach those who needed their aid. At night they slept on mattresses on the floor or spent watchful waiting hours at remote stations to be ready for a sudden call." She stressed that much of the time, Red Cross nurses received no pay, except when they were called for active duty, when their subsistence equaled that of the Army Nurse Corps.

Boardman cited the observations of Red Cross nursing supervisor Mary E. Gladwin, who dispatched teams to the Dayton, Ohio, floods and to battlefields in Belgrade, Yugoslavia. Gladwin extolled the perseverance of weary volunteers who doled out packages of food and clothing to lines of people waiting in the rain. At a school, agency activities turned classrooms into "dormitories, dining room, kitchen, hospital, a recitation room transformed into an accident and first-aid room, drugs and dressings on the teacher's desk; a blue-gowned young woman with the Red Cross on her arm, bandaging cuts and bruises, caring for scores of small ailments and some grave ones" (Boardman 1915, 134). The melange of requests tugged at stout-hearted relief workers, who returned to staff headquarters too overtaxed to tend to their own needs. Gladwin concluded with a salute to a successful effort, "Disheartened, discouraged, depressed, out of sorts with the weather and the general discomfort? Not at all" (Boardman 1915, 134).

In 1909, Jane Arminda Delano, head of nurses at New York's Bellevue Hospital and superintendent of the Army Nurse Corps, organized the Red Cross nursing program, primarily to fight tuberculosis. In 1911, the second annual meeting of the Association for the Prevention of Child Mortality called for the American Red Cross to stem the high rural incidence of tuberculosis, hookworm, fever, and infant and maternal mortality. That same year, a presidential order defined the role of Red Cross workers in border skirmishes resulting from the Mexican Revolution. Reserve nurses were the only volunteers among fighting units stationed along the Rio Grande during border raids by Mexican rebel bandit Pancho Villa.

In rapid order, the organization began the Town and Country Nursing Service, a visiting nurse program in agrarian districts to treat illness and educate people about the necessity of sanitation and personal hygiene. Underwritten by Lillian Wald's funding campaign and superintended by Fannie Clement, the project targeted communities outside the range of municipal roving nurse programs. Within six years, the number of Red Cross public health nurses increased to ninety-seven. Simultaneous with the war on communicable disease was a parallel effort by Charles Lynch and Dr. Matthew Shield to address industrial accidents and other threats to worker health. A corps of traveling instructors carried first aid information across the country by rail and, armed with handbooks in several languages, communicated principles of workplace safety to immigrant laborers.

While President Woodrow Wilson refrained from involving American soldiers in World War I, near the end of 1914, the American Red Cross augmented Allied supplies and personnel with a medical unit dispatched aboard the USS *Red Cross,* carrying two former navy nurses, J. Beatrice Bowman and Katrina Hertzer. Bowman supervised Red Cross nurses at the Royal Navy Hospital outside Portsmouth, England, before moving to the American Women's War Hospital in South Devon. Nurse-anesthetist Faye Fulton reported staff departures on September 13, 1914, aboard a chartered liner in units of fifteen—three doctors and twelve nurses. The ship ferried teams to England, France, Germany, and Russia. Fulton's unit set up in the Pyrenees region between France and Spain to treat wounded from the front. Agency service ended October 1, 1915, because of a shortfall of funds.

The war effort was far from over, however. After Clara Dutton Noyes took charge, she deployed the American Red Cross nurse corps to more than fifty-four wartime hospitals and relief expeditions. Her administration earned her

the Patriotic Service Medal and the Florence Nightingale Medal as well as the French Medal of Honor. In September 1916, navy veteran Katrina Hertzer, liaison officer to the Navy Nurse Corps, began enrolling nurses at Red Cross national headquarters. By October 1917, when Americans filled the trenches of France, more than eight thousand volunteers, twenty-eight base hospitals, 1,250 nurses, and six hundred aides went into action. Among them was nurse Sue Sophia Dauser of the navy hospital in Los Angeles, who headed the nursing staff at a navy hospital handed over by the British Admiralty outside Edinburgh, Scotland. A former poorhouse, it was equipped to accommodate 750 patients, many suffering from Spanish influenza, the deadly conclusion to a disastrous war.

After World War I, Mary Sewall Gardner, author of *Public Health Nursing* (1916), went to Italy as part of the American Red Cross Commission for Tuberculosis. Under the supervision of Jane Delano, Gardner and a staff of fourteen nurses launched a campaign to control contagion through an international consortium on public health and welfare. In primitive medical surroundings, she demonstrated American methods of containing and eradicating tuberculosis by employing a system of rural public health nurses. The program, completed in 1919, earned Gardner a Bronze Decoration from the Genoa provincial authority. Returning to Europe in 1921, she visited Czechoslovakia, Poland, France, and the Balkans as part of a fact-finding mission. On completing the project in 1924, she advised New York's Henry Street Visiting Nurse Service and published a second edition of *Public Health Nursing,* a standard text, which was translated into Spanish, Chinese, Korean, and Japanese to spread its concepts to developing nations. In 1931, she received the Saunders Medal for Distinguished Service in the Cause of Nursing.

The domestic focus of the American Red Cross turned once more to rural care in 1918 with the creation of its Bureau of Public Health Nursing, directed by Mary S. Gardner and Elizabeth Fox. Interwar activities centered on family, tribal, and community welfare. By 1921, thirteen hundred public health nurses were treating tuberculosis, overseeing maternal and child needs, and monitoring chronic illness. Individual projects stood out, particularly first aid and water safety courses and Regina Kaplan's nurse's aide training school for high school girls in Memphis, Tennessee. Of the quality and value of these programs, humorist Will Rogers remarked, "We are so used to the things the Red Cross does that we sometimes just forget to praise them" ("A History," www.redcross.org, 5).

Another outreach of the post–World War I era, the Gray Ladies, mobilized service to institutionalized patients in May 1918 at Washington's Walter Reed Hospital. A volunteer band, they attended to housekeeping, letter writing, entertainment, and shopping. By the 1950s, expansion of services added visitation, crafts, visitors' guides, translation, interpretation, and mobile lending libraries. Today, individual Gray Lady patient contact involves such essential services as teaching aphasic patients to talk, read, and write and serving isolated children as substitute parents.

The challenge of assisting orphans, displaced persons, the homeless, and separated families influenced some of the Red Cross's top interwar priorities. To meet a variety of needs in war and peace, during the 1920s instructors trained volunteers in nursing and trauma response. The drought that created the Dust Bowl, displacement of farm families, and general economic depression of the 1930s created new demands as visiting nurses called on the seedy Hoovervilles where destitute families huddled around campfires in anticipation of the next job. In the late 1930s, the work of collecting, processing, storing, and distributing whole blood called for advanced nursing and administrative skills. In 1941, months before the American entry into World War II, the Red Cross opened its first blood center at New York's Presbyterian Hospital, managed by Dr. Charles Drew, creator of the transfusion process. The connection between rescue and the Red Cross in the American psyche preceded heavy dependence on the agency in the 1940s with war in Europe, Africa, and the Pacific. In addition to three million volunteers, some seventy thousand registered nurses assisted on battlefields and at rehabilitation and civilian reception centers aiding over seventy-five million people.

Today, whether tutoring lifesaving skills, teaching cardiopulmonary resuscitation (CPR), or conducting industrial safety courses, the 1.2 million volunteers of the American Red Cross join 145 national societies and ally with the Magen David Adom Society in Israel to combat suffering in world trouble spots. New needs of AIDS victims and bone and tissue transplant recipients led to more efficient and safe collection and storage of blood and the first centralized bone marrow registry. The focus of the Red Cross's service remains true to its original ideals of humanity, impartiality, neutrality, independence, voluntary service, unity, and universality. To honor the organization, the national headquarters in Washington, D.C., retains items belonging to Clara Barton and depicts Red Cross work in three Tiffany windows. In the garden, a statue celebrates the work of Jane Delano and her professional cadre; an exhibit in the Schuyler Hospital in Montour Falls, New York, contains her personal articles and a glass apple awarded posthumously. Another statue in Arlington National Cemetery depicts Delano, who died in 1919 while serving the Red Cross in France. The statue overlooks graves of nurses who served during World War I.

See also: Barton, Clara

Sources

Abrams, Lynn, and Elizabeth Harvey, eds. *Gender Relations in German History: Power, Agency and Experience from the Sixteenth to the Twentieth Century.* Durham, N.C.: Duke University Press, 1997.

Boardman, Mabel. *Under the Red Cross Flag at Home and Abroad.* London: J. B. Lippincott, 1915.

Brainard, Annie M. *The Evolution of Public Health Nursing.* Philadelphia: W. B. Saunders, 1922.

Griffin, Gerald Joseph, and H. Joann King Griffin. *Jensen's History and Trends of Professional Nursing.* Saint Louis, Mo.: C. V. Mosby, 1965.

"A History of Helping Others." http://www.red-cross.org/pa/lancaste/history.htm.

Hutchinson, John F. *Champions of Charity: War and the Rise of the Red Cross.* Boulder, Colo.: Westview Press, 1996.

Hyman, Paula, and Deborah Dash Moore. *Jewish Women in America.* New York: Routledge, Chapman and Hall, 1997.

Kalisch, Philip, and Beatrice J. Kalisch. *The Advance of American Nursing.* Boston: Little, Brown, 1978.

"Magen David Adom." http://www.mda.org.il/.

McHenry, Robert, ed. *Liberty's Women.* Springfield, Mass.: G. C. Merriam, 1980.

Nelson, Sophie C. "Mary Sewall Gardner." *Nursing Outlook* (January 1954): 37–39.

"Nursing Individuals." http://web.bu.edu/SPECCO/nursind.htm.

Ross, Ishbel. *Angel of the Battlefield.* New York: Harper and Brothers Publishers, 1956.

Sherr, Lynn, and Jurate Kazickas. *Susan B. Anthony Slept Here: A Guide to American Women's Landmarks.* New York: Times Books, 1994.

Sterne, Capt. Doris M. *In and Out of Harm's Way: A History of the Navy Nurse Corps.* Seattle, Wash.: Peanut Butter Publishing, 1996.

Van Devanter, Lynda, and Joan A. Furey, eds. *Visions of War, Dreams of Peace: Writings of Women in the Vietnam War.* New York: Time Warner, 1991.

Wilson, Janet. "Gray Ladies in the Hospital." *Nursing Outlook* (August 1953): 452–453.

Revolutionary War

The role of professional nursing among the thirteen colonies in the 1770s is notable by its absence. Succor of casualties was an essential to the colonial military. During officer training, the development of field care and military strategies became a priority lauded by Baron Friedrich von Steuben, inspector-general and author of *Regulations for the Order and Discipline of the Troops of the United States* (1778–1779). A veteran of the Battle of Yorktown, in 1780, he spoke from experience when he wrote: "There is nothing which gains an officer the love of his soldiers more than his care of them, under the distress of sickness; it is then he has the power of exerting his humanity, and in providing them every comfortable necessity, and making their situation as agreeable as possible" (Wilbur 1997, 47).

After the Battle of Bunker Hill, the Continental Congress created a medical corps called the Hospital for the Army, established on July 27, 1775. The corps drew on the thirty-five hundred colonial medical practitioners, of whom only two hundred were physicians holding medical degrees. The state of medical practice was so riddled with quackery that in 1758, a New York historian bemoaned the small number of qualified health professionals and complained, "Quacks abound like locusts in Egypt" (*Lamps* 1942, 16). Poorly paid, federal doctors were issued no instruments and reported the absence of "jallap [a dried root of the morning glory family used as a purgative], rhubarb, salts, or ipecac" (Cowan 1975, 10). The only way a medical bag could be readied for the battlefield was through the doctor's donation of supplies and equipment.

General George Washington, commander in chief of the Continental army, was a proponent of health care. He deduced that for every death from battlefield wounds, he lost nine soldiers to disease. His staff encountered rampant scurvy and contagion from dysentery, typhus, typhoid, and camp fever. Men on leave returned with viral and bacterial infections contracted at home, including sexually transmitted diseases. As reported at the principal hospital in Bethlehem, Pennsylvania, in 1777, regimental strength teetered precariously from high mortality rates. The main cause of mortal illnesses was a smallpox epidemic exacerbated by appalling sanitation.

At the outbreak of war, military officials posted notices giving few particulars, as found in this Virginia circular: "WANTED for the continental Hospital in Williamsburg, some NURSES to attend the sick. Any such coming well recommended, will have good encouragement by applying to the Director of the hospital" (Spruill 1972, 271). Interviewers hired civilian nurses to staff military hospitals and field dressing stations. Some were relatives who remained with a patient and assisted regular staff surgeons and aides on their rounds. Major William Heth made brief entry of an undisclosed number of female nurses dispatched to each regiment to serve the hospital at the confluence of the Mendham and Black Rivers in New York. On June 14, 1775, Major General Horatio Gates petitioned Washington for female nurses to stem the suffering of soldiers. Upon Washington's request that Congress substantiate a call for matrons and nurses throughout the colonies, on July 27, a budget item supplied the Continental Army with a medical department, which allotted one nurse per ten patients and one matron per one hundred patients. In 1776, the Maryland Council of Safety received notice from nurse Alice Redman that she worked day and night, was allowed no tea or coffee, and earned only $2 a month, from which she had to buy soap and brooms for staff use. By April 7, 1777, the monthly pay for an army nurse reached $8 plus daily rations. Nursing supervisors earned $15 a month. From this tentative beginning, the supervision of the army medical department remained decentralized until the War of 1812.

At Valley Forge, General Washington, fearful of greater loss, ordered his four thousand troops to undergo variolation, an early term for inoculation with live virus. The measure was successful—only one in one thousand died of the serum transfer. In another effort to improve quality care, on June 17, 1777, he recruited female nurses for the hospital in Mendham, New York, an unusual request in the era preceding Florence Nightingale's work in the Crimea. In December, William Livingston, governor of New Jersey and spokesman for the commander, expressed the urgency of health care needs and petitioned Congress for redress before Washington became "a general without an army" (Cowan 1975, 26).

At the end of the colonial era, there were only a few community hospitals, in Bethlehem, Reading, Manheim, Lancaster, and Bristol, Pennsylvania. Hospital care was low on the list of priorities for the sick and wounded, who dreaded mortal contagion in facilities famed for failure. For every two men who died in battle, twenty-five died in hospitals.

One innovator, Dr. James Tilton, designed a log clinic building in Morristown on the model of the American Indian tepee. He placed a fire in the center and sloped the floor outward to the wards to control contamination from runoff. By limiting overcrowding and putrefaction, his creative floor plan limited the spread of disease.

At most facilities, the absence of nurses and deplorable standards of cleanliness in cramped, foul-smelling tents diminished the chances for recovery. Wisely, soldiers shunned care at field hospitals. According to Dr. Benjamin Rush, physician-general of the Continental Army and author of *Medical Inquiries and Observations* (1793), "Hospitals are the sink of human life in an army. They robbed the United States of more citizens than the sword" (Wilbur 1997, 44). Ideally, field hospitals offered a diet of milk, vegetables, barley broth, hardtack, meat, rice, butter, coffee, tea, and wine, but shortages reduced most meals to gruel. There were no antiseptic dressings and no internal surgeries. The only painkillers consisted of opium, wine, and rum. To accommodate the growing casualty list, the medical corps commandeered four private homes in Cambridge, Massachusetts, and three in nearby Roxbury. After the British invaded New York, regimental aides evacuated critical cases to Albany, New York, to a two-story facility comprising forty wards. Farther south, casualties were treated at temporary facilities in the Governor's Palace at Williamsburg, Virginia.

In the face of wartime crisis, nursing became a cottage industry carried out by amateurs. Recent amputees and victims of gunshot wounds and contagious disease were bedded on straw and transported on wagons, sledges, wheelbarrows, handcarts, travois or drags, and litters made from blankets thrown over tree limbs. They took refuge in adjacent buildings and residences to be cared for by housewives, indentured servants, and slaves. Those close to Pennsylvania's religious houses received professional care from nuns and monks at the Uwchlan Meeting House in Lionville, the Single Brethren House Hospital and the five-story Single Brethren House Hospital in Bethlehem, and the Brothers House Hospital of Ephrata, which officials burned in 1778 to rid it of typhus after an influx of army wounded.

For areas without medical facilities or personnel, traditional healing came from nurse-midwives like Margaret Vliet Warne of Washington, New Jersey. A skilled herbalist and practitioner, she remained in practice until her death in 1840. For combat casualties, local women and untrained regimental mates offered limited first aid, as demonstrated by Martha Washington, Lucy Knox, and other wives of officers, who accompanied regiments and tended the sick. Anna Elliott of Charleston, South Carolina, a nonpartisan nurse, comforted unfortunates in prisons and at bedsides, and Kerenhappuch Turner of Greensboro, North Carolina, was honored at Guildford Courthouse National Military Park for her volunteer nursing of patriots. More is known about Esther Gaston Walker, a volunteer nurse at the Battle of Rocky Mount, North Carolina, on July 30, 1770, and the next week at the Battle of Hanging Rock, where she converted a church at Waxhaw into a makeshift hospital.

Individuals cited for tending casualties continued the tradition of Elizabeth Black and Eleanor Felton, who earned £2 per month for bedside care, and of Mrs. Browne, a nurse attached to General Edward Braddock's expeditionary force at Fort Cumberland during the French and Indian Wars. In February 1776, Mrs. Slocumb of Wayne County, North Carolina, volunteered to treat the wounded at the Battle of Moore's Creek. Having no medical kit, she reported: "I looked about and could see nothing that looked as if it would do for dressing wounds but some heart-leaves. I gathered a handful and bound them tight to the holes; and the bleeding stopped. I then went to the others; and—Doctor! I dressed the wounds of many a brave fellow who did good fighting long after that day!" (Clement 1975, 327). On June 14, 1777, Margaret Morris, a Quaker from Burlington, New Jersey, made a journal entry of her treatment of fever suffered by barge operators and their families, who were temporarily lodged at the governor's house. Another impromptu heroine, Mary Ledyard, ministered to thirty-five casualties after the fall of Fort Griswold to Benedict Arnold's band on September 6, 1781, near Groton, Connecticut.

Two names prominent in the revolutionary effort are Margaret Corbin, who operated a gun at the Defense of Fort Washington in 1776, and Mary Ludwig Hays McCauly, dubbed "Molly Pitcher" and "Sergeant Molly," during the Battle of Monmouth on June 28, 1778. A legend in women's history, McCauly earned her more famous sobriquet for carrying a water pitcher to the wounded and exhausted soldiers and for being the only female to receive a military pension. In battle, she rescued a Continental casualty, whom she transported on her back to a safe place, and was performing volunteer aid when her husband, William Hays, fell to the enemy. After her capture, she obtained release from the British and sought treatment for battle wounds at West Point, Maryland, where she was originally buried. At a subsequent grave in Carlisle, Pennsylvania, a flag and cannon commemorate her heroic loading and firing of her husband's cannon. A statue stands at the battle site.

Sources

Blanco, Richard L. *Physician of the American Revolution, Jonathan Potts.* New York: Garland, 1979.

Clement, J., ed. *Noble Deeds of American Women with Biographical Sketches of Some of the More Prominent.* Williamstown, Mass.: Corner House, 1975.

Cowan, David L. *Medicine in Revolutionary New Jersey.* Trenton: New Jersey Historical Commission, 1975.

Dolan, Josephine A., R.N. *History of Nursing.* Philadelphia: W. B. Saunders, 1968.

Fessler, Diane Burke. *No Time for Fear: Voices of American Military Nurses in World War II.* East Lansing: Michigan State University Press, 1996.

"Highlights of the Army Nurse Corps." http://www.army.mil/cmh-pg//anc/Highlights.html.

Lamps on the Prairie: A History of Nursing in Kansas. Emporia: Kansas State Nurses' Association, 1942.

Meier, Louis A. *Healing of an Army, 1777–1778.* Norristown, Pa.: Historical Society of Montgomery County, 1991.

Sherr, Lynn, and Jurate Kazickas. *Susan B. Anthony Slept Here: A Guide to American Women's Landmarks.* New York: Times Books, 1994.

Spruill, Julia. *Women's Life and Work in the Southern Colonies.* New York: W. W. Norton, 1972.

Thatcher, Virginia. *History of Anesthesia, with Emphasis on the Nurse Specialist.* New York: Garland, 1984.

Weatherford, Doris. *American Women's History.* New York: Prentice Hall, 1994.

Wilbur, C. Keith, M.D. *Revolutionary Medicine, 1700–1800.* Old Saybrook, Conn.: Globe Pequot Press, 1997.

Richards, Linda

Revered as the United States' first trained nurse, Linda Richards blended professionalism with religious zeal and a talent for medical administration. Born on a farm near West Potsdam, New York, on July 27, 1841, Melinda Ann Judson Richards, the daughter of Betsy Sinclair and Sanford Richards, a traveling preacher, was named for a missionary, Ann Judson Hasseltine. Resettled in Newbury, Vermont, after a brief sojourn in Wisconsin, the family lived with the Sinclairs after Reverend Richards's death from consumption in 1845. She attended her mother through the disease until her death in 1854. With the assistance of Doc Currier, Richards continued studying medicine informally and entered St. Johnsbury Academy in 1856 for teacher preparation. After three years of classroom work, she was engaged to George Poole in 1860 and worked for the Union Straw Works in Foxboro, Massachusetts. She cared for Poole's wounds for four years after his return from the Civil War until his death in 1869.

Richards moved to Boston in 1870 and, as an unskilled nurse, labored on the staff of Boston City Hospital. The low level of ward nursing compelled her to seek specialized training under Dr. Susan Dimock at the New England Hospital for Women and Children, which issued her the nation's first diploma. While serving New York's Bellevue Hospital as night supervisor, she came under the influence of Sister Helen, a Nightingale nurse, and evolved the first written charting and record-keeping system for nurses. In 1874, Richards headed the Boston Training School, improving its curriculum into a model nursing program. After intensive study at the St. Thomas Hospital in London, she took Florence Nightingale's suggestion and studied at King's College Hospital and the Edinburgh Royal Infirmary.

Upon her return to Boston in 1878, Richards opened a nursing school at Boston College Hospital. As a volunteer to the American Board of Commissioners for Foreign Missions, in 1886, she initiated Japan's first nurse-training program at Doshisha Hospital in Kyoto, Japan, where she remained until poor health forced her return to the United States five years later. After setting up standardized programs in Philadelphia, in 1891 she headed the Visiting Nurse Society of Philadelphia, one of the era's earliest public health projects, which treated the poor along with paying clients.

During Richards's career, she served as superintendent at the Methodist Episcopal Hospital in Philadelphia, New England Hospital for Women and Children, Brooklyn Homeopathic Hospital, Hartford Hospital, University of Pennsylvania Hospital, and Taunton Insane Hospital and Worcester Hospital for the Insane in Massachusetts. Retired from the Michigan Insane Asylum in Kalamazoo, she published a memoir, *Reminiscences of Linda Richards* (1911) and remained active until she was incapacitated by a stroke in 1923. She convalesced at the New England Hospital for Women and Children until her death April 16, 1930. For contributions to the profession and to nursing education, she was inducted into the National Women's Hall of Fame.

Sources

Brainard, Annie M. *The Evolution of Public Health Nursing.* Philadelphia: W. B. Saunders, 1922.

"Linda Richards: America's First Trained Nurse." http://www.northnet.org/stlawrenceaauw/richards.htm.

Webster's Dictionary of American Women. New York: Merriam-Webster, 1996.

Rosado, Luisa

In 1768, Luisa Rosado, a respected practical nurse from Toledo, Spain, competed with male medical doctors with her gentle methods and concern for patient comfort and safety. She resided at the court of King Charles III and worked as a midwife for the Real Colegio de Niños Desamparados (Royal House for Abandoned Children), which sheltered orphans and treated poor and handicapped mothers. Licensed in Zamora in 1765, she completed examination by the Protomedicato, a royal board of regents, and was certified by the Médicos Titulares (Municipal Physicians). Presumably middle-aged and of good family, she was literate and possessed the sterling Christian character required of eighteenth-century practitioners. Her petitions to the king and Council of Castile clarify her ambition to serve women and children.

While working near the Hospital General, in 1770, Rosado began challenging the dominance of *cirujanos-comadrones* (male surgeon-midwives) and establishing her authority on matters of birth and mother and infant care. Omitting any claims to nurse training, she publicized empirical and anecdotal evidence of her practice through handbills, citing a poultice to prevent miscarriage and a painless method of extracting retained placentas as two of her services. The latter was a dire situation in 10 percent of life-threatening deliveries, often resulting in damage to the uterus or patient death. According to former patients, Rosado followed standard medical practice of gentle external massage and manipulation, which retrieved the placenta within six minutes.

A corroborative witness, Dr. Manuel García del Pozal, a Madrid physician at the *Hospital General,* testified that Rosado had intervened in the distress of a woman bearing triplets: "Seeing the patient so afflicted and in great danger of her life due to the repeated distress, sweating, swooning or fainting she was suffering, they called upon Luisa Rosado, who indeed came and helped her to give birth, and made her produce the infants with such skill, art and diligence, that all those who were present were amazed" (Marland 1993, 105). Based on this endorsement, Rosado proclaimed her competence in complicated deliveries, an area usually reserved for obstetrical surgeons.

In March 1770, medical authorities rejected Rosado's first petition for royal certification as unwise competition against professional surgeons. After the king refused her petition in December 1770, she returned with a personal appeal. In June 1771, she tendered a daring offer—to deliver his pregnant daughter-in-law, Princess María Luisa, wife of Crown Prince Charles, heir to the Spanish throne. Because of her obvious self-confidence Rosado obtained a license, but she continued to fight the obstinacy of the medical establishment, which denied her the privileges of bloodletting and purging without supervision of a doctor.

Sources

Marland, Hilary, ed. *The Art of Midwifery: Early Modern Midwives in Europe.* London: Routledge, 1993.

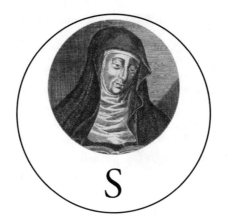

Sanger, Margaret

The United States' standard-bearer for female-controlled contraception, Margaret Sanger advanced the status of women as individuals worthy of sexual autonomy and popularized concepts that have altered family planning. To rescue women from marital misery, crippling, and early death, she championed preventive gynecology, counseling, and infertility services. She sought a discreet environment in which to disseminate reproductive health education and contraceptive devices and, on October 16, 1916, opened the nation's first birth control clinic in the Brownsville section of Brooklyn, New York. For distributing contraceptives among Jewish and Italian immigrant women, she received a jail term. Returning to the front lines of women's struggle for reproductive rights, she protected lower-class immigrant women from the tyranny of the press, Catholic Church, U.S. Postal Service, and Congress.

Born September 14, 1879, in Corning, New York, Margaret Louise Higgins Sanger was the sixth of the eleven children of homemaker Anne Purcell and sculptor Michael Hennessey Higgins. Reared on the importance of charity and selflessness, she witnessed her father's efforts to organize laborers. As the daughter of a controversial social reformer, she was accustomed to being singled out by stares and whispers. A feminist at heart, she embraced the issues of gender equality in her teens. After graduating from Claverick College and the Hudson River Institute, she moved into drama and nourished the ambition to act until she learned that she was too short for a career on the stage.

Sanger taught school for a year and then returned home to nurse her mother, who died from tuberculosis and the burden of bearing and rearing eleven children. After completing nurse's training at White Plains Hospital and a year's study at the Manhattan Eye and Ear Clinic, in 1900, she met and married William Sanger, an architect and political activist. She sidelined her nursing career to raise son Grant and daughter Peggy. Her first medical post after she returned to work in 1910 was as visiting nurse in Lillian Wald's program in the New York City slums, where Sanger observed mothers weakened by bearing too many children and dying from illegal abortions. She refrained from introducing them to contraception because of a legal ban against birth control education. At length, the death of one too many mothers provoked Sanger into answering the pleas of tenement women, who aged before their time from out-of-control childbearing.

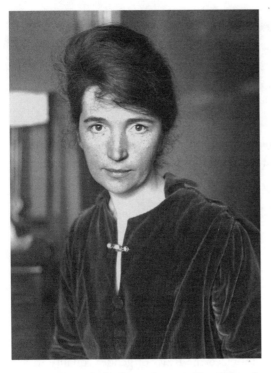

A 1916 photograph of Margaret Sanger in New York as she prepares to defend herself in court (Corbis/Bettmann)

For a year, Sanger researched reproductive history and studied the burgeoning world population and European family-planning methods. She evolved her own goals: to disseminate birth control to women with diseased partners, women endangered by pregnancy or threatened with defective offspring, newlyweds and child brides too young to bear children, and families who couldn't afford children or had several small children. During the pre–World War I unrest in New York in 1914, she began circulating reproductive information and promoted public awareness based on education, organization, and law. With private funds, she intended to offer inexpensive contraceptive devices to the poorest women and adolescent girls. In reference to their life-shortening dilemma, she declared, "I am the partisan of women who have nothing to laugh at" (Chesler 1992, 13).

Sanger battled a congressional bastion of Puritanism, the Comstock Act, which prohibited sending contraceptives and birth control information through the U.S. mail. To make the public aware of high mortality rates from abortion, she published birth control pamphlets and a monthly journal, *The Woman Rebel,* from her apartment. Its slogan rang out her adamant attitude: "No Gods, No Masters!" (Chesler 1992, 13). The editorial content stressed autonomy for women, whom she invited to submit their own articles and commentary. An opening sally launched her protracted war on the status quo, an empty column entitled "What Every Girl Should Know—Nothing; by Order of the U.S. Post Office" (Chesler 1992, 66).

By disturbing patriarchal authority, Sanger acquired sophisticated enemies, notably the Catholic hierarchy, male politicians, and women's suffrage proponents, who maintained that the right to vote superseded birth control in importance. She was dismayed that socialists, like feminists, ignored the plight of women yet campaigned to keep American men out of war. The U.S. Postal Service confiscated certain issues of her magazine, labeling it obscene. On the front cover of the subsequent issue, she wrote in capital letters: "THE WOMAN REBEL FEELS PROUD THAT THE POST OFFICE AUTHORITIES DID NOT APPROVE OF HER. SHE SHALL BLUSH WITH SHAME IF EVER SHE BE APPROVED BY OFFICIALISM OR 'COMSTOCKISM'" ("Margaret Sanger," www.gale.com, 2). Her riposte earned her nine counts of breaking a federal law, which could have resulted in five years each, for a total of forty-five years in prison.

After escaping to London, Sanger armed herself with the theories of Thomas Malthus and John Stuart Mill, both advocates of social enlightenment. Her defense of women found favor with English liberals, who petitioned President Woodrow Wilson on her behalf. While speaking at Fabian Hall in London in 1915, she met English birth control champion Dr. Marie Stopes, who shared ideas and drafted a moving statement on behalf of women: "Have you, Sir, visualized what it means to be a woman whose every fibre, whose every muscle and blood-capillary is subtly poisoned by the secret, ever-growing horror, more penetrating, more long drawn out than any nightmare, of an unwanted embryo developing beneath her heart? . . . What chains of slavery are, have been or ever could be so intimate a horror as the shackles on every limb, on every thought, on the very soul of an unwillingly pregnant woman?" (Rose 1993, 91). In addition to crafting emotional propaganda, Stopes located support for Sanger from novelists Arnold Bennett and H. G. Wells and classicist Gilbert Murray, all pleading with Wilson to pardon Sanger.

Pardoned in 1915, Sanger resumed her crusade in the United States. Her response to federal muzzling was threefold: to found the National Birth Control League, lecture on planned parenthood, and establish clinics to assist poor women in controlling the size of their families to reduce danger to their health. To challenge laws criminalizing contraception, she opened the United States' first birth control clinic on October 16, 1916, in a two-room tenement in the Brownsville section of Brooklyn, New York. With the aid of three staff members—Fania Mindell, a multilingual volunteer from Chicago, Elizabeth Stuyvesant, a social worker, and Sanger's sister, Ethel Higgins Byrne—Sanger opened the doors to hundreds of women lined up along the street and distributed *What Every Girl Should Know* (1916), a patient pamphlet available for a dime in Yiddish and Italian as well as English.

A byproduct of Sanger's crusading was the data she preserved on immigrant family life. Her staff examined clients and began a thorough record-keeping system noting economic status, reproductive health, and number of pregnancies, stillbirths, and miscarriages. The resulting statistics formed the basis for her conclusions about the sad state of women's health. After a plainclothes officer's report launched a police raid, the office closed. Without a means of communicating with poor women, Sanger ended her mission and halted the tabulation of family data. Of all the

indignities she suffered, Sanger was outraged that a female officer, Mrs. Whitehurst, initiated the arrest. Sanger and Byrne faced a judge, who demanded that they observe the law. The duo refused and accepted a thirty-day sentence in a workhouse. After only nine days, the clinic reopened in Sanger's apartment, this time funded by an English philanthropist and staffed by a female doctor.

Sanger was not content to focus on the status of women nationwide. She traveled to Asia to study overpopulation. In Japan, officials denied an entry visa because her native country challenged and spurned the pro-woman crusade. To redirect her advocacy, she peddled her books while lecturing across the United States. Begun in 1921, her *Birth Control Review* remained in publication for five years and garnered over a million letters from subscribers. Her second husband, sewing machine oil magnate J. Noah H. Slee, aided the cause by smuggling rubber-spring diaphragms from Germany for distribution at her clinic. The plight of women trapped in low-paying jobs, tied to large families, or maimed by botched abortions touched her heart. She compiled five hundred personal stories in a book, *Mothers in Bondage* (1928), which pleaded her cause to sympathetic readers. Ignoring the 1930 papal encyclical of Pope Pius XI declaring contraception an offense to God and nature, she lobbied Congress and the American Medical Association (AMA), organized worldwide conferences on family planning, and founded the Clinical Research Bureau of the American Birth Control League to offer safe, inexpensive, and effective sperm blockage. In 1935, she started the *Journal of Contraception* (now *Human Fertility*); by 1938, she had issued eleven books.

Sanger's victories came late in her life, after the death of daughter Peggy from tuberculosis. In 1931, Sanger received the American Women's Association award; five years later, she won a Town Hall award. In 1936, a Supreme Court decision overturning the Comstock Law preceded a reversal of the AMA position on contraceptive distribution to patients and the introduction of birth control to medical school curricula. When the American Birth Control Federation began in 1939, joint efforts with Sanger established a golden age of family planning. In 1942, the federation altered its name to the Planned Parenthood Federation. Widowhood and leukemia compromised Sanger's personal involvement in women's health issues at age 64. She retired to Tucson, Arizona, where she spoke candidly to journalist Lloyd Shearer about events fraught with conflict: "Fifty years ago, what opposition I had: the law, the police, the government, even my own father! He was the most broad-minded Irishman I ever knew—Michael Higgins was his name. But he kept saying, 'Margaret! Get out of it. Get out of it. The kind of nursing you're doing, the kind of project you're involved in— that's no life for a girl!'" (Chesler 1992, 462). At her death on September 6, 1966, her name remained linked with women's fulfillment and control over the forces that impoverished and diminished them.

Sources

Benderly, Jill. "Margaret Sanger." *On the Issues* (spring 1990).

Chesler, Ellen. *Woman of Valor: Margaret Sanger and the Birth Control Movement in America.* New York: Simon and Schuster, 1992.

Felder, Deborah G. *The 100 Most Influential Women of All Time: A Ranking Past and Present.* New York: Citadel Press, 1996.

Gay, Kathlyn, and Martin K. Gay. *Heroes of Conscience.* Santa Barbara, Calif.: ABC-CLIO, 1996.

Kalisch, Philip, and Beatrice J. Kalisch. *The Advance of American Nursing.* Boston: Little, Brown, 1978.

"Margaret Sanger." http://www.gale.com/gale/cwh/sangerm.html.

Reich, Warren Thomas, editor in chief. *Encyclopedia of Bioethics.* New York: Macmillan, 1995.

Rose, June. *Marie Stopes and the Sexual Revolution.* London: Faber and Faber, 1993.

Sherr, Lynn, and Jurate Kazickas. *Susan B. Anthony Slept Here: A Guide to American Women's Landmarks.* New York: Times Books, 1994.

Saunders, Dr. Cicely

An immensely influential figure in the hospice movement, Dame Cicely Saunders wrote *The Management of Terminal Disease* (1967). Both a nurse and doctor, she established St. Christopher's Hospice, a beacon to the terminally ill worldwide. In contrast to the apathy demonstrated by Christian institutions housing the dying, Saunders believed in fighting pain to empower dying people facing their final spiritual quest. Born in 1918 in Barnet, England, she came from upper-middle-class privilege. She attended Oxford University and completed nurse's training before World War II. Disabled by a back injury, she gave up the rigors of bedside nursing to pursue a career as an almoner.

While employed in social work in autumn 1947, Saunders studied the distress that terminal cancer caused one subject, David Tasma, an agnostic emigrant from a Warsaw ghetto. His will earmarked £500 for a memorial window in the hospice that she planned for similar dying patients. She volunteered at St. Luke's Hospice and observed the palliative methods of the sisters, who followed a timed sequence of analgesic dosage rather than on-demand pain management. After studying pharmacology and becoming a medical officer at St. Joseph's Hospice in Hackney, East London, she profited from an era of pharmaceutical progress that introduced tranquilizers, steroids, and antidepressants, all beneficial to the critically ill.

During the rise of the voluntary euthanasia movement, Saunders was influenced by Elisabeth Kübler-Ross's research, later published as *On Death and Dying* (1969). Saunders concluded that a multidisciplinary team of caregivers should respond to the wishes of individual patients with painkillers as well as spiritual affirmation, emotional therapy, preferred foods, massage, and positioning. She advocated the use of radiation therapy and surgery as pain control as well as treatment of disease.

In 1963, Saunders used a grant from Saint Thomas's Hospice in London to tour eighteen American facilities, where she introduced her concept of hospice care. Nurses, ministers, social workers, and support personnel converged to hear her lectures and witness photographic evidence that debilitation and disfigurement were not inevitable. She demonstrated that patients relieved of crushing pain found new hope and a better quality of life for their remaining days. As a result of her initiative, the Douglas Macmillan Fund began opening hospices, creating protocols of palliative treatment, and training caregivers to allay suffering and to reaffirm patient morale with assurances of comfort. Her model countered American technology that prolonged life at any cost with the European concept of death with dignity. Against the American standard of doctors dictating from the top, she encouraged a balanced input of multiple caregivers, including relatives and volunteers.

The result of Saunders's advocacy was the birth of the American hospice movement and more than one hundred facilities and 170 visiting nurse programs for in-home treatment throughout the United Kingdom. Her pragmatic prescription for cheer and hope called for a community of workers and inmates surrounded by pleasant music and art, library carts, videos and training manuals, group activities, comfortable wood and upholstered furnishing, and window views of flower beds and restful scenery. In addition, in 1967, she founded the first modern receiving home for the dying—St. Christopher's Hospice in Sydenham, England—and organized an international hospice network for children and adults.

See also: Hospice

Sources

Corr, C. A., and D. M. Corr. *Hospice Approaches to Pediatric Care.* Annapolis, Md.: Springer, 1985.

"The History of Hospice." http://www.cp-tel.net/pamnorth/history.htm.

"Interview with Florence Wald." http://www.npha.org/intjwald.html, April 22, 1998.

Kastenbaum, Robert. *Death, Society, and Human Experience.* New York: Charles E. Merrill, 1986.

———. *Encyclopedia of Death.* New York: Avon, 1989.

Kübler-Ross, Elisabeth. *On Death and Dying.* New York: Macmillan, 1969.

Levy, M. H. "Pain Control Research in the Terminally Ill." *Omega* (1987–1988): 265–280.

Mor, V. *Hospice Care Systems.* New York: Springer, 1987.

Mor, V., D. S. Gree, and Robert Kastenbaum. *The Hospice Experiment.* Baltimore: Johns Hopkins University Press, 1988.

Mother Frances Domina. "Reflections on Death in Childhood." *British Medical Journal,* no. 294, 108–110.

Saunders, Cicely. *The Management of Terminal Disease.* Hospital Medical Publications, 1967.

Sebba, Anne. *Mother Teresa: Beyond the Image.* New York: Doubleday, 1997.

Siebold, Cathy. *The Hospice Movement: Easing Death's Pains.* New York: Twayne, 1992.

Snodgrass, Mary Ellen. *Celebrating Women's History.* Detroit: Gale Research, 1996.

Twycross, R. G. *Pain Relief and Cancer.* Philadelphia: Saunders, 1984.

Zimmerman, J. *Hospice: Complete Care for the Terminally Ill.* Baltimore: Urban and Schwarzenberg, 1981.

Seacole, Mary Jane

Among the many British citizens to aid the Crimean War effort was Mary Jane Grant Seacole, the bold "doctress" of the Crimea. Born in 1805 of Scottish-Jamaican parentage, she learned Creole medicine and innkeeping from her mother, a mulatta hotelier. Widowed in 1836, Seacole built a boarding house in Kingston, Jamaica, and then traveled in Haiti, Cuba, and the towns of Nassau, Bahamas, and

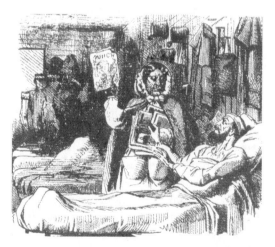

Mary Jane Seacole tending to the sick and wounded as depicted in Punch, *1857 (Library of Congress)*

Cruces, Gatun, Colón, and Escribanos, Panama—all parts of a semicivilized frontier. While running a hotel in Gorgona, Panama, she stitched wounds and nursed islanders during a cholera outbreak. The usually fatal disease cowed native launderers, boatmen, and muleteers, who demanded that priests parade figures of saints through the streets. As the entourage passed, fearful Catholics prostrated themselves to rid the area of contagion. In an energetic pique, she confessed to ousting "the stupid priest and his as stupid worshippers" to set about her healing (Seacole 1988, 33).

According to Seacole, the only hope lay in the "yellow woman from Jamaica with the cholera medicine" (Seacole 1988, 27). Fitting her nostrums to the individual, she applied plasters to neck, heart, and spine; massaged the limbs and trunk with oil, wine, and camphor; and quenched their thirst with cinnamon water and "sugar of lead" but avoided the drowsy release of opiates, which only hastened death. She notes in her memoirs the response of the first patient: "It was a very obstinate case [of cholera], but by dint of mustard emetics, warm fomentations, mustard plasters on the stomach and the back, and calomel, at first in large then in gradually smaller doses, I succeeded in saving my first cholera patient" (Seacole 1988, 25). Writing not only about her successes, she detailed the large numbers of deaths and focused on a small orphan who died in her arms. Her own brush with cholera was slight but left her weak and fatigued.

Back home in Jamaica in 1853, she battled an epidemic of yellow fever, opening her residence to patients transported from ships in Kingston Harbor. Medical authorities hired her to nurse the sick at Up-Park Camp, one mile from Kingston. On a second voyage to Panama to settle her affairs, she advised a surgeon who gave up European medicine to adopt herbal remedies developed from Caribbean plants. Additional experience in Colombia prepared her for the demands of the Crimean War, which began the next year. Seacole volunteered for the British army nurse corps at the London War Office. Nurse recruiter Elizabeth Herbert, wife of the British secretary of war, rejected nonwhites, whom she kept waiting in the hall.

A solitary figure devoid of family protectors, Seacole decided to fend for herself against racial stereotyping with her usual bustling, positive outlook. After assembling recommendations from former patients and doctors, she declared: "I made up my mind that if the army wanted nurses, they would be glad of me, and with all the ardour of my nature, which ever carried me where inclination prompted, I decided that I *would* go to the Crimea; and go I did, as all the world knows" (Seacole 1988, 76).

On her own funds, she traveled east over the Mediterranean Sea aboard the steamer *Hollander* to Malta and Constantinople on the Bosporus Strait. Among the convalescing officers at the army hospital at Scutari, she recognized men she had tended in Panama, who called her "Mother Seacole." While waiting for an audience with Florence Nightingale, Seacole could not resist the urge to spruce up bandages and lift the spirits of men recovering from dysentery and gunshot wounds. She examined the kitchen and found nurses stirring soup, broth, and arrowroot. For the night, Nightingale roomed her with the laundress.

Traveling northeast toward Russia, Seacole edged closer to the combat zone the next day, crossing the Black Sea by steamer to the Crimean coast, where the allies were taking a severe beating. At Balaklava on the southern part of the coast, she arrived at the wharf simultaneously with a load of wounded bound for Scutari and put herself to work for six weeks rebandaging, comforting, and offering pannikins of broth while quartering aboard the ammunition ship *Medora*. With the emotions of the combat nurse, she asked herself: "I wonder if I can ever forget the scenes I witnessed there? Oh! they were heartrending" (Seacole 1988, 98).

At nearby Spring Hill in midsummer, Seacole paid £800 for the British Hotel, which included a rail-side general store, canteen, and dining room for convalescent soldiers, whom she called her English sons. Like a stern parent, she forbade drunkenness and gambling and warred against thieves and pickpockets. For English, French, and Sardinian patients, her kitchens turned out claret punch, hot breads, roast fowl, joints of mutton, and root vegetables and fruits along with hand-mixed cures and tonics. From home base, she ventured regularly to the front for the Battle of Tchernaya on August 16, 1855, and the siege at Sevastopol, which fell the first week of September. In the ruined city ahead of other rescue parties, she countered patrols in an untidy squabble: "I refused positively to dismount, and made matters worse by knocking in the cap of the first soldier who laid hands upon me, with the bell that hung at my saddle. Upon this, six or seven tried to force me to the guard-house in rather a rough manner, while I resisted with all my force, screaming . . . and using the bell for a weapon" (Seacole 1988, 175). There she witnessed a sobering scene of the thousands the retreating Russians had left dead and dying, some hacked beyond recognition.

Overall, Seacole earned her own way through shrewd commerce while nursing casualties and treating cholera, diarrhea, jaundice, and fever. For her patients, she cooked and distributed sickroom delicacies—sponge cake, blancmange, broth, jelly, and sherry. For her ministrations, *Punch* published a tribute that included these lines:

> The sick and sorry can tell the story
> Of her nursing and dosing deeds;
> Regimental M. D. never worked as she,
> In helping sick men's needs.
> (Seacole 1988, 134)

For bravery under fire, she earned the Crimean Medal, the French Legion of Honor, and a Turkish honorarium. At war's end in 1856, she lost her hotel and returned to England. With the combined efforts of *The Illustrated News, Punch,* and the London *Times,* she found enough donors to elude bankruptcy. The next year, she produced an autobiographical best-seller, *Wonderful Adventures of Mrs. Seacole in Many Lands,* which produced an adequate income. Extolled by veterans, she died famous and beloved in 1881 and was buried in Kensal Green, London. Her bust adorns the Institute of Jamaica. In 1990, she acquired the Order of Merit, conferred 134 years after her heroic work.

Sources

Bois, Danuta. "Mary Jane Seacole." http://www.net-srq.com/~dbois/seacole-mj.html.

Carnegie, M. Elizabeth. *The Path We Tread: Blacks in Nursing Worldwide, 1854–1994.* New York: National League for Nursing Press, 1995.

Golding, Jeannette. "Mary Seacole Home Page." http://www.wp.com/internurse/mary.html.

Myers, Pamela. *Building for the Future: A Nursing History 1896–1996.* Chiswick, London: St. Mary's Convent, 1996.

Paquet, Sandra Pouchet. "The Enigma of Arrival: The Wonderful Adventures of Mrs. Seacole in Many Lands." *African American Review* (winter 1992): 1–10.

Parry, Melanie, ed. *Larousse Dictionary of Women.* New York: Larousse, 1996.

Robinson, Amy. "Authority and the Public Display of Identity: Wonderful Adventures of Mrs. Seacole in Many Lands." *Feminist Studies* (fall 1994).

Seacole, Mary. *Wonderful Adventures of Mrs. Seacole in Many Lands.* New York: Oxford University Press, 1988.

Selassíe, Tsahaí Haíle

Among the touching stories of thwarted charity is the nursing career of Ethiopia's beloved Princess Tsahaí Haíle Selassíe. She was born in Addis Ababa on October 13, 1919, and grew up with five siblings in the palace residence known as the Little Gebbi. From her window, she could watch the poor stretch their hands to her father, Tafari Makonnen, the nation's regent, as he made official visits to the empress. She attended an English boarding school at age eight but grew ill in the climate. Her parents transferred her to a school in Switzerland, where she became fluent in French, English, and German. When her father was crowned Emperor Haíle Selassíe in 1930, the outside world castigated the royal family for living far above the subsistence of the nation's poor.

Dressed in Parisian finery and escorted by servants, Tsahaí lived the life of a royal princess but she suffered when her family was separated. In the absence of her married sisters and the empress, who traveled with Prince Sahle, Tsahaí substituted as royal companion and advised her father on plans to improve conditions in Ethiopia. While touring the Seventh-Day Adventist mission hospital, the George Memorial Hospital, staffed by American Presbyterian missionaries, and the clinic run by French nuns, Tsahaí regretted that the nation's capital offered a total of four hundred beds, which accommodated only a small portion of the sick. It distressed her that the majority had to rely on sorcerers, home nursing, and folk cures and that lepers and ailing beggars roamed the bazaars.

As Benito Mussolini and his brown-shirted Fascists menaced Ethiopia in 1935, Tsahaí took an active role in aiding fellow citizens. She sponsored the Ethiopian Women's Welfare Work Association, a volunteer relief agency that supplied soldiers with water, food, tents, and bandages. As a Red Cross worker, she aided director Geuta Herrouy in the difficult period after Italy invaded Ethiopia on October 2. In one of the nation's two ambulances, she tried to assist an army that had no doctors or nurses and no field hospitals. The emperor himself manned a machine gun as Italian bombers dropped their loads on Addis Ababa on December 6.

The pathetic situation of tens of thousands wounded or burned by mustard gas drew Tsahaí to the defense of beleaguered Ethiopians, but enemy strength forced her family into exile. Transferred to Jerusalem and on to England, they lived near Bath, where Tsahaí served as family translator. Against royal tradition, she began nurse training in August 1936 as the only nonwhite probationer at the Great Ormonde Street Hospital for Sick Children in London. Her father took pride in his daughter's goodwill toward Ethiopians and visited her during a staff Christmas party in December of her second year. After her graduation with a degree in pediatric nursing on August

25, 1939, she prepared to open a health service in Ethiopia. She enrolled in postgraduate courses at temporary wartime quarters at Pembury Hospital near Royal Tunbridge Wells, where she tended some victims of the Blitz.

Shortly before completing the final examination, Tsahaí returned to royal duties and escorted her mother home. The hospital matron, Emily MacMannus, noted: "The Princess was very sad about this. She so badly wanted to become a State Registered Nurse of England so that, when she returned to her own country, she could hold an important position in her nation's health service. However, as always, she was her father's most loyal daughter" (Mosley 1964, 264).

Lady Barton, a family friend, raised the question of a suitable emblem to indicate to senior Red Cross volunteers that princess was no mere charity lady but a trained medical professional. Lady Barton suggested that Tsahaí duplicate the Lion of Judah, the royal symbol of the emperor, but the princess chose her mother's crest, the Queen of Sheba. Dressed in the Red Cross uniform with the appropriate patch on the sleeve, nurse Tsahaí and three British colleagues returned to liberated Ethiopia in 1942.

After setting up headquarters at Dese, a town in north-central Ethiopia, the trio conducted general clinics for desert dwellers in Lake Haik and Bartie. On April 26, 1942, Tsahaí interrupted relief work to fulfill a royal obligation to marry Colonel Abiye Ababa, a war hero. Newly settled at Lekemti, where her husband served as governor-general of Eritrea, she mapped out the organization of hospitals and medical care throughout the area. Her hopes for the poor ended on August 16, when she died of hemorrhage caused by a miscarriage. According to custom, a procession of wailers bore her remains to the palace, where the emperor, dressed in mud-stained clothes, mourned the untimely loss of his daughter. A memorial fund underwrote a nurses' training school and the Princess Tsahaí Memorial Hospital, where Ethiopia's poor are treated free of charge. As Tsahaí had hoped, postwar development equalized medical care for all Ethiopians.

Sources

McKown, Robin. *Heroic Nurses.* New York: G. P. Putnam's Sons, 1966.

Mosley, Leonard. *Haile Selassie: The Conquering Lion.* Englewood Cliffs, N.J.: Prentice-Hall, 1964.

Spanish-American War

When the Spanish-American War began with the blockading of Cuban ports on April 22, 1898, along with 200,000 volunteers for the army and navy, thousands of registered nurses signed up for contract posts in both the United States and in the Caribbean. Although the conflict lasted only until mid-August, it dramatized the government's neglect of sanitary measures and medical preparedness. More than 10 percent of American troops suffered preventable contagious diseases, notably typhoid, which infected 20,926 soldiers. After inductees began reporting to southeastern camps, epidemics forced volunteers to set up emergency facilities similar to the crude tent cities of the Civil War era. In contrast to the ready response of the Japanese Red Cross in the Sino-Japanese War of 1894–1895, American war ministers had reason to reflect on obvious failures.

In eight attempts from 1887 to 1900, Clara Barton had advocated the evolving Red Cross model and rode to the front at Siboney, Cuba, in a hay cart as a gesture of humanitarianism and goodwill, yet made no headway in securing federal consent. According to Mabel Boardman's *Under the Red Cross Flag at Home and Abroad* (1915), a history of the agency from its inception to World War I, the effort to aid thousands of civilian men, women, and

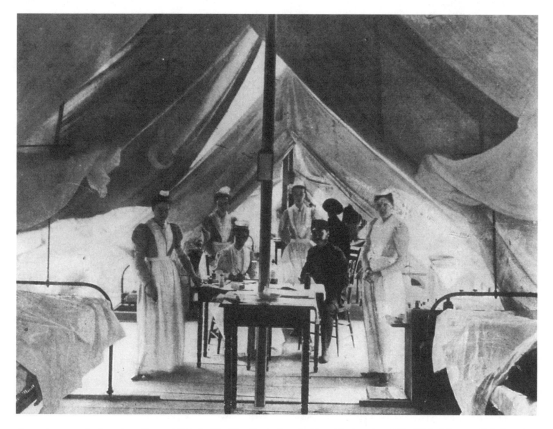

A ward tent at the Sternberg General Hospital in Manila during the Spanish-American War (U.S. Library of Medicine)

children whom the Spanish authorities had interned under guard in barbed-wire enclosures along the coast required the outfitting of a chartered vessel, the *State of Texas*. However, once the Central Cuban Relief Committee had acquired relief supplies, federal authorities prevented their distribution lest they fall into enemy hands. Until the harbor was secure, wretched Cubans received no aid. A second thwarted expedition funded by the American National Red Cross Relief Committee dispatched a load complete with cots, ice plants, ambulances, and nurses aboard a yacht named the *Red Cross,* which turned back to Key West in a storm. Reshipment and misunderstandings foiled this attempt.

In Boardman's poignant description, the debacle was a bitter lesson to the nation. She describes the absurdity of a shipment of abdominal bands to a hospital administrator expecting hospital linens and garments: "Colonel William Cary Sanger felt the tragedy of all this unorganized work while scores of his men lay ill with burning fever and had nothing to wear but their heavy uniforms. In some cases tons of ice were side-tracked and melted away, while the fever-stricken soldiers moaned for ice water" (Boardman 1915, 93). Newspaper headlines expressed outrage at the lack of surgeons, nurses, and supplies for the bungled mission. Meanwhile, Philadelphia, Cleveland, Minnesota, Boston, and the Pacific Coast began their own missions, as did the Woman's National War Relief Association of New York. The good intentions of these floundering expeditions illustrated to President William McKinley the need for a centralized coordination of efforts.

Two public-spirited volunteers proposed solutions to the spiraling crisis. Isabel Hampton Robb offered the government her services as agent for nurses. A former educator at Johns Hopkins School of Nursing, she urged the Nurses' Associated Alumni of the United States and Canada to assist the military in recruiting better personnel. Robb's offer lost out to the unprecedented plan of Dr. Anita Newcomb McGee, the nursing organizer of the

era. The daughter of an admiral and vice president of the Daughters of the American Revolution (DAR), she intrigued Surgeon General George M. Sternberg with a proposal to organize a DAR-led Hospital Corps Committee to augment the services of the Red Cross. Lacking a formal nurse corps, the army had little choice but to accept the plan and draft volunteer or contract nurses.

Recruited and enlisted by McGee, who was made the acting assistant surgeon general, the eight thousand nurses serving during the Spanish-American War proved efficient and loyal. However, like Dorothea Lynde Dix's gargantuan winnowing process during the Civil War, McGee's task of examining them was formidable. In a formal report, she observed: "The work of separating the fit from the unfit was not so simple an accomplishment as it would appear, and the correspondence entailed was enormous. The visitors who made inquiries in person were also numerous. The officers were at their posts daily from 8 A.M. to 11 P.M." (Kalisch and Kalisch 1978, 196). To each applicant, McGee's staff posted a form letter noting that only hospital-trained nurses were considered for duty. Those selected would receive train tickets to their posts and an allotment of $30 and board but no guarantee of lodging. By May 7, 1898, the first four nurses were dispatched to hospital duty in Key West, Florida.

As casualties returned with dysentery, typhoid, diarrhea, and malaria, their depleted state prefaced a late-forming realization that the military medical corps was out of touch with battlefield needs. On May 3, 1898, Surgeon General Sternberg issued a harsh critique to legislators considering the need for a military nursing corps. In his opinion, females were unsuited for war nursing of casualties but might have some minor use in cooking special diets. As of August 31, 1898, the Army Medical Department enlarged the hospital corps from 723 male orderlies and nurses to nearly six thousand men, most of whom were untrained and incapable of meeting wartime emergencies. In a report to the

U.S. War Department dated 1904, Walter Reed, Victor C. Vaughan, and Edward O. Shakespeare stated that corpsmen sloshed the contents of bedpans on beds, floors, ground, and themselves. Without washing or disinfecting their hands, they ate their meals and returned to fevered patients lying in sweaty, soiled linens. As a result of the corpsmen's ineptitude, attendant and patient together contaminated the people and objects they touched. Given the corps's low performance and the mounting need for nurse care to stem the typhoid epidemic, Sternberg, for the first time in American history, began a mass hiring of females.

Nurses' memoirs are filled with the despair and animosity wrought by the misogyny of the Spanish-American War. In Manila, surgical nurse Estelle Hine wrote about the supercilious corpsmen and wardmasters who disdained female nurses at a time when cooperation was crucial. In wretched heat with tents lit by lamps and candles and swathed in mosquito netting, patients arrived in dirty clothing and slept on whatever beds and cots could be found. In stateside camps, the sick suffered needlessly from bedsores, a sign of inadequate sanitation and limited nursing staff. Looking back at this unpromising beginning of military nursing by women, in November 1902, Harriet C. Lounsberry, chief nurse at the Brooklyn Homeopathic Hospital, remembered the era that turned the tide for professionalization. She published an article in the *American Journal of Nursing* recalling the variety of staff from ninety-one training centers all over the country and the pride of nurses displaying graduate badges, caps, and proficiencies.

Nursing cadres sprang up as needed to tend the 30 percent of the 165,000 volunteer soldiers who sickened in stateside camps while waiting to be sent to the front. Kansas native Lucy Shook Huxtable worked at Sternberg General Hospital at Camp Thomas, Chickamauga Park, Georgia, managing the thirteen board huts and infirmary hastily erected in the armory of a Civil War prison. She was appalled by gaping holes chopped in walls to let in light and air with no provision for keeping out flies and mosquitoes. Without staff, she, like matrons of the 1860s, drew on untrained soldiers to contend with abysmal sanitation and fearful contagion. Anna C. Maxwell, director of nursing at New York's Presbyterian Hospital, accepted a request to supervise Sternberg. Her first report bristles with distaste for so primitive a setup: "The laundry work for the camp was contracted for by a firm in Chattanooga, and so little conception had they of the work before them, that they sent a boy with a mule and cart to remove a tent full of soiled linen. I personally listed these clothes (over 800 pieces), the condition of which was indescribable" (Jamieson 1949, 448). Scrubbing with a pound of carbolic and some chloride of lime purchased in Chattanooga, she began disinfecting latrines between tents to battle an army of flies and kill typhoid bacilli.

Another diarist, Red Cross nurse Anne Williamson, a recent graduate of the New York Hospital School of Nursing, embarked from Charleston to Sternberg General Hospital on August 17, 1898. Her memoirs, *50 Years in Starch* (1948), exclaimed over the number of typhoid cases: "Crowded into ambulances—four and sometime six at a time; often after a dreadful stretch of hours without water. They were weak and emaciated, their fever-ridden bodies frequently covered by sores encrusted with dead flies; their lips cracked and swollen so that they could hardly swallow. It was a cruel sight" (Williamson 1948, 124–125). Because of short supplies and staff, nurses had to forgo sponge baths and hose down entire wards. Like others of the auxiliary, Williamson provided her own uniforms in exchange for the small monthly salary and travel expenses to and from each military hellhole. The work was physically and emotionally draining and, on one occasion, terrifying, when she returned to her tent to find a fellow staff member dead at her desk.

In *Leaves from a Nurse's Life's History, 1906,* author Jean S. Edmunds corroborates Williamson's observations by describing her own attention to uniform, orders, and discipline as she worked by lantern light under the command of the exacting Chief Nurse Maxwell. The upgrading of medical care at division hospitals required attention to food, pillows, dishes, instruments, and medications and round-the-clock monitoring of fever victims. The daily routine called for ice baths, regular feedings of broth, constant replacement and airing of soaked bed linens, and medical treatments for delirium. Edmunds had the assistance of one orderly, whom she taught the basics of bed care. She stayed on her feet from 7 A.M. until 9 P.M., taking only twenty minutes twice daily for meals.

Additional details come from a manuscript by nurses Helen B. Schuler and Florence M. Kelly, who coped with patients suffering serious diarrhea and incontinence. Without adequate water or wash basins to maintain clean bedding, the nurses contracted intestinal disease and overran the three staff privies erected 500 feet from their quarters. They concluded, "The majority of the nurses left Sternberg Hospital Service with an intestinal condition which soon became chronic and which we shall suffer from the effects of, until the end of our life" (Kalisch and Kalisch 1978, 203). As of September 13, 1898, twenty-three nurses—twenty of whom were unused to southern heat, humidity, and insects—failed to last out the summer, departing from service because of typhoid, diarrhea, dysentery, and exhaustion. Jane F. Riley recalls staff examinations by Dr. Jesse Lazear, a Cuban specialist in tropical disease, who advised that the army furlough ailing nurses north out of the heat and contagion.

In mid-July, as American forces were winning the war, General William R. Shafter reassigned 729 nurses to Santiago to treat an outbreak of yellow fever. In nurse Lillian Kratz's unpublished writings, the battleship carrying her from New York harbor sped to Santiago in time for passengers to see dead and dying casualties lying on San Juan Hill in the glow of sunset. Nurse Anna Turner reported on the acute nausea and spew of black vomit that bedeviled Spanish and American patients, who writhed pitiably from the intensity of stomach and intestinal distress. The flow of blood from the gums, skin, gut, and kidneys preceded jaundice and a fetid odor peculiar to the disease. Over twelve-hour shifts, staff monitored albumin in the urine and recorded fluid intake. After the crisis, a measured introduction of milk and solid food gradually increased strength in those who weathered the disease. Outside Havana, Turner participated in studies of yellow fever contagion that proved that the disease was not passed from patient to patient, as formerly conjectured. Thus, the brief Spanish-American War ended in military triumph for American forces and a worldwide victory over a formidable disease by linking it to the bite of the *Aedes aegypti* mosquito.

Unfortunately, for many, medical progress came too late. The severity of suffering from yellow fever colored the correspondence of brigade commander Theodore Roosevelt. In a letter to Henry Cabot Lodge, Roosevelt listed his loss of personnel at 24 percent and blamed mismanaged hospital care for terrifying the remaining soldiers. On August 3, 1898, he revealed to the media the contents of a round-robin letter from V Corps addressed to General Shafter warning that the army must be moved from Cuba or else perish from lethal conditions. Within four days, the high command began evacuating men from the tropics to quarantine at Camp Wikoff at Montauk Point, Long Island. The return of the troops again swamped medical facilities. Soldiers lived in tents, slept without bedding, and made do on diminished rations. Of some ten thousand patients, two hundred died. Once more, Surgeon General Sternberg had to mobilize more nurses and doctors.

In an eyewitness account, Nurse Kate M. Walsh summarized the misery of trying to stay clean while tending veterans in a wretched enclosure. Some nurses collapsed from the foul conditions and mid-August heat. The gradual enlargement of facilities and increase in number of beds relieved crowded thirty-bed wards, which often accommodated fifty patients. Another boon was the enlargement of Camp Wikoff's nursing staff to 1,158, bringing the wartime total to 1,563. According to a news item in the September 10, 1898, issue of *Harper's Weekly,* the hastily assembled nursing staff profited from assistance by the Sisters of Charity and the Red Cross. Early release of some patients and the transfer of one thousand others to civilian contagion wards in Philadelphia, Boston, New York, and Providence, Rhode Island, further eased the situation. By October 31, the crisis was over and the camp deserted. In the aftermath, at the cost of great suffering and public embarrassment of the Army Medical Corps, a greater understanding of yellow fever and typhoid improved prevention and treatment.

Investigation continued into 1901, when a committee concluded that 90 percent of the five thousand casualties needlessly died from disease. Blame centered on Secretary of War Russell Alger for unnecessary delays in ordering and transporting supplies, hiring staff, and setting up hospitals. Determined to improve its record, Congress altered the plan of military preparedness with the Army Reorganization Bill, which launched a regular Army Nurse Corps. The new all-female medical wing took shape on February 2, with Dita H. Kinney appointed as supervisor. Another outgrowth of military chaos and the resultant nursing shortage was twofold: the reorganization of the Red Cross and the nucleus of nurse training in Cuba, led by war veterans Lucy Quitard and Eugénie Hibbard.

See also: Hasson, Esther; Red Cross

Sources
Boardman, Mabel. *Under the Red Cross Flag at Home and Abroad.* London: J. B. Lippincott, 1915.
Dodge, Bertha S. *The Story of Nursing.* Boston: Little, Brown, 1965.
Dolan, Josephine A., R.N. *History of Nursing.* Philadelphia: W. B. Saunders, 1968.
Fessler, Diane Burke. *No Time for Fear: Voices of American Military Nurses in World War II.* East Lansing: Michigan State University Press, 1996.
Griffin, Gerald Joseph, and H. Joann King Griffin. *Jensen's History and Trends of Professional Nursing.* Saint Louis, Mo.: C. V. Mosby, 1965.
Hutchinson, John F. *Champions of Charity: War and the Rise of the Red Cross.* Boulder, Colo.: Westview Press, 1996.
Jamieson, Elizabeth, and Mary F. Sewall. *Trends in Nursing History.* London: W. B. Saunders, 1949.
Kalisch, Philip, and Beatrice J. Kalisch. *The Advance of American Nursing.* Boston: Little, Brown, 1978.
Lamps on the Prairie: A History of Nursing in Kansas. Emporia: Kansas State Nurses' Association, 1942.
Sherr, Lynn, and Jurate Kazickas. *Susan B. Anthony Slept Here: A Guide to American Women's Landmarks.* New York: Times Books, 1994.
Williamson, Anne A., R.N. *50 Years in Starch.* Culver City, Calif.: Murray and Gee, 1948.

Stopes, Marie

The inventor of the cervical cap and pioneer of women's health, Dr. Marie Charlotte Carmichael Stopes dedicated her career to providing reliable contraception for women. In her pro-female philosophy, "There is nothing that helps so much with the economic emancipation of woman as a knowledge of how to control her maternity" (Rose 1993, xiii). Vilified by political cartoonists, the Catholic Church, and other conservative groups, she earned support from such influential sources as the Duke of Windsor and authors George Bernard Shaw and Evelyn Waugh and the gratitude of satisfied patrons, both male and female, who acquired some control over family size by applying her principles.

Born October 15, 1880, in Edinburgh, Scotland, Stopes came from a background of strong women. Her mother, intellectual feminist Charlotte Carmichael, met her husband, architect Henry Stopes, at a meeting of the British Association for the Advancement of Science. Tutored at home by her mother, Stopes attended St. George's School in Edinburgh and entered the University College for training in chemistry, geology, and botany. After graduating with honors in 1902, she ob-

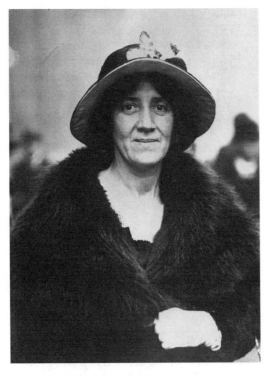

Dr. Marie Stopes, 1923 (Corbis/Bettmann)

tained a doctorate in paleobotany from Munich University's Botanical Institute. As the youngest female science teacher at Manchester University and the youngest scientist with a doctoral degree in Great Britain, she earned a fellowship from the Royal Society, a rare honor for a woman in Edwardian England.

For a decade, Stopes studied ancient flora and published scholarly articles on the formation of coal before encountering a brilliant pioneer who redirected her into a more timely endeavor. In 1915, she attended a lecture by American birth control expert Margaret Sanger, who told of her arrest for opening an illegal birth control clinic among the immigrant tenements of New York City. The two feminists became friends and colleagues, sharing manuscripts and ideas. Following the collapse of Stopes's marriage to Reginald Ruggles Gates, in 1918, she published a manual on human sexuality, *Married Love,* which brought instant name recognition and a host of sophisticated supporters. Oxford Univer-

sity requested a version written for physicians; the Welsh Education Board asked her to head a summer camp to teach children about reproduction. A year later, she joined the National Birth Rate Commission.

A second marriage to publisher Humphrey Verdon Roe, her friend and advocate, increased Stopes's interest in writing books on birth control. A week after the armistice that ended World War I, she published *Wise Parenthood* (1918), a guide to contraception favoring the rubber cervical cap in combination with a quinine pessary, or sponge. She followed with "A Letter to Working Mothers on How to Have Healthy Children and Avoid Weakening Pregnancies," an illustrated, self-published monograph also recommending the cervical cap as a semen block. A boon to working-class families, the innovation provided simple, practical assistance in family planning by halting unwanted pregnancies.

On March 17, 1921, with the aid of her husband, Stopes opened the Mother's Clinic for Constructive Birth Control in Holloway, North London. Her purpose was fourfold: to help the poor with free advice, to survey working-class attitudes toward contraception, to record data on clients' sex lives, and to collect first-person commentary on the type of birth control women preferred. To alleviate patient hesitance, she staffed the facility with female nurse-midwives rather than male doctors. East End visiting nurse Hebbes conducted pelvic exams, fitted each patient with Stopes's original high-domed rubber pessary, and explained the principle of sperm interception. She referred patients with physical anomalies to Dr. Jane Lorrimer Hawthorne, the clinic consultant.

The bold move into one-on-one counseling of wives without their husbands present angered conservative and religious leaders. For a decade, Stopes pursued a lawsuit against Dr. Halliday Sutherland, a Catholic physician who opposed prevention of pregnancy and accused her of experimenting on the poor. The emotionally draining experience precipitated her lifelong antagonism toward the Christian church's meddling in women's lives. Multiple media stories about the seamy court battle buoyed her cause and increased her appeal. That same year, the American version of *Married Love* was published in the United States. The Court of Special Sessions in New York declared it obscene, even after publisher W. J. Robinson purged questionable passages. The decision prefaced a scramble for pirated copies.

The public extolled Stopes's feminist initiatives and packed New York lecture halls in October of 1921 to hear her explain the family's right and obligation to produce only healthy, loved children. Back in England, with additional offices and a horse-drawn mobile clinic, she extended assistance throughout London's suburbs to agencies interested in relieving women of a life shortened by precarious pregnancies too closely spaced for the good of health and family. In 1925, she moved her clinic to central London and began training her own staff of nurses. When officials fired visiting public health nurse E. S. Daniels for dispensing contraceptive information at a maternity center and for referring women to the Mother's Clinic, Stopes agitated for support. With a petition signed by five hundred women, she maneuvered the Ministry of Health into endorsing birth control instruction and published the concession in the September 1930 issue of her *Birth Control News*.

Success freed Stopes to work more openly. She served on England's National Birth Control Council, later called the Family Planning Association, which had opened a dozen clinics modeled on the Mother's Center. Without fear of lawsuit, she published two more books on contraception: *Roman Catholic Methods of Birth Control* (1933) and *Birth Control Today* (1934). Appalled by the Catholic Church's new anticontraception campaign and Sutherland's successful appeal, Stopes was ill-equipped emotionally to recover from a still-birth and difficult delivery of her son Harry and the death of her sister Winnie. With her name bandied by wags and satirists and sung in children's jump rope rhymes, Stopes softened the strident crusade and published a child-centered monograph, *Your Baby's First Year* (1939), as well as poetry and drama. In 1940, the Blitz wrought serious havoc on her headquarters, where two nurses and an office manager continued receiving patients in perilous times. A new location at Norbury Park was also hit by bombs. At the time of her death from breast cancer and brain hemorrhage on October 2, 1958, she had achieved the rank of feminist heroine.

Stopes's mission supporting "children by choice, not by chance" continues to benefit women ("Marie," www.mariestopes.org.uk). Marie Stopes International reaches 1.5 million clients in twenty-five countries throughout Africa, Asia, and South America, including Bosnia, Croatia, Romania, Uganda, South Africa, Malawi, Kenya, Nepal, Indonesia, and Bolivia. Her nursing staff counsels clients in metropolitan areas, outback clinics, mobile units, markets, factories, and workplaces, offering wellness information, health screening, family planning advice, abortion, and male and female sterilization. Late twentieth-century achievements of the New Generation League, the National Abortion Rights Action League (NARAL), Planned Parenthood, Mary S. Calderone's Sex Information and Education Council of the United States (SIECUS), and Judith Widdicombe's Reproductive Health Service owe their existence to Stopes's forthright campaign.

Sources

"Marie Stopes International." http://www.marie-stopes.org.uk/mission.html.

Parsons, Judith. "Marie Stopes." *The Great Scientists.* Danforth, Conn.: Grolier, 1989.

Rose, June. *Marie Stopes and the Sexual Revolution.* London: Faber and Faber, 1993.

Snodgrass, Mary Ellen. *Celebrating Women's History.* Detroit: Gale Research, 1996.

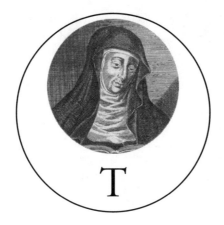

Teresa, Mother

A contemporary of Dr. Cicely Saunders, Lillian Wald, Elisabeth Kübler-Ross, and others transforming care for the dying, Mother Teresa settled in India, became a citizen, and launched a sixty-eight-year career helping the poor, orphans, lepers, and the aged. She established ninety-eight hospice facilities to rescue and comfort terminally ill people among India's marginalized native poor, broadening her ministry to over ninety countries. Unlike the contemporary hospice movement, her outreach reverted to the origins of Christian nursing, which amplified spiritual comfort rather than pain control. Sixty satellite Teresian facilities spread hospice care throughout the world to combat disease, filth, and isolation.

Mother Teresa's humanitarianism began in the dirtiest sections of Calcutta, where she opened a home to wash, feed, and comfort the dying in their final days and hours. Dubbed the "Mother of the Poorest of the Poor" and the "Saint of Calcutta," she did not hesitate to scour garbage heaps for abandoned infants or to embrace wasted bodies crusted with sores. Dressed in her uniform, a white habit and blue-edged neck-to-ankle sari, Mother Teresa shared India's squalor, maintaining a sleeping mat and latrine bucket as her only earthly needs. Her outreach expanded in four directions:

- Medical: dispensaries, leprosy clinics and rehabilitation centers, and orphanages for abandoned children
- Apostolic: catechetical centers, Sunday schools, Catholic action groups, and family and prison ministry
- Educational: primary schools, sewing and commercial classes, handicrafts
- Social: natural birth control clinics, alcoholic rehabilitation, and shelters for the developmentally disabled

Born August 26 (or 27), 1910, the fourth child of Nikola Bojaxhiu, a building contractor and sturdy patriot, and Drana Bojaxhiu, a devout Catholic housewife, Agnes Gonxha was the third child after sister Age and brother Lazer. The family was native to the Serbian town of Skopje in Macedonia, Albania, 200 miles south of Belgrade. After Agnes's father was poisoned in 1921, Drana opened an embroidery and textiles business to feed the family yet maintained Christian charity to the poor. Emulating her mother, Agnes lived her faith daily and was moved by visitors' stories of suffering in India.

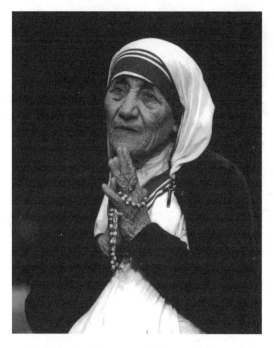

Mother Teresa speaks to a crowd of seventeen thousand in Denver, 20 May 1989. (Corbis/Bettmann-UPI)

At age eighteen, Agnes stood only 5 feet tall but radiated a powerful faith. Under the influence of letters from Balkan Jesuits living in Bengal, she joined the Sisters of Loreto, a branch of the Institute of the Blessed Virgin Mary and founders of a mission to India, and left for the mother house based in an abbey in Rathfarnham, Ireland. As a postulant, she slept in a cold, damp stone building while she learned Gaelic, English, and the silence expected of Christ's handmaidens. After six weeks of indoctrination, she left with Sister Magdalene aboard the *Marchait* for a five-week voyage to Darjeeling, India, a resort near the Himalayas. As a novice, she studied Hindi and Bengali and worked at St. Mary's Entally Convent compound. On May 4, 1932, she took the tripartite vow of poverty, chastity, and obedience, the preface to a holy life as Sister Mary Teresa, a bride of Christ, ministering to the poor of Calcutta.

At the convent's school, Sister Teresa was within a whiff of the Moti Jheel bustee (slum). While teaching three hundred Bengali girls catechism, geography, and history and nursing them through minor illnesses, she felt stymied by the peaceful rhythms of upper-class India and yearned for more involvement with destitute Indians. After her final vows in 1937, she dedicated herself to the school, over which she became principal, then superior of an order of sisters, the Daughters of St. Anne. As leader of the Sodality of Mary, she led young Christian, Hindu, and Muslim members to street ministry and visited the Silratan Sakor Hospital.

Sister Teresa's first breach of the settled life occurred the night she brought Granny, an elderly beggar, to her own cell for feeding and rest. In obedience to personal philosophy, Sister Teresa initiated her famous one-on-one ministry with a single patient. Mother Cenacle encouraged an experiment by which Sister Teresa brought twenty slum children to the convent for care, but all but two slipped away from the strangeness of the compound to the familiarity of their tattered homes. The constraints of World War II forced more of the poor into a desperate search for food and flight from postwar violence.

On a retreat in September 1946, Sister Teresa sat on the night train to Darjeeling and pondered the young and old suffering in Moti Jheel. A year after proposing a mission to the Archbishop of Calcutta, she could wait no longer. With the blessing of Mother Gertrude, on August 16, 1948, she donned sandals, uniform sari, and a small cross pinned at the shoulder. With the assistance of the Medical Mission Sisters of Mother Dengal at Holy Family Hospital in Patna, near the sacred Ganges River, she learned to nurse the squalid street poor, who suffered malnutrition, intestinal parasites, leprosy, and other contagion. Mother Dengal cautioned Sister Teresa to eat more than a handful of rice to keep herself as fit for the job as possible.

On December 21, 1948, Sister Teresa arrived at her mission field with 5 rupees and high hopes of making a difference. Her first project was an open-air school, where she taught illiterate children the Bengali alphabet by scratching letters in the dust with a stick.

She expanded to a mud hut where she demonstrated the basics of hygiene for children unused to regular bathing. Friends offered soap, paper, and stools. With a few medical supplies, she established an infirmary to clean and bandage the sick and dispense medicines.

No longer sheltered by the convent, Sister Teresa had to locate closer to work. At 14 Creek Lane, she roomed rent-free at the three-story home of teacher Michael Gomes, an admirer of her spunk. To her thinking, the upstairs quarters paralleled the Cenacle, or Upper Room used by Christ. She acquired the aid of helper and cook Charur Ma and welcomed a Bengali volunteer and first disciple, Shubashini Das, renamed Sister Agnes. Three others—sisters Gertrude, Bernard, and Frederick—joined the vigorous order. Sister Teresa instructed them on the importance of humility, confidence, peace, optimism, and charity. Her simple rooms expanded to a quarantine ward, where she treated sisters with infectious diseases. The nascent order soon occupied the second floor, a separate bath, and an annex. By October 7, 1950, the archbishop had blessed the mission of a new and fully recognized order, the Missionaries of Charity.

A devout Muslim donated a house, where in February 1953, India's acclaimed Mother Teresa established a Christian hospice soon known the world over. With the assistance of a police officer, the staff scrubbed a two-room rest house at the back of Kalighat, a temple to Kali, the Hindu goddess of death. Renamed the Nirmal Hriday, or Place of the Immaculate Heart, it welcomed the dying. The mission was not without its critics, including Gilly Burn, a crusading nurse who disagreed with Mother Teresa on the need for more analgesia for terminal cancer patients. Dr. Jack Preger advocated record keeping and the isolation of tubercular patients and restriction of their linens and cutlery from those of other inmates. Dr. Marcus Fernandes objected to the assumption that all inmates would die and strongly advocated vitamins and nutrients for curable patients suffering malnutrition, a pro-

tocol Mother Teresa rejected as against God's plan. Hindus protested the defilement of Kali's temple and the violation of karma, a philosophy based on fate, and threatened to kill her, but she shrugged off their threats.

Mother Teresa's treatment of a Hindu priest dying of cholera impressed native detractors. Now supporters of her nonsectarian mission, they helped with the washing and feeding of patients and rounded up clothing, linens, mattresses, pillows, and food. Volunteer doctors offered their time and solicited drugs, medical equipment, and supplies. Ann Blaikie, an English supporter, organized a volunteer sisterhood called the Marian Society to collect toys and clothes for an annual Christmas party. Mother Teresa requested donations of shoes, money for lepers, knitted garments, and bandages, thus involving Blaikie's volunteers as a full-time support staff. Named the International Co-Workers of Mother Teresa, the Marian Society spread to Poland, Japan, and the Arctic Circle. In 1955, the outpouring enabled Mother Teresa to open the Shishu Bhavan orphanage at 54A Lower Circular Road near the mother house, where children rescued from heaps of offal slept in clean nightgowns on packing boxes and floor mats.

A master organizer and manipulator of the media, Sister Teresa drew resources and volunteers from Indian society but acquired a reputation for intransigence and disdain for the middle and upper classes. Adoring features in the *Statesman*, the BBC's *Meeting Point, Amrita Bazar Patrika, Time*, and the *Illustrated Weekly* spread her message to readers while concealing critics' annoyance at her dogmatic rejection of divorce, contraception, and abortion. In Egypt, she ignored the government's attempt to curb overpopulation and urged mothers to produce more children. She found adoptive homes among Catholics who never practiced birth control and denied adoptions to prospective parents from the United States as a means of driving up demand for children as a deterrent to abortion on demand. Among her foundlings, she sponsored marriages and advanced schooling and vocational training on a gender-biased system: girls received necessary dowries and boys a proper education. Her high school kept troubled children off the streets and out of crime.

Mother Teresa's project turned into a full-scale siege against neglect and want. Her food service distributed bananas, dal, and rice to itinerant beggars. Near the railroad tracks of Titagarh in 1957, despite a stoning from neighbors, she opened Shanti Nagar, or the Place of Peace, a leper refuge, sponsored in part by an American utilities company. Father Alfred Schneider of Catholic Relief Services in Delhi gave her money for a van, which she transformed into a mobile clinic, the first of a fleet of six hundred. Her intervention in the early stages of leprosy enabled many to lead useful lives and to avoid the shunning and ignorance that forced lepers from society. In the late 1980s, she mobilized Teresan sisters to aid international disaster areas, including the Chernobyl nuclear meltdown and Armenian earthquake. Some of her hostels met with controversy, such as a homeless center for women in London that burned to the ground, killing nine women in a structure exempt from ordinances requiring fire escapes.

As her posture grew stooped and her skin wrinkled, Mother Teresa became a familiar sight among India's poor. In 1963, she established the Missionary Brothers of Charity, a network of monks led by Father Ian Travers-Ball, to ferry patients to the hospital. The Pope visited the order and donated a white Lincoln Continental, which she raffled off to support the leprosarium. She visited the scene of mass rape of Muslim women in Pakistan and refused to soften her antiabortion stance toward women left to bear children sired by their attackers. Philanthropists in the United States, Bombay and Delhi, Taiwan, Hong Kong, Macao, Papua New Guinea, Harlem, New York, Belfast, Ireland, Amman, Jordan, Caracas, Venezuela, Rome, Italy, Melbourne, Australia, London, England, Lima, Peru, Yemen, and Tanzania launched Teresan services, including the rescue of mentally ill children in Beirut, Lebanon, the Gift of Love, an AIDS hospice in New York's Greenwich Village, a soup kitchen in the Bronx, and a shelter for women and newborns in Washington, D.C. Gradually, Mother Teresa advanced her ministry in these foreign locales, beginning with a handful of sisters to open a shelter, school, or hospital. On visits to these outposts, she gathered more medicines, food, and clothing. After learning that she volunteered to serve as an airline stewardess in exchange for free passage, Indira Gandhi arranged for a permanent pass aboard Air India.

In old age, Mother Teresa earned the nickname "Mother of the World" in the same era when the most pointed criticism assailed her for unsanitary conditions, reuse of disposables, religious fanaticism, and treatment bordering on the impersonal. Columnist Christopher Hitchens, echoing the complaint of Debasis Bhattachariya of the Indian Science and Rationalists Association, accused her of exploiting the simple and humble. Nonetheless, with prize money from the Magsaysay Award for International Understanding, Pope John XXIII's Peace Prize, Templeton Award for Progress in Religion, John F. Kennedy International Award, Good Samaritan Award, Jewel of India, Jawaharlal Nehru Award for International Understanding, Order of Merit, and honoraria from university degrees, she bankrolled more convents and community missions.

The pinnacle of Mother Teresa's influence occurred at age sixty-nine. While the world photographed and interviewed her, she traveled to Oslo, Norway, with sisters Agnes and Gertrude to receive the 1979 Nobel Peace Prize of $193,000 and a gold medal inscribed *Pro Pace et Fraternitate Genitium* (For Peace and the Brotherhood of Nations). Before addressing a gathering of monarchs, prime ministers, and academic dignitaries with a simple, ecumenical call to love others as God loved humankind, she asked that the $7,000 dinner be canceled and the money spent on feeding the poor. To the dismay of feminists, Planned Parenthood, and liberal foundations, her speech was pointedly antichoice: "Many people are very, very concerned with the children of India, with the children of Africa, where quite a number die maybe of malnutrition and hunger and so on, but millions are dying deliberately by the will of the mother" (Sebba 1997, 1960). She asserted that abortion destroys peace and spreads the concept of killing as a viable solution to human ills. Poignantly, she concluded with a stark claim concerning evil and good: "There is nothing in between."

Following her plunge into international renown as a Nobel Peace Prize recipient, press coverage spread Mother Teresa's face and loving ministry throughout the globe. Her intent remained steady: "We serve Jesus in the poor. We nurse him, feed him, clothe him, visit him, comfort him in the poor, the abandoned, the sick, the orphans, the dying. But all we do, our prayer, our work, our suffering is for Jesus" (Le Joly 1983, flap copy). By her seventies, she had established more than 600 missions and 180 receiving centers in 130 countries staffed by 275 brothers, 4,000 nuns, and 120,000 volunteers.

Mother Teresa's final years regularly found their way into telecasts. When her heart began to fail in 1989 from fatigue, vascular obstruction, and long-term malarial and pneumonia infections, the press followed as she underwent surgery and installation of a pacemaker. Although willing to retire, she admitted that she had not groomed a successor. In 1992, Glenda Jackson played the part of the living saint in a film, *City of Joy.* Christopher Hitchens's critical British documentary, *Hell's Angel,* aired November 8, 1994, on the BBC to a chorus of complaints that broadcaster Tariq Ali had denigrated a contemporary icon of goodness. In this season of public controversy, Mother Teresa published eight books: *Loving Jesus* (1991), *Seeking the Heart of God: Reflections on Prayer* (1993), *Total Surrender* (1993), the best-selling *The Simple Path* (1995), *My Life for the Poor* (1996), *Mother Teresa: In My Own Words* (1996), *The Blessings of Love* (1996), and *Joy in Loving: A Guide to Daily Living with Mother Teresa* (1997). In 1996, in separate incidents, she broke a clavi-

cle and foot and cracked her skull in a fall from bed. Four months before her death in Calcutta on September 5, 1997, she countenanced the selection of Sister Nirmala, a Hindu convert to Catholicism, as successor and head of the Missionaries of Charity.

Sources

"Angel of Mercy." http://home1.pacific.net.sg/~alquek/teresa1.htm.

Felder, Deborah G. *The 100 Most Influential Women of All Time: A Ranking Past and Present.* New York: Citadel Press, 1996.

Gay, Kathlyn, and Martin K. Gay. *Heroes of Conscience.* Santa Barbara, Calif.: ABC-CLIO, 1996.

Giff, Patricia Reilly. *Mother Teresa: Sister to the Poor.* New York: Viking Kestrel, 1986.

Le Joly, Edward, S.J. *Mother Teresa of Calcutta.* San Francisco: Harper and Row, 1983.

Lee, Betsy. *Mother Teresa: Caring for All God's Children.* Minneapolis, Minn.: Dillon Press, 1981.

"Mother Teresa Books." http://www.catholic.net/RCC/people/mother/teresa/books.html.

Pace, Eric. "Mother Teresa, Hope of the Despairing, Dies at 87." *New York Times,* September 6, 1997.

Sebba, Anne. *Mother Teresa: Beyond the Image.* New York: Doubleday, 1997.

Siebold, Cathy. *The Hospice Movement: Easing Death's Pains.* New York: Twayne, 1992.

Twentieth-Century Nursing

Nursing in the late twentieth century bears little resemblance to the wearying housekeeping, feeding, and laundering performed by Florence Nightingale's wartime team. Evolving over an era that saw phenomenal advancement in medical care, including telemetry, organ transplant, laser and neurosurgery, and the abatement or defeat of trachoma, diabetes, influenza, polio, hepatitis, cholera, AIDS, birth defects, and numerous types of cancer, the field of nursing has placed more demands on medical education to produce staff equal to technology and medical protocols. The star performers of the profession hold doctorates in administration and research and publish their clinical studies and online impressions of ward nursing, intensive care, and mobile army surgical hospital (MASH) units in combat.

In a period that has witnessed fewer ambulatory patients, more critical care needs involve

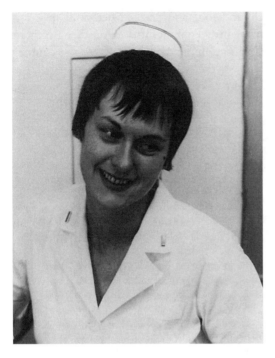

Lt. Dolores "Dee" O'Hara, nurse to the astronauts, 1963 (NASA)

quality of care. At the First and Second Convention of the American Society of Superintendents of Training Schools for Nursing in 1897, Sophia Palmer lauded an organized effort as the only way for the profession to function. In 1900, as the premier editor of the *American Journal of Nursing,* she established the aim of the periodical to present a monthly progress report, nursing news, and "the most progressive thought," along with the nursing questions of the day. In 1918, she stated, "Do not let it go down in history that when the young men of our country were called into service in defense of democracy . . . the nurses held back . . . because they shirk from the hardships of war service" ("Voices," www.ana.org, 2).

Globally, a focus on medical proficiency guided improvements. Guam, Samoa, the Virgin Islands, and the Philippines profited from military hospitals, which trained local women in nursing and midwifery. In Canada, a Permanent Army Medical Corps Nursing Service, headed by Captain Georgina F. Pope in 1904, awarded rank to nurses and allied with the Red Cross for emergency preparedness. The English formed a similar corps, the Queen Alexandra Imperial Military Nursing Service. The Mexican General Hospital opened in 1905 with sixteen hundred beds and a training school under the supervision of Mary J. McCloud. In Israel in 1918, Henrietta Szold, who launched Hadassah, a women's Zionist society, established maternity nursing at Rothschild Hospital. South America, too, made advances. Beginning in 1921, Chile boasted a donor-endowed training facility, the Carlos Van Buren School in Valparaiso. In Brazil, the Anna D. Nery School opened in Rio de Janeiro with a handful of students in 1923.

nurses in philosophical and ethical issues, such as alternative medicine, pain control, living wills, and the right to die. In practice, bed care is less onerous than in previous generations. Intravenous hydration, nutriment, and medication has replaced the spoon-feeding and injections of the past with a steady flow into a single port in the arm. Flexible, impermeable gloves are a standard for practitioners in even the simplest hands-on procedure, thanks in part to nurse Caroline Hampton, a surgical nurse for whom the Goodyear Rubber Company made two pairs of gloves in 1890 to relieve her allergy to disinfectants. Progressive care groups critical patients in private, high-tech units. Beds and cribs have acquired technical wizardry from the National Aeronautics and Space Administration (NASA) to weigh, massage, and monitor patients and to feed results to screens at a central station, where blood volume meter, drug cart, hypothermic unit, respirator, and crash truck await emergencies.

From early in the century, military and public service and education boosted the

Ireland contributed its own brand of nurses during the pervasive unrest that preceded civil war against Britain. One of the heroines of the war, Annie Smithson, worked for Sinn Fein in 1918 and nursed wounded volunteers. Arrested while tending casualties at the siege of Moran's Hotel, she was forced out of the

Queen's Nurses Committee. During the 1940s, she helped establish the Irish Nurses' Union and published her memories of an active life in *Myself and Others* (1944). Her contemporary, Linda Kearns of Dromard, trained at Baggot Street Hospital and operated a Red Cross field hospital during the 1916 uprising. As a rebel nurse doubling as arms smuggler, she opened a safe house in 1918 and was arrested and tried in Belfast. Transferred from Walton Prison, Liverpool, to Mountjoy Prison in Dublin, she escaped and resumed her heady career, which evolved from revolution to feminism. After serving as a senator, she returned to nursing and opened a convalescent home at Kilrock in 1945. Before her death in 1951, the International Committee of the Red Cross presented her the Florence Nightingale Medal.

Another spirited Irish rebel, Bridget Dirrane, a native of Inishmore, grew up in the Aran Islands and migrated to Dublin in 1919

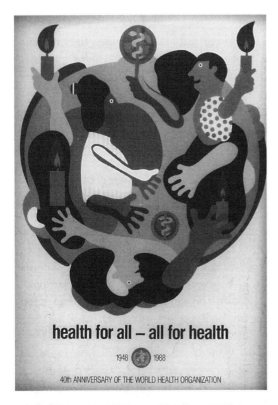

health for all – all for health

1948   1988

40th ANNIVERSARY OF THE WORLD HEALTH ORGANIZATION

A poster designed by P. Davies, published in 1986 in celebration of the fortieth anniversary of the World Health Organization (U.S. Library of Medicine)

to train at St. Ultan's Children's Hospital at Ballsbridge. With the war of independence raging, she lived and worked on the grounds but maintained covert contacts with underground factions. After her arrest and incarceration at the Mountjoy Jail and transfer to Bridewell Prison, she kept up a hunger strike until her release by Dublin's lord mayor. During the worst of Ireland's civil war, she returned to private duty and, in 1927, emigrated to Boston, Massachusetts. She found plenty of private duty and visiting nurse posts around the Dorchester neighborhood and, in 1943, earned a certificate of appreciation for her stint as the plant nurse for McCulloch Manufacturing. While working for the military, she diagnosed and treated soldiers at Keesler Field, Biloxi, Mississippi.

Early in the century, metropolitan areas dispatched itinerant nurses and public health teams to outlying areas, such as the rural sod huts beyond Hutchinson, Kansas, attended by Edith Stanforth and her Comanche assistant. A fellow Kansan, Mennonite sister Frieda Kaufman, traveled by milk wagon to one patient and treated the poor free of charge. Public health nurses began combating the intestinal parasites, sexually transmitted diseases, and congenital heart ailments that military doctors found in the rural poor while examining them for military duty during World War I. By the 1920s, public health education was improving, aided by such crusaders as Clara Barton, Dr. Marie Stopes, Lillian Wald, Margaret Sanger, and Emma Goldman. A major contribution to public awareness and nurse training was Josephine Goldmark's research into the conditions under which women and children worked in American factories. From her studies came four valuable works: *Child Labor Legislation Handbook* (1907), *Fatigue Efficiency* (1912), *A Case for the Shorter Workday and Women and Industry* (1916), and *Nursing and Nursing Education in the United States* (1923), a Rockefeller Foundation publication.

A campaign to reduce Hawaii's infant mortality rate caused participants to study the is-

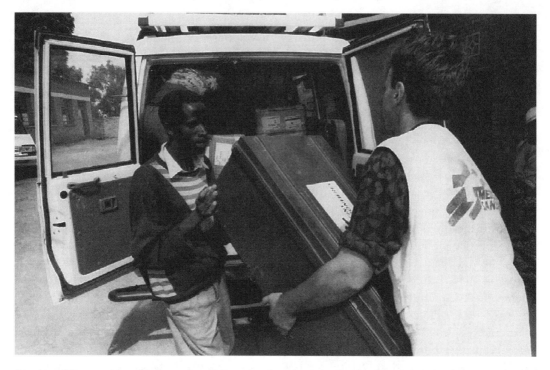

Members of Doctors without Borders pack up their goods to leave Rwanda after the government ordered representatives of all nongovernmental organizations to leave, 14 December 1995. (Reuters/Cedric Galbe/Archive Photos)

lands' topography, economy, religions, culture, and traditions. The blend of ethnic groups combined Filipino witchcraft, Chinese patriarchy, and Christianity with the herbalism of the *kahuna hanau* (lay practitioners who supervised childbirth). In 1952, premature birth was the central factor in 65.5 percent of neonatal deaths. The transfer of weak infants from home births to hospital neonatal wards and the purchase of more incubators improved the chances of survival. Under the instruction of Ethel Tschida, supervisor of premature infant nursing at New York Hospital, the Children's Bureau began a campaign to raise the survival rate. In conjunction with the Honolulu County Medical Society, nursing institutes held in 1953 demonstrated techniques and practice at St. Francis and Kapiolani Hospitals. The focus of the program was the individualization of care for each baby. Tschida demonstrated improvised suction apparatus and gavage for abdominal feeding and established procedures for resuscitation and temperature and infection control.

Among Australia's aborigines, the Little Sisters of the Poor, assisted by a pilot known as the "Flying Doctor," continued the frontier projects of the nineteenth century by operating clinics among isolated tribes. According to Norma Cappaert, community health service superintendent to Kalgoorlie and other outback villages, tribes suffered the typical complaints of a primitive lifestyle, notably malnutrition, perforated eardrum and ear discharge, chronic foot irritations, alcoholism, scabies, and poor hygiene. After white citizens recognized their duty to Australia's aboriginal poor, they integrated hospital wards. For the first time, aboriginal patients received European-style care and enjoyed such luxuries as sleeping in beds on pristine linen and balanced meals served on trays.

In Canada, the loose affiliation of nurse-training programs was restructured under the Canadian Association of University Schools of Nursing as a means of upgrading and standardizing programs and outcomes. Led by known professionals Margaret Hart and

Mona MacLeod of the University of Manitoba, Catherine Aikin of the University of Western Ontario, Helen Niskala of the University of Alberta, and Sister Denise Lefebvre of Institut Marguerite d'Youville, the new federation increased credibility. In collaboration with the Canadian Nurses Association, they formulated new standards for accrediting agencies, baccalaureate entry into practice, and doctoral education. These alterations boosted Canadian nursing from the frontier privations of the Yukon gold rush to modern proficiency.

Bolstering a worldwide nursing endeavor, the World Health Organization (WHO), begun in 1946 in Geneva as a United Nations initiative, targeted a global effort, "the attainment by all peoples of the highest possible level of health" (Baly 1995, 360). The organization appointed a Nightingale nurse, Olive Baggallay, as head of its vast system, with regional offices in Manila, New Delhi, Brazza-ville, Copenhagen, Washington, D.C., and Alexandria, Egypt. In 1954, Canadian nurse Lyle Creelman advanced to chief of WHO's nursing sector. A veteran of public health work in Canada, she applied her observations and experience to international situations.

In 1952, nursing educator Dr. Hildegard Elizabeth Peplan, the "mother of psychiatric nursing," published *Interpersonal Relations in Nursing: A Conceptual Framework for Psychodynamic Nursing*. Her approach pioneered a one-on-one relationship that she developed after service in the Army Nurse Corps during World War II. She directed graduate programs at Columbia University and Rutgers, and served as president and executive director of the American Nursing Association while lecturing and publishing articles in the fundamentals of interpersonal nursecare.

President John F. Kennedy's call for a Peace Corps in 1961 created an independent agency to uplift struggling nations with professional

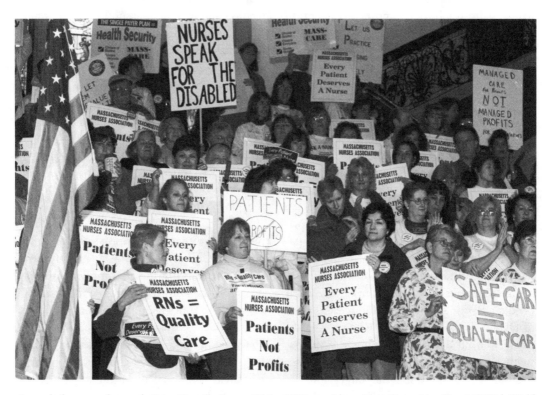

A crowd of nurses gathers at the State House in Boston, 6 May 1996, to celebrate Nurse Recognition Day. (AP Wide World Photos/Susan Walsh)

volunteers. The method was simple: to introduce developing nations to concepts already in place in industrialized nations. In 1968, Marie Manthey, instructor for the Peace Corps and vice president for nursing at Yale–New Haven Hospital, proposed the concept of primary nurse care, a one-on-one focus that bonded patient with nurse. Functioning as patient advocate, the nurse coordinated all phases of treatment, monitored diet, accompanied patients to a convalescent center or nursing home, and judged emotional health. Unusual difficulties, such as transfusing members of Jehovah's Witnesses with whole blood or plasma and gaining rights to treat the children of Christian Scientists, illustrate the core role of the primary caregiver as patient advocate, who educates associate health professionals on individual strictures. In some settings, discharged patients telephoned primary nurses to discuss adverse reactions to medication, problems with an incision or prosthesis, or the absence of home care. The increase in nurse morale slowed career drift from job to job and raised retention rates, one of the criteria of quality employment standards.

A parallel centralization of hospital care launched by Pat Baskin, senior nurse at Sir Charles Gardner Hospital in Perth, Australia, challenged the fragmentation of nurse care. Focusing on the problem-solving approach of community nursing, the project examined shared responsibility and accountability. Essentials of the model called for assignment of each patient to a specific general nurse for the length of the hospital stay. It became the primary nurse's responsibility to assess the patient on admission, construct a care plan, tend daily needs, and direct team members, who assumed responsibility when the caregiver was off duty. Baskin's concept prefigured the work of Dr. Cicely Saunders and the hospice movement. Central to both paradigms was the patient, who identified goals and assumed responsibility for selecting the target level of physical function. The patient's family or visiting staff joined the model as the patient re-

turned home or departed to a rehabilitation facility.

By the late 1970s, primary nurse care had become an essential. In 1976, Virginia Henderson addressed Commonwealth University in Richmond, Virginia, on the essence of nursing. Her well-worded assertions championed primary care by warning of the dangers of fragmentation: "No one category of health worker should stake out a claim to their share of the burden—say they will do this but not that—without reference to the shares claimed by other workers and the effect on human welfare if some essential tasks involved in health care are disclaimed or shunned, by all" (Henderson 1979, 2012). Henderson's focused, patient-centered nursing and decision-making called for a regrouping of traditions and new initiatives to suit a changing medical environment. While aiding patients, her speech also lifted nurses' morale and salvaged some on the brink of leaving the profession.

Unfortunately, the liberation of nurses from wearying, repetitive tasks such as hand-feeding and manual measurement of temperature and blood pressure did not end the profession's periods of shortages. Between 1945 and 1947, the growing need for nurses meant that practical nurses took on more duties. In the 1990s, the problems spawned legal and illegal importation of foreign nurses, often with suspect or bogus credentials. Adding to the era's problems was the disparity between metropolitan facilities and those in the boondocks. In the mid-1960s, Dr. Henry Silver of the University of Colorado School of Medicine initiated a project dispatching pediatric public health nurse-practitioners to carry vaccination, sight and hearing tests, emergency treatment, and routine examination and diagnosis to rural and tribal areas. With $500,000 from New York's Commonwealth Fund, established by Mrs. Stephen V. Harkness in 1918, he began a four-month pediatric training program before assigning nurses to high-risk areas. Bilingual nurse Susan Stearly, the first of his trainees, treated underserved Latino patients in Trinidad, Colorado, in the

1960s, covering routine childhood complaints and referring more complex needs to doctors. The concept remained in place a decade later. In a wellness clinic in Horseshoe Bend, Idaho, in the mid-1970s, nurse-practitioner Eleanora Fry treated a community of five hundred, offering X rays, lab tests, and medication along with family-centered counseling, education, and comfort.

A contributing factor to contemporary healing practices is the high ratio of registered and specialty nurses to practical nurses and aides. The concept of functional nursing, or nursing teams, arose from the doctoral dissertation of nursing instructor Dr. Eleanor C. Lambertsen. A New Jersey native and head of nursing education at Teachers College of Columbia University from 1961 to 1970, she advanced to the posts of dean and associate director of Cornell University–New York Hospital School of Nursing. Centering on individual patient needs, she brought together a variety of nurse specialists into working units led by registered nurses and doctors and augmented by practical nurses, aides, and physical and occupational therapists. With documentation of needs and responsibilities, she evolved a practical model to make the best use of ward personnel. Her idea, published by Teachers College Press as *Nursing Team Organization and Functioning,* spread to government facilities and professional organizations. She demonstrated the project among cancer patients at Francis Delafield Hospital in Manhattan. In 1970 and 1984, the American Nurses Association lauded Lambertsen for distinguished service and innovation through investigative study.

In the last quarter of the century, feminism, activism, and unionism began raising the consciousness of the female-dominated profession to think of themselves as valued, if underrated, medical professionals. As of 1980, the 1.4 million U.S. nurses constitute the largest segment of health professionals but seethed with turmoil and discontent, as demonstrated by grumbling, turnover, burnout, hassles with administrators, and low morale. Reporting to *Ms.* magazine in 1983, Diana Mason, founder of an independent nursing practice, targeted the dehumanized treatment in hospitals: "Most hospitals strip you of your control from the time you walk in the door. You are a patient. You must take off your clothes; you must wear their wristband, you cannot take your children, your family, or your friends with you" (Moccia 1983, 104).

In a mounting shift in power since World War II, the practice of medicine as big business downgraded nursing from patient care to a factory mentality. By 1965, Medicare and Medicaid sealed the fate of patients and staff as part of a growth industry intent on cost cutting. The result was militant, frustrated nurses moving from job to job in search of respect and satisfying patient contact. Sondra Clark, vice president of the National Union of Hospital and Health Care Employees, reduced the fault of modern medicine into a single image—the hurried nurse bypassing psychological needs to keep up with paperwork and an overprogrammed medical assembly line.

Worsening issues of autonomy, strikes and sex discrimination cases focused attention on the gap in pay between doctor and underling. Predominantly, the earnings of male personnel dwarfed those of females, at times as high as one hundred to one. Radical restaffing in the medical hierarchy forced more nurses from patriarchal, doctor-centered establishments into independent nurse-run clinics. Although the American Medical Association disdained ancillary care to patients without the consultation of a physician, storefront offices immediately found a clientele eager for good service, personal attention, and fees ranging from 80 to 85 percent of what doctors charged. Staffed by a fraction of the nation's seventy thousand nurse-practitioners, these medical clearinghouses profit from the work of the registered nurse who has added two years of graduate school after completing a four-year degree and hospital experience. Clinics typically concentrate on wellness and offer routine blood, urine, and pregnancy tests, treatment of home accidents and minor ills, and advice on stress, diet, exercise, and over-the-counter preparations. In forty-nine U.S. states, nurse-practitioners can prescribe mild drugs.

The success of the nurse-practitioner model was immediate. From home base at Chicken Soup Plus in Sacramento, California, Mary Baker made house calls and provided pre-employment physicals at half the fee doctors charged. A similar reduction of costs marked a parallel effort, Community Nursing Services for the Elderly in Elmyra, New York, run by Jean Sweeney-Dunn. To enhance the offerings of nursing clinics, Joanne Gersten's Erie Family Health Center in Chicago acquired nine staff physicians. In 1982, Kansas City nurse Elizabeth Dayani began a new trend in decentralized health care, American Nursing Resources, a financially promising employment referral service specializing in dietitians, therapists, and nurses.

Similar programs tailored nurse clinics to the community. Winner of the 1984 Wonder Woman Foundation award, Betty Baines Compton, one of the first nurse-practitioners to graduate from the University of North Carolina School of Medicine, operated a clinic in rural Orange County, North Carolina. Among her accomplishments were lobbying efforts to alter overprotective statutes hampering the work of field nurses, particularly in the areas of trauma, prenatal care, pediatrics, and adolescent health. In 1997, the success of a city clinic in midtown Manhattan was the subject of the *New York Times*'s critical review of the phenomenon. On the positive side, proponents and health maintenance organizations (HMOs) praised the quality and economy of providing primary care for minor complaints such as stomach upset, colds, and flu and monitoring such chronic conditions as diabetes, hypertension, and asthma.

The growth of space exploration created the need for a new breed of professional—the space nurse. An outstanding pioneer, Idaho native Dolores "Dee" O'Hara, managed NASA's human research office at the Ames Research Center. On loan from the U.S. Air Force Nurse Corps, she saw service in 1961 as administrative flight nurse at the Johnson Space Center and prepped astronauts for Project Mercury. While mediating between astronauts and biomedical investigators, O'Hara became the first woman in a key role in a space program. She gathered medical data on the effects of weightlessness on human anatomy, a job featured in the film *The Right Stuff* (1983). Along with nurse Shirley Sineath, she witnessed the successful launch of *Freedom 7* on May 1, 1961. She oversaw medical details of the next flight, which took Gus Grissom into space aboard *Liberty Bell 7* on July 21, 1961. On September 11, 1991, in Washington D.C., O'Hara received the Women in Aerospace Lifetime Achievement Award, which brought tributes from former astronauts John Glenn, Wally Schirra, and Deke Slayton.

Simultaneous with the growth of nursing in the space program, the military groomed its twentieth-century methods into a paradigm of flexibility. Following successes in the Korean and Vietnam wars, the MASH unit made no changes in basic setup and operation in the Gulf War. For the field soldier, the Department of Defense maintained its standard training of all soldiers in evaluating and treating casualties. With the threat of nerve agents looming from Iraqi threats to launch biological weapons as allied soldiers approached from Kuwait, all recruits learned to render first aid as well as perform the basic field treatments: to clear the throat of obstruction; perform cardiopulmonary resuscitation (CPR), field dress a limb or apply a tourniquet, dress abdominal, chest, and head wounds, prevent shock, splint fractures, and treat burns, heat stroke, and frostbite. For evacuating casualties to aid stations, they practiced the over-the-shoulder or fireman's carry as well as litter transport.

Rescue missions adapted the mobile hospital concept worldwide to treat epidemics, trauma, and malnutrition. In 1988, a volunteer-based field hospital operation placed the

Israeli Defense Force in Armenia to treat 2,400 earthquake victims. A second deployment in July 1994 provided three relief teams to 3,500 Rwandan refugees in Gama, Zaire. Essential to the missions was the training of corpsmen in first aid. In Zaire, the team effort required 21 nurses and paramedics to staff triage, a pediatric unit, and medical and surgical facilities. Nurses tracked patients, returned children to parents, and assigned unidentified children to orphanages. For ease of identification, nurses marked patient numbers on the skin with colored pens.

A brief return to war nursing in 1990 resurrected the MASH unit, which was officially introduced in Korea in 1950 and refined in the protracted Vietnam conflict. On December 8, as the army mobilized for Operations Desert Shield and Desert Storm, the Army activated the 807th MASH, led by Colonel Bradford Mutchler. The team's 188 members assembled in Paducah, Kentucky, three days later for transport from Fort Campbell by the 101st Airborne Division. Grown to 245 members, the staff underwent intensive briefing on nuclear, chemical, and biological warfare under desert conditions and issuance of gas masks and immunization for plague, cholera, and tetanus before deployment in Iraq. Wounded began arriving on February 25, and, in a one-hundred-hour ground war, the effort culminated in the treatment of seventy-six casualties, of whom two died, both dismembered from cluster bomb explosions after the cease-fire. By March 10, 1991, staff received the injured from burning oil refineries in Kuwait along with refugees and civilians injured from more cluster bombs, which killed six children. By April 10, the team had treated 1,007 patients and performed 122 surgeries. In all, there were eight deaths and four births.

Many of the heroic efforts in nursing in the last half of the twentieth century have occurred in certified specialties, including psychiatry, cardiac care, renal dialysis, gerontology, respiratory disease, burns, and trauma. One example of upgrading is the replacement of a two-year program with four-year training at the St. Francis School of Nursing in Hartford, Connecticut. Graduates who earn the title of advanced practice registered nurse enjoy a collegiality with doctors, with whom they team to practice psychiatry, cardiology, trauma, neonatology, and other demanding specialties. In a baccalaureate address, Patricia N. Grady, director of nursing research at the National Institutes of Health in Bethesda, Maryland, outlined the crucial role of nursing in the twenty-first century's demand for specialized and accessible health care.

One highly publicized example of specialty nursing, the treatment of crime victims, marked the violence of the age. Society has come to expect miracles from nurses in what author Dorothy Canfield Fisher wryly termed as putting "scrambled eggs back into the shell" (Maggio 1996, 186). During the mid-1990s, the subject of trauma nursing was the focus of the women's tribunal at the United Nations human rights conference. In Tulsa, Oklahoma, sexual assault nurse examiners (SANE) launched a novel program in 1995 to combat the nation's 100,000 annual rapes. The management concept quickly passed to Kingston, New York, Portland, Oregon, Tucson, Arizona, Anchorage, Alaska, and the entire states of Massachusetts and New Jersey.

As explained by clinical director Jessie Dragoo, forensic nurses remain on call to treat emergencies and to administer a seventeen-step rape exam. The SANE nurse typically undresses the victim over a large sheet of paper to preserve evidence, swabs the mouth, anus, and vagina, collects blood samples, and takes a cervical culture. To isolate exterior matter, she scrapes nails on each hand, combs the body for foreign hairs, and surveys for semen with ultraviolet light. She takes photographs with a colposcope to magnify cuts and bruises in the vagina and places evidence—hair, blood, semen, saliva, nails, skin—in the seventeen envelopes that come with each rape kit. The exam ends with counseling about human immunodeficiency virus (HIV) and a prescription for morning-after contraceptives and antibiotics to counter sexually transmitted diseases. A veteran of sixty exams, the nurse specialist, rather than a doctor, provides courts with expert witness as to the condition of the female pelvis, inside and out. The intent of SANE's careful preservation and presentation of evidence is to change a badly flawed investigative system that arrests only a third of rapists and convicts fewer than half of those charged with rape.

Response to disaster is another area of violence that has forged new resolve among nurses. According to Linda A. Williams, R.N., director of education at Oklahoma City's Presbyterian Hospital, the bomb blast that destroyed the Alfred P. Murrah Federal Building on April 19, 1995, underscored the need for planning and allocation of nurses and emergency workers. The organizational model that emerged from Oklahoma City's crisis is primed for the next multiple demand on treatment centers, whether from explosives or deployment of poison, nerve gas, or other terrorist methods. Personnel will wear color-coded armbands to identify nurses, physicians, and respiratory therapists. In addition to crowd control, communication, and supply, personnel will anticipate needs in triage, computerized axial tomography (CAT) and magnetic resonance imaging (MRI), surgery, shock and burns, and outpatient care. On-the-scene measures such as pinning patient information to clothing should alleviate problems with documenting treatment and prognosis. Disaster packets will contain preprinted and numbered identification bracelets and stickers for labeling X rays and lab specimens. For the sake of the staff, three-stage stress management to demobilize, defuse, and debrief will protect nurses from post-traumatic depression and malaise.

Mixed reviews of New Age healing brought controversy to Dolores Krieger, R.N., originator of therapeutic touch (TT), a mobilization of the body's own invisible electrical charge. Working with theosophist, or mystic, Dora Van Gelder Kunz, Krieger evolved the technique in the 1970s while teaching at the nursing school at New York University. Akin to Reiki, faith healing, and reflexology, the concept places the nurse-practitioner in active focus on a human energy field, a dynamic power source thought to maintain somatic balance and well-being. Nursing theorist Martha Rogers corroborated TT's effect based on a notion of the science of unitary human beings, a pan-dimensional theory that human beings share substance and power with environmental fields. As demonstrated by Linda Degnan at a lecture held on January 25, 1995, at Frankford Hospital in Philadelphia, the practitioner uses touch to differentiate between a tension headache and migraine. Nurses can learn the alternative healing skill in an eight-hour workshop. Support for TT is widespread in the nursing profession but largely anecdotal. The unsubstantiated method, which tens of thousands of TT proponents employ to comfort, relax, and relieve patients, ostensibly alters blood chemistry and repatterns the body's inner strength to promote healing. Members of the Rocky Mountain Skeptics protest use of hospital staff for a bizarre methodology that many in the medical community consider flawed and empirically untestable.

To prevent drug and alcohol abuse, Rutgers University sponsors Live for Life, a continuing cross-country nurse fellowship program begun in 1988 and aimed at facilitating the job of the school nurse. Essential to the consortium is a prioritizing of activities that enable the school nurse to learn about the community and school, to identify early signs of recreational and problem substance abuse, and to intervene in instances that threaten the at-risk adolescent. Adjunct programs assist students in conflict resolution and in dealing with the drug and alcohol dependency of their parents. Additional impetus for school nurse–led programs comes from National Alcohol and Drug Addiction Recovery Month programs. Held in September, the opening month of traditional school schedules, the school nurse's preteen and teen focus concentrates on decreasing criminal behaviors and treatment and recovery programs.

Overall, women's health came into its own from 1970 to 1990. The focus on abortion rights and HMOs made possible the profitability of gender-specific health centers. Aimed at middle-income women, these centers involved nurses, nurse-practitioners, and nurse-midwives at a high and sustained level of involvement and showcased empathetic attention as opposed to less specific gynecological care of traditional family practice. Essential to the staff-patient relationship were collaborative approaches, team-oriented problem solving, and education-centered prevention programs, the most successful being self-examination of breasts, mammograms, ultrasound, and Pap smears. Into the 1990s, a growing concentration on wellness and prevention also encouraged alternative procedures, including massage, herbal cures, diet and nutrition counseling, acupuncture, and holistic treatment as part of a comprehensive continuity of care.

A prospectus from WHO, "Nursing Beyond the Year 2000" (1994), anticipates the needs of the twenty-first century. As has been true throughout history, it is women and children who suffer the greatest lack of nursing care. Each year, 500,000 women die from neglect, abuse, or victimization. Their deaths accrue from female infanticide, genital mutilation, malnutrition, anemia, too early marriage, childbirth, unsafe abortion, sexually transmitted diseases, and domestic and random violence, rape, and incest. According to United Nations statistics, more than 80 percent of deliveries in sub-Saharan Africa are unmonitored by professional midwives or nurses. As a consequence of haphazard birthing or nonexistent health care, black women in sub-Saharan Africa are seventy-five times more likely to die than their contemporaries in western Europe.

WHO's tabulation of health care workers worldwide identifies most as nurses and midwives, especially in remote areas. Studies show that using these agents is cost-effective; however, because their tasks are labeled "women's work," governmental agencies and private or religious missions offer low pay and diminished status. Thus, the nurse-midwife's daily fare consists of substandard education, poor conditions, primitive facilities, no opportunity for advancement, and social ranking equivalent to unskilled laborers. In their subservient role, it is not surprising that they are in short supply in 95 percent of developing countries and in rural and tribal areas of 83 percent of the industrialized nations.

A philanthropic adjunct to native medicine can be found in the nurses and doctors of Médicins sans Frontières (Doctors without Borders), a Belgian-based mission that flies staff to distant areas in crisis. One volunteer, Norwegian midwife Kristin Liland, began serving Chitembo, Angola, in 1983 during civil unrest. Teaming with a Swedish doctor and logician, she managed problem pregnancies and births and instructed native nurse-midwives in current methodology, which was intended to upgrade the current record of seven surviving children out of every ten births. At work from dawn to sundown, she expected nighttime calls and traveled by plane to patients in isolated villages and refugee compounds. A compatriot, Dutch nurse Simon Van Den Berg, combated the civil strife, disasters, and epidemics of southern Sudan, which were fueled by drought and chronic hunger. Of her work among the world's poorest people, she said, "The situation is terrible. Mothers have no food. . . . We give them supplementary food. Every day recently two children die in our therapeutic feeding center" ("Doctors without Borders," www.dwb.org, 1).

As these trends illustrate, the future of nursing was already evident in the late 1990s. Increased demands on medical care resulted in more preventive measures, alternative approaches to care, and increased technological services, particularly dialysis and respiratory treatment. Among Native American healers, a proliferation of naturalists, counselors, herbalists, aroma therapists, and masseurs attests to a growing demand for Indian methods, not surprisingly, as a counter to the curtailment of treatment under tight HMO restrictions. In Zimbabwe in 1999, nurse midwives, such as Amie Bishop of the Program for Appropriate Technology in Health, offered a simple test for uterine cancer, a vinegar swab that increases the chances of cancer detection for women who are seldom screened. In service to all people, the nurses of the future will form the front line of caregivers aiding refugees, the homeless, the chronic mentally ill, and the vast population of AIDS patients worldwide, especially in Africa, Russia, parts of South America, and Indonesia. According to the consortium of contributors to the WHO report—Anne J. Davis and Margretta Madden Styles, University of California; Ruth Stark, Fiji; Nelly Garzon, National University of Columbia; and R. Margaret Truax, WHO nurse scientist—ominous trends reflect that "the vulnerable are becoming more vulnerable," a fact that is as old as human history ("Nursing Beyond" 1994, 16). The hope for the poorest nations is fuller collaboration of the health community and a sensitivity to the growing disparity between the ideal and the real.

See also: African-American Nurses; Cadet Nurse Corps; Cavell, Edith; Christian Nursing; Communism, Nursing under; *Curandera;* Disease; Farmborough, Florence; Galard, Geneviève de; Gender Issues in Nursing; Hale, Clara; Hasson, Esther; Hospice; Kenny, Elizabeth; Korean War; Lubic, Ruth; Midwifery; Native American Nursing; Navy Nurse Corps; Nazi Nurses; Nutting, M. Adelaide; Paget, Dame Mary Rosalind; Sanger, Margaret; Saunders, Dr. Cicely; Selassíe, Tsahaí Haíle; Spanish-American War; Stopes, Marie; Teresa, Mother; Vietnam War; World War I; World War II

Sources

Anteau, Carlene M., R.N., and Linda A. Williams, R.N. "What We Learned from the Oklahoma City Bombing." *Nursing* (March 1998): 52–55.

Baly, Monica E. *Nursing and Social Change.* New York: Routledge, 1995.

Black, James T. "North Carolina's Super Nurse." *Southern Living* (May 1984): 165.

Byerly, Dr. W. Grimes, personal interview, August 18, 1998.

Castro, Janice. "Florence Nightingale Inc." *Time,* July 14, 1986, 47.

"Doctors without Borders USA, Inc." http://www.dwb.org/index.htm.

"Does a Terminal Patient Have the Right to Die?" *Good Housekeeping* (May 1984): 81–84.

Dolan, Josephine A., R.N. *History of Nursing.* Philadelphia: W. B. Saunders, 1968.

"807th MASH." http://www.iglou.com/law/mash.htm.

"For 'New Nurse': Bigger Role in Health Care." *U.S. News and World Report,* January 14, 1980.

Freudenheim, Milt. "As Nurses Take on Primary Care, Physicians Are Sounding Alarms." *New York Times,* September 30, 1997.

Glickman, Robert, R.N. "Nurse Martha Rogers, a Critical Look." http://www.voicenet.com/~eric/tt/rogers.htm.

Glickman, Robert, R.N., and Ed. J. Gracely. "Therapeutic Touch: Investigation of a Practitioner." *The Scientific Review of Alternative Medicine* (spring/summer 1998): 43–47.

The Grolier Library of Women's Biographies. Danbury, Conn.: Grolier Educational, 1998.

Henderson, Virginia. "Preserving the Essence of Nursing in a Technological Age." *Nursing Times,* November 22, 1979, 2012–2013.

Heron, Echo. *Condition Critical: The Story of a Nurse Continues.* New York: Ivy Books, 1994.

———. *Intensive Care: The Story of a Nurse.* New York: Ivy Books, 1987.

Heyman, Samuel N. "Airborne Field Hospital in Disaster Area: Lessons form Armenia and Rwanda." *Prehospital and Disaster Medicine,* January–March 1998, 14–28.

Higham, Robin, and Carol Brandt, eds. *The U.S. Army in Peacetime.* Manhattan, Kans.: Military Affairs/Aerospace Historian Publishing, 1975.

Jamieson, Elizabeth, and Mary F. Sewall. *Trends in Nursing History.* London: W. B. Saunders, 1949.

Jaroff, Leon. "A No-Touch Therapy." http://www.pathfinder.com/time/magazine/archive/1994/941121/941121.health.html.

Kilborn, Peter T. "Nurses Get New Role in Patient Protection." *New York Times,* March 26, 1998.

Kirkpatrick, Mary K., R.N. "Women's Issues and Wellness." *Health Values* (March-April 1989): 38–39.

Koblinsky, Marge, Judith Timyan, and Jill Gay, eds. *The Health of Women: A Global Perspective.* Boulder, Colo.: Westview Press, 1993.

Kraegel, Janet, and Mary Kachoyeanos. *Just a Nurse.* New York: Dell Books, 1989.

Kratz, Dr. Charlotte. "Letter from Australia: The Aborigines." *Nursing Times,* November 22, 1979, 2042–2043.

———. "Letter from Australia: Primary Nursing." *Nursing Times,* October 18, 1979, 1790–1791.

Lamps on the Prairie: A History of Nursing in Kansas. Emporia.: Kansas State Nurses' Association, 1942.

Langewiesche, Wolfgang. "ICU—Newest Thing in Nursing." *Reader's Digest* (November 1964): 208–214.

Looker, Patty. "Women's Health Centers: History and Evolution." *Women's Health Issues* (summer 1993): 95–100.

Mackey, Robert. "Discovery of the Healing Power of Therapeutic Touch." *American Journal of Nursing* (April 1995): 27–33.

MacMillan, Patricia. "Si tibi deficiant medici. . . ." *Nursing Times,* August 2, 1979, 1298–1299.

Maggio, Rosalie, ed. *The New Beacon Book of Quotations by Women.* Boston: Beacon Press, 1996.

Magner, Lois N. *A History of Medicine.* New York: Marcel Dekker, 1992.

Marshall, Marilyn. "Nursing: Not for Women Only." *Ebony* (December 1981): 48–51, 54.

McDonnell, Virginia B., R.N. *Dee O'Hara: Astronauts' Nurse.* Edinburgh: Rutledge Books, 1991.

"Medicine Women." http://www.powersource.com/powersource/gallery/womansp/medwomen.html.

"Médicins sans Frontières Volunteer Profiles." http://www.msf.org/aboutyou/vols/profiles/1nor.htm.

Meehan, T. C. "Therapeutic Touch and Post-Operative Pain: A Rogerian Research Study." *Nursing Science* (summer 1993): 69–78.

Milgram, Gail Gleason. "School Nurses: Counselors' Overlooked Allies?" *The Counselor* (July-August 1998): 10–11.

Miller, Floyd. "A Celebration for Mary Donnelly." *Reader's Digest* (October 1973): 122–127.

Miller, Virginia. "Characteristics of Intuitive Nurses." *Western Journal of Nursing Research* (June 1995): 305–316.

Moccia, Patricia. "If Nurses Had Their Way." *Ms.* (May 1983): 104–106.

"Nurse! Nurse!" *Time,* April 12, 1954, 79–80.

"Nursing Beyond the Year 2000." Geneva: WHO, 1994.

O'Ceirin, Kit, and Cyril O'Ceirin. *Women of Ireland: A Biographical Dictionary.* Galway: Tir Eolas Newtownlynch, 1996.

O'Connor, Rose, and Jack Mahon, eds. *A Woman of Aran: The Life and Times of Bridget Dirrane.* Dublin: Blackwater Press, 1997.

Patchett, Ann. "The Comfort of Strangers." *Vogue* (October 1995): 90–94.

Plum, Sandra D. "Nurses Indicted: Three Denver Nurses May Face Prison in a Case That Bodes Ill for the Profession." *Nursing* (July 1997): 34–35.

"Qualification and Utilization of Nursing Personnel Delivering Health Services in Schools." http://www.aap.org/policy/01584.html.

Quintero, Carmen. "Blood Administration in Pediatric Jehovah's Witnesses." *Pediatric Nursing* (January-February 1993): 46–48.

Raybould, Elizabeth. "An Opportunity Within Our Grasp." *Nursing Times,* August 16, 1979, 1389–1390.

"Rebellion Among the 'Angels.'" *Time,* August 27, 1979, 62–63.

Richardson, Sharon L. "Transformation of the Canadian Association of University Schools of Nursing." *Western Journal of Nursing Research* (August 1995): 416–434.

Roberts, Marjory. "Hands-On Healers." *U.S. News and World Report,* August 5, 1991.

Rubbelke, Leona. "Hawaii Studies the Problems of Its Smallest Citizens." *Nursing Outlook* (November 1954): 568–571.

Rubin, Rita. "Study: Vinegar Could Screen for Cervical Cancer." *USA Today,* March 12, 1999, p. 9A.

Saxon, Wolfgang. "Eleanor C. Lambertsen, 82; Introduced Use of Nurse Teams." *New York Times,* April 10, 1998.

———. "Hildegard Elizabeth Peplar, 89, Developer of Psychiatric Medicine." *New York Times,* March 28, 1999, p. 51.

Schorr, Thelma M., R.N., and Anne Zimmerman, R.N., eds. *Making Choices, Taking Chances: Nurse Leaders Tell Their Stories.* St. Louis: C. V. Mosby, 1988.

Schweitzer, Jane, R.N. *Tears and Rage: Nursing Crisis in America.* Fair Oaks, Calif.: Adams-Blake, 1995.

Seelye, Katharine Q. "U.S. Strikes at Smuggling Ring That Exploited Foreign Nurses." *New York Times,* January 15, 1998.

The Soldier's Manual of Common Tasks. Washington, D.C.: Headquarters Department of the Army, October 3, 1983.

"Special Award for Dee O'Hara." *Astrogram.* NASA, Ames Research Center, September 27, 1991, 1.

Spingarn, Natalie Davis. "Primary Nurses Bring Back One-on-One Care." *New York Times Magazine,* December 26, 1982, 26.

"Therapeutic Touch." http://www.therapeutic-touch.org/html/touch.html.

"Voices from the Past . . . Visions of the Future." http://www.ana.org/centenn.htm.

"Where Doctors Don't Reach." *Time,* July 22, 1966, 71–72.

Witteman, Betsy. "Transitions at St. Francis's Century Mark." *New York Times,* July 6, 1997.

Zalumas, Jaqueline. *Caring in Crisis: An Oral History of Critical Care Nursing.* Philadelphia: University of Pennsylvania Press, 1995.

Zungolo, Eileen, R.N. "A Study in Alienation: The Nurse Practitioner." *Nursing Forum* (1968): 38–49.

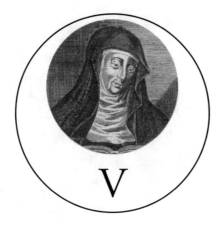

V

Vietnam War

From the Tonkin Gulf Resolution in August 1964 and President Lyndon Baines Johnson's order of Marines into Da Nang in 1965 to troop withdrawal in 1973, the Vietnam War was the United States's longest and bitterest struggle. The rigorous task of nursing in Vietnam derived from the devastating wounds inflicted on American personnel and indigenous civilians by automatic weapons, land mines, and napalm, a gasoline-based gel causing catastrophic burns. Many casualties were so peppered with shrapnel from mortars, rockets, and AK-47 fire that teams of professionals x-rayed whole bodies and then worked together to remove shards to save the patient from receiving additional anesthesia. In addition to battle wounds, treatment of skin ulcers, attention to paraplegics, and preoperative and postoperative procedures, nurses encountered such tropical diseases as cholera, malaria, bubonic plague, and jungle rot as well as tetanus and bites from snakes, spiders, and monkeys. Some devoted off-hours to volunteer work at orphanages, refugee centers, and the Qui Nhon leprosarium near the 67th Army Evacuation Hospital. The wisest eased the weight of daily sorrows with good humor, such as jokes about helmets that wouldn't fit over hair curlers and beds too low to accommodate a full-busted nurse in flak jacket during an alert.

The Vietnam War was a high-water mark for battlefield survival. The combined efforts of corpsmen, MedEvac helicopter crews, combat nurses, specialists, and surgeons reduced mortality to below 2 percent, which contrasted with the World War I rate of 5 percent, World War II's rate of 3.3 percent, and the Korean War's rate of 2.7 percent. The steady drop did what Florence Nightingale predicted in the previous century—diminished fear of dying in the field boosted morale and military efficiency. Obviously, saving lives of trained soldiers was a win-win situation in terms of victories, cost reduction, and lives. Mobile army surgical hospital (MASH) units (Figure 3), engineered for amphibious landings near the end of World War II, offered a miniature medical army composed of general practitioners, general surgeons, neurosurgeons, orthopedists, thoracic and urologic surgeons, anesthesiologists, internal medicine specialists, and nurses.

Among the most difficult jobs was triage, the French word for the process of selecting which patients to treat, which to delay, and which to let die. In tight situations, abandoning the third category freed personnel and equipment to save those most likely to sur-

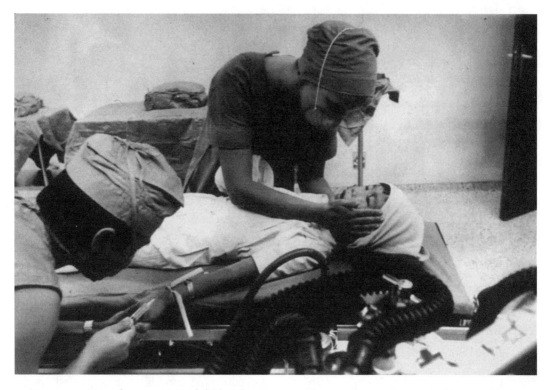

An American nurse comforts a war-injured child while a Vietnamese doctor applies anesthesia at the Center for Plastic and Reconstructive Surgery, Saigon. (Archive Photos)

vive. According to Elizabeth Norman's *Women at War: The Story of Fifty Nurses Who Served in Vietnam* (1990, 37), nurses "concentrated on keeping some men alive and did not think about those who might die. The pace was fast and the judgments mechanical." Nursing staff faced the added moral dilemma of treating soldiers alongside Vietcong wounded, including the enemy women and children recruited as saboteurs. The method was the inverse of the egalitarian method used back home in civilian hospitals, as was the unwritten policy to treat Americans first.

Reception of incoming wounded began with a quick study of the dog tag, which gave the particulars of name, blood type, and religion, and evaluation of the first aid checklist that corpsmen wired to casualties detailing morphine, plasma, packing, and other measures initiated in the field. Within antiseptic, well-lighted, air-conditioned suites, each patient received care, medication, and sterile dressings in a setting that guaranteed the best chance of recovery. Fearful sights and smells assaulted the staff, as in the treatment of a soldier seared by napalm: "By now, he was covered with a sickly blue-green slime, called pseudomonas, a common bacterial infection among severely burned patients. I could barely look at the kid while we scraped away the infected dead tissue, trying to get down to a viable area so he might have some chance of healing" (Van Devanter 1983, 93).

Stabilized patients passed from frontline MASH units to a total of sixteen hundred military beds in the facilities of Guam, the Philippines, and Japan or to navy hospital ships, the *Sanctuary* and the *Repose*. The doomed, such as those with massive head wounds, died untended behind screens of a receiving ward as staff raced to save the salvageable. These hard choices of war forged a tight camaraderie among nurses, doctors, corpsmen, and evacuation pilots.

Losses derived from Red Cross data specify people killed in Vietnam and honored at the national Vietnam Veterans Memorial in Washington, D.C., a moving remembrance known as "The Wall," which names the 58,183 dead in order by date of death, first to last. Among the nurses who died are these:

- Pennsylvanian Carol Ann Drazba and Elizabeth Ann Jones of South Carolina were killed in a helicopter crash near Saigon on February 18, 1966, along with pilot Charles Honour, Jones's fiancé.

- Nurses Eleanor Grace Alexander, Jeremy Olmstead, Hedwig Diane Orlowski, and Kenneth Shoemaker died in a plane crash November 30, 1967, outside Qui Nhon.

- Nurses dying of disease include Pamela Dorothy Donovan of Massachusetts, who succumbed to an Asian virus and pneumonia July 8, 1968, in Qui Nhon, and North Carolinian Annie Ruth Graham, a veteran of World War II and the Korean War, who was felled by a stroke in Tuy Hoa and died August 14, 1968.

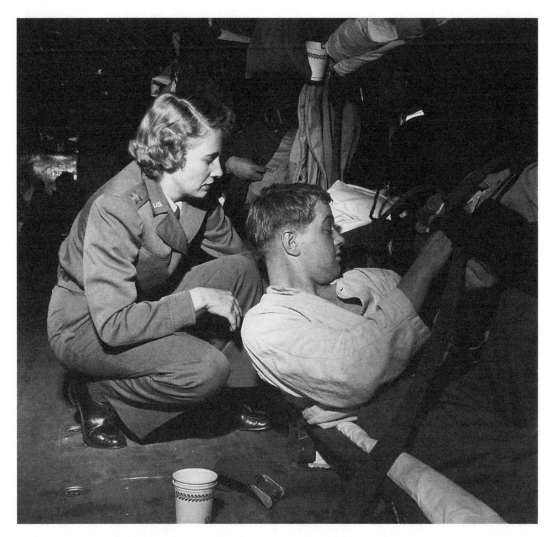

A U.S. army nurse cares for wounded soldiers aboard one of the many aircraft turned hospitals during the Vietnam War.
(Corbis/Genevieve Naylor)

- Captain Mary Therese Klinker of Indiana, along with 243 Vietnamese children, died in a plane crash during Operation Babylift April 9, 1975, shortly before the fall of Saigon.
- Sharon Ann Lane of Canton, Ohio, is the only nurse to die of enemy fire, incurred at the 312th Evacuation Hospital in Chu Lai on June 8, 1969, when a Vietcong rocket exploded shortly before 6:00 A.M. A bronze monument at Aultman Hospital School of Nursing, Canton, Ohio, depicts her. Her medals include the Purple Heart, Vietnamese Gallantry Cross, and Bronze Star.

Another tribute to these victims and to the eleven thousand nurses serving during the conflict came from nurse Diane Carlson Evants, who solicited donors for the Vietnam Women's Memorial adjacent to the Wall. Composed of four figures atop sandbags and sculpted by Glenna Goodacre in 1993, the depiction of a nurse tending a fallen soldier along with two sister nurses is the first official honor the nation has paid to U.S. women in the military.

In the war's aftermath, first-person writing bore little resemblance to the memoirs of the Civil War, Spanish-American War, Korean War, or the two world wars. In 1985, Keith Walker's compendium *A Piece of My Heart: The Stories of Twenty-Six American Women Who Served in Vietnam* highlighted the eyewitness accounts of women in war. Head Nurse Rose Sandecki of the 12th Evac Hospital at Cu Chi took as her personal creed the Medical Corps's motto: "Preserve the Fighting Strength" (p. 9). In memory of the twenty thousand patients passing through the wards, she explained the necessity of putting up an emotional wall to numb the feelings and keep body and mind operational. Maureen Walsh, a navy nurse at U.S. Naval Support Activity Hospital, Da Nang, recalled a specific moment—turning just in time to prevent a female prisoner of war from stabbing her with a fork. Dot Weller, a rehabilitation volunteer with the American Friends Service Commit-

tee, carried home nightmares and flashbacks of multiple atrocities and the sufferings of everyone involved.

After Walker's anthology came more unburdening. Shirley Lauro composed *A Piece of My Heart* (1992), an adaptation for stage. Opening at the Manhattan Theatre Club in 1991, it earned the Barbara Derning Foundation award for its compelling study of combat nursing. A brutally impersonal introduction from head nurse Whitney welcomes protagonist Martha to Vietnam: "'Red Alert' means you are in immediate danger—a direct rocket hit. Or a sapper attack. When the enemy penetrates our perimeter. If you're off-duty you crawl immediately into a bunker. If you're on duty, put on flak jackets, helmets, and put the mattresses *over* all your patients, then take cover yourself, while someone guards the door" (Lauro 1991, 38).

The motet of voices interweaves Whitney's orders with the naiveté and curiosity of Martha, Sissy Maryjo, and Leeann, who blanch at the growing intensity of incoming wounded. Among them are two Vietnamese children with their hands lopped off. In Act II, Martha, a Vet Center counselor, turns her postwar energies to counseling student nurses. Boldly, she asserts, "It will *not* be your glorious childhood dream of Florence Nightingale come true! It will be hell on earth! You will *never* get over it afterwards! So get ready! Get set!" (Lauro 1991, 118). In the final scene, Leeann, perusing the Wall by candlelight, receives a lei of yellow ribbons from a "double amp" who salutes her with, "This is for you! Welcome home!" (Lauro 1991, 124).

In 1992, North Carolinian Winnie Smith, an idealistic captain in the Army Nurse Corps, published *American Daughter Gone to War: On the Front Lines with an Army Nurse in Vietnam,* a Book-of-the-Month Club alternate selection. A witness to the carnage of Pleiku, she spoke passionately of the horrific job of nursing at the front. Before her introduction to Vietnam, she absorbed the horror of wounds with a daily round of duties at Fort Dix, New Jersey, particularly care of infections: "Squirting syringes of sterile solution into the cavity flushed out pus, and its sickly sweet smell permeated the room as it drained into a basin. Men with such wounds stared in stony silence as the foul secretions spilled out of them" (Smith 1992, 19).

In the intensive care unit of Saigon's Third Field Hospital and Long Binh's 24th Evac, tropical heat and battle fatigue exaggerated the burden of colostomies, decerebrates and decorticates, cardiac arrests, phosphorus flare and napalm burns, and the "expectants" dying behind yellow screens. As casualties arrived from combat to the helicopter pad, a steady flow of wounded kept her ever on edge. She deliberately numbed her brain as her language degenerated to the "fuck," "goddamn," and "shit" of frontline grunts, an emotional outlet not countenanced in her family back home.

In the emotional slide that permeates the book, Smith grows morbid. At one point she yells for surgeons while treating a profound wound—"squash meat," hospital slang for a limb so crushed by tank treads that it undulates like a Slinky toy: "It's a bloodbath, blood pouring from everywhere. The dressings are soaked with crimson blood; the fatigues are clotted with burgundy blood. Puddles of it ooze over the gurney. More runs from bottles into both arms, but anyone can see they won't be enough" (Smith 1992, 131). Smith later experienced a shelling at An Khe, which, in its peremptory outburst, was less terrible than silent moments in the intensive care unit (ICU) with men too shot up to survive.

Beset by nausea, depression, hysteria, and flashbacks, Smith reacquainted herself with home. Among an apathetic nation that devalued her service, like so many others she felt misplaced and sought invisibility in April 1975, at war's end. Postwar trauma dogged her grasps at normality until a suicide attempt in spring 1983. It was the writing of Lynda Van Devanter in *Home before Morning: The Story of an Army Nurse in Vietnam* (1983) that began the process of silencing ghosts, granting absolution for a war she could not halt. Smith's uneasy truce with sorrow and rage began with nightmares of the Mekong Delta and alcohol and marijuana desensitizing her heart, but the long cure ended with peace in 1984 among fellow veterans. At a Veterans Day ceremony in Washington, D.C., she wept at the Wall, her fingers caressing letters carved in granite in tribute to death in a far-off land. When President Ronald Reagan thanked the men who had given their all in the war, Smith led the call, "What about the women?" (Smith 1992, 326).

Two contemporaries of the era of unburdening, Lynda Van Devanter and Joan A. Furey, published *Visions of War, Dreams of Peace: Writings of Women in the Vietnam War* (1991) as a voice for women who had been largely overlooked in other war compendia. A salute to the "woman veteran," the poems introduced women's accomplishments during a terrifying conflict. By expressing women's place in the domain of men, the work enlarged on the wartime contributions of fifteen thousand military nurses, USO staff, Red Cross volunteers, and logistical and altruistic staff. By ending the silence, the collection offered comfort at the same time that it conferred honor and dignity. Along with Gloria Emerson's *Winners and Losers: Battles, Retreats, Gains, Losses, and Ruins from the Vietnam War* (1992), Frances Fitzgerald's Pulitzer Prize–winning *Fire in the Lake: The Vietnamese and the Americans in Vietnam* (1972), Lady Borton's *After Sorrow: An American among the Vietnamese* (1995), and Wendy Wilder Larson and Tran Thi Nga's *Shallow Graves: Two Women in Vietnam* (1986), the poetry collection took its place within the male-dominated tradition of war reflection and reportage.

In the preface to *Visions of War,* the editors cite Florence Nightingale's obsession with war and explode the myth that women have no reason to create war literature. They comment: "For centuries women have gone to war. Frequently they have disguised themselves as men, often not had their true identities known. If thought of at all, they were usually thought of as saints or as sinners. And, almost always, they have been dismissed as unimportant after the war is over" (Van Devanter and Furey, 1991, xxi).

To express the poignant realities of women's memories of service amid harsh, unrelenting conditions, the collection returns repeatedly to the experience of nurses:

- Sharon Grant, a member of the Army Nurse Corps from 1970 to 1971, recalled work as an operating room nurse in Pleiku and Qui Nhon. To her, the press of work blended into "Tuesdaywednesdaythursdayfriday—saturdaysunday" (Van Devanter and Furey, 1991, 5).
- To Kathleen Trew at the 93rd Evacuation Hospital in Long Binh from 1969 to 1970, Saigon was a fetid stench and bustle that had supplanted the beauty of a city once called the "Oriental Pearl." In "Pre-Op," she envisioned the death of a doorgunner, who is already moribund as she wipes dust from his forehead. "Road Show" recaptured the wounded as "broken puppet soldiers" (Van Devanter and Furey, 1991, 61).
- Twenty years after service, Kathleen F. Harty, veteran emergency room and ICU nurse at the 36th Evacuation Hospital at Vung Tau, composed "One Small Boy," a searing memory of a child dying on a gurney.
- From service at the 24th Evacuation Hospital in Long Binh, Mary Beyers Garrison also carried a memory two decades. In "Recovery," she observed a flirtatious patient who regretted that he could no longer work as a steeplejack.
- From memories of Da Nang Naval Hospital from 1969 to 1970, Marilyn McMahon reprised the role of listener and counselor to wounded men. In "The Kid" and "In This Land," she recreated the horror of a body floating nearby and the death of a man suffering inoperable brain stem damage. "Wounds of War" imagined the rage of patients who can never heal.

- The terror took shape clearly in the words of Lady Borton, a Quaker veteran of three volunteer tours who recalled amputees learning to walk and lauds Vo Thi Truong, who resided under a hospital bed in the paraplegic ward to nurse her mother, a victim of a bullet to the spinal cord. Of the effects of napalm, Bolton reported:

  He had no nose,
  only two holes in the middle of his face.
  His mouth was off to the side.
  One eye was gone;
  There was a hollow in his forehead above
     the other.

  (Van Devanter and Furey, 1991, 13)

- With "In Memoriam," Joan Parrot Skiba, an emergency room nurse at the 18th Surgical Hospital in Camp Evans and the 71st Evacuation Hospital in Pleiku, relived triage and the fateful winnowing out of those too far gone to save.
- Linda Spoonster Schwartz, a nurse at the U.S. Air Force Hospital in Tachikawa, Japan, described drama in "Images at the Wall," a montage of protest, Agent Orange, and a nation's apathy at veterans returning from an unpopular war.
- In "Death Speaks" and "Tears," Norma J. Griffiths dredged up suppressed sorrows of the 67th Evacuation Hospital in Qui Nhon, which she served as emergency room and triage nurse.
- Helen DeCrane Roth, Navy operating room nurse on the USS *Sanctuary,* relived person-to-person contact with "Eyes," in which she treated a man whose face was destroyed. She spoke of shared humanity and a mask that hid her pity for a brutal wound that couldn't be repaired.
- Another volunteer, Bobbie Trotter, recalled Red Cross work with starving war babies whose survival depended on the next supply shipment, which arrived too late for one child.

- From work with the Red Cross at Cam Rahn Bay, Cu Chi, Quang Tri, and II Field Force, Penni Evans composed "Left Behind," a paean to her emotional maiming from seeing so much human suffering.
- In "Dark Angel," Joan Arrington Craigwell, a flight and triage nurse in Cam Ranh Bay and the 26th Casualty Staging Unit, gamely claimed "it don't mean nothin'/'cause us black gals are tough," a self-serving boast that salves her sanity (Van Devanter and Furey, 1991, 76).
- "Where Are They Now?" captured the ambivalence of Margaret Flatt, a nurse with the 36th Evacuation Hospital in Vung Tau.
- In "Our War," Diane Carlson Evans, nurse at Pleiku's 71st Evacuation Hospital and Vung Tau's 36th Evacuation Hospital, tackled the issue of the women whose service was discounted or ignored.
- A veteran of the neurosurgical ICU at the 24th Evacuation Hospital in Long Binh, Diane C. Jaeger's "My War" recounted the callous antiwar spirit of American citizens. Thirteen years after returning home, she felt that part of her lay buried in Vietnam.
- Dana Shuster, who worked in the operating room, emergency room, and ICU during two tours of duty with the Army Nurse Corps, dramatized contact with severely wounded men in "Mellow on Morphine"; in "Like Emily Dickinson," she nicknamed "Lonnie from Tennessee," "Danny from LA," "Chief the Ute," and "Pocho from Arizona" (Van Devanter and Furey, 1991, 73). In "Like Swans on Still Water," she relived "a crazy-shift morning,/when I've worked through the night and I'm too tired to care" (Van Devanter and Furey, 1991, 17).
- Editor Joan Furey, a postoperative/ICU nurse at Pleiku's 71st Evacuation Hospital, spoke of a "Vigil," a parade of men reduced to maimed stumps that pushed her compassion to the limit of tolerance. "Some Days" recalled the eighteen years that anger and regret coursed through her psyche.
- Penny Kettlewell, a veteran of tours at the 67th Evacuation Hospital in Qui Nhon and the 24th Evacuation Hospital in Long Binh, observed a nun in "Sister Mary," a tribute to tenderness and prayer. In "The Coffee Room Soldier," Kettlewell retreated beyond emotion after coming upon a shattered corpse on the coffee room floor.
- With "Saving Lives," Mary O'Brien Tyrrell, head nurse at the D2 Air Evac Ward at a naval hospital on Guam, spoke of a medic called "Doc" whose name she found on the Wall. In "Unseen," she recalled the Tet offense and the aftermath of burns, broken bones, and severed arteries.
- Sara J. McVicker's tour with the 71st Evacuation Hospital undergirded "Montagnard Bracelets," a stark image of blood that corrodes the metal, and "Crying," a vignette of suppressed emotion.
- Bernadette Harrod of the Army Nurse Corps served in the operating room at Phu Bai's 22nd Surgical Hospital. In "Even Now," she told of two decades of feeling abandoned and forgotten.
- Writing seventeen years after the war, Mary Pat O'Connor, a Red Cross volunteer at Camp Kue Army Hospital in Okinawa, unleashed bitter accusations in "Seventeen Summers after Vietnam."
- Janet Krouse Wyatt, veteran of ICU and emergency room service at the 71st Evacuation Hospital in Pleiku, recalled nurses' isolation in "Our Own Parade." She spoke in tight parallels in "We Went, We Came," a tribute to the healing engendered by the Wall.
- Joyce A. Merrill, Air Force nurse with the critical care unit at Cam Ranh Bay, asked that observers "Look Into my Eyes and See," a plea for compassion for forgotten veteran nurses.

- In "Cheated," Mary Lu Ostergren Brunner, veteran of Pleiku's 71st Evacuation Hospital, saw a "very long year" as a progression of victims about whom she must remain cool and objective (Van Devanter and Furey, 1991, 45).
- Lou McCurdy Sorrin, who served in the ICU at Cu Chi's 12th Evacuation Hospital and Qui Nhon's 67th Evacuation Hospital, guarded personal pain and isolation in "Confessional," which begged a blessing after two decades of private grief.
- In March 1999, LeAnn Thieman recalled a more hopeful war effort. In April 1975, she participated in "Operation Babylift," an adoption program that airlifted one hundred infants to the United States. Aboard a C-5A cargo jet, she and eight other attendants anchored babies in twenty-two cardboard boxes for the chancy flight through enemy territory. As the heavy load exited the danger zone, the nurses cheered.

Sources

Byerly, Dr. W. Grimes, personal interview, August 18, 1998.

Emergency War Surgery. Washington, D.C.: Department of Defense, 1958.

Lauro, Shirley. *A Piece of My Heart.* New York: Samuel French, 1992.

Norman, Elizabeth. *Women at War: The Story of 50 Military Nurses Who Served in Vietnam.* Philadelphia: University of Pennsylvania, 1990.

"Operation Babylift." *Newsweek,* March 8, 1999.

Sherr, Lynn, and Jurate Kazickas. *Susan B. Anthony Slept Here: A Guide to American Women's Landmarks.* New York: Times Books, 1994.

Smith, Winnie. *American Daughter Gone to War: On the Front Lines with an Army Nurse in Vietnam.* New York: William Morrow, 1992.

Van Devanter, Lynda. *Home before Morning: The Story of an Army Nurse in Vietnam.* New York: Warner Books, 1983.

Van Devanter, Lynda, and Joan A. Furey, eds. *Visions of War, Dreams of Peace: Writings of Women in the Vietnam War.* New York: Time Warner, 1991.

Walker, Keith. *A Piece of My Heart: The Stories of Twenty-Six American Women Who Served in Vietnam.* Novato, Calif.: Presidio, 1985.

"The War: Working against Death." *Time,* December 31, 1965, 62–63.

Vincent de Paul, Saint

An apostle of charity and originator of Christian nurse care among beggars in the seventeenth century, Vincent de Paul, a saint of the Reformation era, founded the order of Lazarists or Vincentians. He was born of humble origin on April 24, 1581, in Pouy, France, and attended boarding school with the Franciscan Fathers at D'Acqs. While tutoring aristocratic children, he completed his education at the College de Foix of the University of Toulouse and took priestly vows on September 23, 1600. After capture by North African pirates in 1605 on a voyage from Marseilles to Toulouse, he was sold into slavery in Tunis to a Christian who released him after two years' service. The ordeal instilled a sympathy in Vincent de Paul for the most wretched and hopeless human beings. He rose to the post of royal chaplain at the court of Henry IV under Queen Margaret of Valois, whose connections with Count Philip de Gondi's family brought Vincent a tutoring job in 1609.

While tending to parish work in Châtillon-les-Dombes in 1617, Vincent realized that dispatching food parcels to the hungry was not enough. The work required trained hands to hand-feed, examine, bandage, and nurse suffering peasants who had nowhere else to turn. To carry out this work, he drew on funds from the Countess de Gondi and formed the Confraternity of Charity, a circle of lay nurses who served the public. In 1624, he became the principal of the mother house, named Saint-Lazare.

In 1629, Vincent sought the assistance of Louise de Gras, later known as St. Louise de Marillac, a Parisian widow educated at the Dominican Convent at Poissy who dedicated her life to religious service. As supervisor of the 130 branches of charity nurses, she systematized the distribution of food and clothing at Montmirail and traveled from station to station stocking dispensaries with medicines and herbs. A tenderhearted woman, Louise served as head nurse and carried out Vincent's injunction to bathe, nourish, and comfort the suffering in person. For her ministrations, she and her order earned the thanks of the lowly.

Within four years, Louise's followers assembled in Paris on November 29, 1633, to Father Vincent's newly commissioned Daughters of Charity. Clad in blue-gray tunics, simple woolen aprons, and white collars, they topped their serviceable habit with the flared *cornette,* a winged cap that distinguished the order. According to Vincent's direction, they ranged beyond the confines of headquarters at Saint-Lazare to live in rented quarters along city streets and to serve in hospital wards, where they watched by bedsides. One of the prefatory stages in the evolution of nursing, Vincent's sisters placed themselves in service to doctors and remained obedient and respectful of medical orders. The concept spread worldwide, forming the first official network of religious nurses, whose reputation grew during the Napoleonic wars, in the Crimea, and on the battlefields of the American Civil War.

In 1634, Vincent established Les Dames de Charité (Ladies of Charity), another cadre of

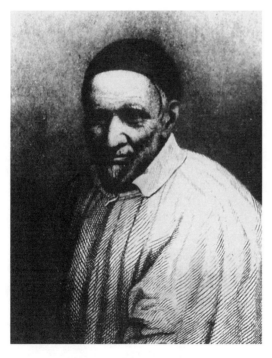

St. Vincent de Paul (U.S. Library of Medicine)

aristocratic women who served the sisters as an auxiliary force. With headquarters at the Hôtel Dieu, Paris's hospice for the poor, these literate women read from the Bible and provided spiritual comfort as well as monetary assistance to charitable works. The symbiosis of religious nurses and women's auxiliary worked well to carry out Vincent's intent of channeling supplies, money, and good works to the places they were most needed. Among galley slaves and veterans of the Thirty Years War (1618–1648) and in prisons, workhouses, and asylums for the infirm and insane, the sisters extended the love of the Vincentians.

Upon learning the wretched conditions in which unwanted babies were treated, Vincent reorganized La Couche, a French foundling center, to halt the practice of selling poor children into slavery or turning them into clever street beggars. With the combined efforts of Louise de Marillac, the Daughters of Charity, and the Ladies of Charity, he rescued abandoned waifs, spirited them away by night in closed wagons, and parceled them out to foster parents or to his own orphanages. After Louise's death on March 15, 1660, Father Vincent maintained his mission until his death.

In 1737, Vincent de Paul was declared a saint. His statue was the only one to survive the violence of mobs who desecrated Paris's Pantheon during the French Revolution. In 1833, Frederic Ozanam, under the tutelage of Sister Rosalie Rendu, founded the St. Vincent de Paul Society, which remains a strong arm of Catholic benevolence with three thousand chapters in Europe, Asia, Africa, and North America. Pope Leo XIII named St. Vincent the patron of charities in 1885. Louise de Marillac was canonized March 11, 1934.

See also: Christian Nursing; Civil War; Public Health Nursing

Sources

Baly, Monica E. *Nursing and Social Change.* New York: Routledge, 1995.

Bentley, James. *A Calendar of Saints.* London: Little, Brown, 1993.

Cohn-Sherbok, Lavinia. *Who's Who in Christianity.* Chicago: Routledge, 1998.

Griffin, Gerald Joseph, and H. Joann King Griffin. *Jensen's History and Trends of Professional Nursing.* Saint Louis, Mo.: C. V. Mosby, 1965.

Hallam, Elizabeth, general ed. *Saints: Who They Are and How They Help You.* New York: Simon and Schuster, 1994.

McKown, Robin. *Heroic Nurses.* New York: G. P. Putnam's Sons, 1966.

Ranft, Patricia. *Women and the Religious Life in Premodern Europe.* New York: St. Martin's Press, 1996.

"St. Vincent de Paul." http://www.catholic.org/saints/saints/vincentdepaul.html.

"Vincent de Paul and Louise de Marillac, Compassionate Servants and Saints." http://www.cptryon.org/vdp/vdp-ldm/index.html.

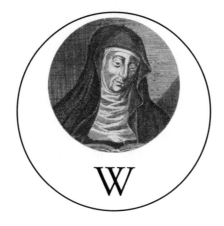

Wald, Florence

The developer of the Yale Study Group that brought the United States into the hospice movement, Florence Wald, a 1998 inductee of the National Women's Hall of Fame, is best known for pragmatic work sessions with nurses, attendants, physical therapists, and other caregivers to relieve the feelings of isolation and helplessness among the dying. In an April 1998 interview with Jane Kolleeny, a researcher into the Connecticut Department of Correction's care of terminally ill patients, Wald defined the hospice philosophy succinctly: "Hospice is an interdisciplinary comfort-oriented care that allows terminally ill patients to die with dignity and humanity with as little pain as possible in an environment where they have mental and spiritual preparation for the natural process of dying" ("Interview," www.npha.org, 3). Wald considers it appropriate that numerous professionals—doctors, nurses, counselors, chaplains, social workers, and volunteers—work together to deliver "palliative care, symptom management, and family support." Reflecting on poor people surviving in crumbling neighborhoods and alienated from the more affluent, she estimated the importance of hospice to a terminally ill person not in pain-free days or hours but in the boost to self-value and self-image.

In 1963, Wald invited Dr. Cicely Saunders to join her staff at the Yale School of Nursing, where Wald had served as dean since 1958. Two years later, Wald resigned to study in Europe. By spending a sabbatical at St. Christopher's Hospice in Sydenham, England, she absorbed the groundwork already done in the European movement to humanize care for the dying. In 1969, Elisabeth Kübler-Ross's best-selling *On Death and Dying* was published, providing over five hundred interviews with terminal patients, a sobering, enlightening source for Wald's project, which she hoped would assist visiting nurses and facilitate home monitoring and treatment for patients who chose to die at home among family.

As a model, Wald established an interdisciplinary team. With a grant in 1969 to analyze the needs of the dying, she coordinated a two-year study of twenty-two patients through Yale–New Haven Hospital, enhanced by frequent consultations with Saunders. Commenting on success in overcoming patient tentativeness and fear, Wald lauded the lighter moments the team created: "I admire the nurses who, through music or a phrase, can get a whole group of people—patients, families, nurses—into a dialogue. It's a constant dance, in a way, of getting a sense of what's going on and then taking risks" ("Interview," www.npha.org, 6).

Most of the patients Wald encountered remained at home until their final three months of life and were stable enough to make decisions for themselves. According to her observations, the newfound autonomy was difficult for physicians, who were not accustomed to this reversal of the power structure or to the collective input of patient, family, and staff. She published "The Interdisciplinary Study for Care of Dying Patients and Their Families" (1971), a perceptive analysis of the wishes of the terminally ill. The work assisted the legislative initiative of Senators Frank Church and Frank E. Moss, who, in 1974, launched a bill to provide federal funds for hospice care.

Although the request for congressional funding failed, Wald's study group triggered a tremendous response nationwide. Accounting for the groundswell, she noted, "People had experience in their lives of cancer patients being bombarded with intensive treatment, where the families and patients were suffering. . . . The families, by seeing how death could be handled, were able to keep their relationships open with the patient in a way that they couldn't before" ("Interview," www. npha.org, 2).

Wald attributes the project's popularity to its ability to educate frightened families, especially those of dying prison inmates, a growing segment of society. She remarked on prisoners' "tremendous regret or renunciation, or maybe anger, discontentment and unwillingness to accept bitterness," all feelings exaggerated by their confinement. By offering a humanistic approach—patience, listening, compassion, forgiveness—in an era of faceless, mechanized health management systems, Wald's natural approach links death to the span of human experiences—being born, maturing, rearing a family, and coping with end-of-life dilemmas.

Sources

"The History of Hospice." http://www.cp-tel.net/ pamnorth/history.htm.

"Interview with Florence Wald." http://www.npha. org/intjwald.html, April 22, 1998.

Siebold, Cathy. *The Hospice Movement: Easing Death's Pains.* New York: Twayne, 1992.

Wald, Lillian D.

A blend of nurse and social worker, Lillian D. Wald, a practical idealist, devoted her career to treating people she characterized as "hyphenated Americans," the poor immigrants of New York City. Among her many social betterment projects, she established the Henry Street Settlement to serve Italian, Hungarian, and black tenement dwellers and promoted the creation of the federal Children's Bureau, the watchdog agency over child labor and health. She became an activist for nonviolence, trade unions, feminism, education, and civil rights and influenced other projects aimed at social change.

Born in Cincinnati, Ohio, to merchant Marcus D. "Max" Wald and homemaker Minnie Schwarz Wald, on March 10, 1867, Wald was the progeny of two Jewish families who fled European revolutions in 1848. She grew up in Rochester, New York, in a warm, loving extended family. In public school, she enjoyed art, literature, math, and science, a balance that served her well in adulthood. While observing her older sister Julia in childbirth, Wald determined to train as a nurse. Because Vassar College rejected her at age sixteen, she studied at New York Hospital, completed her training in 1891, and worked in the New York Juvenile Asylum, an orphanage for young children. In 1892, she took postgraduate course work at the Women's Medical College.

As a public health nurse, a term she coined in 1893, Wald hoped to improve hygiene, preventive care, and wellness in the city's Lower East Side, where poor immigrants lived in misery. Amid broken pavement and steps, reeking toilets, dirty furnishings, and curbside refuse, she entered the pathetic dwellings that housed large families and their boarders. Of her first home visit, she commented: "That morning's experience was a baptism of fire. Deserted were the laboratory and academic work of college. I never returned to them. . . . I rejoiced that I had training in the care of the sick that in itself would give me an organic relationship to the neighborhood in which this awakening had come" ("Lillian Wald," www.JWA.org). Like other visiting district or public health nurses, she accepted each home situation as the best the family could do and earned only what clients were able to pay.

The late 1890s buoyed Wald's idealism. With the assistance of colleague Mary Brewster, a graduate of New York Hospital, in 1893 Wald established the Visiting Nurse Service. Two years later, she received from mentor Jacob Schiff the gift of a settlement house at 265 Henry Street, an address known through nursing histories as the site where community health service began. Her firsthand experience preceded a lecture series at Columbia University in 1899, the impetus to the school's permanent nursing and health department. By 1903, the district system was treating forty-five hundred patients annually in eighteen districts. Total one-on-one visitations produced 35,035 home visits, 3,524 convalescent calls, and 28,869 first aid treatments. In a 1907 speech on district nursing, she proclaimed that district nursing "has been used since the beginning of history to carry propaganda as there has been always an enthusiastic belief in the possibility of the nurse as teacher in religion, cleanliness, temperance, cooking, housekeeping, etc." (Coss 1989, 66). The impact of localized care for the poor called for standards and the creation of the National Organization of Public Health Nurses, with Wald as its first president. The program received a subsidy from Metropolitan Life Insurance Company in 1909, when Wald's staff began treating policyholders.

Along with teaching public health principles and practicing medicine among the needy, Wald enlarged her Henry Street Settlement House by adding a convalescent center, summer field trips, a library, vocational training, insurance partnerships, and a savings bank. The Henry Street meeting room was the setting of the 1909 National Negro Conference, forerunner of the National Association for the Advancement of Colored People. At the 1914 women's peace parade to keep the United States out of war in Europe, Wald declined a position of honor, but countenanced a marching contingent of Henry Street nurses dressed in their familiar blue uniforms. She recruited Governor Charles Evans Hughes to investigate the exploitation of the poor in public works projects. Her notes on workplace hazards led to the formation of the State Bureau of Industries and substantial workplace reform under the Joint Board of Sanitary Control, which monitored factory ventilation, pollution, lighting, sanitation, and fire protection.

With the improvement in economic conditions for workers and families, Wald turned her attention to public education, which she characterized as the stronghold of democracy. In addition to neighborhood humanitarianism, she pressed for school lunches and the hiring of Lina L. Rogers as the city's first public school nurse. In an address to the 1915 graduates of Vassar College, Wald summarized the life of Florence Nightingale as an ennobling portrait of the nurse: "Florence Nightingale lifted the vague, casual, though kindly and devoted, *feeling* of women into organized, efficient, and invaluable service; she enlarged the nurse's visitation to sympathy for great groups outside her family or particular tribe" (Coss 1989, 81).

Wald published *The House on Henry Street* (1915), a testimonial to her settlement mission, which provided children with a safe play yard and attention to their social and physical needs. As a result of her innovation, New York City established a system of municipal playgrounds. The intense concern for children involved her in the public schools, where she advocated special education instruction for learning-disabled and handicapped students. The school board complied by adding a department of special education and hiring Elizabeth Farrell as its first special needs teacher.

By the end of her life, Wald had shouldered a number of crusades. Skilled at organization and publication, she distributed antiwar and disarmament handbills, supported antiwar socialist Emma Goldman, and offered the Henry Street building as wartime headquarters for the Red Cross and Food Council. She promoted women's suffrage and spearheaded the Children's Bureau Baby Saving Campaign. As a lobbyist, she championed prohibition and pursued federal funding for home nursing. Along with Harriet Knight, Irene Lewisohn, and Yssabella Waters, she toured Hong Kong, China, Russia, and Japan to study the social systems of other nations. In 1918, she halted some of her crusades to treat victims of the Spanish influenza outbreak and to recruit volunteers and attended the 1920 Red Cross conference in Cannes, France.

Housebound in Connecticut by a stroke in 1925, Wald composed *Windows on Henry Street* (1934), a reflection on social and economic changes published in 1934. A consummate friend maker, she welcomed pacifists and idealists of the caliber of Albert Einstein, Jane Addams, Sylvia Pankhurst, and Eleanor Roosevelt. By 1933, ill health forced Wald to pass supervision of the Henry Street Settlement to Helen Hall, who was later honored with Helen House, a residence for single mothers with toddlers.

In 1937, at the Henry Street celebration of Wald's seventeenth birthday, Sara Delano Roosevelt read a letter from her son, President Franklin Roosevelt, praising Wald's unselfish devotion to human worth and dignity. At Wald's death from cerebral hemorrhage on September 1, 1940, eulogist Paul Kellogg, writing for the *New York Times,* noted, "Every nation in Europe was represented among the people that found the way to the house on Henry Street" (Coss 1989, 14). From Wald's work came the American Union against Militarism, American Civil Liberties Union, International Conference of Women for Peace, and League of Nations Child Welfare Division. For creativity, dedication, and courage, Wald earned the accolades of social leaders at a posthumous testimonial at Carnegie Hall, where the mayor, governor, and president's encomiums honored four decades of humanitarianism.

Sources

Brainard, Annie M. *The Evolution of Public Health Nursing.* Philadelphia: W. B. Saunders, 1922.

Coss, Clare. *Lillian Wald: Progressive Activist.* New York: Feminist Press, 1989.

Daniels, Doris Groshen. *Always a Sister: The Feminism of Lillian D. Wald.* New York: Feminist Press, 1995.

Kraut, Alan. *Silent Travelers: Germs, Genes, and the "Immigrant Menace."* New York: Basic Books, 1994.

"Lillian D. Wald." http://www.JWA.org/exhib98/wald/lwbio.htm.

———. http://www.netsrq.com/~dbois/wald.html.

McHenry, Robert, ed. *Liberty's Women.* Springfield, Mass.: G. C. Merriam, 1980.

Sherr, Lynn, and Jurate Kazickas. *Susan B. Anthony Slept Here: A Guide to American Women's Landmarks.* New York: Times Books, 1994.

Yost, Edna. *American Women of Nursing.* Philadelphia: J. B. Lippincott, 1947.

World War I

The most mechanized conflict in history, World War I inflicted cataclysmic disease, wounds, permanent disability, and death as a result of global hostilities. The advent of the machine gun, aerial warfare, and mustard gas altered the type and severity of wounds, which afflicted officers and enlisted men alike. To combat need on an unprecedented scale, war departments recruited, trained, and dispatched medical personnel. Owing to the foresight of those who created the Voluntary Aid Detachments (VAD) in 1909 and to nursing organizer Ethel Gordon Fenwick in setting standards for registered nurses, England was able to assign 276 territorial, or community, nurses to the front as early as June 1915. General hospitals rapidly expanded capacity to five and six times the normal patient load. At home, patriotic women supplanted those professionals who left domestic posts to go to the front. Overall, the ratio of trained nurses to beds was one to sixteen for the military but dropped to one to nineteen for civilian facilities.

World war found the United States in a state of preparedness. Unlike the abysmal fail-

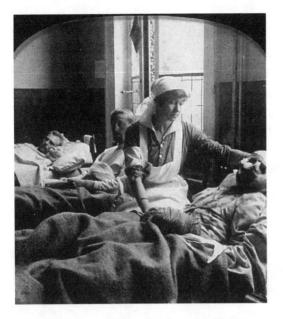

A nurse cares for wounded soldiers during World War I at a hospital in Antwerp, Belgium. (Archive Photos)

ure accompanying the Spanish-American War, the military drew on the four-hundred-member Army Nurse Corps, established in 1901 by Dr. Anita Newcomb McGee, who sought to end the prejudice against female nurses that Dorothea Dix, Dr. Elizabeth Blackwell, Clara Barton, Kate Cumming, and others had encountered during the Civil War. Additional staff came from the Navy Nurse Corps, which Paul Hamilton, secretary of the navy, had proposed in 1810, but which was formally begun in 1908. The Red Cross mobilized in 1914 when hostilities began in Europe and appointed Helen Scott Hay to supervise nurses in the Balkans and Lucy Minnigerode to the Polytechnic Institute in Kiev, Russia, where Czar Nicholas II presented her the Cross of St. Anne. Nurse Emily Simmons, a highly decorated English staff member at Roosevelt Hospital in New York, was the first U.S.-trained nurse to aid the Allied cause. She volunteered as a Red Cross nurse in 1914 and left England for Serbia, later serving as inspector of European hospitals. The European headquarters, later managed by Hay, was already sorting a deluge of requests to treat, feed, clothe, and house refugees, displaced persons, orphans, and military prisoners.

On the American home front, by 1917, the American Red Cross, under the command of Jane A. Delano, director of nurses, profited from an overnight growth of local chapters and volunteer nurses. A meeting of the Committee on Nursing on June 24, 1917, found Adelaide Nutting organizing the stars of the profession: Dr. Winford H. Smith and Annie Warburton Goodrich, representing the American Hospital Association; Lillian Clayton, president of the National League of Nursing Education; Dora Thompson, chief of the Army Nurse Corps; pacifist and social reformer Lillian Wald; and Delano, Red Cross spokesperson. The steering committee advanced to federal recognition on August 2 as it estimated the number and classification of nurses already available at 200,000 and drafted a system of keeping the reserves at maximum levels to accommodate the military, which projected its need for nurses at thirty-five thousand.

The war gave female nursing professionals an opportunity to influence both military and public health. In February 1918, Annie Goodrich, president of the American Nurses Association and associate professor of nursing at Columbia University, accepted the job of chief inspector of United States Army hospitals and named Elizabeth C. Burgess as her assistant. By May 25, the two completed a plan of action to increase proficiency of bedside caregivers by halting the practice of rotating corpsmen in wards and instituting the primary nurse care found in civilian hospitals. To ensure the best in military ward nursing, Goodrich tabulated a survey of national nursing resources, which unanimously proposed an army training center. Her competence and leadership impressed the secretary of war, who named her dean of the Army School of Nursing in 1919. A colleague, Isabel Maitland Stewart, published recruitment pamphlets for the Nursing Council on National Defense as well as *Developments in Nursing Education*

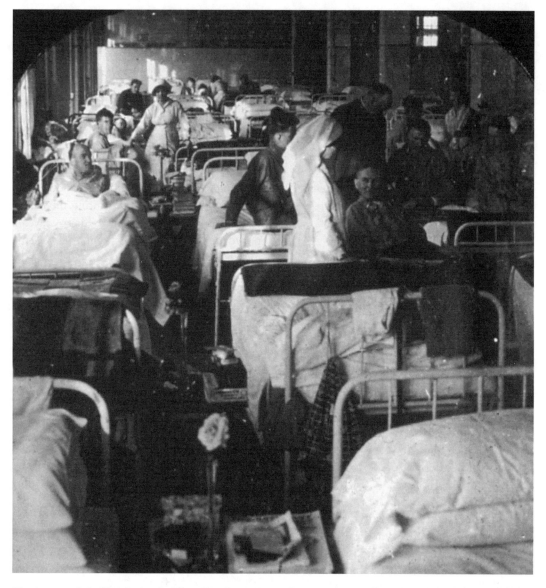

Nursing wounded soldiers back to health at Convalescent Hospital No. 5 in New York. (Archive Photos)

since 1918 (1921) and *A Short History of Nursing* (1920), coauthored by Lavinia L. Dock.

Initially, more than ten thousand nurses enlisted to work in Europe, China, Puerto Rico, Hawaii, and the Philippines. A major recruiter of nursing staff, Anne A. Williamson, a veteran of the Spanish-American War and author of *50 Years in Starch* (1948), answered a crisis call for staff to combat the flu epidemic. She justified lowering her usually high standards for Red Cross nurses this way: "It was no time to be too particular, and those who applied were put on duty to be watched over carefully by the head nurses" (Williamson 1948, 197). There were many sick and one fatality among the women she selected to staff Navy Base No. 3 in Scotland.

The workload ranged to eighteen-hour days with no time off from tending up to nine thousand patients in each facility, for a grand total of 184,000. Exacerbating conditions were poison gas alerts, when all personnel had to don helmets and masks until the danger of chlorine, phosgene, and mustard fumes had passed. By the end of the fighting, three hundred nurses had died, the majority from fatigue, pneumonia, and Spanish influenza. Only five succumbed to shells and explosions. One, Helen Fairchild, who died in France on January 18, 1918, of liver failure caused by mustard gas after reportedly giving her mask to a soldier, was honored with a military funeral and interred at the Somme American Cemetery, Bony, France.

Diarist Maude Mortimer remarked on the odors of ether, blood, and sickness blended with the steam of sterilizing agents. Her account, *A Green Tent in Flanders* (1918) captured the drama of a night of "bad cases." She focused a taut, objective memory on a boy who appeared dead from a gut wound. "They do all they can to bring him round. He revives. They chloroform him, open the abdominal cavity. Floods of dark blood well out. We are too late" (Kalisch and Kalisch 1978, 316). Another nurse, Shirley Millard, composed *I Saw Them Die* (1936), a hellish phantasm of muddy puttees, fetid field dressings, bayonet gashes streaming with intestinal matter, buckets of detached limbs, and a double thigh wound left to drain into sphagnum moss. To Millard, the scenes ehoed Dante's *Inferno*. On the Serbian front, war produced disgruntlement in Mary Gladwin, a decorated Red Cross nurse from Akron, Ohio, who saw the human frailty of armed conflict. She muttered, "War will end when youth is taught what war really means—the conflict of the greedy" (Sherr and Kazickas 1994, 353). In retrospect, Red Cross nurse Florence Farmborough wrote of her experience at the Russian front: "Will they be remembered? But who could remember all those many thousands and thousands?" (Van Devanter and Furey, 1991, 72).

A slender memoir from France, *Mademoiselle Miss* (1916), glimpsed the daily activities of an anonymous young girl at a French hospital on the front line near the Marne River. She praised an orderly named Gaston for performing the minutiae of a nurse's chores—cutting cottons, folding compresses, stocking bandages, and polishing instruments as well as changing linens and hurriedly shifting patients from ambulance to bed. Unaccustomed to trauma nursing, she described an operating room scene during which she extracted shrapnel and bits of cloth from a deep wound and bragged about contriving two boards and gauze thongs to bind a soldier's crippled feet into normal position. On November 28, 1915, she detailed the "living skeleton with wounds in back and hands and shoulder that they brought me filthy and nearly dead from another pavilion. . . . I diagnosed him as a case of neglect and slow starvation, and treated him accordingly—malted milk, eggs, soap, and alcohol to the fore" (Cabot 1916, 47).

In treating him, she worked an hour and a half daily at his dressing and fed him drop by drop. Jubilant at his survival, she exulted, "He's *saved,* and that makes up for much" (Cabot 1916, 48). By February 27, 1916, her spirits sank as the war moved to Verdun. She remarked, "We know nothing except that every frontier town is crowded with wounded, and the battle rages. . . . The suspense is agonizing" (Cabot 1916, 69).

To the nursing staff, authorities doled out a haphazard allotment of war decorations and honors. Among exceptional volunteers was Amelia Greenwald, a public health nurse from Gainesville, Alabama, and organizer of a farm women's program for the National Council of Jewish Women, who served the Red Cross in the Meuse-Argonne sector and earned the Victory Medal for battlefield nursing at Verdun. Others' rewards were less tangible. Mary Margaret Robinson Godfrey, a troop ship nurse aboard the largest transport, *Leviathan,* reported General John J. Pershing's respect for military nurses aboard ship. When he bowed his head toward their table, she said, "That's for all nurses, not just us" (Sterne 1996, 54). It was not until 1944 that military nurses earned the rank, rights, and privileges of officers, and nurses also acquired retirement and disability benefits.

In a study of gender roles among German nurses of World War I, Regina Schulte notes that female attendants were anomalous, being neither male heroes nor stereotypical *hausfraus*. Of the ninety-two thousand nurses and assistant nurses employed by the Imperial Commissar and Military Inspector, the prominent figures were 19,703 Red Cross volunteer nurses and the "Empress's Army," members of the Vaterländische Frauenvereine (Women's Associations), founded by Queen Augusta in 1866 after the Austro-Prussian War. Additional staffing came from sisters from Lutheran mother houses, Orders of St. John, Silesian and Rhenish-Westphalian Knights of Malta, Royal Bavarian Knights of St. George, Sisters of Mary, and Grey Sisters of St. Elizabeth in Breslau. Diarists Emmy von Rüdgisch and Bertha von der Schulenburg attest to the pro-war patriotism that impelled these German women to the front.

Experience changed the German gung-ho anticipation to immediate shock, as stated by Minna Stöckert: "The wounded they bring us are almost all dying. All of them very young men. I am seeing mass death for the first time. Horrifying!" (Abrams and Harvey 1997, 129). She listed the inconvenience of overcrowding, with casualties packed four deep on sacks and straw. Inadequate supplies required her and other nurses to take down curtains and cut them into bandages. Rations tapered down to water and dry army bread. The flow of wounded from the doctors' tables at the tent door continued through the night, leaving Stöckert to murmur, "So many died in the night. It is so terribly cold and frightful here." The resultant rebellion of nurses at the rudeness and arrogance of doctors won out in the face of the women's solidarity and self-confidence.

Postwar emotions were mixed. Overall, German nurses valued the Iron Cross award; in *Frontschwestern: Ein Deutsches Ehrenbuch, 1936* (The Western Front: A German Paean, 1936), Elfriede von Pflugk-Harttung named as her highest reward the name "sister," which

men and officers called all nurses. Yet, the double burden of humiliation and defeat overshadowed demobilization, raising feelings of scorn and contempt. In *Kamerad Schwester 1914–1919* (Comrade Sister) (1934), veteran Helene Mierisch wrote: "How differently we had imagined our homecoming and reception! . . . This cannot possibly be the end of such a heroic struggle" (Abrams 1997, 134). A veteran of the Russian front, Elfreide Schulz, clenched her teeth and mourned the nation's shattered ideals and loss of honor.

One Canadian nurse, Emily Long of Saskatoon, demonstrated the patriotism and verve of a Red Cross hero. A graduate of nurse training in Iceland, she had emigrated to Canada in the early 1900s and retrained at Neepawa, Manitoba, before volunteering for the war effort. From a hospital on England's Channel coast, she advanced to superintend the home of Lady Willingdon of Wales, who offered her residence as auxiliary wards for the overflow from overcrowded hospitals. Honored by the Canadian League and by Queen Alexandra, the queen mother, Long earned praise for adaptability to a war that put new and unforeseen demands on British subjects. On return to Wadena, she duplicated her wartime flexibility by establishing the Wynyard Hospital in a former hotel and a cottage hospital in a small residence as well as running Edam Hospital at Kerrobert.

In reflection, Chief Nurse Julia Catherine Stimson, author of *Finding Themselves* (1918), developed an unshakable faith in nurses, who had met the wartime demands and proved themselves worthy. In her estimation, the steamy atmosphere, ether, filth, and operating room odor was not so onerous as the hands-on experience of "sewing and tying up and putting in drains while the doctor takes the next piece of shell out of another place. Then after fourteen hours of this with freezing feet, to a meal of tea and bread and jam, then off to rest if you can, in a wet bell tent in a damp bed without sheets, after a wash with a cupful of water" ("Nurse Helen Fairchild," http://raven.cc.ukans.edu).

The army's first female major, Stimson headed the Army Nurse Corps until 1937, providing competent management and growth into the pre–World War II period. The achievements of combat nurses brought out boosterism in Frances Payne Bolton, who helped found the Army School of Nursing and, in 1923, endowed the Frances Payne Bolton School of Nursing at Western Reserve University in Cleveland, Ohio. She remained a friend to the profession throughout the interwar era, when, as a member of Congress, she kept the importance of nurse care in the forefront of legislation.

See also: Farmborough, Florence; Kenny, Elizabeth
Sources

Abel-Smith, Brian. *A History of the Nursing Profession.* London: Heinemann, 1960.

Abrams, Lynn, and Elizabeth Harvey, eds. *Gender Relations in German History: Power, Agency and Experience from the Sixteenth to the Twentieth Century.* Durham, N.C.: Duke University Press, 1997.

Cabot, Dr. Richard C. "Introduction." *Mademoiselle Miss.* Boston: W. A. Butterfield, 1916.

Dodge, Bertha S. *The Story of Nursing.* Boston: Little, Brown, 1965.

Dolan, Josephine A., R.N. *History of Nursing.* Philadelphia: W. B. Saunders, 1968.

Farmborough, Florence. *With the Armies of the Tsar: A Nurse at the Russian Front, 1914–1918.* New York: Stein and Day, 1974.

Fessler, Diane Burke. *No Time for Fear: Voices of American Military Nurses in World War II.* East Lansing: Michigan State University Press, 1996.

Fraser, Evelyn G., R.N. *Fifty Years of Service: History of the School of Nursing of the Roosevelt Hospital, New York City.* New York: Alumnae Association of the Roosevelt Hospital School of Nursing, 1946.

Griffin, Gerald Joseph, and H. Joann King Griffin. *Jensen's History and Trends of Professional Nursing.* Saint Louis, Mo.: C. V. Mosby, 1965.

Gudmundson, Darrell. "Pioneer of Saskatoon, Emily Long, Pioneer Nurse." http://www.nyherji.is/~halfdan/westward/emily.htm.

Hyman, Paula, and Deborah Dash Moore. *Jewish Women in America.* New York: Routledge, Chapman and Hall, 1997.

Kalisch, Philip, and Beatrice J. Kalisch. *The Advance of American Nursing.* Boston: Little, Brown, 1978.

Lamps on the Prairie: A History of Nursing in Kansas. Emporia: Kansas State Nurses' Association, 1942.

McHenry, Robert, ed. *Liberty's Women.* Springfield, Mass.: G. C. Merriam, 1980.

"Nurse Helen Fairchild: My Aunt, My Hero." http://raven.cc.ukans.edu/~kansite/ww_one/medical/MaMh/MyAunt.htm.

"Salute to the Military." *Daughters of the American Revolution Magazine* (November 1990): 852–853.

Sterne, Capt. Doris M. *In and Out of Harm's Way: A History of the Navy Nurse Corps.* Seattle, Wash.: Peanut Butter Publishing, 1996.

Van Devanter, Lynda, and Joan A. Furey, eds. *Visions of War, Dreams of Peace: Writings of Women in the Vietnam War.* New York: Time Warner, 1991.

Williamson, Anne A., R.N. *50 Years in Starch.* Culver City, Calif.: Murray and Gee, 1948.

Yost, Edna. *American Women of Nursing.* Philadelphia: J. B. Lippincott, 1947.

World War II

In the late 1930s, Hitler's assault on Czechoslovakia brought civil defense and air raid plans for England and a call for soldiers, medical staff, and civilian volunteers. Trained and assistant nurses formed the Civil Nursing Reserve, later augmented by the British Red Cross Society and St. John's Ambulance Brigade. Within six years, the figures rose dramatically: Queen Alexandra Imperial Military Nursing Service went from 640 to 12,000; Queen Alexandra Royal Navy Nursing Service from 78 to 1,341; and Princess Mary Royal Air Force Nursing Service from 171 to 1,215.

American nursing authorities, led by Julia C. Stimson, Stella Goostray, Grace Ross, Mary Beard, and Mary Roberts, met in New York on July 29, 1940, to study the prewar situation. The group formed the Nursing Council on National Defense, a massing of forces that enlisted nursing associations, military nurse corps, the Children's Bureau, the Department of Indian Affairs, and the Veterans Administration. Aided by President Franklin D. Roosevelt's push for clinics, nursing homes, and hospitals, the national alert reduced the surprise of American entry into global combat seventeen months later.

At the beginning of the war, the staffing of segments of the army's medical service put

Figure 3: The organization of medical services during World War II, from aid stations to hospitals

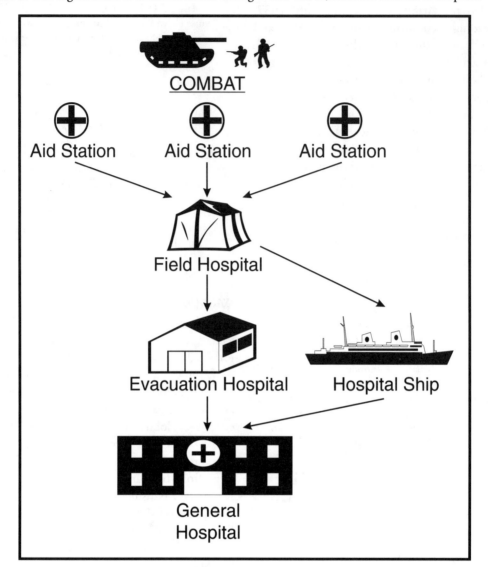

women as far back from heavy fighting as possible. Within the first twenty-four to forty-eight hours after a wound was inflicted, corpsmen from the same division treated the casualty at an aid station within 1–3 miles of the front in range of gunfire. For minor colds, cuts, sprains, and bruises, the application of first aid often put the soldier back in action and spared the division the trouble of ordering a replacement. For more serious illnesses or wounds requiring transfusion, suturing, and minor surgery, aids bore the casualty by litter to an ambulance and then to a field hospital located 5–8 miles behind the front. Staffed by doctors, nurses, and orderlies, these tent receiving centers offered rapid diagnoses and treatment but afforded the patients only a modicum of hospital comfort. The most pressing medical and surgical cases were transported or airlifted away from combat to an evacuation hospital on land or ship for stabilization and immediate care and on to a general hospital for more sophisticated surgery, such as amputation, treatment of a major organ, or repair of multiple facial or skull fractures.

In the first weeks of mobilization, casualties were disarmingly low, but winter brought bron-

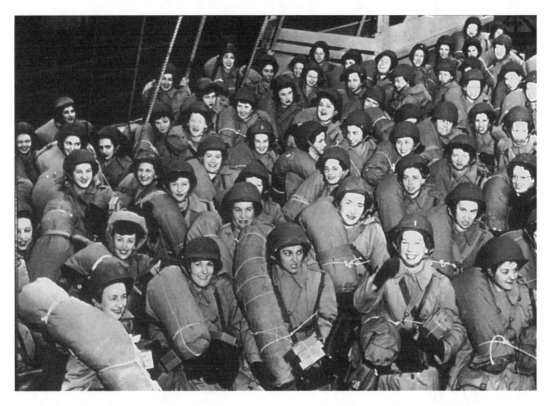

U.S. Army nurses, helmeted and wearing full field dress, arrive in England via transport ship after having crossed the Atlantic Ocean. (Archive Photos/Imperial War Museum)

chitis and pneumonia. While recruiting nurses, Major Julia Stimson, the army's first female major, warned probationary nurses: "War is three-quarters waiting and boredom and tiresomeness, and it is one quarter of the hardest work you ever heard of in your life or ever dreamed of" (Cowdrey 1994, 106). Her prophecy proved grimly true after the tide of war turned following the evacuation of British forces from Dunkirk and successive dive-bombings by German planes. Treatment stations struggled with the load of soldiers and refugees as the German blitzkrieg sharpened its claws on the vulnerable. In one of the last groups to be evacuated were a World War I veteran, Matron Jean Mitchell of Dundee, Scotland, and thirteen nurses, who waited on the dunes of Krouhelse, Belgium, for the minesweeper *Oriel* to carry them to safety. Mitchell survived to set up a field hospital in Caserta, Italy, during the attack on Monte Cassino.

As the toll of fighting favored the Allies, German forces abandoned their casualties, leaving them for British ambulance crews. Staff offered beds and care to all, enemy or domestic, and parceled out treasured stores of penicillin without regard to nationality. Ambulance crews transported critical cases to the nearest facility, regardless of its original purpose. Thus, adults could regain consciousness at London's Great Ormond Street hospital for sick children. Families were often separated as ambulance teams ferried the wounded to whatever hospital had space. Lying-in wards recommended that mothers retreat to the country from the nightly air raids at least a month before delivery to ready them for motherhood.

In the Suez Canal zone, which was ringed with predators, headquarters dispatched more medical staff to manage casualties. Although there were only a few gunshot wounds from snipers at the frontiers, diseases, predominantly dysentery, polio, and diphtheria, weakened the regiments in the Middle East. Sporadic cases of bubonic plague and smallpox called for stringent quarantine, creating both staff and bed shortages. The British victory over Benito Mussolini at Sidi Barrani deluged facilities with Italian prisoners of war.

A contingent of British sisters treated forces near Kiffissia, Greece, in winter 1940. Slow evacuation of casualties over craggy mountain slopes worsened an onslaught of fleas and lice. Patients with frostbite also suffered from gangrene and underwent crude field amputations. At Christmas, peasants brought the sisters into their homes and churches for celebration and thanksgiving. When the tide of battle favored Nazi reinforcements, Joan Wilson, with the aid of Louis MacPherson, an Australian ambulance orderly who rose from his sickbed to help, worked a ward overwhelmed by Greek casualties. After the fall of Yugoslavia in mid-April 1941, MacPherson refused to leave Wilson. On April 25, MacPherson evacuated nineteen walking wounded as German forces menaced their position and turned over the remains of her ward to Greek nurses. She survived to take the job of night superintendent in Helmieh, Egypt, in 1942.

On Malta, nurse Alice Elliott, a civilian volunteer, reported the terror of enemy bombs late in 1940: "Like nasty black flies, dropping their eggs on Valetta. The sky was full of flak and the noise was dreadful" (McBryde 1985, 50). After treating some of the three thousand civilian refugees in underground granaries during the bomb runs of January 1941, she was bicycling to limited shelters aboveground when a bomber ranged overhead: "Our ack-ack guns opened up with a terrific noise, firing at enemy planes overhead. Searchlights swung over my head and sickly yellow flares were dropping all around me. Suddenly, one of the enemy planes dived. . . . He dropped his load of bombs but he missed me" (McBryde 1985, 51). With spirited insouciance, she added, "I lived to tell the tale." Transferred to Imtarfa, she learned

to dismiss night raids as nuisances and cheered the downing of Germans as the texture of the island turned to pocked craters and empty walls and civilians died from malnutrition and inadequate medicines and infant formula. In August 1942, German planes sank a convoy of blockade runners, but three merchant ships bobbed to life, rescuing Elliott's charges from starvation. She moved to the hospital ship *Oranji* and to a postwar assignment among Germany's displaced persons.

At Gibraltar Military Hospital, officials assigned Zena Potter a burn unit. To allay the panic on the faces of men anticipating the agony of fresh dressings, she stocked her cart with champagne, which brightened patients as it dulled their pain. An influx of disaster victims from the wreck of the carrier *Eagle* in August 1942 tied her to the ward, where she ate and rested only when time permitted and conducted regular evacuation drills in case the hospital had to move underground. In retrospect, she regretted that penicillin, which was not then available, would have spared many seamen.

The Pacific theater involved medical staff in direct confrontation with the enemy after the Japanese captured St. Albert's Convent in Hong Kong in December 1941. Two days before Christmas, brusque soldiers with fixed bayonets nabbed Matron Mary Currie, tied her hands with telephone wire, and struck her with a rifle butt. She refused to be intimidated and informed her captors of the Geneva Conventions regarding hospital personnel. To convince one English-speaking officer that British staff were not savages, she led him to the mortuary to uncover the corpse of an officer she had treated, then dressed in medals and national flag after his death. The display made little impression. The officer forced her to undress wounds to prove that all patients were not faking hospitalization. For her courage and cool leadership, Currie earned the Royal Red Cross Medal.

Conditions worsened for staff as Japanese invaders of Hong Kong lorded their victory over female staff and turned St. Albert's into a prisoner of war (POW) infirmary. Dysentery patients rapidly declined from a diet of rice, spinach, turnips, and chrysanthemum leaves. The Japanese hid boxes of serum that might have saved many from an epidemic of diphtheria. By August, captors closed the facility and transported nurses to Stanley Internment Camp on Hong Kong island. Nurse Kathleen Thomson salvaged names and addresses of next of kin by hiding a thin roll of paper in the bottom of her talcum tin. On return to England, she was able to share with relatives the final moments of loved ones who had died in the POW camp and to confide that each coffin was decorated with local hibiscus and blessed by an army padre. Although Canadian army nurses May Waters and Kay G. Christie were repatriated in 1943, fourteen British nurses remained in confinement among two thousand civilian prisoners.

The fall of the Third Reich put British army and Red Cross nurses at the heart of Hitler's extermination unit at Belsen in West Germany. On April 17, 1945, staff members were perplexed by the emotionless German nurses and doctors who observed sixty thousand skeletal prisoners and a carpet of corpses in grotesque contortions. According to one Red Cross worker observing survivors at Ravensbrück: "They had sunken cheeks, distended bellies and swollen ankles. Their complexion was sallow. All of a sudden, a whole column of those starving wretches appeared. In each row a sick woman was supported or dragged along by her fellow-detainees" (Gilbert 1993, 227). The Herculean task of tending, feeding, and cleansing the frail survivors pressed Allied medical crews to the limit of their strength and supplies.

While officers scouted the countryside for food, nurse Mary Sands joined the base staff in evacuating the sickest, disinfecting and delousing the camp, and settling patients into comfortable billets. A case-by-case diagnosis found multiple ills ranging from malnutrition to tuberculosis, typhus, typhoid, diphtheria, polio, and heart and kidney disease. Patients became unruly and embittered. Some sick-

ened from the richness of a diet of powdered milk, oatmeal, and sugar; others died of stress, disease, malnutrition, and exhaustion at the rate of three hundred a day. Sands wrote, "It was a grisly task and reminded me of dreadful stories of the Black Death in the Middle Ages and the cries of 'Bring out your Dead!'" (McBryde 1985, 184).

The initiation of Americans into wartime nursing began on the morning of December 7, 1941. Like most of the citizenry, nurses aboard the *Solace* in Pearl Harbor, Hawaii, were as unprepared for attack as the military. Chief Nurse Lieutenant Grace Lally and a staff of twelve were immediately swamped with wounded as the waters rocked and spurted with depth charges to protect the ship from Japanese submarines. Nurse Agnes Shurr began receiving patients almost immediately as sailors on liberty took boats through the harbor to pick up wounded men from the water. At Schofield Barracks, Mildred Irene Clark Woodman worked nonstop to treat severe chest and spinal wounds, cranial and abdominal surgeries, and amputations. At the request of patients, she recited the Twenty-third Psalm and prayers while assisting in surgery. She prayed for courage, hope, and cheer and the understanding and compassion of her forebears.

On shore at the Sick Officers' Quarters, stretcher-bearers removed patients to the basement to free up space for the wounded and burned, who soon filled the beds and rows of mattresses in the hall. Nurses worked twenty-four-hour shifts as the first wave engulfed all facilities. Nelli Osterlund despaired at triage, which drew her away from hopeless burn victims to men who could survive. Ann Davidson and Catherine Richardson took turns sleeping for an hour before returning to an exhausting schedule of hustling men into and out of surgery. Phyllis Dana and Valera Vaubel Wiskerson, a navy dietitian, recalled the terrible smell of burn victims, many without eyelids, ears, and noses. Lenore Terrell Rickert praised ambulatory patients who gave up their beds to incoming wounded. Helen Entrikin helped rig a dressing room as an auxiliary operating theater. Her twin, Sarah Entrikin, was one of seven nurses at Hickam Field, where staff relied on local drivers to ferry patients to Tripler General Hospital. Gelane Matthews Barron worked alongside hospital volunteers, among whom was a mismatch of inactive nurses, service wives, friends, and even Honolulu prostitutes. Head Nurse Ann Leah Fox, who was wounded in the bombing, became the first woman to receive a Purple Heart.

As the war grew lethal, the European theater high command moved nurses through dangerous waters and air space and into military units. One north Atlantic convoy carrying Bostonian Mary Ann Sullivan and other nurses was torpedoed. The women survived lifeboat rescue in icy waters with minor frostbite before being transported to Iceland. At Second General Hospital, Chief Nurse Marjorie Peto and her staff endured constant German and American planes overhead and air raid sirens wailing into the night. During a lull, she accepted an invitation to meet the royal family at Buckingham Palace. On June 6, 1944, she, Caroline Renski, Frances Slanger, and others joined the D day landing party at Normandy, France, and set up field hospitals close enough to the fighting to feel rains of shrapnel through tent walls. A hospital ship was named for Slanger, who died in predawn shelling October 21.

In London, hospitals prepared for a flood of air raid casualties. Nurse trainee Beatrice Jobbins and hundreds of fellow staff worked under unstable conditions—sleeping in hallways, foraging for food supplies, and sharing cramped toilets. As doctors began entering the military, nurses took more responsibility for the deluge of patients. Medical staff gave functional lectures to civilian stretcher-bearers and ambulance teams. Supplies of rubber gloves were patched and repatched to extend their use. Razor blades were scarce, as were uniform hose.

American women received no reprieve from jostling and heavy loads. Esther Edwards of the 10th Field Hospital departed for Oran, Algeria, with a full load:

- blue uniforms
- white uniforms
- blue seersucker shirtwaist uniforms
- overcoats with zipper linings
- navy blue capes lined with red
- duty caps
- dress uniform caps
- clothing to wear in case of gas attack, including one-piece underwear and coveralls with a cap that protected the head and neck
- two musette bags with shoulder strap, one for clothes and the other for carrying cosmetics, toothbrushes, and so on
- bedroll, a piece of canvas that could be used as a ground cover for sleeping . . . two army blankets, rolled tightly (Fessler 1996, 132)

For the service of women like Edwards, the government beefed up the monthly pay of $150 by 10 percent for overseas duty. When the 48th Surgical Unit boarded a train for an eighteen-hour ride, Chief Nurse Theresa Archard and her nurses slept wherever there was space, then loaded musettes and bedrolls onto a ship. Knowing nothing of their destination, they were shifted to North Africa on November 8, 1942, as American ships bombarded German forces entrenched on the desert. The women approached the beach in small boats and remained on the alert in case they were forced back into the Mediterranean or assailed by sniper fire.

As the Allied invasion forces moved inland, the 48th Surgical accompanied them. Nurses Ruth Haskell, Phyllis MacDonald, and Edna Atkins traveled through unsecured territory near Arzeu, Algeria, to a decrepit hospital building filled with the odor of filth and bloody casualties waiting for aid. Under primitive conditions, she and her comrades sterilized instruments over an alcohol lamp and began the lengthy process of surgery. For three days, they shared a small ration of water for drinking only, ate cold rations, and swatted flies. The work was grueling, the uniform functional, and the boots often caked with mud and gore. The women had no bathing facilities for four months. By May 1943, the invasion had secured North Africa.

In the waters off Salerno, Sicily, nurses exemplified noncombatant valor. At 5:00 A.M. on September 9, 1943, those aboard the *Newfoundland* sustained a hit by a German bomb. Three American women were wounded and six British nurses killed. The *St. Andrew* evacuated survivors to North Africa. After two weeks, the women returned to assist the 95th Infantry. In *They Called It Purple Heart Valley*, Margaret Bourke-White, a photographer for *Life* and *Fortune* magazines, recorded the ingenuity and courage of Chief Nurse Hallie Almond and her staff. Suffering fatigue neurosis, the women maintained their composure for the good of patients. In reference to Kentuckian Betty Cook and nine other surgical nurses at the 11th Field Hospital, Bourke-White noted: "These girls were working closer to the battle line than American women had ever worked before in this or any other war. . . . A short stroll in the wrong direction would bring one right into German territory" (Bourke-White 1944, 123). Despite the danger, the crisis demanded immediate care for cerebral, chest, and belly wounds that were too chancy to transport to the rear. For her work, Cook earned the first Bronze Star and the first Purple Heart awarded to a nurse in the Italian theater.

On November 8, 1943, a transport plane bound from Catania, Sicily, to Bari, Italy, met impenetrable fog and landed in occupied Albania. Agnes Jensen Mangerich, Ann Kopcso, Lois Watson McKenzie, and ten others managed to elude capture until German troops won a skirmish against American insurgents. Three nurses—Wilma Lytle, Ava Maness, and Helen Porter—disappeared from the party. The rest crossed the mountains in a fall blizzard and, after two months of dodging Germans, connected with a British ship on the Adriatic coast. The remaining three hid until Albanians disguised them as locals and drove them to British secret service agents. On March 22, 1944, after an eighteen-week ordeal, they reunited with the other nurses.

At the war's crux, sustained heavy fighting hammered Anzio, a 7-by-15-mile beachhead in southwestern Italy where thirty-three thousand American and fifteen thousand British casualties entered care in a span of four months. Among the fallen buried at Anzio are six nurses. Under round-the-clock German artillery fire, nurses moved operations to tents set up in an open field. Working on swampy land, the medical staff treated a steady stream of wounded, who were quickly stabilized, evacuated by ambulance down Purple Heart Drive to small boats, and ferried to a hospital ship. Offshore, the British hospital ship *St. David* was bombed and sunk. Two medics died; nurses Ruth Hindman and Anna Bess Berrett survived. On February 7, 1944, a German bomber, fleeing two British spitfires, dumped five bombs on a ward tent of the 95th Evacuation Hospital. The massive blow killed patients, doctors, corpsmen, Chief Nurse Blanche Sigman, Carrie Sheetz, and Marjorie Morrow and wounded nurses Ruth Buckley, Fern Wingerd, and sixty-two others. After the war, an army hospital ship was named in honor of Sigman.

As the staff of the 95th Evacuation Hospital was departing the area, their replacement, the 33rd Field Hospital, came under nighttime assault. Chief Nurse Mary Roberts collapsed from the concussion of the bombing, then rallied. As she groped for light to assist the wounded in the burning tents, she set a good example by remaining calm and focused during a hellish night of shelling, fires, and a generator explosion. By morning, a count of the damage included one wounded nurse and two dead, Chief Nurse Glenda Spelhaug and LaVerne Farquhar. The hospital continued its work. Three of its nurses earned Silver Stars—Mary Roberts, Elaine R. Roe, and Virginia Rourke—the first women to be so honored for bravery and leadership.

General George Patton's last plunge into northern Europe produced some of its bloodiest fighting in December 1944, when Bernice Tansy of the 140th General Hospital performed distinguished service. Of work at the

8th Field Hospital, Grace G. Peterson recalled receiving eight hundred wounded in one day and counted seventeen hundred patients shipped out. The total for that six-month engagement was seventy-five hundred. In Arlon, Belgium, in February 1945, Mary Ferrell earned a Bronze Star and five campaign stars for meritorious service, which Ernest O. Hauser reported in a March 10, 1945, feature for the *Saturday Evening Post*. Of her work in the "Chamber of Horrors" of battlefield trauma, he surmised: "If the mothers of these . . . boys could have seen Mary Ferrell standing by their sons, keeping them silent company through that long cruel night, and escorting them gently up to the threshold of the last, wide-open portal—if their mothers could have caught a glimpse of it, I think it might have made them feel just a little better about it all" (Hauser 1945, 50). Such reporting in the popular press put faces and names on the largely anonymous heroism of medical workers and communicated to citizens that American soldiers received the best possible care.

Postwar reflections preserved the difficulty of maintaining quality medical care. Lieutenant Helen Hubbard Cross described a nomadic caravan of tents carrying her and sixty other nurses in the University of Illinois's 27th Evacuation Hospital as it rumbled from Casablanca to Oran, then across the Mediterranean to Naples, Italy, and into France and Germany. More than fifty years after the fact, she recalled: "The worst injuries you ever saw is when the guys would accidentally run into a mine field. They just, oh . . . They just tear the flesh to pieces" (Schmich 1998, 1). In an effort to be explicit, she added, "It's not like a bullet wound. It's really a mess. It's hard to prep when the flesh is in such a mess." Working twelve-hour days, she and tent mates Gail Young and Ruth Steinkamp faced an endless row of men awaiting surgery. The roving hospital remained free of German raids, primarily because the staff occasionally treated enemy casualties.

Australian combatants, totaling 900,000 men and women, suffered their share of hard-

ship. At the beginning of the war, the Australian Army Nursing Service had thirty-five hundred members. In Malaya before the fall of Singapore, a band of 118, assigned to the 8th Division Australian Imperial Force and staffing a makeshift hospital in a Chinese school and guest house, boarded ships to safety. On February 11, 1942, one group sailing on the *Empire Star* reached Batavia (now Djakarta), Indonesia, on the way to Australia. The second group, composed of sixty-five nurses, left the next day aboard the *Vyner Brooke*, which the Japanese sank off Banka Island on February 14. Of the fifty-three who survived, the Japanese murdered twenty-one and took thirty-two prisoner.

Betty Jeffrey's first-person record of the nurses' story, *White Coolies* (1954), includes the women's physical and mental anguish in a Pelambang prison and the standout courage of Sister Vivian Bullwinkel, sole survivor of the Banka Island massacre. Jeffrey comments on the brutal machine-gunning of noncombatants: "All were killed outright but Vivian. A bullet passed through her left side just above her hip and sent her headlong into the water. She floated there for some minutes, then, when the Japanese had gone away, was able to struggle ashore" (Jeffrey 1954, 23). Bullwinkel salvaged one English soldier, treated him in the jungle for ten days, and fled down a road. The man died, but she survived after incarceration in a Japanese jail. By August 18, 1945, three days after the Japanese surrendered, the remaining prisoners from the *Vyner Brooke* had shrunk to twenty-four. Jeffrey commented: "When people die the women have to carry them out of the camp to a small Chinese cemetery in the jungle not far from here. We have a special corner for the people of this camp. . . . The missionaries or the nuns always take the service at the grave side. The cemetery is in a very pretty spot on the hillside, with a profusion of wild jungle flowers everywhere" (Jeffrey 1954, 144).

After three and a half years of journal-keeping, Jeffrey exulted in reunion with white soldiers, both English and Dutch. Still in camp on September 13, 1945, they thrilled to parcels of bread dropped from planes. Airlifted on September 17 and welcomed by the Red Cross in Singapore, she and her fellow POWs reveled in hot baths, poached eggs, and cups of tea.

In Medan, Sumatra, Dutch nurse Janna Nienhuys and her first aid team treated local bombing victims and aided the village hospital as Japanese soldiers began to take control of the Dutch East Indies. In April 1942, she and her daughters were ordered to join a prison train, which marched them to a deserted rubber plantation. Under severe limitations, she treated cuts, infection, and cases of diabetes and polio and delivered infants of inmates. Over the next year, many children died. Nienhuys and other volunteers vaccinated all against a typhus epidemic. Resettled after a long train ride, they battled starvation in a squalid concentration camp beset by bedbugs. After the British liberated survivors in August 1945, Nienhuys and her daughters reunited with her husband and, in late January 1946, returned to Holland.

To the north of Malaya, the Philippines produced its own challenge. Jeanne Quint Benoliel, a graduate at the beginning of the Pacific war, joined the Army Nurse Corps in 1943 and traveled to Milne Bay, New Guinea, with the 80th General Hospital. She was ambivalent about her wartime experience, which contained its share of casualties plus patients suffering from malaria, dengue fever, and tsutsugamushi disease, a form of typhus. In Thelma M. Schorr and Anne Zimmerman's *Making Choices, Taking Chances: Nurse Leaders Tell Their Stories* (1988, 17), Benoliel remarked: "My memories of that time are full of 18- and 19-year-old kids with psychiatric breakdowns and other emotional problems resulting from soldiering in a jungle where the enemy could not be seen." When the army evacuated its military personnel from the Philippines shortly before Christmas 1941, Dorothy Davis, a civilian nurse, remained behind at Sternberg Hospital to care for several hundred casualties. Blackouts left her without

power, telephones, and transportation until New Year's Day, 1942, when she was interned with other nurses at Santo Tomás University, a prison camp in Manila.

At Bataan on the Philippine island of Luzon, nurses scrubbed old barracks into shape at Limay to receive five hundred close-spaced cots and readied Number Two, a jungle hospital. Limay received sixteen hundred patients, who shared double and triple bunk beds. Under heavy bombing, nurses dressed in khaki, steel helmets, and GI boots and suffered from food shortages, which reduced their numbers rapidly. Lieutenant Juanita Redmond, an army surgical nurse and author of *I Served on Bataan* (1943), doled out rations to soldiers who had been living on bananas and lizards and snakes captured in the jungle. When Dakin's solution (a disinfectant) and sulfa ran low, she assisted in treating gangrene, which spread from the heavy concentration of anaerobic bacteria on the island: "The wound is cut open, perhaps the entire leg laid open to the bone if it is that far gone, and the infected tissue removed. Then, after being swabbed with peroxide, the morbid area is left uncovered except for mosquito netting, while the exposure to sunrays and oxygen destroys the bacteria" (Redmond 1943, 61–62). After an extended period of such primitive treatments for serious war wounds, she confided that seeing people torn and dying in large numbers cracked something inside her that could never be repaired.

During the worst of the siege of Corregidor, Redmond reported on the tight quarters in the tunnel labyrinth, where hospital work continued during bombardment. Under orders from General Jonathan Wainwright, Bataan's commander, every able inmate worked. Nurses treated patients who were stacked on double and triple bunk beds. Echoes of shelling and stale air made the underground atmosphere miserably oppressive. Food poisoning exacerbated the inmates' condition and filled the stale air with the smell of vomit and feces. Evening strollers near the gates suffered a direct hit; a second shell struck the crowd that rushed to their aid. The resulting casualties needed injections, surgery, and amputations. Nurses and corpsmen worked through the night to sterilize instruments, bandage wounds, and comfort those who could not be saved.

When the front moved too close, nurses and corpsmen evacuated the wounded south down the peninsula to Little Baguio on ambulances, trucks, and cars. Food supplies dwindled to stringy water buffalo, then no meat at all. Make-do rations turned from horse meat to wild monkey, pig, and snake. Nurses contended with scurvy and beriberi and combated amoebic dysentery and diarrhea from the impure water of nearby ponds and creeks. Acute shortages of quinine meant less control of malaria, which threatened thousands daily. Bombers demolished 90 percent of the beds. Three wounded nurses were evacuated to Corregidor, an island 2 miles west of Manila.

Aboveground, battle fatigue, anemia, and hysteria weakened men who badly needed a break from combat. On the emperor's birthday, Bataan sustained fourteen air raids and numerous shellings. At the height of bombardment, triage teams assisted the wounded aboveground until litter bearers could evacuate the men to the tunnels. Belowground, medical staff breathed gritty air, gasped at the smoke, and steadied themselves and their breakables from jarring and concussion. Superintended by Chief Nurse Josephine Nesbitt, nurses were evacuated to Middleside Hospital on April 8, 1942, leaving patients behind with doctors and corpsmen. In the background they could see U.S. troops destroying supplies to keep them out of enemy hands. The move did not spare the nursing staff from constant Japanese MIGs overhead or the threat of a bitter hand-to-hand fight for Corregidor, the last American holdout. Meanwhile, nurses treated a steady stream of casualties in the hospital tunnel, an airless, malodorous makeshift ward.

Upon receiving evacuation orders to Melbourne, Australia, Nurse Redmond remarked, "I was leaving the Islands, I was leaving a losing battle—a lost battle" (Redmond 1943, 151). After a fearful, island-hopping flight, her convoy arrived at Port Melbourne Hospital on May 5, 1942, only a day before General Wainwright's American insurgents surrendered Corregidor to the Japanese. Redmond described her fellow nurses as "thin as famine victims, hungry-eyed, and shivering." Postbattle treatment restored stamina with liver extract, vitamins, tonic, and bed rest.

The aftermath of Bataan centered the world's attention on courage and fortitude under the worst of conditions. Reporters and families stalked survivors to gather information about soldiers imprisoned by the Japanese or killed in the final assault. Rose Van Hoorebeck Hawkins of the 35th General Hospital treated survivors of the Bataan Death March, whom she had to scrub and spoon-feed liquids and soft foods until they recovered from their bad treatment. Pearl Will Haugland Bach of the 133rd General Hospital worked twenty-four-hour shifts and, in July 1945, was among the first to treat patients with penicillin, the era's wonder drug. At a ceremony in Washington, D.C., Eleanor Roosevelt and Nursing Director Mary Beard of the American Red Cross honored the six U.S. army nurses who had escaped from Bataan: Dorothea Daley, Eunice Hatchitt, Harriet G. Lee, Mary G. Lohr, Florence Mac-Donald, and Juanita Redmond.

Other theaters in the Pacific tested the mettle of nurses. After serving with the 153rd Station Hospital in Brisbane, Australia, Edith Vowell and her fellow nurses saw similar duty in a corrugated iron building in Port Moresby, New Guinea. Living near the equator in tents and grass huts as the first women to arrive since the evacuation of civilians, they braved sucking mud, mosquitoes, and stunning heat as they followed General Douglas Mac-Arthur's troops northwest up the coast. Nearby units at New Caledonia, Efate, Espiritu Santo, Guadalcanal, Tulagi, and other South Sea locales battled rats and vermin while absorbing the wounded from land battles in the Solomon Islands. Althea Williams treated "scrub typhus," a deadly sickness among patients on the islands of Biak and Owi in the Dutch East Indies. Rosanna Comes Jones worked in a tin hospital on Guam, where she improvised dressings from packing and rags. Audrey Lampier with the 362nd Station Hospital recalled nurses who had to be sent home because of the miseries of Milne Bay, New Guinea. Also in Milne Bay, the 268th Station Hospital received one of the first contingents of fifteen black nurses, including Prudence Burns Burrell, a Red Cross nurse and recruiter for the Army Nurse Corps, which segregated black staff members for meals and private quarters and designated black blood supplies with an "A" for African American.

Captain Catherine Acorn and Marie Pirl were among the staff following MacArthur's troops into the Philippines in October 1944 and performed splendidly under the leaky roof of the operating theater. Off Iwo Jima on February 19, 1945, the *Samaritan* rode at anchor as barges maneuvered alongside to unload the wounded. Recovering from an unexploded shell that ripped through two decks and lodged in a ventilator, the ship continued to Saipan in the Marianas with nurses, corpsmen, and surgeons working without rest. On land, Julia Polchlopek Scott of the 369th Station Hospital topped cots with mattresses to protect bedfast patients from bombing and strafing and, in a pinch, received five minutes of instruction on giving intravenous treatment. Flight nurse Jane Kandeigh helped load wounded on transport planes bound for Ulithi, Saipan, and Guam. Unlike hospital ship staff, who were always near fighting, she and her fellows flew in and out of danger, transferring casualties to Pearl Harbor and the United States before returning to hot war zones. During one flight, Lieutenant Dorothy Shikoski suffered injury when the plane crashed in the sea, where she continued supervising the wounded and positioning them in life rafts.

Captured in the tunnels of Corregidor, nurses Ruth Stoltz and Minnie Breese shared cramped space and limited raffia beds at Santo Tomás University with some four thousand British and American civilian and military prisoners of war. Dorothy Davis canvassed thirty-five hundred inmates to determine who had medical training. She located staff from mission hospitals in India, China, and Hong Kong and obtained iron beds, basins, and bedpans from Manila's Red Cross Emergency Unit. Two Filipino nurses took over night duty. Within a month, the camp infirmary acquired a Bunsen burner for heating water, a few drugs from nearby medical clinics, and equipment for a makeshift physiotherapy suite and dental clinic. With the influx of navy and army nurses, Chief Army Nurse Maude Davison superintended the camp infirmary, where staff treated rheumatic fever, gastroenteritis, amoebic dysentery, and parasites. Nurse Dorothy Still Danner survived a camp appendectomy without infection. Captors transported those requiring more complicated surgeries to a Filipino hospital in Manila, where compassionate care proved natives loyal to the American military.

To combat tedium, inmates played cards and taught courses in architecture, geology, Spanish, English literature, anthropology, and other subjects. Carrie Edwina Todd collected volumes for a lending library. The Red Cross delivered a few letters, which Japanese guards sometimes detained for months. Tropical diseases such as dengue fever, dysentery, malaria, and jungle rot depleted the inmates along with tuberculosis, plague, typhoid, and beriberi, a result of poor nutrition. Food shortages reduced daily meals from three to two, augmented by sparse Red Cross packages. Surviving on mush, rice, soybean soup, and occasionally caribou meat, the nurses parceled out the few potatoes to the most fragile—the elderly, sick, and young. At Baguio, Beatrice Chambers witnessed brutal beatings and the capricious killing of a child with a motorcycle; Evelyn Whitlow Greenfield saw a nurse fend off a would-be rapist.

When American planes arrived September 21, 1944, the Japanese stepped up discipline by forcing plane watchers to stand at attention in the sun all day without food or water. The hospital death rate worsened from starvation and despair. Nurse Margaret Nash, infected with tuberculosis, recalled January 1945, when prisoners were living a day at a time, hoping that the war would end in time to save them. On February 3, 1945, when tanks and amtracs approached Santo Tomás, seventeen prisoners died in the fighting. Nash and Edwina Todd fled the firing with newborns in their arms.

The U.S. First Cavalry liberated all. Medical teams turned Bilibid Prison into a hospital to treat the weakest internees. Three weeks later, authorities learned of two thousand prisoners at Los Baños and freed them. Chief Nurse Laura Cobb and other former POWs were soon at work treating the wounded. When the sixty-eight army nurses were being shipped home, Charlotte McFall Mallon, a wounded veteran and recipient of an Air Medal, was among the nurses greeting them on a brief stop at Saipan in the Marianas. She and Jane Simons Silva of the 829th Medical Air Evacuation Squadron also assisted in airlifting skeletal soldiers who survived the Bataan Death March.

With the invasion of Okinawa, Japan, on April 1, 1945, kamikaze attacks inflicted mayhem on the American fleet. Nurse Lee Hurley was among the crew of the *Bountiful,* which weathered a typhoon while ferrying casualties from Okinawa to a base hospital at Ulithi in the Caroline Islands. On April 28, the *Comfort* suffered a direct hit by a Japanese plane, which struck the operating room, killing twenty-three, including six surgical nurses. Survivors added the staff wounded to their roster of casualties as the ship limped its way to Saipan.

The end of the conflict brought nurses together in a mutual celebration and memorial. Esther Edwards of the 10th Field Hospital spent a month at Dachau as the military sorted out guards and prisoners, many of whom died of typhus, dysentery, cholera, tuberculosis, and starvation. Sad to leave a formidable medical team, she remarked on her unit's seven battle stars, the most for any hospital in the war. On August 6, 1945, after mud, blood, snakes, and an earthquake, Dorothy Wood Angerer of the 58th Evacuation Hospital in Leyte shared the playing of "When the Lights Go on Again All over the World," a poignant anthem to peace.

The liberation intensified the ward work of LaVonne Telshaw Camp, an army nurse and veteran of Burma and China assigned to the 142nd General Hospital in Calcutta, India. She had already taken action on an official report from the surgeon general, Thomas Parran, about milk contaminated with ditch water, abattoirs clouded with dust and dried manure, dogs and vultures snatching at entrails, and vegetables sprinkled with human excrement. She declared, "Asepsis and isolation technique was one nursing function in which I was highly proficient" (Camp 1997, 133). Among prisoners of the Japanese released from Burma, Malaysia, and the Valley of the Kwai, she confronted listlessness, rampant malaria, missing teeth, and pitiable emaciation. Before her departure in 1946, she commented, "I was keenly aware of these prisoners' reluctance to talk, so kept a respectful silence as I ministered to their bodies" (Camp 1997, 134). She noted that, when the men did speak, they said nothing of hatred for their captors. Their thoughts turned universally to home.

Overall, the American experience in World War II was a boost for some forty-two thousand nurses, of whom fifteen thousand were assigned to the European theater of operations. They proved themselves capable of joining soldiers in pickup games of softball, dancing to Glenn Miller's "String of Pearls," dodging shells, and wading in muck and body fluids to attend distressing wounds and disease. When doctors were short-staffed, some nurses performed medical procedures and surgeries, earning the trust and admiration of their superiors. According to Brigadier

General Connie L. Slewitzke, more than fifty-seven thousand army nurses served in World War II, in a variety of locales at home and in combat zones, including in hospitals, on trains and planes, and at clearing stations. Of their total, sixteen hundred received decorations for heroism; two hundred died. By war's end, the nurses *were* soldiers, some decorated for bravery and leadership, others buried with honor in military cemeteries alongside the men they had bathed, comforted, and bandaged.

At a turning point in world history, the example of women in service established the need for frontline nursing. Likewise, the American Red Cross stepped up the search for qualified personnel. In 1942, the navy saw the wisdom of issuing a standard uniform. The military authorized officer's rank for nurses in February 1942 and dispatched nurses to war zones on hospital ships, in transport planes, and at ground installations in England, Australia, India, North Africa, and the Pacific; by 1943, under the supervision of Army Nurse Corps superintendent Florence A. Blanchfield, special training facilities readied nurses for the battlefield and wartime nursing duties. To speed up recruitment, the government established the Cadet Nurse Corps, headed by Lucile Petry, which drew sixty-five thousand trainees the first year with promises of R.N. degrees and commissions in the army or navy. In March 1945, the need for nurses was so great that a bill in the U.S. House of Representatives sought a draft for graduate nurses, but the end of the war preceded a vote on the controversial issue of sending women into combat zones. The availability of tuition funds through the GI Bill helped veteran nurses to complete their training with higher degrees. Some were still in service during the Korean and Vietnam Wars.

The war effort produced a host of standout nurses. After safely airlifting five patients from India to Washington, D.C., Lieutenant Elsie S. Lott Mandot of the 803rd Medical Air Evacuation Squadron was the first flight nurse and the first woman to earn an Air Medal for meritorious achievement. From the same squadron, Audrey Rodgers McDonald, a veteran of action in Burma, earned a Purple Heart and Air Medal. Florence Jacobs won a Bronze Star for her work in Russia. Jean Yunker Johnson and Roberta Ross of the 821st Medical Air Evacuation Squadron were among nurses receiving the Distinguished Flying Cross for heroism in Burma and India; a fellow nurse, Aloha Drennan Sanchez, was awarded the Air Medal and Bronze Star. Wilma Vinsant Shea, killed while serving the 806th Medical Air Evacuation Squadron, was the impetus for an annual flight nurse award. Kathleen Dial Coile, a heavily decorated war veteran of the 804th Medical Air Evacuation Squadron, earned an Air Medal for a sea rescue and a Purple Heart and Distinguished Flying Cross after suffering head and shoulder injuries in a plane crash at Port Moresby while ferrying eighteen psychotic patients to the United States. Marcella R. LeBeaut, a Cheyenne River Sioux from Promise, South Dakota, won a medal from the Belgian government in 1944 for service to the Army Nurse Corps. Colonel Irene Clark Woodman, a veteran of the bombing of Pearl Harbor, rose to the position of chief of the Army Nurse Corps, which she held from 1963 to 1967. For her service in war- and peacetime, she received an outstanding alumni citation from the University of Michigan School of Nursing and induction into the Michigan Women's Hall of Fame.

In the war's aftermath, nations worldwide struggled to rehabilitate civilian and military casualties. In a war memoir, *So Far from the Bamboo Grove* (1986), Yoko Kawashima Watkins, daughter of a Japanese attaché, relived a childhood memory of the war. Dressed in a kimono costume and accompanied by koto and shamisen players, she sang and danced for veterans at a military hospital in Nanam, Korea, where her family lived in 1945. Through the curtains of the auditorium she caught her first glimpse of "wounded soldiers, wearing white hospital gowns. Some wore slings, some walked with crutches, some, their eyes bandaged, were led by nurses. Some had no arm, or no leg." The most poignant sight of all was "a man on a stretcher who had no arms or legs" (Watkins 1986, 10).

Virginia M. Ohlson, one of four nurses assigned to the Public Health and Welfare sector of the Supreme Command of Allied Powers, advanced to General Douglas MacArthur's headquarters in Japan in 1947. Working with Japanese nurses to rebuild Japan's health care system, she surveyed pathetic medical facilities and poor educational and working conditions for nurses. In her words, "They were malnourished; many had no shoes, and their feet and hands were covered with chilblains. All metal in public and private buildings had been stripped and used to make weapons and other implements of war. There were no glass panes left in any windows, no central heating or cooking facilities" (Schorr and Zimmerman 1988, 284). After working as chief nurse of the U.S. occupation force to raise standards for nursing, midwifery, and public health, she joined the Atomic Bomb Casualty Commission in 1951 at Hiroshima's research center as consultant to Japanese nurses at Tokyo's Institute of Public Health. For her commitment to bicultural understanding, she received an honorary doctorate and membership in the Japanese Nursing Association.

See also: Cadet Nurse Corps; Nazi Nurses; Red Cross

Sources

Anderson, Owannah. *Ohoyo One Thousand: A Resource Guide of American Indian/Alaska Native Women.* Washington, D.C.: U.S. Department of Education, 1982.

Blassingame, Wyatt. *Combat Nurses of World War II.* New York: Random House, 1967.

Bourke-White, Margaret. *They Called It Purple Heart Valley.* New York: Simon and Schuster, 1944.

Camp, LaVonne Telshaw. *Lingering Fever: A World War II Nurse's Memoir.* Jefferson, N.C.: McFarland, 1997.

Cowdrey, Albert E. *Fighting for Life: American Military Medicine in World War II.* New York: Free Press, 1994.

Emergency War Surgery. Washington, D.C.: Department of Defense, 1958.

Fessler, Diane Burke. *No Time for Fear: Voices of American Military Nurses in World War II.* East Lansing: Michigan State University Press, 1996.

Hauser, Ernest O. "Shock Nurse." *Saturday Evening Post,* March 10, 1945, 12–13, 48–50.

Jeffrey, Betty. *White Coolies.* Sydney: Angus and Robertson, 1954.

Kalisch, Philip, and Beatrice J. Kalisch. *The Advance of American Nursing.* Boston: Little, Brown, 1978.

Longmate, Norman, ed. *The Home Front: An Anthology of Personal Experience, 1938–1945.* London: Chatto and Windus, 1981.

Gilbert, Martin. *Atlas of the Holocaust.* New York: William Morrow, 1993.

McBryde, Brenda. *Quiet Heroines: Nurses of the Second World War.* London: Hogarth Press, 1985.

McHenry, Robert, ed. *Liberty's Women.* Springfield, Mass.: G. C. Merriam, 1980.

McKown, Robin. *Heroic Nurses.* New York: G. P. Putnam's Sons, 1966.

Read, Phyllis J., and Bernard L. Witlieb. *The Book of Women's Firsts.* New York: Random House, 1992.

Redmond, Juanita. *I Served on Bataan.* Philadelphia: J. B. Lippincott, 1943.

"Salute to the Military." *Daughters of the American Revolution Magazine* (November 1990): 852–853.

Sherr, Lynn, and Jurate Kazickas. *Susan B. Anthony Slept Here: A Guide to American Women's Landmarks.* New York: Times Books, 1994.

Schmich, Mary. "Heroic War Nurses Saved Thousands of Private Ryans." *Chicago Tribune,* August 9, 1998, sect. 4, p. 1.

Schorr, Thelma M., R.N., and Anne Zimmerman, R.N., eds. *Making Choices, Taking Chances: Nurse Leaders Tell Their Stories.* St. Louis: C. V. Mosby, 1988.

Sterne, Capt. Doris M. *In and Out of Harm's Way: A History of the Navy Nurse Corps.* Seattle, Wash.: Peanut Butter Publishing, 1996.

Stewart, Charles Fyfe, M.D. *The Ninth Evac: Experiences in a World War II Tent Hospital in North Africa and Europe.* New York: Vantage Press, 1990.

Van Devanter, Lynda, and Joan A. Furey, eds. *Visions of War, Dreams of Peace: Writings of Women in the Vietnam War.* New York: Time Warner, 1991.

Vedder, James S. *Combat Surgeon: On Iwo Jima with the 27th Marines.* Novato, Calif.: Presidio, 1984.

Watkins, Yoko Kawashima. *So Far from the Bamboo Grove.* New York: Puffin Books, 1986.

Wheal, Elizabeth-Anne, Stephen Pope, and James Taylor, eds. *Encyclopedia of the Second World War.* Edison, N.J.: Castle Books, 1989.

Yost, Edna. *American Women of Nursing.* Philadelphia: J. B. Lippincott, 1947.

Timeline of Landmarks in Nursing

3000 B.C.	Egyptian papyri described medical treatment through magic and worship.
2650 B.C.	Imhotep reigned as the Egyptian god of medicine.
	Emperor Shen Nung founded Chinese medicine.
1700 B.C.	Egyptian midwives preferred birthing chairs.
1500 B.C.	Midwives studied at Heliopolis, Egypt.
	The Ebers Papyrus preserved ancient Egyptian spells, incantations, and eight hundred simples.
1134 B.C.	Greek plague victims received care in quarantine huts.
800 B.C.	A Jewish midwife attended Rachel, Jacob's favorite.
7th century B.C.	An Assyrian cuneiform tablet preserved 250 healing remedies.
600 B.C.	Aesculapius became a Greek cult figure.
Ca. 401 B.C.	Greek historian Thucydides described nursing care during an epidemic in *The Peloponnesian War.*
300 B.C.	Shen Nung, a Chinese herbalist, wrote *Pen Tsao,* a guide to one thousand herbal compounds.
3rd century B.C.	Agnodice became the first midwife in the Western world.
1st century	A bas-relief at Ostia depicted a two-woman team caring for a Roman woman in childbirth.
	Christian nurses supplanted the Roman system of slave nurses tending the sick.
2nd century	Soranus of Ephesus wrote *Concerning Women's Disease,* the first identified text on midwifery.
120	Hindu healers published *Charaka,* a standard medical text.
3rd century	St. Helena opened a nursing home for the elderly in Rome.
325	The Council of Nicaea planned hospices in religious houses.
350	St. Ephrem of Syria superintended a three-hundred-bed hospital for critically ill plague victims at Edessa in northern Greece.
370	St. Basil of Caesarea and his sister Macrina founded a hospital and leprosarium and hired visiting nurses to transport the sick.
ca. 380	The first nursing instructor, St. Marcella, converted her Aventine palace into a monastery to tend the sick in Rome.
385	St. Paula sailed to Bethlehem to establish a hospice for pilgrims.
390	St. Fabiola opened the first Christian hospital in Rome.

	Flacilla worked in a Byzantine hospital.
	St. Zoticus established a hospital in Constantinople.
5th century	King Clovis claimed to cure scrofula by a royal touch.
	Lepers sought out St. Bridget's abbey in Kildare, Ireland.
	St. Alexis opened a hospital that served as a medical school's clinic.
432	St. Patrick, patron saint of Ireland, treated lepers.
6th century	In Gaul, Clothilde and Radegonde pioneered modern nursing.
	St. Scholastica fought plague at her convent near Monte Cassino, Italy.
542	In Lyons, King Childebert I opened the Hôtel Dieu, the oldest hospital in continuous service.
650	St. Fiacre of Ireland opened a hospice in France.
8th century	St. Walburga founded hospice for plague victims in Hildesheim, Germany.
9th century	Caliph Harun al-Rashid founded Baghdad's first hospital.
10th century	Caliph al-Muktadir opened the second Islamic hospital.
910	The Islamic healer Rhazes published *A Treatise on the Small Pox and Measles.*
925	Rhazes recorded patient histories in *The Compendium.*
936	England's first leprosarium was founded at York by King Aethelstan.
962	At St. Bernard's Augustinian hospice in the Italian Alps, dogs sniffed out lost travelers.
1025	Avicenna completed the *Canon of Medicine,* a comprehensive medical encyclopedia.
1050	The Knights Hospitallers of St. John opened St. John of Jerusalem, a one-thousand-bed hospital.
1060	Constantinus Africanus transported valuable Islamic medical texts to Salerno, Italy.
1095	The Order of Antonines treated erysipelas throughout Europe.
12th century	Moses Maimonedes practiced medicine in Spain.
	Herrade of Landsburg served a hospice on Mt. St. Odelia in the Vosges Mountains in Alsace.
1117	Queen Matilda established St. Giles's Hospital as a leprosarium.
1145	The Holy Ghost Hospital opened at Montpellier, France, and sponsored additional hospices in Europe.
1147	St. Hildegard of Bingen formed a visiting nurse team.
1180	St. Hugh of Lincoln opened his priory in Witham, Somerset, to lepers.
1184	The Béguines renounced a secular life to nurture the poor.
1197	The Order of Trinitarians carried first aid to casualties of war and domestic outbreaks of plague.
13th century	St. Clare founded the Poor Clares.
	Juliana of Cornillon, France, occupied an Augustinian cloister, cared for the sick, and tended lepers.
	The Hôtel Dieu in Paris, home of the oldest ward in continuous use, set aside a women's ward.
1203	St. Hedwig of Bavaria opened a hospice for female lepers at Neumarkts.
1222	The Grey Sisters opened a hospice in France.
1226	Abbess Euphemia of England established innovative sanitation at a Benedictine house in Hampshire.
1232	Fachtna of Kilcolgan, Ireland, kept a guest house for lepers.
1244	The Misericordia, a masked band of Italian laymen, initiated an ambulance and first aid service.
1249	On a mission to the Holy Land, Hersend and Guillamette de Luys served the staff of Louis IX of France as royal midwife.
1250	In Egypt during the Mamluk dynasty, midwives celebrated births.
1320	Jacoba Felicie was charged in Paris for practicing medicine without a license.

1326	Sarah of St. Gilles, a Jewish healer in Marseilles, France, received royal permission to train an apprentice.
1346	St. Bridget of Upland, patron saint of Sweden, founded the Bridgettine order at Vadstena.
1348	The Alexian brotherhood opened its European beggar houses.
1367	St. Catherine of Siena, patron saint of Italy, treated victims of epidemics.
1368	St. Roch of Montpellier, France, focused his care on the plague victims of Piacenza, Italy.
15th century	Frances of Rome and her sister-in-law, Vannozza, served as visiting nurses.
	In Milan, St. Charles of Borromeo set up a hospice for plague victims.
	Queen Isabella of Spain invented the first movable hospitals.
	St. Catherine of Bologna taught the Poor Clares.
	St. Catherine of Genoa treated plague.
1439	Elysabeth Keston earned a stipend as nurse in Warwick, England.
16th century	Damián Carbón and Juan Alonso de loy Ruyzes published birthing handbooks in Castilian.
	Candida purchased land for a foundling home in China.
1519	Hernán Cortés reported on Aztec drugs.
1522	An Aztec herbal listed botanical formulae.
1524	Cortés established the first European hospital in the Americas.
1528	Álvar Núñez Cabeza de Vaca recorded treatment of infections among American Indians.
1531	St. Jerome Emiliani cared for children orphaned when the plague swept Venice.
1537	St. John of God set up treatment centers for poor plague victims in Granada, Spain.
1540	Spaniards learned herbal techniques from Kansas Indians.
1553	A shipwreck in the Gulf of Mexico brought Texas its first European nurse, Fra Juan de Mena, a Dominican friar.
1560	The Damsels of Charity established a visiting nurse society.
1584	St. Camillus de Lellis, patron of nurses, founded the Society of Servants of the Sick in Naples, Italy.
1591	St. Aloysius Gonzaga, a Jesuit healer of Castiglione, Italy, died while treating plague victims in Rome.
1605	St. Francis de Sales and St. Jeanne-Françoise de Chantal of Dijon began the Congregation of the Visitation of Holy Mary.
	The first European nurse in the Americas, Marie Rollet Hébert Hubou, joined the Jesuit colonial hospital at Port Royal, Nova Scotia.
1609	Louyse Bourgeois published an obstetrical textbook, the first scientific handbook published by a woman.
1617	St. Vincent de Paul formed the Confraternity of Charity.
1629	St. Louise de Marillac supervised 130 organized branches of charity nurses at Montmirail, France.
1633	Calancha of Peru described cinchona, a natural pain remedy.
	St. Vincent de Paul and St. Louise de Marillac founded the Daughters of Charity.
1634	Peter Chamberlen, the inventor of forceps, tried to unionize English midwives.
	Vincent de Paul established the Ladies of Charity.
1637	Anne Marbury Hutchinson, a practicing midwife in the Massachusetts Bay Colony, was ousted for delivering and burying a monstrous fetus.
1644	In September, Jeanne Mance, the New World's first lay hospital nurse-missionary, founded the Hôtel Dieu of Montreal.
	Priests shipped cinchona bark to Europe.
1649	Quaker sisters were expelled from Anglican hospitals.

1651	Fernando Hernández compiled *A Treasury of Medicine of New Spain, or a History of Mexican Plants, Animals, and Minerals.*
1658	America's first hospital began in a sailor's shed set up in New York by the West India Company.
1662	A court in Stockport, England, harassed midwives Ann Shield and her daughter Constance.
	The Act of Uniformity ended the power of barber-surgeons over licensing rights and placed midwives under the control of bishops of the Church of England.
1665	During the Great Plague of London, attendants refused to risk infection by handling the sick and dying.
1679	On October 26, midwife Elizabeth Cellier was linked to the Meal Tub Plot.
18th century	Surgeons began ousting female midwives from the tasks of autopsy and investigation of infanticide.
1700	In June, Elizabeth Haddon Estaugh, a Quaker nurse in Newtown, New Jersey, opened her home to patients.
1703	Sisters of the Hôtel Dieu died treating smallpox.
1710	Sisters of the Hôtel Dieu died treating yellow fever.
1720s	Elizabeth Harrison underwent smallpox vaccination and survived nursing a hospitalized victim.
1727	Mother Marie Tranchepain de St. Augustin set up the Ursuline Academy hospital in New Orleans.
1730	Sister Anne Leroy established Maidens of the Good Savior of Caen as visiting nurses to the homebound sick and elderly.
1737	Marguerite d'Youville, the first Canadian to be canonized, organized the Gray Sisters.
1759	On October 19, Louis XV appointed Angélique du Coudray France's first and only itinerant specialist in midwifery.
1766	Male physicians and barber-surgeons encouraged the use of forceps.
1770	On June 14, Margaret Morris made a journal entry of her treatment of fever.
	On July 30, Esther Gaston Walker served as a volunteer nurse at the Battle of Rocky Mount, North Carolina, and the next week at the Battle of Hanging Rock.
1771	Luisa Rosado served the court of King Charles III as royal midwife.
1775	On June 14, 1775, Major General Horatio Gates petitioned Commander in Chief George Washington for female nurses to attend sick soldiers.
	On July 27, Congress supplied the Continental Army with a medical department.
1776	Nurse Alice Redman petitioned the Maryland Council of Safety for better working conditions.
	In February 1776, Mrs. Slocumb of Wayne County, North Carolina, volunteered to treat the wounded at the Battle of Moore's Creek.
1777	On June 17, female nurses were recruited for a hospital in Mendham, New York.
1778	Officials burned the Brothers House Hospital of Ephrata to rid it of typhus after an influx of army wounded.
1781	On September 6, Mary Ledyard ministered to thirty-five casualties after the fall of Fort Griswold near Groton, Connecticut.
1785	Midwife Martha Moore Ballard began a twenty-seven-year journal of her experiences.
1789	Isabella Graham and Sarah Ogden Hoffman formed the Widow's Society.
1793	Absalom Jones, Richard Allen, Mary Scott, Sarah Bass, and Caesar Cranchal cared for yellow fever victims during an outbreak in Philadelphia.
1795	Midwife Manuela Matiana de Lara served as an expert witness.
1798	In June, John Wall became the first naval corpsman.
	Valentine Seaman organized a midwifery training program.
19th century	The Tolcha treated paralysis with hot packs.

1800	Marie Boivin of Montreuil, France, set up L'Hospice de la Maternité and studied fetal heartbeat.
1804	On May 20, José Antonio Cavellero ordered a general inoculation against smallpox in Texas.
1806	On May 19, Meriwether Lewis treated Indians.
1809	Elizabeth Seton founded the American Sisters of Charity of St. Joseph in Baltimore.
	In Nacogdoches, Texas, *curandera* María Benítez intervened in the beating of slave Lorenzo Marets.
1813	Stephen Decatur employed nurses Mary Allen and Mary Marshall aboard the frigate *United States.*
1816	Bellevue Hospital was established.
1818	On April 14, Congress created a modern medical corps.
1828	Male midwives dominated birthing at University College in England.
1832	Dr. Joseph Warrington organized the Lying-in Charity for Attending Indigent Women in Their Homes.
1833	The one-thousand-bed Royal Hospital opened in Baghdad, Iraq.
1835	Dr. Peter Parker set up a mission hospital in Canton, China.
1836	At the fall of the Alamo in San Antonio, Texas, Andrea Candelaria and Suzanna Dickerson treated casualties.
1839	Dr. Joseph Warrington launched the Philadelphia Nurse Society.
1840	Elizabeth Fry organized London's Quaker Nursing Sisters, who influenced bedside care across Europe.
	Margaret Barrett Prior visited the sick in Sing Sing Prison.
1843	Charles Dickens's *Martin Chuzzlewit* ridiculed London's workhouse nurses.
1844	During the Irish famine, Mother Jane Francis supervised the Sisters from Limerick in establishing a mission to the sick and starving.
1849	In January, Dr. Elizabeth Blackwell became the United States's first female physician.
1850	Sarah Paschal treated yellow fever in Texas.
1853	In Jamaica, Mary Jane Seacole battled an epidemic of yellow fever.
1854	On October 21, Florence Nightingale and her team of thirty-eight nurses sailed for Scutari, Turkey during the Crimean War.
1855	After the Battle of Tchernaya in the Crimea on August 16, Mary Jane Seacole treated allied casualties at the battlefront.
1856	In July, Florence Nightingale returned to Lea Hurst, England, an international idol.
	In August, Congress authorized the appointment of hospital stewards from noncommissioned male enlistees.
1857	Florence Nightingale launched a campaign to establish sanitary measures in India.
1859	Florence Nightingale published *Notes on Nursing: What It Is and Is Not.*
	Mary Agnes Jones established district nursing in England.
	William Rathbone instituted a district nursing project in Liverpool and set up a nursing school at the Liverpool Royal Infirmary.
	In June, Jean-Henri Dunant, a Genevan philanthropist, was inspired to create the Red Cross after seeing wounded on the battlefield of Solferino.
1860	Hanna Sandusky charged no fee for midwifery in Pennsylvania.
	In February, Dr. Elizabeth Blackwell's "Letter to Young Ladies Desirous of Studying Medicine" advised aspiring medical students to serve as hospital nurses as a means of learning about disease.
	On June 15, the first ten Nightingale nurses entered training.
1861	During the Civil War, Dorothea Lynde Dix was appointed superintendent of female nurses of the United States Sanitary Commission.
	Mary McCray fled slavery and volunteered as a Union nurse in Nashville, Tennessee.
	In April, Clara Barton became battle nurse to the Sixth Massachusetts Regiment.

On April 18, at Harpers Ferry, Virginia, Catholic sisters staffed abandoned hotels and chapels and readied warehouses for casualties.

On June 8, Union nurse Mary Ann Bickerdyke began work.

In July, Kady Brownell attended the casualties at Manassas, Virginia, where she was wounded in action.

On July 21, "Cap'n Sally" Tompkins converted her Richmond residence into the twenty-two-bed Robertson Hospital.

The U.S. War Department sought Florence Nightingale's advice on setting up medical installations.

1862   After the Battle of Shiloh in spring 1862, Sallie Chapman Gordon Law expanded the twelve-bed Southern Mothers' Hospital in Memphis, Tennessee.

Civil War nurses began staffing floating hospitals in February 16.

During the Union siege of the Confederate stronghold at Galveston, Texas, the Ursulines susters opened a hospital.

On May 31, while retrieving casualties from the field of battle, Juliet Ann Opie Hopkins suffered a permanent handicap. To honor her the state of Alabama placed her likeness on coins and paper money.

On June 19, Mother Paul Lennon established a treatment center at a looted hotel in Beaufort, North Carolina.

On July 14, the surgeon general's office set up an all-female nurse corps under superintendent Dorothea Lynde Dix.

On July 30, Sister Mary Consolata Conlon succumbed to fever while praying for dying patients at Point Lookout, Maryland.

In late August, Harriet P. Davie served at the Second Battle of Bull Run and was captured by Confederate forces.

At the Second Battle of Bull Run in August, Clara Barton and Almira Fales treated three thousand wounded.

On September 6, Sisters of Charity superintended a federal hospital in Frederick, Maryland.

At the Battle of Antietam on September 17, Clara Barton helped treat twenty-three thousand casualties.

In December, Walt Whitman managed a trainload of wounded bound for Washington.

Beginning in December, Louisa May Alcott worked night duty to treat casualties of the Battle of Fredericksburg.

Mother Angela Gillespie served aboard the steamer *Red Rover* at the height of the Civil War.

The navy commissioned the *Red Rover* as its first official hospital ship.

Under fire at Fort Ridgely in Fairfax, Minnesota, Eliza Muller nursed refugees and soldiers after the Sioux Indian Outbreak.

On December 31, Kate Cumming treated casualties from the Battle of Stone River at Murfreesboro, Tennessee.

1863   In January, Mary Ann Bickerdyke superintended the army pest house at Fort Pickering outside Memphis, Tennessee. In May, Anna Blair Etheridge was wounded in battle.

In early July, near Gettysburg, Pennsylvania, the St. Joseph's convent of the Daughters of Charity tended casualties at a Catholic church.

In September, the navy established a military hospital in a Memphis hotel headed by Sister St. John.

While smuggling opiates, Mary Kate Patterson Davies was arrested but returned to her job of nursing southern casualties.

1864	Clara Barton assumed the title of superintendent of the Department of Nurses for the Army of the James.
	In January, Dr. Mary Edwards Walker, the only woman during the Civil War to receive the Congressional Medal of Honor for Meritorious Service, was appointed assistant surgeon of the 52nd Ohio Infantry.
	In January, Felicia Grundy Porter organized the Women's Relief Society of the Confederate States.
	The Sisters of Charity opened Kansas's first civilian hospital in Leavenworth.
1865	On March 11, President Abraham Lincoln appointed Clara Barton as supervisor of the office of missing soldiers, making her the first woman to operate a U.S. government bureau.
	On April 9, 1865, Mary Ann Bickerdyke began mustering out 90 percent of two thousand Civil War convalescents.
	On May 24, Mary Ann Bickerdyke paraded with the Union Army before White House reviewing stands.
	While serving with the U.S. Christian Commission on the Ohio River, Isabella Morrison Fogg permanently injured her spine in a fall on the hospital ship *Jacob Strader.*
1866	Kate Cumming's *A Journal of Hospital Life in the Confederate Army of Tennessee from the Battle of Shiloh to the End of the War* particularized the carnage of the Battle of Shiloh, Tennessee.
1868	Mother Mary Baptist Russell headed St. Mary's Hospital in San Francisco, the West Coast's first Catholic facility.
1870s	Pilar Jáuregui published articles in the 1870s in *The Spanish Medical Amphitheatre.*
1870	Francisca Iracheta of Madrid published the first medical textbook issued by a Spanish woman.
1872	Dr. John Berry established the International Hospital in Kobe, Japan.
	Linda Richards evolved the first written charting and record-keeping system for nurses.
1873	New England Hospital for Women and Children graduated the first American registered nurse, Linda Richards.
	Father Damien volunteered as nurse-missionary to Hawaii's leper colony.
	Mother Marianne devoted her life to the leper colony of Molokai, Hawaii.
	The navy altered the title of nurse to bayman.
1877	Count Sano proposed the *Hakuiaisha,* the Japanese Red Cross Society.
	Frances Root became New York's first official visiting nurse.
	Lottie Moon, a Baptist missionary to Tengchow, observed relief efforts among sick peasants during a famine.
	Sister Henrietta began a one-year on-the-job training program at Kimberley, South Africa.
1878	Franciscan nuns opened the General Hospital of Colombo, Sri Lanka.
	Linda Richards opened a nursing school at Boston College Hospital.
1879	Sister Mary Aikenhead of the Irish Sisters of Charity spearheaded the establishment of Our Lady's Hospice.
	The first civilian black nurse, Mary Eliza P. Mahoney, graduated from training.
1880	Aldonza Eltrich and Vanossa Woenke taught classes in anesthesiology at St. John's Hospital in Springfield, Illinois.
1881	The Royal Prince Alfred Hospital in Sydney, Australia, reorganized under the Nightingale model.
1882	The United States formally chartered the Red Cross.

	In March, the United States signed the Geneva Convention, promising to care for the sick during war.
	On May 20, Clara Barton became the first president of the American Red Cross.
1884	Alice Fisher and Edith Horner established Philadelphia General Hospital.
1885	The Lady Dufferin Fund opened Western schools to female trainees in India.
1886	Dr. Mary Cutler established the East Gate Hospital for Women in Seoul, Korea.
	Elizabeth Pratt Jenks founded a visiting nurse project in Philadelphia.
	Eloisa Vílchez was appointed as resident midwife at the maternity home in Granada, Spain.
	Linda Richards initiated Japan's first nurse training program in Kyoto, Japan.
	Mary Cyrilla Erhard taught anesthesiology in Hawaii.
	On February 8, Boston's District Nursing Association hired its first nurse, Amelia Hodgkiss.
1887	Sister Mary Bernard pioneered nurse-anesthesiology at St. Vincent's Hospital in Erie, Pennsylvania.
1888	The Siriraj Hospital opened in Bangkok.
1889	Queen Victoria chartered the Jubilee Institute for Nurses.
	The Catholic Sisters of St. Francis, led by Sister Mary Joseph Dempsey, completed St. Mary's Hospital, a segment of the renowned Mayo Clinic.
	Susan La Flesche Picotte practiced medicine in Nebraska.
1890	The Goodyear Rubber Company made two pairs of gloves for nurse Caroline Hampton.
1891	Linda Richards headed the Visiting Nurse Society of Philadelphia.
	The U.S. government classified nurses of the Indian Health Service as civil service workers.
	William Hoare initiated the Hostel of God.
1892	Frances Watkins Harper wrote *Iola Leroy: Or, Shadows Uplifted,* which details the adventures of a mixed-blood Civil War nurse.
1893	Lillian Wald coined the term "public health nurse." Wald also open the Henry Street Settlement House during this same year.
	Alice Magaw established anesthesiology at the Mayo Clinic.
1894	The first national nursing organization began as the American Society of Superintendents of Training.
	Shimidzu led the Japanese Red Cross in training uniformed physicians, nurses, pharmacists, and corpsmen.
1895	Ada Mayo Stewart became the nation's first company visiting nurse.
	Pilar Ortiz Grimaud and Cristina Martín served the Casa de Socorro as official midwives.
	Rose Hawthorne Lathrop treated cancer patients at Blackwell's Island charity hospital in New York City.
1896	The first professional nurses in South Africa were German Red Cross staff at Windhoek.
1897	At the First and Second Convention of the American Society of Superintendents of Training Schools for Nursing, Sophia Palmer lauded nursing unions.
1898	Dr. Anita Newcomb McGee organized the Daughters of the American Revolution to lead a Hospital Corps Committee to augment the services of the Red Cross during the Spanish-American War.
	Emmy Krigar Suren became the first trained midwife in South Africa.
	Five female graduates of the Tuskegee Institute served in Cuba, and one black male nurse served in the Philippines during the Spanish-American War.
	In July, Namahyoke Curtis searched New Orleans for nurses who were immune to yellow fever to care for victims of the disease.

In mid-July, General William R. Shafter reassigned 729 nurses to Santiago de Cuba to treat an outbreak of yellow fever.

As of September 13, twenty-three ailing nurses had been furloughed home from the Spanish-American War.

Lady Ishbel Marjoribanks Aberdeen launched the Victorian Order of Nurses.

Nurses staffed the navy's first Red Cross hospital ship, the *Solace.*

1899	Ethel Baxter became the first nurse-anesthetist in the South.
1900s	Jessie Pettigrew, the first trained nurse assigned by the Baptist Foreign Mission Board, served in Hwanghsien, China.

Rose Kaplan set up a nursing settlement among Jewish refugee camps in Alexandria, Egypt.

1900   During the Boxer Rebellion, Japanese nurses treated the wounded of both sides.

On October 3, Jessie Sleet Scales became the United States' first black public health nurse.

Sophia Palmer edited the *American Journal of Nursing.*

1901   Agnes P. Mahoney began a ministry in Liberia.

After the Army Reorganization Bill launched a regular Army Nurse Corps on February 2, Dita H. Kinney was appointed supervisor.

On August 24, Clara Louise Maass died during a yellow fever study.

1902   Dame Mary Paget led the campaign for nursing registry in England.

The memoirs of Susie Baker King Taylor preserved the only written account of a black female participant in the Civil War.

1903   Adelaide Nutting led the Maryland State Nurses Association in a campaign for nursing regulations.

The first tuberculosis nurse in the United States, Reiba Thelin, worked at Johns Hopkins University Hospital.

1904   Canada's Army Medical Corps Nursing Service, headed by Captain Georgina F. Pope, awarded rank to nurses.

On June 16, Clara Barton resigned the presidency of the American Red Cross to Mabel T. Boardman.

Japan's St. Luke's Hospital thrived under the management of Araki San, its U.S.-trained superintendent of nurses.

1905   Jane Van Zandt supervised a Beirut nursing school.

The Mexican General Hospital opened under the supervision of Mary J. McCloud.

Margaret Edmunds opened Korea's first nursing school.

1906   Toronto acquired Canada's first tuberculosis nurse, Christina Mitchell.

1907   Dr. Sara Josephine Baker, the first woman to receive a Ph.D. in public health, joined the successful search for "Typhoid Mary" Mallon.

The first lying-in clinic, Elizabeth Haus, opened in Rehobeth, South Africa.

1908   The Sisters of Charity opened a nursing school in Panama City.

On August 18, Esther Hasson was appointed chief of the U.S. Navy Nurse Corps.

1909   Jane Delano organized the Red Cross nursing program.

The Henry Street Settlement House was the setting of the National Negro Conference, forerunner of the National Association for the Advancement of Colored People.

1910   Elizabeth Kenny initiated a hot pack treatment for polio.

Baltimore's board of health appointed Ellen La Motte as superintendent of visiting tuberculosis nurses.

1911   In Toronto, Eunice Henrietta Dyke became Canada's first tuberculosis nurse.

1912   Catholic officials established Lourdes.

The Siamese Red Cross established a nursing school.

1913   Carolyn Van Blarcom became the first licensed midwife in the United States.

On August 15, Hélène Bresslau Schweitzer assisted at the first surgery at Lambaréné, Gabon.

1914   China's first college-trained nurse, Elizabeth McKechnie, organized the China Nurses' Association.

The American Red Cross dispatched a medical unit aboard the USS *Red Cross.*

The Red Cross appointed Helen Scott Hay to supervise nurses in the Balkans and dispatched Lucy Minnigerode to the Polytechnic Institute in Kiev, Russia.

Emily Simmons was the first U.S.-trained nurse to aid the Allied cause in World War I.

1915   A memorial at the Andersonville National Cemetery in Georgia was the first to honor a civilian volunteer.

In June, England dispatched its Voluntary Aid Detachments to the front.

On October 12, German forces executed English nurse Edith Cavell for helping Allied soldiers to escape.

1916   Linda Kearns operated a Red Cross field hospital during the Irish uprising against British occupation of Northern Ireland.

Mademoiselle Miss, an anonymous nurse's memoir, portrayed the daily activities of World War I.

On October 16, Margaret Sanger opened the first U.S. birth control clinic.

1917   American Red Cross nurses formed a special black World War I unit at Camp Sherman.

On June 24, Adelaide Nutting organized the military nursing program for World War I.

In August, Frances Ban Ingen supervised nurses aboard the *Henderson* during World War I.

1918   Albertina M. Walker supervised an emergency center for flu victims in Windhoek, South Africa.

Annie Smithson, a nurse for Sinn Fein, treated wounded volunteers during the Irish rebellion.

In February Annie Goodrich was named chief inspector of United States Army hospitals.

In May, the Gray Ladies were mobilized at Walter Reed Hospital in Washington, D.C.

Beginning in September, patient load in England doubled from an end-of-war epidemic of Spanish influenza.

As of November 11, 1918, four corps nurses earned the Navy Cross.

Dr. Marie Stopes published *Married Love* and *Wise Parenthood.*

In Israel, Henrietta Szold, founder of Hadassah, established maternity nursing at Rothschild Hospital.

Mary Sewall Gardner and Elizabeth Fox directed the Red Cross Bureau of Public Health Nursing.

On September 22, United States Navy nurse Maude Coleman died of influenza. She was buried in Arlington National Cemetery, the first navy nurse to receive that honor.

The Maternity Center Association, the first nurse-midwife school, opened in New York City.

Mary Anne Nelson, who dropped dead in the ward at Aus, Namibia, was the only civilian nurse in southern Africa to be buried in a military cemetery with full honors.

1919   Mary Sewall Gardner received a Bronze Decoration from the Genoa, Italy, provincial authority for initiating public health nursing to eradicate tuberculosis.

Sadie Stewart Hobday of St. Helena Island became the first black nurse–social worker.

1920	Isabel Maitland Stewart and Lavinia L. Dock published *A Short History of Nursing.*
	The Indian Red Cross Society was founded.
1921	Leo and Jessie Halliwell carried their Seventh-Day Adventist medical mission to Brazil's Amazon Basin.
	Mother Mary Martin of Glenageary, Ireland, volunteered for the Catholic mission in Calabar, Nigeria.
	On March 17, Dr. Marie Stopes opened the Mothers' Clinic in Holloway, North London.
	The Carlos Van Buren School in Valparaiso, Chile, began the nation's first nurse-training program.
1923	Frances Payne Bolton endowed the Frances Payne Bolton School of Nursing at Western Reserve University.
	In Uganda, Teresa Kearney began a birthing service.
	The Anna D. Nery school opened in Rio de Janeiro, Brazil.
1924	Mary Sewall Gardner published a second edition of *Public Health Nursing.*
	Miss E. S. E. Perala of Helsinki, Finland, was the first South African midwife qualified in instrument deliveries.
1925	On Mary 28, Mary Breckinridge established the Frontier Nursing Service in Leslie County, Kentucky.
1926	Laura M. Bayne was the only African-American nurse in central Africa.
	Sister Mary Rose established the Servants of Relief.
	Pauline Bray Fletcher, Birmingham's first black registered nurse, opened a tuberculosis camp in Kelly Ingram Park.
1927	Carrie E. Bullock, president of the National Association of Colored Graduate Nurses, edited and published the monthly *National News Bulletin.*
1928	Lady Stanley organized the Association for Promoting Nursing as a Profession in Sri Lanka.
1930s	In Nazi Germany, health leader Leonardo Conti called for euthanasia of defective infants.
1932	Rose McNaught opened the first U.S. nurse-midwife training program.
1933	Elizabeth Kenny established a polio clinic in Queensland, Australia.
	Méiní O'Shea Dunlevy served the Blasket Islands, Ireland, as the only midwife.
1934	Only 9.2 percent of Germans joined the "Red Swastika nurses."
	The Australian government sponsored the Kenny Clinic and Training School.
1935	Karin Kirn of Owamboland published *Theory and Practice of Nursing* in the Oshindonga language.
	Margaret Sanger started the *Journal of Contraception.*
	Naomi Deutsch was named director of the United States Public Health Department.
	On September 15, the Nuremberg Laws were passed to enforce sterilization of second-class German citizens.
1939	On August 25, Princess Tsahaí Haíle Selassíe earned a degree in pediatric nursing to aid Ethiopia's poor.
1940s	Annie Smithson helped establish the Irish Nurses' Union.
1940	Elizabeth Kenny demonstrated polio treatment at the Minneapolis General Hospital.
1941	In July, the Bishop of Munster rebuked Hitler for his euthanasia program.
	Margaret Thomas directed the Tuskegee School of Nurse Midwifery, which opened on September 15.
	On December 7, aboard the *Solace,* Grace Lally retrieved victims aboard the *Arizona,* which sank in Pearl Harbor.
	The Japanese imprisoned eleven navy nurses.
	In New York, the Red Cross opened its first blood center.
1942	On January 5, the navy petitioned for fifty thousand nurses.

	In February, the U.S. military authorized officer's rank for nurses.
	In April, Allied troops dispatched nurses to safety before the surrender of Bataan.
	On July 3, Congress authorized ranks for nurses.
	On July 10, Nazi medical staffs began human experimentation at Auschwitz.
	In December, Sue Dauser headed the U.S. Navy Nurse Corps.
	Tsahaí Haíle Selassíe set up a public health headquarters in Ethiopia.
1943	A black nursing administrator and educator, Estelle Massey Riddle, advised the National Nursing Council for War Service.
	Navy nurses entered training as flight nurses.
	On June 14, the U.S. Congress passed the Bolton Act, setting up the Cadet Nurse Corps.
	On September 9, six British nurses aboard the *Newfoundland* were killed when the ship was bombed.
	On November 8, nurses Wilma Lytle, Ava Maness, and Helen Porter were lost in occupied Albania after a forced landing.
	Sisters M. Helen Herb and M. Theophane Shoemaker opened Santa Fe's Catholic Maternity Institute and School for Nurse-Midwifery.
1944	Eleanor Roosevelt christened the *Liberty Ship Harriet Tubman.*
	Ethel M. Greathouse consolidated a volunteer staff called the "Miracle of Hickory."
	On February 7, a German bomber killed allied patients, doctors, corpsmen, and three nurses at Anzio.
	On March 22, three nurses lost in Albania were recovered alive.
	On June 5, following the D day landing in Normandy, France, nurses set up field hospitals.
	Ruth Council alerted the Red Cross to a polio epidemic in Hickory, North Carolina.
1945	Lucile Petry recruited 135,000 volunteers for the U.S. Cadet Nurse Corps.
	On January 25, the U.S. Navy Nurse Corps admitted its first black nurse, Phyllis Mae Daley.
	On January 6, President Franklin D. Roosevelt asked Congress to draft nurses into the military.
	On February 23, the army recovered eleven captive navy nurses.
	On April 17, Allied rescuers observed sixty thousand skeletal prisoners at Auschwitz.
1946	Ilma Kaisa Esteri Laitenen became South Africa's first official nurse instructor.
	In Kakata, Liberia, Ellen Miama Moore set up the Samuel Grimes Maternal and Child Welfare Center.
	Mother Cabrini was canonized as the first American saint and patron of refugees and immigrants.
	The United Nations launched the World Health Organization.
1947	Nurses of the Supreme Command of Allied Powers helped to rebuild Japan's health care system.
	The Red Hook Experiment combined the missions of New York City's Department of Health with Brooklyn's Visiting Nurse Association to treat inner-city poor.
1948	On December 21, Mother Teresa began mission work among the poor of India.
1949	Yukon public health nurse Amy V. Wilson opened a clinic at Whitehorse.
1950s	Rosina Binte Karim traveled Malaysia as its first public health nurse.
1950	Beginning in June, 260 army nurses served in the Korean War.
	In July, the Air Force Nurse Corps was officially begun.
	On October 7, Mother Teresa launched the Missionaries of Charity.
	The MASH unit was officially introduced in Korea.
	The U.S. Navy Nurse Corps staffed three hospital ships.
1952	Ethel Tschida began a campaign to raise the survival rate of Hawaiian infants.
	Sister Dulce became a volunteer street nurse in Salvador de Bahía, Brazil.

Dr. Hildegard Elizabeth Peplau, the "mother of psychiatric nursing," published *Interpersonal Relations in Nursing: A Conceptual Framework for Psychodynamic Nursing,* which pioneers the notion of a one-on-one relationship between nurses and patients.

1954   On March 28, Geneviève de Galard earned the French Legion of Honor award for her service during the fall of Dien Bien Phu, Vietnam.

Canadian nurse Lyle Creelman headed WHO's nursing sector.

1955   On April 12, thousands of March of Dimes volunteers celebrated the Salk vaccine.

1960s   Bilingual nurse Susan Stearly treated underserved Latino patients in Trinidad, Colorado.

Dr. Connie Redbird Pinkerman-Uri established Los Angeles's first Indian Free Clinic.

Sabinita Herrera of Truchas, New Mexico, selected and administered herbs at the Truchas Medical Clinic.

1960   Annie Wauneka taught health through radio broadcasts at Gallup, New Mexico.

1962   Ruth Bronson won the Oveta Cult Hobby Award for medical service.

1965   Magrieta Airaksinen wrote an illustrated text in the Owambo language.

1966   On February 18, Carol Ann Drazba and Elizabeth Ann Jones were killed in a helicopter crash during the Vietnam War.

1967   Dr. Cicely Saunders founded the first modern receiving home for the dying and organized an international hospice network for children and adults.

Florence Wald launched the American concept of hospice.

On November 30, Eleanor Grace Alexander, Jeremy Olmstead, Hedwig Diane Orlowski, and Kenneth Shoemaker died in a plane crash outside Qui Nhon.

1968   On February 1, Betty Ann Olsen, a staff nurse for the Christian Missionary Alliance, was captured in Vietnam.

On September 29, Betty Ann Olsen died in prison.

Marie Manthey proposed the concept of primary nurse care for use in the Peace Corps.

Richard Hooker's *MASH* (1968) immortalized the MASH nurse of the Korean War.

1969   Dr. Elisabeth Kübler-Ross published *On Death and Dying.*

Florence Wald established an interdisciplinary team to analyze the needs of the dying.

On June 8, Sharon Ann Lane became the only nurse to die from enemy fire during the Vietnam War.

The Indian Health Service lowered mother and infant morality rates in Alaska by hiring a midwife.

1970s   Eleanora Fry treated an Idaho community of five hundred.

Ida M. Martinson completed a national model on home care for the dying child.

Dolores Krieger originated therapeutic touch.

1970   Betty Jumper treated the sick on the Seminole Reservation in Florida.

Dr. Eleanor C. Lambertsen proposed nursing teams.

1971   Florence Wald published "Interdisciplinary Study for Care of Dying Patients and Their Families."

1973   In the United States, abortion on demand was legalized on January 22 after the Supreme Court overturned a severe Texas law in the case of *Roe v. Wade.*

1975   On April 9, Mary Therese Klinker and 243 Vietnamese children died in a plane crash during Operation Babylift.

1977   Faye Wattleton of Planned Parenthood led the fight against the Right to Life initiative during an antichoice backlash.

1979   Hazel Winifred Johnson became the first black female general.

Mother Teresa received the Nobel Peace Prize.

1980s   Helen Miramontes volunteered to test an AIDS vaccine.

1980	The 1.4 million U.S. nurses made up the largest segment of health professionals.
1982	Elizabeth Dayani established American Nursing Resources.
	In November, Sister Frances Dominica launched Helen House in Oxford, England.
1983	Médicins sans Frontières dispatched Kristin Liland to upgrade midwifery in Chitembo, Angola.
	Ann Armstrong Dailey founded Children's Hospice International.
	Drs. Françoise Barre-Sinoussi and Luc Montagnier of the Pasteur Institute in Paris officially named AIDS.
1984	Betty Baines Compton received the Wonder Woman Foundation award.
1985	Dr. Ruth Watson Lubic was named March of Dimes nurse.
	On February 16, President Ronald Reagan proclaimed Clara Hale an American hero for sheltering babies born with drug addiction and AIDS.
1987	Brigadier General Clara Mae Leach Adams-Ender, the first woman to earn an Army Expert Field Medical badge, headed the Army Nurse Corps.
1988	Rutgers University sponsors Live for Life to aid school nurses.
1989	On November 16, Los Angeles declared Biddy Mason Day, to honor the former slave who became midwife to a whole community.
	The American Nurses Association acknowledged an abortion clinic patients' right to privacy.
1990	On December 8, the 807th MASH began training for nuclear, chemical, and biological warfare under desert conditions.
1992	On June 12, Margarethe Cammermeyer challenged the U.S. Army Nurse Corps for giving her a summary discharge on the grounds of homosexuality.
	There were sixteen arsons, thirteen attempted arsons or bombings, and one bombing, with damages amounting to more than $2 million, at U.S. abortion clinics.
1993	Glenna Goodacre sculpted the Vietnam Women's Memorial, the first official honor the nation paid to U.S. women in the military.
	Author Alice Walker reported on interviews with midwives who performed female genital mutilation.
1994	WHO published "Nursing Beyond the Year 2000."
	Cuban nurse Raynaldo Soto Hernández won a poetry prize for *Habitaciones*.
1995	Brenda Pratt Shafer contested the controversial procedure called partial birth abortion.
	In April, Ebola killed a nurse in Kikwit, Zaire.
	Jesse Dragoo launched the Sexual Assault Nurse Examiners.
	On January 25, 1995, Linda Degnan demonstrated therapeutic touch.
1997	In April, Roussel Uclaf halted U.S. distribution of RU-486.
1998	Canada's first registered midwives practiced in British Columbia.
	Cynthia Gorney published *Articles of Faith: A Frontline History of the Abortion Wars,* a dialectic that balanced opposing points of view.
	On January 29, a security guard was killed and nurse Emily Lyons crippled by a bomb blast at Birmingham's New Woman All Women Health Care Center.
	In June 1998, doctors, nurses, and midwives in the Third World were accused of sterilizing women with the untested drug quinacrine.

Works by and about Healers

An Account of the Principal Lazarettos of Europe, John Howard, 1789

American Daughter Gone to War: On the Front Lines with an Army Nurse in Vietnam, Winnie Smith, 1992

American Red Cross Textbook on Home Hygiene and Care of the Sick, Jane Delano, 1918

And They Shall Walk, Elizabeth Kenny, 1943

Aphorism, Hildegard of Bingen, ca. 1160

Beulah, Augusta Jane Evans Wilson, 1869

Birth Control Today, Dr. Marie Stopes, 1934

The Blessings of Love, Mother Teresa, 1996

Book of Healing Herbs, Hildegard of Bingen, ca. 1150

Book of Medical Treatment and Causes and Cures, Hildegarde of Bingen, ca. 1150

A Case for the Shorter Workday and Women and Industry, Josephine Goldmark, 1916

Castaways, Cabeza de Vaca, 1528

A Century of Nursing with Hints toward the Organization of a Training School, Abby Woolsey, 1876

Child Labor Legislation Handbook, Josephine Goldmark, 1907

Childbearing: A Book of Choices, Ruth Lubic and Gene R. Hawes, 1988

Christ's Poor, Rose Hawthorne Lathrop, 1901

Comrade Sister, Helene Mierisch, 1934

Concerning the Cure of Diseases, Trotula of Salerno, ca. 1100

Concerning Women's Disease, Soranus of Ephesus, early 2nd century

Curing Women's Diseases, Trotula of Salerno, ca. 1100

Developments in Nursing Education since 1918, Isabel Maitland Stewart, 1921

Dialogues on the Soul and the Body, St. Catherine of Genoa, late 15th century

Fatigue Efficiency, Josephine Goldmark, 1912

50 Years in Starch, Anne Williamson, 1948

Finding Themselves, Julia Catherine Stimson, 1918

Gleaning from the Southland, Kate Cumming, 1866

A Green Tent in Flanders, Maude Mortimer, 1918

Habitaciones, Reynaldo Soto Hernández, 1994

A Handbook of Nursing for Family and General Use, Georgeanna Woolsey, 1879

Harmonic Symphony of Heavenly Revolutions, Hildegard of Bingen, 1147

The History and Progress of District Nursing, William Rathbone, 1890

Home Before Morning: The Story of an Army Nurse in Vietnam, Lynda Van Devanter, 1983

Hospital Days, Jane Stuart Woolsey, 1870

Hospital Sketches in *Commonwealth,* Louisa May Alcott, May 22–June 26, 1863

The House on Henry Street, Lillian Wald, 1915

How to Talk to Your Child about Sex, Faye Wattleton, 1986

"The Hygiene of a Midwife," Soranus of Ephesus, early 2nd century

I Saw Them Die, Shirley Millard, 1936

I Served on Bataan, Juanita Redmond, 1943

Instruction of Midwives, Francisca Iracheta, 1870

"The Interdisciplinary Study for Care of Dying Patients and Their Families," Florence Wald, 1971

Iola Leroy: or, Shadows Uplifted, Frances Watkins Harper, 1892

Journal of Hospital Life in the Confederate Army of Tennessee from the Battle of Shiloh to the End of the War, Kate Cumming, 1866

Joy in Loving: A Guide to Daily Living with Mother Teresa, Mother Teresa, 1997

Lamps on the Prairie: A History of Nursing in Kansas, Kansas State Nurses' Association, 1942

The Last Ninety Days of the War in North Carolina, Cornelia Phillips Spencer, 1866

The Laws of Life with Special Reference to the Physical Education of Girls, Dr. Elizabeth Blackwell, 1852

Leaves from a Nurse's Life's History, 1906, Jean S. Edmunds, 1906

"Letter to Young Ladies Desirous of Studying Medicine" in *The English Woman's Journal,* Dr. Elizabeth Blackwell, February 1860

Loving Jesus, Mother Teresa, 1991

Mademoiselle Miss, anonymous, 1916

Making Choices, Taking Chances: Nurse Leaders Tell Their Stories, Thelma M. Schorr and Anne Zimmerman, 1988

The Management of Terminal Disease, Dr. Cicely Saunders, 1967

A Manual of Nursing, Dr. Victoria White, 1878

Married Love, Dr. Marie Stopes, 1918

Memoranda During the War, Walt Whitman, 1876

Memories, Fannie Beers, 1888

A Memory of Solferino, Henri Dunant, 1862

Method Versus Muddle and Waste in Charitable Work, William Rathbone, 1890

The Midwife in England, Carolyn C. Van Blarcom, 1913

A Midwife's Tale: The Life of Martha Ballard, Based on Her Diary, 1785–1812, Laurel Thatcher Ulrich, 1990

The Midwives Book, or the Whole Art of Midwifery Discovered, Directing Childbearing Women How to Behave Themselves in Their Conception, Bearing and Nursing of Children, J. Sharp, 1671

Mother and Child Saved: The Memoirs of the Frisian Midwife Catharina Schrader, 1693–1745, Catharina Schrader, 1745

Mother Teresa: In My Own Words, 1996

Mothers in Bondage, Margaret Sanger, 1928

My Life for the Poor, Mother Teresa, 1996

My Story of the War, Mary A. Livermore, 1887

Myself and Others, Annie Smithson, 1944

No Time for Prejudice: A Story of the Integration of Negroes in Nursing in the United States, Mabel Doyle Keaton Staupers, 1961

Notes on Hospitals, Florence Nightingale, 1859

Notes on Matters Affecting the Health, Efficiency and Hospital Administration of the British Army, Florence Nightingale, 1857

Notes on Nursing: What It Is and Is Not, Florence Nightingale, 1859

Nurse and Spy in the Union Army, Sarah Emma Evelyn Edmonds, 1865

A Nurse in the Yukon, Amy V. Wilson, 1965

Nursing and Nursing Education in the United States, Josephine Goldmark, 1923

Nursing the Sick, Florence Nightingale, 1882

Observations in Midwifery, Percival Willughby, ca. 1670

Our Army Nurses, Mary A. Gardner, 1896

The Path We Tread: Blacks in Nursing, 1854–1984, Mary Elizabeth Lancaster Carnegie, 1986

The Person with AIDS: Nursing Perspectives, Jerry D. Durham and Felissa L. Cohen, 1987

Physica St. Hildegardis, Hildegard of Bingen, 16th century

A Piece of My Heart (drama), Shirley Lauro, 1991

A Piece of My Heart: The Stories of Twenty-Six American Women Who Served in Vietnam, Keith Walker, 1985

The Practice of Midwifery or Memoirs and Selected Observations, Marie Anne Victoire Boivin and Marie-Louise Lachapelle, ca. 1800

Prisons and Prison Discipline, Dorothea Lynde Dix, 1845

Public Health Nursing, Mary Sewall Gardner, 1916

Recollections of Workhouse Visiting and Management During Twenty-Five Years, Louisa Twining, 1880

Reminiscences of Linda Richards, 1911

Reminiscences of My Life in Camp, Susie Baker King Taylor, 1902

Reminiscences of the Life of a Nurse in Field, Hospital and Camp during the Civil War, Anna P. Erving, 1904

Roman Catholic Methods of Birth Control, Dr. Marie Stopes, 1933

Scivias, Hildegard of Bingen, 1152.

Seeking the Heart of God: Reflections on Prayer, Mother Teresa, 1993

A Short History of Nursing, Isabel Maitland Stewart and Lavinia L. Dock, 1920

A Short Practical Handbook, Trotula of Salerno, ca. 1100

Sick Nursing and Health Nursing, Florence Nightingale, 1893

The Simple Path, Mother Teresa, 1995

South after Gettysburg: Letters of Cornelia Hancock, 1863–1868, Cornelia Hancock, 1956

A Southern Woman's Story, Phoebe Yates Pember, 1879

Specimen Days and Collect, Walt Whitman, 1883

A Story of Courage, Rose Hawthorne Lathrop, 1894

Story of My Childhood, Clara Barton, 1907

Story of the Red Cross, Clara Barton, 1904

A Summary of the Art of Midwifery, Angélique du Coudray, 1759

Theory and Practice of Nursing, Karin Kirn, 1935

Total Surrender, Mother Teresa, 1993

Training of Nurses, Florence Nightingale, 1882

Tuberculosis Nurse, Ellen La Motte, 1915

Under the Care of the Japanese War Office, Ethel McCaul, 1905

Under the Guns: A Woman's Reminiscences of the Civil War, Annie T. Wittenmyer, 1895

Under the Red Cross Flag at Home and Abroad, Mabel Boardman, 1915

Visions of War, Dreams of Peace: Writings of Women in the Vietnam War, Lynda Van Devanter and Joan A. Furey, 1991

Wide Neighborhood: A Story of the Frontier Nursing Service, Mary Breckinridge, 1952

Windows on Henry Street, Lillian Wald, 1925

With the Armies of the Tsar: A Nurse at the Russian Front, 1914–1918, Florence Farmborough, 1974

Women at War: The Story of Fifty Nurses Who Served in Vietnam, Elizabeth Norman, 1990

Wonderful Adventures of Mrs. Seacole in Many Lands, Mary Jane Seacole, 1857

Your Baby's First Year, Dr. Marie Stopes, 1939

Bibliography

Books

Abel-Smith, Brian. *A History of the Nursing Profession.* London: Heinemann, 1960.

Abrams, Lynn, and Elizabeth Harvey, eds. *Gender Relations in German History: Power, Agency and Experience from the Sixteenth to the Twentieth Century.* Durham, N.C.: Duke University Press, 1997.

Aikman, Lonnelle. *Nature's Healing Arts: From Folk Medicine to Modern Drugs.* Washington, D.C.: National Geographic, 1966.

Allen, Catherine B. *The New Lottie Moon Story.* Nashville, Tenn.: Broadman Press, 1980.

Amico, Eleanor B., ed. *Reader's Guide to Women's Studies.* Chicago: Fitzroy Dearborn, 1998.

Anaya, Rudolfo A. *Bless Me, Ultima.* Berkeley, Calif.: TOS Publications, 1972.

Anderson, Peggy. *Nurse.* New York: St. Martin's Press, 1978.

Anderson, Owannah. *Ohoyo One Thousand: A Resource Guide of American Indian/Alaska Native Women.* Washington, D.C.: U.S. Department of Education, 1982.

Annas, George J., and Michael A. Grodin. *The Nazi Doctors and the Nuremberg Code.* New York: Oxford University Press, 1992.

Apple, Rima D., ed. *Women's Health, Health and Medicine in America: A Historical Handbook.* New Brunswick, N.J.: Rutgers University Press, 1992.

Armstrong, Dorothy Mary. *The First Fifty Years: A History of Nursing at the Royal Prince Alfred Hospital, Sydney, from 1882–1932.* Sydney: Royal Prince Alfred Hospital Graduate Nurses' Association, 1965.

Augur, Helen. *An American Jezebel: The Life of Anne Hutchinson.* New York: Brentano's, 1930.

Austin, Anne L. *The Woolsey Sisters of New York.* Philadelphia: American Philosophical Society, 1971.

Backhouse, Frances. *Women of the Klondike.* Vancouver: Whitecap Books, 1995.

Baker, Rachel. *The First Woman Doctor.* New York: Scholastic Books, 1987.

Baly, Monica E. *Nursing and Social Change.* New York: Routledge, 1995.

Bataille, Gretchen M., ed. *Native American Women: A Biographical Dictionary.* New York: Garland, 1993.

Battis, Emery. *Saints and Sectaries: Anne Hutchinson and the Antinomian Controversy in the Massachusetts Bay Colony.* Chapel Hill: University of North Carolina Press, 1962.

Baugh, Albert C., ed. *A Literary History of England.* New York: Appleton-Century-Crofts, 1948.

Bell, Irvin Wiley. *Embattled Confederates.* New York: Harper and Row, 1964.

Bell, Robert E. *Dictionary of Classical Mythology.* Santa Barbara, Calif.: ABC-CLIO, 1982.

———. *Women of Classical Mythology: A Biographical Dictionary.* Santa Barbara, Calif.: ABC-CLIO, 1991.

Bentley, James. *A Calendar of Saints.* London: Little, Brown, 1993.

Berrill, Jacquelyn. *Albert Schweitzer: Man of Mercy.* New York: Dodd, Mead, 1956.

Blain, Virginia, Patricia Clements, and Isabel Grundy. *The Feminist Companion to Literature in English.* New Haven, Conn.: Yale University Press, 1990.

Blanco, Richard L. *Physician of the American Revolution, Jonathan Potts.* New York: Garland, 1979.

Blassingame, Wyatt. *Combat Nurses of World War II.* New York: Random House, 1967.

Boardman, Mabel. *Under the Red Cross Flag at Home and Abroad.* London: J. B. Lippincott, 1915.

Bourke-White, Margaret. *They Called It Purple Heart Valley.* New York: Simon and Schuster, 1944.

Bowder, Diana, ed. *Who Was Who in the Roman World.* New York: Washington Square Press, 1980.

———. *Who Was Who in the Greek World.* New York: Washington Square Press, 1982.

Boylston, Helen. *Clara Barton.* New York: Random House, 1955.

Bradley, S. A. J., ed. *Anglo-Saxon Poetry.* London: J. M. Dent, 1995.

Brainard, Annie M. *The Evolution of Public Health Nursing.* Philadelphia: W. B. Saunders, 1922.

Breckinridge, Mary. *Wide Neighborhood: A Story of the Frontier Nursing Service.* New York: Harper and Row, 1952.

Brooke, Elisabeth. *Women Healers: Portraits of Herbalists, Physicians, and Midwives.* Rochester, Vt.: Healing Arts Press, 1995.

Brown, Jordan. *Elizabeth Blackwell.* New York: Chelsea House, 1989.

Brown, Michael. *Nurses, the Human Touch.* New York: Ivy Books, 1992.

Bryant, Arthur. *The Medieval Foundation of England.* Garden City, N.Y.: Doubleday, 1967.

Buck, Claire, ed. *The Bloomsbury Guide to Women's Literature.* New York: Prentice Hall, 1992.

Bullough, Vern L., Olga Maranjian Church, and Alice P. Stein. *American Nursing: A Biographical Dictionary.* New York: Garland, 1988.

Burke, Helen. *The Royal Hospital Donnybrook.* Dublin: Royal Hospital Donnybrook, 1993.

Burleigh, Michael. *Death and Deliverance: Euthanasia in Germany, 1900–1945.* Cambridge: Cambridge University Press, 1994.

Bushman, Claudia Lauper, and Richard Lyman Bushman. *Mormons in America.* New York: Oxford Press, 1998.

Butler, Alban. *Lives of the Saints.* New York: Barnes and Noble, 1997.

Cabeza de Vaca, Álvar Nuñez. *Castaways.* 1528. Berkeley: University of California Press, 1993.

Cabot, Dr. Richard C. "Introduction." *Mademoiselle Miss.* Boston: W. A. Butterfield, 1916.

Camp, LaVonne Telshaw. *Lingering Fever: A World War II Nurse's Memoir.* Jefferson, N.C.: McFarland, 1997.

Campbell, Marie. *Folks Do Get Born.* New York: Rinehart, 1946.

Carnegie, Mary Elizabeth Lancaster. *The Path We Tread: Blacks in Nursing Worldwide, 1854–1994.* New York: National League for Nursing Press, 1995.

Cavendish, Richard, ed. *Man, Myth and Magic.* New York: Marshall Cavendish, 1970.

Chesler, Ellen. *Woman of Valor: Margaret Sanger and the Birth Control Movement in America.* New York: Simon and Schuster, 1992.

Clarke, Richard F., S.J. *Lourdes, Its Inhabitants, Its Pilgrims, and Its Miracles.* New York: Benziger Brothers, 1888.

Cleaveland, Agnes Morley. *No Life for a Lady.* Lincoln: University of Nebraska Press, 1941.

Clement, J., ed. *Noble Deeds of American Women with Biographical Sketches of Some of the More Prominent.* Williamstown, Mass.: Corner House, 1975.

Clores, Suzanne. *Native American Women.* New York: Chelsea House, 1995.

Cohn-Sherbok, Lavinia. *Who's Who in Christianity.* Chicago: Routledge, 1998.

Corr, C. A., and D. M. Corr. *Hospice Approaches to Pediatric Care.* Annapolis, Md.: Springer, 1985.

Cosner, Sharon. *War Nurses.* New York: Walker, 1988.

Coss, Clare. *Lillian Wald: Progressive Activist.* New York: Feminist Press, 1989.

Cousins, Norman. *Albert Schweitzer's Mission: Healing and Peace.* New York: W. W. Norton, 1985.

Cowan, David L. *Medicine in Revolutionary New Jersey.* Trenton: New Jersey Historical Commission, 1975.

Cowdrey, Albert E. *Fighting for Life: American Military Medicine in World War II.* New York: Free Press, 1994.

Crichton, Jennifer. *Delivery: A Nurse-Midwife's Story.* New York: Warner Books, 1986.

Crystal, David, ed. *The Cambridge Biographical Dictionary.* Cambridge: University of Cambridge, 1996.

Cumming, Kate. *A Journal of Hospital Life in the Confederate Army of Tennessee from the Battle of Shiloh to the End of the War.* Louisville, Ky.: John P. Morton, 1866.

Cunningham, H. H. *Doctors in Gray: The Confederate Medical Service.* Baton Rouge: Louisiana State University Press, 1986.

Current Biography. New York: H. W. Wilson, 1985.

Curtis, Edith. *Anne Hutchinson.* Cambridge, Mass.: Washburn and Thomas, 1930.

Cushman, Karen. *The Midwife's Apprentice.* New York: HarperTrophy, 1995.

Daniels, Doris Groshen. *Always a Sister: The Feminism of Lillian D. Wald.* New York: Feminist Press, 1995.

Davidson, Cathy N., and Linda Wagner-Martin. *The Oxford Companion to Women's Writing.* New York: Oxford University Press, 1995.

Day, A. Grove. *Hawaii and Its People.* New York: Duell, Sloan and Pearce, 1960.

Day, James. *The Black Death.* New York: Bookwright Press, 1989.

de Leeuw, Adele, and Cateau. *Nurses Who Led the Way.* Racine, Wis.: Whitman Publishing, 1961.

Deen, Edith. *Great Women of the Christian Faith.* Westwood, N.J.: Barbour, 1959.

Defoe, Daniel. *A Journal of the Plague Year.* New York: New American Library, 1960.

Delehaye, Hippolyte. *The Legends of the Saints.* Dublin: Four Courts Press, 1955.

Denney, Robert E. *Civil War Medicine: Care and Comfort of the Wounded.* New York: Sterling Publishing, 1995.

DeVoto, Bernard, ed. *The Journals of Lewis and Clark.* Boston: Houghton Mifflin, 1953.

Dickens, Charles. *Martin Chuzzlewit.* New York: Signet Classic, 1965.

Dictionary of National Biography, 1941–1950. New York: Oxford University Press, 1959.

Dock, Lavinia, and Isabel M. Stewart. *A Short History of Nursing.* New York: G. P. Putnam's Sons, 1959.

Dodge, Bertha S. *The Story of Nursing.* Boston: Little, Brown, 1965.

Dolan, Josephine A., R.N. *History of Nursing.* Philadelphia: W. B. Saunders, 1968.

Donahue, M. Patricia. *Nursing, the Finest Art.* St. Louis: C. V. Mosby, 1985.

Duby, Georges, and Michelle Perrot, general eds. *A History of Women in the West.* Cambridge, Mass.: Belknap Press, 1992.

Duncan, Louis C. *The Medical Department of the United States Army in the Civil War.* Washington: Surgeon General's Office, 1914.

Durant, Will. *The Life of Greece.* New York: Simon and Schuster, 1939.

Durham, Jerry D., and Felissa L. Cohen, eds. *The Person with AIDS: Nursing Perspectives.* New York: Springer, 1987.

Eagle, Dorothy, and Meic Stephens, eds. *The Oxford Illustrated Literary Guide to Great Britain and Ireland.* New York: Oxford University Press, 1992.

East, Charles, ed. *Sarah Morgan: The Civil War Diary of a Southern Woman.* New York: Touchstone, 1991.

Edmonds, S. Emma. *Nurse and Spy in the Union Army: The Adventures and Experiences of a Woman in Hospitals, Camps, and Battlefields.* Philadelphia: W. S. Williams, 1865.

Ehrenreich, Barbara, and Deirdre English. *Witches, Midwives, and Nurses: A History of Women Healers.* New York: Feminist Press, 1995.

Ehrlich, Eugene, and Gorton Carruth. *The Oxford Illustrated Literary Guide to the United States.* New York: Oxford University Press, 1982.

Ekstrom, Reynolds R. *The New Concise Catholic Dictionary.* Mystic, Conn.: Twenty-Third Publications, 1995.

Elkon, Juliette. *Edith Cavell, Heroic Nurse.* New York: Julian Messner, 1956.

Ellis, Peter Berresford. *Celtic Women: Women in Celtic Society and Literature.* Grand Rapids, Mich.: William B. Eerdmans, 1995.

Emergency War Surgery. Washington, D.C.: Department of Defense, 1958.

Emert, Phyllis Raybin, ed. *Women in the Civil War: Warriors, Patriots, Nurses, and Spies.* New York: Discovery Enterprises, 1995.

The Encyclopedia of World Biography. New York: McGraw-Hill, 1973.

Euripides. *Hippolytus* in *Greek Tragedies,* vol. 1. David Grene and Richmond Lattimore, eds. Chicago: Phoenix Books, 1960.

Evans, Barrie. *O.R.: The True Story of a Nurse Anesthetist.* New York: Dell, 1982.

Ewen, Jean. *China Nurse, 1932–1939.* Toronto: McClelland and Stewart, 1981.

Faber, Doris. *Anne Hutchinson.* Champaign, Ill.: Gerrard Publishing, 1970.

Fall, Bernard B. *Hell in a Very Small Place: The Siege of Dien Bien Phu.* New York: Vintage Books, 1966.

Farmborough, Florence. *With the Armies of the Tsar: A Nurse at the Russian Front, 1914–1918.* New York: Stein and Day, 1974.

Farmer, David Hugh. *The Oxford Dictionary of Saints.* Oxford: Oxford University Press, 1992.

Felder, Deborah G. *The 100 Most Influential Women of All Time: A Ranking Past and Present.* New York: Citadel Press, 1996.

Fessler, Diane Burke. *No Time for Fear: Voices of American Military Nurses in World War II.* East Lansing: Michigan State University Press, 1996.

Flanagan, Lyndia. *One Strong voice: The Story of the American Nurses Association.* New York: ANA, 1976.

Franck, Irene, and David Brownstone. *Women's World: A Timeline of Women in History.* New York: HarperPerennial, 1995.

Fraser, Evelyn G., R.N. *Fifty Years of Service: History of the School of Nursing of the Roosevelt Hospital, New York City.* New York: Alumnae Association of the Roosevelt Hospital School of Nursing, 1946.

Fraser, Gertrude. *African American Midwives in the South.* New York: Cambridge University Press, 1998.

Gale, Dr. Robert Peter, and Thomas Hauser. *Final Warning: The Legacy of Chernobyl.* New York: Warner Books, 1988.

Garraty, John A., ed. *Dictionary of American Biography.* New York: Charles Scribner's Sons, 1955.

Gay, Kathlyn, and Martin K. Gay. *Heroes of Conscience.* Santa Barbara, Calif.: ABC-CLIO, 1996.

Gelbart, Nina. *King's Midwife: A History and Mystery of Madame du Coudray.* Berkeley: University of California Press, 1998.

Gian, Richard V. N. *The History of the U.S. Army Medical Service Corps.* Washington, D.C.: Offices of the Surgeon General and Center of Military History of the U.S. Army, 1997.

Gibbon, John Murray. *Three Centuries of Canadian Nursing.* Toronto: Hunter-Rose, 1994.

Giff, Patricia Reilly. *Mother Teresa: Sister to the Poor.* New York: Viking Kestrel, 1986.

Gilbert, Martin. *Atlas of the Holocaust.* New York: William Morrow, 1993.

Gino, Carol. *The Nurse's Story.* New York: Bantam Books, 1982.

Gollaher, David. *Voice for the Mad: The Life of Dorothea Dix.* New York: Free Press, 1995.

Goodnow, Minnie. *Nursing History.* London: W. B. Saunders, 1942.

———. *Outlines of Nursing History.* Philadelphia: W. B. Saunders, 1940.

Gorney, Cynthia. *Articles of Faith: A Frontline History of the Abortion Wars.* New York: Simon and Schuster, 1998.

Gragg, Rod, ed. *The Illustrated Confederate Reader.* New York: Harper and Row, 1989.

Greenbie, Marjorie Barstow. *Lincoln's Daughters of Mercy.* New York: G. P. Putnam's Sons, 1944.

Gridley, Marion E. *American Indian Women.* New York: Hawthorn Books, 1974.

Griffin, Gerald Joseph, and H. Joann King Griffin. *Jensen's History and Trends of Professional Nursing.* Saint Louis, Mo.: C. V. Mosby, 1965.

Griffin, Lynne, and Kelly McCann. *The Book of Women: 300 Notable Women History Passed By.* New York: Bob Adams, 1992.

Grmek, Mirko D. *History of AIDS: Emergence and Origin of a Modern Pandemic.* Princeton, N.J.: Princeton University Press, 1990.

The Grolier Library of Women's Biographies. Danbury, Conn.: Grolier Educational, 1998.

Gutman, Israel, editor in chief. *Encyclopedia of the Holocaust,* vol. 3. New York: Macmillan, 1990.

Hall, David D., ed. *The Antinomian Controversy, 1636–1638: A Documentary History.* Middletown, Conn.: Wesleyan University Press, 1968.

Hallam, Elizabeth, general ed. *Saints: Who They Are and How They Help You.* New York: Simon and Schuster, 1994.

Halliwell, Leo. *Light in the Jungle.* New York: David McKay, 1959.

Hammond, N. G. L., and H. H. Scullard, eds. *The Oxford Classical Dictionary.* Oxford: Clarendon Press, 1992.

Harris, Robert, and Jeremy Paxman. *A Higher Form of Killing: The Secret Story of Chemical and Biological Warfare.* New York: Hill and Wang, 1982.

Hastings, James, ed. *Encyclopedia of Religion and Ethics.* New York: Charles Scribner's Sons, 1951.

Heron, Echo. *Condition Critical: The Story of a Nurse Continues.* New York: Ivy Books, 1994.

———. *Intensive Care: The Story of a Nurse.* New York: Ivy Books, 1987.

Higham, Robin, and Carol Brandt, eds. *The U.S. Army in Peacetime.* Manhattan, Kans.: Military Affairs/Aerospace Historian Publishing, 1975.

Hine, Darlene Clark. *Black Women in White.* Bloomington: Indiana University Press, 1989.

Hine, Darlene Clark, Elsa Barkley Brown, and Rosalyn Terborg-Penn, eds. *Black Women in America: An Historical Encyclopedia.* Bloomington: Indiana University Press, 1993.

Hollister, C. Warren. *Medieval Europe: A Short History.* New York: McGraw-Hill, 1994.

Hospice and Hemlock. Eugene, Ore.: Hemlock Society U.S.A., 1993.

Howatson, M. C., ed. *The Oxford Companion to Classical Literature.* New York: Oxford University Press, 1989.

Hufton, Olwen. *The Prospect before Her: A History of Women in Western Europe, 1500–1800.* New York: Vintage Books, 1995.

Hume, Edgar Erskine. *Victories of Army Medicine.* Philadelphia: J. B. Lippincott, 1943.

Hurd-Mead, Kate Campbell. *A History of Women in Medicine: From the Earliest Times to the Beginning of the Nineteenth Century.* Haddam, Conn.: Haddam Press, 1938.

Hurmence, Belinda. *Before Freedom: 48 Oral Histories of Former North and South Carolina Slaves.* New York: Mentor Books, 1990.

Hutchinson, John F. *Champions of Charity: War and the Rise of the Red Cross.* Boulder, Colo.: Westview Press, 1996.

Hyginus. *Hygini Fabulae.* Leyden, Holland: A. W. Sythoff, 1933.

Hyman, Paula, and Deborah Dash Moore. *Jewish Women in America.* New York: Routledge, Chapman, and Hall, 1997.

The International Who's Who, 1987–1988. London: Europa Publications, 1987.

The Interpreter's Dictionary of the Bible. New York: Abingdon Press, 1962.

James, Peter, and Nick Thorpe. *Ancient Inventions.* New York: Ballantine Books, 1994.

Jamieson, Elizabeth, and Mary F. Sewall. *Trends in Nursing History.* London: W. B. Saunders, 1949.

Jeffrey, Betty. *White Coolies.* Sydney, Aust.: Angus and Robertson, 1954.

Jensen, Deborah MacLurg, Gerald Joseph Griffin, and H. Joanne King Griffin. *The History and Trends of Professional Nursing.* St. Louis: C. V. Mosby, 1985.

Jones, Katherine M. *Heroines of Dixie.* Indianapolis, Ind.: Bobbs-Merrill, 1955.

Jordan, Denise. *Susie King Taylor.* Orange, N.J.: Just Us Books, 1994.

Kalisch, Philip, and Beatrice J. Kalisch. *The Advance of American Nursing.* Boston: Little, Brown, 1978.

Kastenbaum, Robert. *Death, Society, and Human Experience.* New York: Charles E. Merrill, 1986.

Kastenbaum, Robert, and Beatrice Kastenbaum, eds. *Encyclopedia of Death.* New York: Avon, 1989.

Kater, Michael H. *Doctors under Hitler.* Chapel Hill: University of North Carolina Press, 1989.

Kauffman, Christopher J. *Tamers of Death: The History of the Alexian Brothers.* New York: Seabury Press, 1976.

Kenny, Elizabeth. *And They Shall Walk.* North Stratford, N.H.: Ayer, 1980.

Kent, Jacqueline C. *Women in Medicine.* Minneapolis, Minn.: Oliver Press, 1998.

Kerr, Janet, and Jannetta MacPhail. *Canadian Nursing: Issues and Perspectives.* Toronto: McGraw-Hill Ryerson, 1988.

Koblinsky, Marge, Judith Timyan, and Jill Gay, eds. *The Health of Women: A Global Perspective.* Boulder, Colo.: Westview Press, 1993.

Koonz, Claudia. *Mothers in the Fatherland.* New York: St. Martin's Press, 1981.

Kraegel, Janet, and Mary Kachoyeanos. *Just a Nurse.* New York: Dell Books, 1989.

Kraut, Alan. *Silent Travelers: Germs, Genes, and the "Immigrant Menace."* New York: Basic Books, 1994.

Kübler-Ross, Elisabeth. *On Death and Dying.* New York: Macmillan, 1969.

Kuykendall, Ralph S., and A. Grove Day. *Hawaii, a History.* Englewood Cliffs, N.J.: Prentice-Hall, 1961.

Lacey, Candida Ann, ed. *Barbara Leigh Smith and the Langham Place Group.* New York: Routledge and Kegan Paul, 1987.

La Motte, Ellen N. *The Tuberculosis Nurse.* 1915. New York: Garland, 1985.

Lamps on the Prairie: A History of Nursing in Kansas. Emporia: Kansas State Nurses' Association, 1942.

Landells, E. A., ed. *Military Nurses of Canada.* White Rock, B.C.: Co-Publishing, 1995.

Latham, Jean L. *Elizabeth Blackwell: Pioneer Woman Doctor.* Champaign, Ill.: Gerrard, 1975.

Laurence, Leslie, and Beth Weinhouse. *Outrageous Practices: How Gender Bias Threatens Women's Health.* New Brunswick, N.J.: Rutgers University Press, 1997.

Lauro, Shirley. *A Piece of My Heart.* New York: Samuel French, 1992.

Le Joly, Edward, S.J. *Mother Teresa of Calcutta.* San Francisco: Harper and Row, 1983.

Leavitt, Judith Walzer. *Brought to Bed: Childbearing in America 1750–1950.* Cambridge, Mass.: Oxford University Press, 1986.

Lee, Betsy. *Mother Teresa: Caring for All God's Children.* Minneapolis, Minn.: Dillon Press, 1981.

Lee, Gerard A. *Leper Hospitals in Medieval Ireland.* Dublin: Four Courts Press, 1996.

Lee, W. Storrs. *The Islands.* New York: Holt, Rinehart, and Winston, 1966.

Lefkowitz, Mary. *Women's Life in Greece and Rome.* Baltimore: Johns Hopkins University Press, 1992.

Lewis, Lionel Smithett. "The Celtic Church." In *St. Joseph of Arimathaea at Glastonbury.* London: James Clarke, 1955.

Ligate, Ontario: A Canadian Nursing Sister's Tale. Belleville, Ont.: Mika Publishing, 1981.

Loftin, Robert Jay. *The Nazi Doctors.* New York: Basic Books, 1986.

Longmate, Norman, ed. *The Home Front: An Anthology of Personal Experience, 1938–1945.* London: Chatto and Windus, 1981.

Lopez, Robert S. *The Birth of Europe.* New York: M. Evans, 1967.

Love, Harold. *The Royal Belfast Hospital for Sick Children.* Belfast: Blackstaff Press, 1998.

Lowry, Thomas P. *The Story the Soldiers Wouldn't Tell: Sex in the Civil War.* Mechanicsburg, PA: Stackpole Books, 1994.

Lyons, Albert S., M.D., and R. Joseph Petrucelli, M.D. *Medicine: An Illustrated History.* New York: Abrams, 1987.

Mackenzie, Ross, and Todd Culbertson, eds. *Eyewitness: Writing from the Ordeal of Communism.* New York: Freedom House, 1992.

Maggio, Rosalie, ed. *The New Beacon Book of Quotations by Women.* Boston: Beacon Press, 1996.

Magic and Medicine of Plants. Pleasantville, N.Y.: Reader's Digest, 1986.

Magner, Lois N. *A History of Medicine.* New York: Marcel Dekker, 1992.

Magnusson, Magnus, general ed. *Cambridge Biographical Dictionary.* New York: Cambridge University Press, 1990.

Mantinband, James H. *Dictionary of Latin Literature.* New York: Philosophical Library, 1956.

Marcus, Jacob R. *Communal Sick-Care in the German Ghetto.* Cincinnati, Ohio: Hebrew Union College Press, 1947.

Marinacci, Barbara. *O Wondrous Singer! An Introduction to Walt Whitman.* New York: Dodd, Mead, 1970.

Marks, Geoffrey, and William K. Beatty. *Women in White.* New York: Charles Scribner's Sons, 1972.

Marland, Hilary, ed. *The Art of Midwifery: Early Modern Midwives in Europe.* London: Routledge, 1993.

Marland, Hilary, and Anne Marie Rafferty. *Midwives, Society and Childbirth: Debates and Controversies in the Modern Period.* London: Routledge, 1997.

Marshall, George, and David Poling. *Schweitzer.* Garden City, N.Y.: Doubleday, 1971.

Martino, John. *I Was Castro's Prisoner: An American Tells His Story.* New York: Devin-Adair, 1963.

Marvell, William. *Andersonville: The Last Depot.* Chapel Hill: University of North Carolina Press, 1994.

Masson, Madeline. *A Pictorial History of Nursing.* Twickenham, Middlesex: Hamlyn, 1985.

Mathews, Basil. *The Book of Missionary Heroes.* New York: George H. Doran, 1922.

Matson, Leslie. *Méiní the Blasket Nurse.* Dublin: Mercier Press, 1996.

Mays, James L., general ed. *Harper's Bible Commentary.* San Francisco: Harper and Row, 1988.

McBryde, Brenda. *Quiet Heroines: Nurses of the Second World War.* London: Hogarth Press, 1985.

McCall, Andrew. *The Medieval Underworld.* New York: Dorset Press, 1979.

McClain, Carol Shepherd. *Women as Healers: Cross-Cultural Perspectives.* New Brunswick, N.J.: Rutgers University Press, 1989.

McDonnell, Virginia B., R.N. *Dee O'Hara: Astronauts' Nurse.* Edinburgh: Rutledge Books, 1991.

McHenry, Robert, ed. *Liberty's Women.* Springfield, Mass.: G. C. Merriam, 1980.

McKown, Robin. *Heroic Nurses.* New York: G. P. Putnam's Sons, 1966.

McNeill, William. *Plagues and People.* New York: Anchor Books, 1977.

Meier, Louis A. *Healing of an Army, 1777–1778.* Norristown, Pa.: Historical Society of Montgomery County, 1991.

Meigs, Cornelia, Elizabeth Nesbit, Anne Eaton, and Ruth Hill Viquers. *A Critical History of Children's Literature.* New York: Macmillan, 1953.

Meisner, Maurice. *Mao's China: A History of the People's Republic.* New York: Free Press, 1977.

Mellish, J. M. *A Basic History of Nursing.* Durban, South Africa: Butterworths, 1984.

Melosh, Barbara. *The Physician's Hand: Work, Culture and Conflict in American Nursing.* Philadelphia: Temple University Press, 1982.

Michalczyk, John H., ed. *Medicine, Ethics and the Third Reich.* Kansas City, Mo.: Sheed and Ward, 1994.

Monette, Paul. *Borrowed Time: An AIDS Memoir.* New York: Avon Books, 1988.

Moore, Frank. *Women of the War: Their Heroism and Self-Sacrifice.* Hartford, Conn.: S. S. Scranton, 1866.

Moore, Judith. *A Zeal for Responsibility: The Struggle for Professional Nursing in Victorian England, 1868–1883.* Athens: University of Georgia Press, 1988.

Mor, V. *Hospice Care Systems.* New York: Springer, 1987.

Mor, V., D. S. Gree, and Robert Kastenbaum. *The Hospice Experiment.* Baltimore: Johns Hopkins University Press, 1988.

Mosley, Leonard. *Haile Selassie: The Conquering Lion.* Englewood Cliffs, N.J.: Prentice-Hall, 1964.

Murphy, Claire Riddle, and Jane G. Haigh. *Gold Rush Women.* Anchorage: Alaska Northwest Books, 1997.

Murray, James P. *Galway: A Medico-Social History.* Galway: Kenny's Bookshop and Art Galleries Ltd., n.d.

Myers, Pamela. *Building for the Future: A Nursing History 1896–1996.* Chiswick, London: St. Mary's Convent, 1996.

Native American Women. New York: American Indian Treaty Council Information Center, 1975.

Nelson, Mary Carroll. *Annie Wauneka.* Minneapolis, Minn.: Dillon Press, 1972.

Newlin, George, ed. and comp. *Everyone in Dickens,* Vol. 1. Westport, Conn.: Greenwood, 1995.

Nicholson, G. W. L. *Canada's Nursing Sisters.* Toronto: Hakkert, 1975.

Nikiforuk, Andrew. *The Fourth Horseman: A Short History of Epidemics, Plagues, Famine and Other Scourges.* Toronto: Penguin, 1992.

Nixon, Pat Ireland, M.D. *The Medical Story of Early Texas, 1528–1853.* Lancaster: Lancaster Press, 1946.

Norman, Elizabeth. *Women at War: The Story of 50 Military Nurses Who Served in Vietnam.* Philadelphia: University of Pennsylvania, 1990.

Oates, Stephen B. *Woman of Valor: Clara Barton and the Civil War.* New York: Free Press, 1994.

O'Ceirin, Kit, and O'Ceirin, Cyril. *Women of Ireland: A Biographical Dictionary.* Galway: Tir Eolas Newtownlynch, 1996.

O'Connor, Rose, and Jack Mahon, eds. *A Woman of Aran: The Life and Times of Bridget Dirrane.* Dublin: Blackwater Press, 1997.

O'Croinin, Daibhi. *Early Medieval Ireland, 400–1200.* London: Longman, 1995.

Ofer, Dalia, and Lenore J. Weitzman. *Women in the Holocaust.* New Haven, Conn.: Yale University Press, 1998.

Oldstone, Michael B. A. *Viruses, Plagues, and History.* New York: Oxford University Press, 1998.

Ott, Katherine. *Fevered Lives: Tuberculosis in American Culture since 1870.* Cambridge, Mass.: Harvard University Press, 1996.

Paor, Liam de. *Saint Patrick's World.* Dublin: Four Courts Press, 1996.

Parry, Melanie, ed. *Larousse Dictionary of Women.* New York: Larousse, 1996.

Patterson, Lotsee, and Mary Ellen Snodgrass. *Indian Terms of the Americas.* Englewood, Colo.: Libraries Unlimited, 1994.

Paull, Nancy B. *Capital Medicine: A Tradition of Excellence.* Encino, Calif.: Jostens, 1994.

Perrone, Bobette, H. Henrietta Stockel, and Victoria Krueger. *Medicine Women, Curanderas, and Women Doctors.* Norman: University of Oklahoma Press, 1989.

Plutarch. *Lycurgus* in *Lives of the Noble Greeks.* Edmund Fuller, ed. New York: Laurel Classic, 1959.

Powell, J. H. *Bring Out Your Dead: The Great Plague of Yellow Fever in Philadelphia in 1793.* New York: Time, 1965.

Proctor, Robert N. *Racial Hygiene: Medicine under the Nazis.* Cambridge, Mass.: Harvard University Press, 1988.

Pryor, Elizabeth Brown. *Clara Barton: Professional Angel.* Philadelphia: University of Pennsylvania Press, 1987.

Raby, F. J. E., ed. *A History of Christian-Latin Poetry.* Oxford: Clarendon Press, 1953.

Radice, Betty, ed. *Who's Who in the Ancient World.* New York: Penguin Books, 1973.

Ranft, Patricia. *Women and the Religious Life in Premodern Europe.* New York: St. Martin's Press, 1996.

Rawcliffe, Carole. *Medicine and Society in Later Medieval England.* Gloucestershire: Alan Sutton Publishing, 1995.

Read, Phyllis J., and Bernard L. Witlieb. *The Book of Women's Firsts.* New York: Random House, 1992.

Redmond, Juanita. *I Served on Bataan.* Philadelphia: J. B. Lippincott Co., 1943.

Reich, Warren Thomas, editor in chief. *Encyclopedia of Bioethics.* New York: Macmillan, 1995.

Rice, David Talbot, ed. *The Dawn of European Civilization: The Dark Ages.* New York: McGraw-Hill, 1965.

Rivers, J. *Dame Rosalind Paget: A Short Account of Her Life and Work.* London: Midwives' Chronicle, 1981.

Roberts, Mary M., R.N. *American Nursing.* New York: Macmillan, 1959.

Rose, June. *Marie Stopes and the Sexual Revolution.* London: Faber and Faber, 1993.

Ross, Ishbel. *Angel of the Battlefield.* New York: Harper and Brothers Publishers, 1956.

———. *Child of Destiny: The Life Story of the First Woman Doctor.* New York: Harper, 1949.

Rostenberg, Leona. *Literary, Political, Scientific, Religious and Legal Publishing: Printing and Bookselling in England 1551–1700.* New York: Burt Franklin, 1965.

Rowland, Mary Canaga. *As Long as Life: The Memoirs of a Frontier Woman Doctor.* Seattle, Wash.: Storm Peak Press, 1994.

Royce, Marion. *Eunice Dyke, Health Care Pioneer.* Toronto: Dundurn Press, 1983.

"Ruth Watson Lubic." *Current Biography Yearbook.* New York: Bowker, 1996, 328–332.

Sabin, Francene. *Elizabeth Blackwell: The First Woman Doctor.* Mahwah, N.J.: Troll Associates, 1982.

Sage, W. D. M. *Battlefield Nurse.* Vancouver: Sage Family, 1994.

St. Pierre, Mark, and Tilda Long Soldier. *Walking in the Sacred Manner: Healers, Dreamers and Pipe Carriers—Medicine Women of the Plains Indians.* New York: Simon and Schuster, 1995.

Saunders, Cicely. *The Management of Terminal Disease.* Hospital Medical Publications, 1967.

Saxton, Martha. *Louisa May: A Modern Biography of Louisa May Alcott.* Boston: Houghton Mifflin, 1977.

Saywell, John T., ed. *The Canadian Journal of Lady Aberdeen, 1893–1898.* Toronto: Champlain Society, 1960.

Schlissel, Lillian, Vicki L. Ruiz, and Janice Monk, eds. *Western Women: Their Land, Their Lives.* Albuquerque: University of New Mexico Press, 1988.

Schorr, Thelma M., R.N., and Anne Zimmerman, R.N., eds. *Making Choices, Taking Chances: Nurse Leaders Tell Their Stories.* St. Louis: C. V. Mosby, 1988.

Schroeder-Lein, Glenna R. *Confederate Hospitals on the Move: Samuel H. Stout and the Army of Tennessee.* Columbia: University of South Carolina Press, 1994.

Schweitzer, Jane, R.N. *Tears and Rage: Nursing Crisis in America.* Fair Oaks, Calif.: Adams-Blake, 1995.

Seacole, Mary Jane. *Wonderful Adventures of Mrs. Seacole in Many Lands.* 1857. New York: Oxford University Press, 1988.

Sebba, Anne. *Mother Teresa: Beyond the Image.* New York: Doubleday, 1997.

Sharpe, William D. "Introduction." *Confederate States Medical and Surgical Journal.* Metuchen, N.J.: Scarecrow Press, 1976.

Shearer, Benjamin F., and Barbara S. Shearer. *Notable Women in the Life Sciences.* Westport, Conn.: Greenwood Press, 1996.

Sherr, Lynn, and Jurate Kazickas. *Susan B. Anthony Slept Here: A Guide to American Women's Landmarks.* New York: Times Books, 1994.

Shoemaker, Sister M. Theophane. *History of Nurse-Midwifery in the United States.* New York: Garland Publishing, 1984.

Shroff, Farah. *The New Midwifery.* Toronto: Women's Press, 1997.

Shura, Mary Frances. *Gentle Annie: The True Story of a Civil War Nurse.* New York: Scholastic, 1991.

Siebold, Cathy. *The Hospice Movement: Easing Death's Pains.* New York: Twayne, 1992.

Sills, David L., ed. *International Encyclopedia of the Social Sciences.* New York: Macmillan and Free Press, 1968.

Sink, Alice E. *The Grit behind the Miracle.* Lanham, Md.: University Press of America, 1998.

Smaridge, Norah. *Hands of Mercy: The Story of Sister-Nurses in the Civil War.* New York: Benziger Brothers, 1960.

Smith, Jesse Carney. *Epic Lives: One Hundred Black Women Who Made a Difference.* Detroit: Visible Ink, 1993.

———. *Notable Black American Women.* Detroit: Gale, 1992.

Smith, Winnie. *American Daughter Gone to War: On the Front Lines with an Army Nurse in Vietnam.* New York: William Morrow, 1992.

Snodgrass, Mary Ellen. *Celebrating Women's History.* Detroit: Gale Research, 1996.

———. *Crossing Barriers: People Who Overcame.* Englewood, Colo.: Libraries Unlimited, 1993.

———. *Encyclopedia of Frontier Literature.* Santa Barbara, Calif.: ABC-CLIO, 1997.

———. *Encyclopedia of Satirical Literature.* Santa Barbara, Calif.: ABC-CLIO, 1996.

———. *Encyclopedia of Southern Literature.* Santa Barbara, Calif.: ABC-CLIO, 1997.

———. *Late Achievers: Famous People Who Succeeded Late in Life.* Englewood, Colo.: Libraries Unlimited, 1992.

———. *Voyages in Classical Mythology.* Santa Barbara, Calif.: ABC-CLIO, 1994.

The Soldier's Manual of Common Tasks. Washington, D.C.: Headquarters Department of the Army, October 3, 1983.

Solzhenitsyn, Alexander. *Cancer Ward.* New York: Farrar, Straus and Giroux, 1968.

Spence, Jonathan D. *The Search for Modern China.* New York: W. W. Norton, 1990.

Spencer, Cornelia Phillips. *The Last Ninety Days of the War in North Carolina.* New York: Watchman Publishing, 1866.

Spruill, Julia. *Women's Life and Work in the Southern Colonies.* New York: W. W. Norton, 1972.

Steer, Diana. *Native American Women.* New York: Barnes and Noble, 1996.

Steinberg, S. H., ed. *Cassell's Encyclopaedia of World Literature.* New York: Funk and Wagnalls, 1953.

Steiner, Stan. *The New Indians.* New York: Delta Books, 1968.

Stephen, Sir Leslie, and Sir Sidney Lee. *The Dictionary of National Biography.* London: Oxford University Press, 1922.

Sterne, Capt. Doris M. *In and Out of Harm's Way: A History of the Navy Nurse Corps.* Seattle, Wash.: Peanut Butter Publishing, 1996.

Stewart, Charles Fyfe, M.D. *The Ninth Evac: Experiences in a World War II Tent Hospital in North Africa and Europe.* New York: Vantage Press, 1990.

Straubling, Harold E. K. *In Hospital and Camp: The Civil War through the Eyes of Its Doctors and Nurses.* Harrisburg, Pa.: Stackpole Books, 1993.

Strehlow, Wighard, M.D., and Gottfried Herzka, M.D. *Hildegard of Bingen's Medicine.* Santa Fe: Bear and Company, 1988.

Sutherland, Daniel E., ed. *A Very Violent Rebel: The Civil War Diary of Ellen Renshaw House.* Knoxville: University of Tennessee Press, 1996.

Thatcher, Virginia. *History of Anesthesia, with Emphasis on the Nurse Specialist.* New York: Garland, 1984.

Thoms, Adah B. *Pathfinders: A History of the Progress of Colored Graduate Nurses.* New York: Kay Printing House, n.d.

Thucydides. *The Peloponnesian Wars.* New York: Washington Square Press, 1963.

Trager, James. *The Women's Chronology.* New York: Henry Holt, 1994.

Tuchman, Barbara W. *A Distant Mirror: The Calamitous 14th Century.* New York: Alfred A. Knopf, 1978.

Twain, Mark. *Life on the Mississippi.* New York: Oxford University Press, 1990.

Twycross, R. G. *Pain Relief and Cancer.* Philadelphia: Saunders, 1984.

Tyrmand, Leopold. *The Rosa Luxemburg Contraceptives Cooperative: A Primer on Communist Civilization.* New York: Macmillan, 1972.

Ullmann, Manfred. *Islamic Medicine.* Edinburgh: University Press, 1978.

Ulrich, Laurel Thatcher. *A Midwife's Tale: The Life of Martha Ballard, Based on Her Diary, 1785–1812.* New York: Alfred A. Knopf, 1990.

Underwood, J. L. *Women of the Confederacy.* New York: Neale Publishing, 1906.

Underwood, Larry D. *Love and Glory: Women of the Old West.* Lincoln, Neb.: Media Publishing, 1991.

van der Peet, Rob. *The Nightingale Model of Nursing.* Edinburgh: Campion Press, 1995.

Van Devanter, Lynda. *Home Before Morning: The Story of an Army Nurse in Vietnam.* New York: Warner Books, 1983.

Van Devanter, Lynda, and Joan A. Furey, eds. *Visions of War, Dreams of Peace: Writings of Women in the Vietnam War.* New York: Time Warner, 1991.

van Dyk, Agnes. *A History of Nursing in Namibia.* Windhoek: Gamsbert Macmillan, 1997.

Van Olphen-Fehr, Juliana. *The Diary of a Midwife.* Westport, Conn.: Greenwood Press, 1998.

Vedder, James S. *Combat Surgeon: On Iwo Jima with the 27th Marines.* Novato, Calif.: Presidio, 1984.

Vigil, Evangelina. *Woman of Her Word: Hispanic Women Write.* Houston, Tex.: Arte Publico Press, 1987.

Waldman, Carl. *Who Was Who in Native American History: Indians and Non-Indians from Early Contacts through 1900.* New York: Facts on File, 1990.

Walker, Keith. *A Piece of My Heart: The Stories of Twenty-Six American Women Who Served in Vietnam.* Novato, Calif.: Presidio, 1985.

Ward, Fred. *Inside Cuba Today.* New York: Crown Publishers, 1978.

Washington, Mary Helen. *Invented Lives: Narratives of Black Women, 1860–1960.* New York: Anchor, 1987.

Watkins, Yoko Kawashima. *So Far from the Bamboo Grove.* New York: Puffin Books, 1986.

Weatherford, Doris. *American Women's History.* New York: Prentice Hall, 1994.

Webster's Dictionary of American Women. New York: Merriam-Webster, 1996.

Werminghaus, Esther A. *Annie W. Goodrich: Her Journey to Yale.* New York: Macmillan, 1950.

Wertz, Richard W., and Dorothy C. Wertz. *Lying-In: A History of Childbirth in America.* New Haven, Conn.: Yale University Press, 1989.

Wheal, Elizabeth-Anne, Stephen Pope, and James Taylor, eds. *Encyclopedia of the Second World War.* Edison, N.J.: Castle Books, 1989.

Who's Who in America, 1978–1979. New Providence, N.J.: Marquis Who's Who, 1979.

Wigginton, Eliot, ed. *Foxfire 2.* Garden City, N.Y.: Anchor Books, 1973.

———. *Foxfire 9.* Garden City, N.Y.: Anchor Books, 1986.

Wilbur, C. Keith, M.D. *Revolutionary Medicine, 1700–1800.* Old Saybrook, Conn.: Globe Pequot Press, 1997.

Williams, Marty Newman, and Anne Echols. *Between Pit and Pedestal: Women in the Middle Ages.* Princeton, N.J.: Markus Wiener Publishers, 1994.

Williamson, Anne A., R.N. *50 Years in Starch.* Culver City, Calif.: Murray and Gee, 1948.

Wilson, Amy V., R.N. *A Nurse in the Yukon.* New York: Dodd, Mead, 1965.

Wilson, Charles Reagan, and William Ferris, eds. *Encyclopedia of Southern Culture.* Chapel Hill: University of North Carolina Press, 1989.

Woodham-Smith, Cecil. *Florence Nightingale.* New York: McGraw-Hill, 1951.

Woodward, C. Vann, ed. *Mary Chesnut's Civil War.* New Haven, Conn.: Yale University Press, 1981.

Woodward, Kenneth L. *Making Saints.* New York: Simon and Schuster, 1990.

Woolsey, Jane Stuart. *Hospital Days: Reminiscence of a Civil War Nurse.* 1870. Edinburgh, Scotland: Edinburgh Press, 1996.

Wu, Harry. *Troublemaker: One Man's Crusade against China's Cruelty.* New York: Times Books, 1996.

Yost, Edna. *American Women of Nursing.* Philadelphia: J. B. Lippincott, 1947.

Young, Carrie. *Nothing To Do but Stay: My Pioneer Mother.* New York: Delta, 1991.

Zalumas, Jaqueline. *Caring in Crisis: An Oral History of Critical Care Nursing.* Philadelphia: University of Pennsylvania Press, 1995.

Zimmerman, J. *Hospice: Complete Care for the Terminally Ill.* Baltimore: Urban and Schwarzenberg, 1981.

Zinsser, Hans. *Rats, Lice and History.* New York: Black Dog and Leventhal Pubs., 1963.

Articles, Interviews, Films, and Monographs

Ailinger, Rita L., and Maria Elena Causey. "Health Concept of Older Hispanic Immigrants." *Western Journal of Nursing Research* (December 1995): 605–613.

Allen, A. "Old Enemies Practice Teamwork . . . Health Problems That Exist in Russia." *Journal of Post-Anesthesia Nursing* 9, no. 4 (1994): 247–249.

Amstey, Marvin S., M.D. "The Political History of Syphilis and Its Application to the AIDS Epidemic." *Women's Health Issues* (spring 1994): 16–19.

"Another Robinson Pioneer." *Ebony* (December 1982): 106–107.

Anteau, Carlene M., R.N., and Linda A. Williams, R.N. "What We Learned from the Oklahoma City Bombing." *Nursing* (March 1998): 52–55.

Anthony-Tkach, C. "Nursing and Health Care in the Soviet Union." *Nursing Forum* 22, no. 2 (1985): 45–52.

Baj, R. "Integrating the Russian Émigré Nurse into U.S. Nursing." *Journal of Nursing Administration* 25, no. 3 (1995): 43–47.

Baker, Nina Brown. "Cyclone in Calico." *Reader's Digest* (December 1952): 141–162.

Baldinger, Pamela. "Training the Care Givers." *China Business Review* (July-August 1992): 34–36.

Barritt, Evelyn R., R.N. "Florence Nightingale's Values and Modern Nursing Education." *Nursing Forum* (1973): 7–47.

Bean, William B., M.D. "Medicine's Forgotten Man—the Patient." *Nursing Forum* (1963): 46–69.

Benderly, Jill. "Margaret Sanger." *On the Issues* (spring 1990).

Benshoof, Janet. "Beyond *Roe,* After *Casey:* The Present and Future of a 'Fundamental' Right." *Women's Health Issues* (fall 1994): 162–168.

Bernal, H., et al. "Community Health Nursing in a Former Soviet Union Republic: A Case Study of Change in Armenia." *Nursing Outlook* 43, no. 2 (1995): 78–83.

Bidel, Susan. "When Mom's a Hard Act to Follow." *Woman's Day,* May 22, 1990, 88.

Black, James T. "North Carolina's Super Nurse." *Southern Living* (May 1984): 165.

Bragg, Rick. "Despite Bombing, Clinic Goes On." *Charlotte Observer,* June 20, 1998, 2A.

Breeden, James O. "Confederate General Hospitals." *North Carolina Medical Journal* (February 1992): 110–119.

Buckley, William F. "A Visit to Lourdes To Be a Pilgrim." *National Review,* August 9, 1993, 33.

Byerly, Dr. W. Grimes, personal interview, August 18, 1998.

"Calling for a Nursing Revolution in Eastern Europe." *World Health* (November-December 1993): 28–37.

"Canadian Nursing Professionals Help Update Ukraine's Health Care." *Ukrainian Weekly,* June 23, 1996, 9.

Carcaterra, Lorenzo. "Mother Hale of Harlem Has Saved 487 Drug-Addicted Babies with an Old Miracle Cure: Love." *People,* March 5, 1984, 211–214.

Carr, Mary. "Kindness and Consideration." *Nursing Mirror,* November 2, 1983, 26–28.

Castledine, George. "Proud Sunset over Leningrad." *Nursing Mirror* 156, no. 7 (1983): 22.

Castro, Janice. "Florence Nightingale Inc." *Time,* July 14, 1986, 47.

Cheers, D. Michael. "Nurse Corps Chief." *Ebony* (June 1989): 64–66.

Chen, Kaiyi. "Quality versus Quantity: The Rockefeller Foundation and Nurses' Training in China." *Journal of American-East Asian Relations* (spring 1996): 77–105.

"Cincinnati Woman Now National Nursing Head." *Cincinnati Time Star,* January 5, 1936, 15.

"Clara Hale To Get Truman Award for Public Service." *Jet,* March 20, 1989, 23.

Codling, Karen. "Letters." *Ms.* (September-October 1998): 7–8.

Cohen, I. Bernard. "Florence Nightingale." *Scientific American* (March 1984): 128–132.

Collins, Huntley. "Mission for the Millennium: Choke Out Remains of Polio." *Charlotte Observer,* March 14, 1999, 1A, 10A.

Constable, Pamela. "India Making Big Gains in Battle against Leprosy." *Charlotte Observer,* October 4, 1998, 28A.

Dempsey, Patricia, and Theresa Gesse. "Beliefs, Values, and Practices of Navajo Childbearing Women." *Western Journal of Nursing Research* (December 1995): 591–604.

Dennis, L. I. "Soviet Hospital Nursing: A Model for Self-Care." *Journal of Nursing Education* 28, no. 2 (1989): 76–77.

Deutsch, Naomi, personal correspondence. Nursing Archives, Boston University, Massachusetts.

Dobson, R. B. "Gilbert of Sempringham and the Gilbertine Order: ca. 1130–ca. 1300." *English Historical Review* (February 1998): 147–149.

"Does a Terminal Patient Have the Right to Die?" *Good Housekeeping* (May 1984): 81–84.

Dorff, Elliot. "Judaism and Health." *Health Values* (May-June 1988): 32–36.

Dyer, Brainard. "The Treatment of Colored Union Troops by the Confederates, 1861–1865." *The Journal of Negro History* (July 1935): 273–286.

Edmonds, Patricia. "Harlem's 'Mother Hale' Dies; Took in 1,000 Babies." *USA Today,* December 21, 1992, 2A.

Erickson, John. "Night Witches, Snipers, and Laundresses." *History Today* (July 1990): 29–36.

"$50,000 Rehab House for Cocaine-Addicted Babies." *Jet,* January 25, 1988, 23.

Fischer-Kamel, Doris Sofie. "The Midwife in History with Special Emphasis on Practice in Medieval Europe and in the Islamic World." University of Arizona, 1987.

"For 'New Nurse': Bigger Role in Health Care." *U.S. News and World Report,* January 14, 1980.

Freedman, Alix M. "Disputed Third World Sterilization Drug Rooted in N.C." *Charlotte Observer,* June 20, 1998, 1A, 19A.

Freudenheim, Milt. "As Nurses Take on Primary Care, Physicians Are Sounding Alarms." *New York Times,* September 30, 1997.

Furnas, J. C. "The House That Saves Lives." *Saturday Evening Post,* May 16, 1953.

Garey, Diane, and Lawrence R. Hott. *Sentimental Women Need Not Apply: A History of the American Nurse* (film). New York: Florentine Films, 1988.

Garloch, Karen, "Lean on Me." *Charlotte Observer,* December 7, 1998, 1E, 4E.

"Gen. Adams-Ender Now Top Woman in Army as Head of Ft. Belvoir in Va." *Jet,* October 21, 1991, 8.

"The General Is a Lady." *Ebony* (February 1980): 44–47.

Ginsburg, Ann M., M.D. "The Tuberculosis Epidemic." *Public Health* (March-April 1998).

Gioiella, E. C. "Russia: The Soviet Health Care System for the Aged." *Journal of Gerontological Nursing* 9, no. 11 (1983): 582–585.

Glickman, Robert, R.N., and Ed. J. Gracely. "Therapeutic Touch: Investigation of a Practitioner." *The Scientific Review of Alternative Medicine* (spring-summer 1998): 43–47.

Grimes, D. et al. "An Epidemic of Antiabortion Violence in the United States." *American Journal of Obstetrics and Gynecology* (1991): 1266.

Hacker, Kathy. "Mother Hale: A Savior and Her Growing Mission." *Philadelphia Inquirer,* May 7, 1986.

"Hale Receives $1.1 Million to Expand Home for Babies." *Jet,* May 19, 1986, 26.

Halpin, Tony. "Cover Story: Disaster and Recovery; Two Years Later, a Shattered Nation Picks Up the Pieces at a Crawling Pace." *Armenian International Magazine,* January 31, 1991, 8.

Hannam, June. "Rosalind Paget: Class, Gender, and the Midwives' Institute." *History of Nursing Society Journal* 5 (1994–1995): 133–149.

Hauser, Ernest O. "Shock Nurse." *Saturday Evening Post,* March 10, 1945, 12–13, 48–50.

Heath, Melanie. "Nurses for LIFE." *Nursing Times,* December 13, 1979, 2145–2146.

Henderson, Virginia. "Preserving the Essence of Nursing in a Technological Age." *Nursing Times,* November 22, 1979, 2012–2013.

Heyman, Samuel N. "Airborne Airfield Hospital in Disaster Area: Lessons from Armenia and Rwanda." *Prehospital and Disaster Medicine,* January-March 1998, 14–28.

"In Praise of Women." *Ms.,* April/May 1999, 62–71.

"Jewels in the Crown." *New Internationalist* (May 1998): 27–29.

Johnson, Herschel. "Clara (Mother) Hale: Healing Baby 'Junkies' with Love." *Ebony* (May 1986): 58–61.

Kahl, Jurgen. "Psychology Comes to China." *World Press Review* (November 1992): 48.

Kalnins, Irene, and Zaiga Priede Kalnins. "Latvian Nurses Depart from Soviet Ways." *Nursing Outlook* (March-April 1991): 64–68.

Kalnins, Zaiga Priede. "Nursing in Latvia from the Perspective of Oppressed Theory." *Journal of Transcultural Nursing* 4, no. 1 (1992): 11–16.

Karim, Rosina Binte Haji Abdul. "Missi Ubat—the Malayan Medicine Miss." *Nursing Outlook* (April 1959): 224–225.

Karosas, L. M. "Nursing in Lithuania as Perceived by Lithuanian Nurses." *Nursing Outlook* 43, no. 4 (1995): 153–157.

Kelly, Katy. "Doc Lehman Is a Bridge to Divergent Worlds." *USA Today,* June 9, 1998.

Kent, Heather. "Canada-China Hospital Being Developed." *Canadian Medical Association Journal,* November 15, 1997.

Kilborn, Peter T. "Nurses Get New Role in Patient Protection." *New York Times,* March 26, 1998.

Kirkpatrick, Mary K., R.N. "Women's Issues and Wellness." *Health Values* (March-April 1989): 38–39.

Kratz, Dr. Charlotte. "Letter from Australia: The Aborigines." *Nursing Times,* November 22, 1979, 2042–2043.

———. "Letter from Australia: Primary Nursing." *Nursing Times,* October 18, 1979, 1790–1791.

Langewiesche, Wolfgang. "ICU—Newest Thing in Nursing." *Reader's Digest* (November 1964): 208–214.

Lanker, Brian, and Maya Angelou. "I Dream a World." *National Geographic* (August 1989): 206–226.

Lepper, Elisabeth. "Midwifery Services in Holland." *Nursing Times,* November 29, 1979, 2084–2087.

Levy, M. H. "Pain Control Research in the Terminally Ill." *Omega* (1987–1988): 265–280.

Lewis, Dale. "Woman Is Medicine: An Interview with CheQweesh Auh-Ho-Oh." *Woman of Power* (winter 1987).

Light, Louise. "Health Watch." *New Age,* March/April 1999, 30.

Livingston, M. Christine. "The Victorian Order of Nurses for Canada." *Nursing Outlook* (January 1958): 42–44.

Looker, Patty. "Women's Health Centers: History and Evolution." *Women's Health Issues* (summer 1993): 95–100.

Lyon, Joseph L. "Mormon Health." *Health Values* (May/June 1988): 37–44.

Mackey, Robert. "Discovery the Healing Power of Therapeutic Touch." *American Journal of Nursing* (April 1995): 27–33.

MacMillan, Patricia. "Si tibi deficiant medici. . . ." *Nursing Times,* August 2, 1979, 1298–1299.

Martin D. L. "The Development of the Profession of Nursing in Kyrgyzstan." *Journal of Multicultural Nursing and Health* 3, no. 1 (1997): 6–10.

McCain, Nancy L, and David F. Cella. "Correlates of Stress in HIV Disease." *Western Journal of Nursing Research* (April 1995): 141–155.

McGregor, Deborah Kuhn. "'Childbirth-Travells' and 'Spiritual Estates': Anne Hutchinson and Colonial Boston, 1634–1638." *Caduceus* (1989): 1–33.

McKeegan, Michele. "The Politics of Abortion: A Historical Perspective." *Women's Health Issues* (fall 1993): 127–131.

Meehan, T. C. "Therapeutic Touch and Post-Operative Pain: A Rogerian Research Study." *Nursing Science* (Summer 1993): 69–78.

Milgram, Gail Gleason. "School Nurses: Counselors' Overlooked Allies?" *The Counselor* (July-August 1998): 10–11.

Miller, Floyd. "A Celebration for Mary Donnelly." *Reader's Digest* (October 1973): 122–127.

Miller, Virginia. "Characteristics of Intuitive Nurses." *Western Journal of Nursing Research* (June 1995): 305–316.

Miramontes, Helen, telephone interview, June 12, 1998.

Moccia, Patricia. "If Nurses Had Their Way." *Ms.* (May 1983): 104–106.

Moody, Linda E. "Glasnost, Perestroika, and Health Problems of the 1990s." *Journal of Holistic Nursing* (March 1992): 47–62.

Mother Frances Domina. "Reflections on Death in Childhood." *British Medical Journal,* no. 294: 108–110.

"Mother Hale Appears on NBC-TV's 'Amen' Series." *Jet,* February 19, 1990.

"Mother Hale Honored." *Jet,* July 10, 1989, 22.

"Mother Hale's Help." *Jet,* May 25, 1987, 36.

Muina, Natalia. "To Make Whole." *Woman of Power* (winter 1987).

"Named to U.S. Post: Miss Deutsch to Head Nurses." *Oakland Chronicle,* December 15, 1935, n.p.

"Naomi Deutsch." *Pacific Coast Journal of Nursing* (September 1934): 487–488.

Nayeri, Kamran. "The Cuban Health Care System and Factors Currently Undermining It." *Journal of Community Health* (August 1995): 321–335.

Nelson, Sophie C. "Mary Sewall Gardner." *Nursing Outlook* (January 1954): 37–39.

Nimmons, David. "The Santa Claus Awards." *Ladies' Home Journal* (December 1986): 122–129, 168.

"Nurse! Nurse!" *Time,* April 12, 1954, 79–80.

"Nursing Beyond the Year 2000." Geneva: WHO, 1994.

"Operation Babylift," *Newsweek,* March 8, 1999.

"Ordinary Women of Grace: Subjects of the 'I Dream a World' Photography Exhibit." *U.S. News and World Report,* February 13, 1989, 54.

Pace, Eric. "Mother Teresa, Hope of the Despairing, Dies at 87." *New York Times,* September 6, 1997.

"Paid Blood Donors Banned with AIDS Spreading Fast." *Seattle Post-Intelligencer,* October 1, 1998.

Paquet, Sandra Pouchet. "The Enigma of Arrival: The Wonderful Adventures of Mrs. Seacole in Many Lands." *African American Review* (winter 1992): 1–10.

Parsons, Judith. "Marie Stopes." *The Great Scientists.* Danforth, Conn.: Grolier, 1989.

Pasquali, Elaine Anne. "Santeria." *Journal of Holistic Nursing* (December 1994): 380–391.

Patchett, Ann. "The Comfort of Strangers." *Vogue* (October 1995): 90–94.

Plum, Sandra D. "Nurses Indicted: Three Denver Nurses May Face Prison in a Case That Bodes Ill for the Profession." *Nursing* (July 1997): 34–35.

Quintero, Carmen. "Blood Administration in Pediatric Jehovah's Witnesses." *Pediatric Nursing* (January-February 1993): 46–48.

Radford, Barbara. "Antiabortion Violence: Causes and Effects." *Women's Health Issues* (fall 1993): 144–151.

Raybould, Elizabeth. "An Opportunity within Our Grasp." *Nursing Times,* August 16, 1979, 1389–1390.

"Reagan Cites Clara Hale as a 'Hero' in Union Address." *Jet,* February 25, 1985, 6.

"Rebellion among the 'Angels.'" *Time,* August 27, 1979, 62–63.

"Rebirth for Midwifery." *Time,* August 29, 1977, 66.

"Return of the Midwife." *Time,* November 20, 1972, 56–57.

Richardson, Sharon L. "Transformation of the Canadian Association of University Schools of Nursing." *Western Journal of Nursing Research* (August 1995): 416–434.

Roberts, Marjory. "Hands-On Healers." *U.S. News and World Report,* August 5, 1991.

Robinson, Amy. "Authority and the Public Display of Identity: Wonderful Adventures of Mrs. Seacole in Many Lands." *Feminist Studies* (fall 1994).

Rubbelke, Leona. "Hawaii Studies the Problems of Its Smallest Citizens." *Nursing Outlook* (November 1954): 568–571.

Rubin, Rita. "Study: Vinegar Could Screen for Cervical Cancer," *USA Today,* March 12, 1999, 9A.

Ryan, T. Michael, and Ray Thomas. "Trends in the Supply of Medical Personnel in the Russian Federation." *Journal of the American Medical Association,* July 24, 1996, 339–342.

Sado, Monica. "The Good, the Bad and the Different." *Nursing Mirror,* November 2, 1983, 24–26.

Safran, Claire. "Mama Hale and Her Little Angels." *Reader's Digest* (September 1984): 49–54.

"Salute to the Military." *Daughters of the American Revolution Magazine* (November 1990): 852–853.

Samuels, Gertrude. "With Army Nurses Somewhere in Korea." *New York Times Magazine,* April 15, 1951, 14, 33–34.

Saxon, Wolfgang. "Eleanor C. Lambertsen, 82; Introduced Use of Nurse Teams." *New York Times,* April 10, 1998.

———. "Hildegard Elizabeth Peplan, 89, Developer of Psychiatric Nursing." *New York Times,* March 28, 1999, 5J.

Schmich, Mary. "Heroic War Nurses Saved Thousands of Private Ryans." *Chicago Tribune,* August 9, 1998, sect. 4, p. 1.

Schwab, Peter. "Cuban Health Care and the U.S. Embargo." *Monthly Review* (November 1997): 15.

Scouller, Alison, Mary Smith, and Barbara Nelson. "Nurses for a Woman's Right to Choose." *Nursing Times,* December 13, 1979, 2144–2145.

Seelye, Katharine Q. "U.S. Strikes at Smuggling Ring That Exploited Foreign Nurses." *New York Times,* January 15, 1998.

Sheldon, Kathryn. "A Brief History of Black Women in the Military." *Precinct Reporter,* April 18, 1996, 2–6.

Smith, Dean. "A Persistent Rebel." *American History Illustrated* (January 1981): 28–36.

"Special Award for Dee O'Hara." *Astrogram,* NASA, Ames Research Center, September 27, 1991, 1.

Spingarn, Natalie Davis. "Primary Nurses Bring Back One-on-One Care." *New York Times Magazine,* December 26, 1982, 26.

Spiritual Wonders of Europe (video). British Virgins: Palm Plus Produkties, 1997.

Spry, Cynthia C. "A Western OR Delegation to the People's Republic of China." *AORN Journal* (March 1996): 525–533.

Stoddard, Marthe. "Program Delivers Birth Support." *Lincoln Star,* June 23, 1995, 1, 8.

Stringer, Marian. "Junk Bay Bus to Hope." *Nursing Mirror,* November 2, 1983, 38–39.

"The Stubborn Sister." *Time,* December 8, 1952, 80–81.

Titus, Harold. "The Return of the Practical Nurse." *Saturday Evening Post,* May 28, 1949, 39.

"Transition." *Newsweek,* December 8, 1952, 67.

Trevelyan, J. "Bringing Hope: Hospice Care in the Soviet Union." *Nursing Times,* January 16, 1991, 16–17.

———. "Nursing Sisters." *Nursing Times,* May 30, 1990, 16–17.

Turton, Pat. "After Chernobyl." *Nursing Times,* May 28, 1986, 27.

Tylee, Claire M. "The Spectacle of War: Photographs of the Russian Front by Florence Farmborough." *Women: A Cultural Review,* 8(1997):65–80.

Waitzen, Howard, Karen Weld, Romina Kee, Ross Davidson, and Lisa Robinson. "Primary Care in Cuba: Low- and High-Technology Developments Pertinent to Family Medicine." *Journal of Family Practice* (September 1997): 250–259.

"The War: Working against Death." *Time,* December 31, 1965, 62–63.

Ward, Geoffrey C. "Queen Barton." *American Heritage* (April 1988): 14–15.

Watanabe, Myrna E. "Science, Policy Issues Put AIDS Vaccine on Slow Track." *The Scientist,* November 10, 1997, 1, 4–5.

Wei Ke. "Chinese Hospitals Get U.S. Loans." *China Daily,* June 23, 1998.

Weiner, Lynn Y. "Reconstructing Motherhood: The La Leche League." *Journal of American History* (March 1994): 1–12.

"Where Doctors Don't Reach." *Time,* July 22, 1966, 71–72.

Widdicombe, Judith, telephone interview, April 22, 1998.

Wienke, Kay. "Health Care Chinese Style." *Orthopaedic Nursing* (May-June 1996): 39–48.

Wilson, Janet. "Gray Ladies in the Hospital." *Nursing Outlook* (August 1953): 452–453.

Winter, Annette. "Spotlight." *Modern Maturity* (October-November 1988): 18.

Witteman, Betsy. "Transitions at St. Francis's Century Mark." *New York Times,* July 6, 1997.

"Women in the Military." *Essence* (April 1990): 44–45.

Zungolo, Eileen, R.N. "A Study in Alienation: The Nurse Practitioner." *Nursing Forum* (1968): 38–49.

Internet

"ACLU Urges FDA to Approve Mifepristone for Early Medical Abortion." http://www.aclu.org/news/n071996a.html.

Adamson, Peter. "Commentary: A Failure of Imagination." http://www.unicef.org/pon96/womfail.htm.

"A. J. Wright." http://eja.anes.hscyr.edu/anes/anest–1/1992/92_01.txt.

Allen, Lisa. "Lesbian Congressional Candidate Visits Indy." http://www.starnews.com/news/election/98/104/0417SN_cammermeyer.html.

"Alumni Information." http://www.temple.edu/education/alumni/REDLT.HTM.

"American Assembly for Men in Nursing." http://www.nursingcenter.com/people/nrsorgs/aamn.

"Angel of Mercy." http://home1.pacific.net.sg/~alquek/teresa1.htm.

"Ann Armstrong Daily." http://www.wic.org/bio/adailey.htm.

"Antietam Aftermath: The Stern Reality of Want." http://www.state.me.us/sos/arc/archives/military/civilwar/foggyarn.htm.

"The Army Nurse Corps in World War II." http://www.island.net/~times/timesdir/T4/nurses.htm.

"Aunt Lizzie Aiken from Peoria." http://www.rsa.lib.il.us/~ilwomen/files/03/htm1/aiken.htm.

Bing, Elisabeth. "Lamaze Childbirth: Then and Now." http://www.lamaze-childbirth.com/bingart.html.

Boeynaems, Libert H. "Father (Joseph de Veuster) Damien." *Catholic Encyclopedia,* http://www.knight.org/advent/cathen/04615a.htm.

Bois, Danuta. "Mary Eliza Mahoney." http://www.netsrq.com/~dbois/mahoney-me.html.

———. "Mary Jane Seacole." http://www.netsrq.com/~dbois/seacole-mj.html.

———. "Trotula of Salerno." http://www.netsrq.com/~dbois/trotula.html.

Brooks, Diane. "Cammermeyer Says She's Ready to Run." http://www.seattletimes.com/extra/browse/html97/camm_111197.html.

Burgess, Barbara. "The Puritan Exiles the Separatists." http://www.naccc.org/congregationalist/Volume157/Number4/exile.html.

"The Cadet Nurse: 'The Girl with the Future.'" http://www.armstrong.son.wisc.edu/~son/dean/alumni/vol6cad.html.

"Caring about People with Enthusiasm." http://cause-www.colorado.edu/information-resources/ir-library-abstracts/vic0027.html.

"The Catholic Encyclopedia." http://www.knight.org/advent/cathen.html.

"Catholic Online Saints." http://www.catholiconline.com/saints.html.

"Civil War Nurses." http://www.wayne.esu1.k12.ne.us/civil/morris.html.

"Clara Adams-Ender." http://www.army.mil/cmh-pg/anc/18_Ender.html.

"Clara Barton." http://www.redcross.org/hec/pre1900/cbarton.html.

Cole, Wendy. "None But the Brave." *Time,* October 6, 1997. http://www.pathfinder.com/time/magazine/1997/dom/97001/science.none_but_the_.html.

"Condition Upgraded for Nurse Severely Injured in Bombing." http://www.boston.com/dailynews/wirehtml/033/Condition_upgraded_for_nurse_severe.htm.

"Dien Bien Phu." http://www.ecr.mu.oz.au/~npl/vn5.htm.

"Discovered Historical Documents Uncover the First Official Missing Persons Investigator, Clara Barton." http://www.pimall.com/nais/n.barton.html.

DISCovering Multicultural America, http://www.galenet.gale.com.

"Doctors Without Borders USA, Inc." http://www.dwb.org/index.htm.

"Edith Cavell." http://www.thehistorynet.com/BreitishHeritage/articles/1997/05972_text.htm.

"18th Medcom Nursing." http://www.seoul.amedd.army.mil/nursing/18121dnm.htm.

"807th Mash." http://www.iglou.com/law/mash.htm.

"Elisabeth Kübler-Ross." http://www.wic.org/bio/eross.htm.

"Ethnopharmacology of Ska Maria Pastora." http://dog.net.uk/salvia.html.

Falcoff, Mark. "Is It Time to Rethink the Cuban Embargo?" *Latin American Outlook.* http://www.aei.org/lao/lao8875.htm.

"Famous Belgians: Lambert le Bègue." http://ourworld.compuserve.com/homepages/tielemans/hp67marc.htm.

"Father Damien de Veuster." http://www.damien.edu/damien/father.html.

"Female Genital Mutilation." http://www.albany.net/~crystal/GG1/Naturopath/FGM.html.

———. http://www.amnesty.org/ailib/intcam/femgen/fgm1.htm.

———. http://www.int/inf-fs/en/fact153.html.

Finnegan, Rachel. "The Professional Careers: Women Pioneers and the Male Image Seduction." *Classics Ireland.* http://www.ucd.ie/~classics/Finnegan95.html.

"First!" http://www.bluejacket.com/first.htm.

"Florence Nightingale." http://www.dnai.com/~borneo/nightingale//38.htm.

"Freedom of the Press, an Annotated Bibliography." http://www.lib.siu.edu/cni/leter-c1.html.

"The Frontier Nursing Service." http://www.achiever.com/freehmpg/kynurses/fns.html.

"Frontier School History." http://www.midwives.org/history.htm.

Galloway, Paul. "Book Turns Down Volume to Look at America's Sometimes-Uncivil War over Abortion." http://www.arlingtonnet/news/doc/1047/1:BPAGE13/1:BPAGE13020198.html.

Glickman, Robert, R.N. "Nurse Martha Rogers, a Critical Look." http://www.voicenet.com/~eric/tt/rogers.htm.

Golding, Jeannette. "Mary Seacole Home Page." http://www.wp.com/internurse/mary.html.

"Gravesites of Prominent Nurses." http://users.aol.com/NsgHistory/Index.html.

Guash-Melendez, Adam. "The Truth about the Testimony of Nurse Brenda Pratt Shafer." http://www.cais.net/agm/main/nurse.htm.

Gudmundson, Darrell. "Pioneer of Saskatoon, Emily Long, Pioneer Nurse." http://www.nyherji.is/~halfdan/westward/emily.htm.

Hanson, Jillian. "Choosing a Childbirth Educator." http://pregnancytoday.com/reference/articles/simkin-choose.htm.

"Harriet Tubman." http://www.acusd.edu/!jdesnet/tubman.html.

———. http://www.davison.k12.mi.us/projects/women/tubman.htm.

———. http://www.techline.com/~havelokk/harriet.html.

"Hazel W. Johnson." http://www.army.mil/cmh-pg/anc/18-Johnson.html.

"Highlights of the Army Nurse Corps." http://www.army.mil/cmh-pg//anc/Highlights.html.

"Histoire brève de Marguerite d'Youville." http://www.sgm.qc.ca/FRmmy1.htm.

"Histories of the School of Nursing." http://www.rush.edu/Departments/Archives/Nursing/index.html.

"A History of Helping Others." http://www.redcross.org/pa/lancaste/ history.htm.

"The History of Hospice." http://www.cp-tel.net/pamnorth/history.htm.

"History of Nurse Anesthesia Practice." http://www.aana.com/information/infohistory.htm.

"History of Nurse-Midwifery in the U.S." http://www.acnm.org/educ/fenmhist.htm.

"The History of Nursing." http://www.lib.auburn.edu/madd/docs/unionlist/h24.html.

"The History of St. Giles." http://www.oxford.anglican.org/Parishes/stgilesoxford/history.htm.

"The History of the Frontier Nursing Service." http://www.barefoot.com/fns/fns.html.

Humphry, Dick. "Films Dealing with Dying and Euthanasia." http://www.rights.org/~deathnet/ergo-films.html, 1995.

"Images from the History of the Public Health Service." http://ftp.nlm.nih.gov/exhibition/phs_history/137.html.

"In Honor of Sister Dulce." http://psg.com/~walter/irmadulc.html.

"Interview with Florence Wald." http://www.npha.org/intjwald.html, April 22, 1998.

Jaroff, Leon. "A No-Touch Therapy." http://www.pathfinder.com/time/magazine/archive/1994/941121/941121.health.html.

"Johns Hopkins Hospital Centennial." http://hopkins.med.jhu.edu/BasicFacts/hundred.html.

"Kate Cumming." http://www.glue.umd.edu/~cliswp/Bios/kcbio.html.

Kidder, Nicole. "'Serving in Silence' Author Margarethe Cammermeyer Shares Her Life Story." http://www.seattleu.edu/student/spec/02–20–97/news01.html.

Kirsch, J. P. "St. Dymphna." http://www.madnation.org/Heroine.htm, 1999.

Knuth, Elizabeth T. "The Beguines." http://www.users.csbsju.edu/~eknuth/xpxx/beguines.html, December 1992.

Lago, José F. "A First Approximation Design of the Social Safety Net for a Democratic Cuba." http://info.lanic.utexas.edu/la/cb/cuba/asce/cuba4/healsys2.html.

"Lillian D. Wald." http://www.JWA.org/exhib98/wald/lwbio.htm.

———. http://www.netsrq.com/~dbois/wald.html.

"Linda Richards: America's First Trained Nurse." http://www.northnet.org/stlawrenceaauw/richards.htm.

Longfellow, Henry Wadsworth. "Santa Filomena." *Atlantic Monthly* (November 1857). http://www.theatlantic.com/atlantic.html.

"Louisa Lee Schuyler." http://www.allsouslnyc.org/UUsofnote/Louisa-Lee-Schuyler.html.

"Mabel Keaton Staupers." http://www.nursingworld.org/hof/staumk.htm.

"Magen David Adom." http://www.mda.org.il/.

"Margaret Sanger." http://www.gale.com/gale/cwh/sangerm.html.

"Marie Stopes International." http://www.mariestopes.org.uk/mission.html.

"Mary Breckinridge, 1881–1965." http://www.ana.org/hof/brecmx.htm.

"Mary Edwards Walker." http://www.northnet.org/stlawrenceaauw/walker.htm.

———. " http://www.wayne.esu1.k12.ne.us/civil/mary.html.

"Mary Eliza Mahoney." http://www.netsrq.com/~dbois/mahoney-me.html.

———. http://www.njrsingworld.org/hof/mahome.htm.

McSkimming, Sammy. "The Coming of Saint Columba." http://www.dalriada.co.uk/Archives.columba.htm, 1992.

"Medical Corps." http://www.army.mil/cmh-pg/books/korea/22_1_5.htm.

"Medicine Women." http://www.powersource. com/powersource/gallery/womansp/ medwomen.html.

"Médicins sans Frontières Volunteer Profiles." http://www.msf.org/aboutyou/vols/profiles/ 1nor.htm.

"Medieval Sourcebook: Life of St. Goderic." http://www.fordham.edu/halsall/source/goderi c.html, 1996.

Montgomery, Lori. "Despite Popularity, RU-486 May Disappear." http://www.bergen.com/ morenews/475861997062807.htm.

"Mother Angela Gillespie." http://women. eb.com/women/articles/Gillespie_Mother_ Angela.html.

"Mother Teresa Books." http://www.catholic.net/ RCC/people/mother/teresa/books.html.

"NARAL Factsheet—Mifepristone (RU 486) and the Impact of Abortion Politics on Scientific Research." http://www.naral.org/publications/ facts/ru486fin.html.

"Notes on Advanced Nursing." http://www. search.com/Infoseek/1,135,0,0200.html.

"Nurse Helen Fairchild: My Aunt, My Hero." http://raven.cc.ukans.edu/~kansite/ww_one/ medical/MaMh/MyAunt.htm.

"Nurses and Human Rights." http://www. amnesty.org/ailib/aipub/1997ACT/ A7500297.htm.

"Nursing Individuals." http://web.bu.edu/ SPECCO/nursind.htm.

Olson, Christopher G. "Historical Nursing Leader: Florence Nightingale." http:// www.internurse.com/flo.htm.

"One Nurse's Experience on Partial Birth Abortion." http://www.fril.com/~buchanan/ dorie/abrtpage.htm.

"On the Frequency Distribution of Recent Time Cost Studies." http://www.lib.ncsu.edu/stacks.

"The Opening Statement of the Prosecution of Brigadier General Telford Taylor, 9 December 1946." http://www.ushmm.org/research/ doctors/telfptx.htm.

"The Order of Trinitarians." http://www.knight. org/advent/cathen/15045d.htm.

"Position Statements." http://www.ana.org/ readroom/position/social/screpr.htm.

"Post WWII and Korea." http://userpages.aug. com/captbarb/femvets6.html.

"Prehistory." http://www.geocities.com/Athens/ Forum/6011/sld003.htm.

"A Prison Hospice Model for the Future." http:// www.npha.org/ftworth.html.

"Psautier de 'Lambert le Bègue.'" http://www.ulg. ac.be/libnet/enlumin/en10302.htm.

"Qualification and Utilization of Nursing Personnel Delivering Health Services in Schools." http://www.aap.org/policy/ 01584.html.

Rau, Elizabeth. "Anne Hutchinson: Courage Ahead of Her Time." http://www.projo.com/ horizons/elect96/229spr1.htm.

Rodriguez, Raymond. "Folk Cures of My Youth Gaining Respectability." http://www.latinolink. com/opinion/opinion97/1228hi1e.htm.

Rogers, Jay. "America's Christian Leaders: Anne Hutchinson." http://www.forerunner.com/ forerunner/X0193_Anne_Hutchinson.html.

Rogers, Nicole. "Wimmenspeak on Midwifery Lore." http://www.murdoch.edu.au/elaw/ issues/v2n3/rogers.txt.

Schreiber, Bernhard. "The Men behind Hitler: A German Warning to the World." http:// homepages.enterprise.net/toolan/hitler/htm.

Shafer, Brenda. "Nurse Is Eyewitness to Horrifying Partial-Birth Abortion Procedure." http://www.fc.net/~garti/newsletter/sep95/ nurse.html.

Soltis, Andy. "Cop Killed and Nurse Hurt in Bombing at Alabama Abortion Clinic." http:// www.nypostonline.com/news/3345.htm.

Sponselli, Christina. "Vaccine Volunteer." http://www.nurseweek.com/features/97–11/mi ramontes.html.

"St. Columba." http://www.heritagehouse.uk. com/columba.thm.

———. http://www.reformation.org/ vol2ch20.html.

"St. Elizabeth Ann Seton." http://www.catholic. org/saints/saints/elizabethannseton.html.

———. http://www.knight.org/advent/cathen/ 137391a.htm.

"St. Gilbert." http://www.hullp.demon.co.uk/ SacredHeart/saint/StGilbertS.htm.

"St. Vincent de Paul." http://www.catholic.org/ saints/saints/vincentdepaul.html.

"Statement Concerning Mifepristone." http:// www.now.org/foundationreproduc/ ru486tes.html.

Stuber, Irene. "Women of Achievement and Herstory Calendar." http://www.city- net.com/~lmann/women/history/cal4.html.

"Surge in Political Power." http://www.umsl.edu/services/library/womenstudies/1990s.htm.

"Therapeutic Touch." http://www.therapeutic-touch.org/html/touch.html.

Thornhill, Gill. "Trotula of Salerno." http://www.amazoncity.com/technology/museum/trotula.html.

Thornton, Fr. James. "Defying the Death Ethic." http://www.execpc.com/~jfish/na/052697n1.txt.

"Two Brave Women." http://www.sunlink.net/~bud/dak8f.htm.

"Under the Knife: A History of Medicine." http://must.jhu.edu/demo/performing_arts_journal/18.2skipitares.html.

Valdes, Leander J. III, Jose Luis Diaz, and Ara G. Paul. "Ethnopharmacology of Ska Maria Pastora." http://dog.net.uk/salvia.html.

"Vincent de Paul and Louise de Marillac, Compassionate Servants and Saints." http://www.cptryon.org/vdp/vdp-ldm/index.html.

"A Visit to the Curandera." http://www.dreamagic.com/stan/00000058.html.

"Voices from the Past . . . Visions of the Future." http://www.ana.org/centenn.htm.

Wallin, Rev. Msgr. Kevin. "A Visit to Lourdes." http://www.spirituality.org/issue10/10page04.html.

"Wherwell." http://www.hants.org.uk/localpages/north_west/andover/wherwell/about.html.

White, Julia. "Susan La Flesche, Omaha." http://www.powersource.com/powersource/gallery/womansp/omaha.html.

"The Wichita Black Nurses Association." http://www.wichitawellness.org/wbna.html.

"Women in Medicine." http://www.med.virginia.edu/hs-library/historical/antigua/stext.htm.

"Women's Philanthropic and Charitable Work." http://www.harpweek.com.

"Zapata." http://ocean.st.usm.edu/~wsimkins/zapata4.html.

Index